Veterinary Nutrition and Health

Veterinary Nutrition and Health

Editors:
S.P. Tiwari
and
P.K. Sanyal

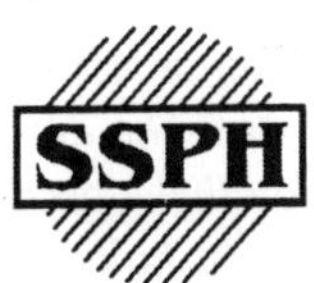

SATISH SERIAL PUBLISHING HOUSE
403, Express Tower, Commercial Complex, Azadpur, Delhi-110033 (India)
Phone : 011-27672852, Fax : 91-11-27672046
E-mail :info@satishserial.com, hkjain1975@yahoo.com
Website : www.satishserial.com

Published by :

SATISH SERIAL PUBLISHING HOUSE
403, Express Tower, Commercial Complex, Azadpur, Delhi-110033 (INDIA)
Phone : 011-27672852 Fax : 91-11-27672046
E-mail : info@satishserial.com, hkjain1975@yahoo.com

Proceedings of Symposium of Indian Academy of Veterinary Nutrition and Animal Welfare

ISBN 978-93-81226-06-3

Typeset at: Harminder for Laxmi Art Creation
Printed at: Salasar Imaging Systems, Delhi-110035

Preface

Good nutrition is the fundamental requirement of all animals and birds and is considered one of the biggest contributors to animal welfare. Malnutrion and improper nutrition adversely affect animal productivity, health, behaviour and in turn, welfare of animals. As safety of foods of animal origin is affected by poor animal welfare activity due to close linkage between poor nutrition and diseases, poor nutrition can increase susceptibility of various infectious, non-infectious food-borne diseases. Control of those diseases in food producing animals is primarily attempted by the frequent and indiscriminate use of antimicrobial and anti-parasitic drugs in animals reared in intensive and semi-intensive management systems. In recent decades, the dependence on drugs to cure the animals has led to the development of drug resistant microbial and parasite strains, pest resurgence, environmental pollution, drug residues in food and food products and uneconomic animal production. All these problems are particularly severe in developing countries, like India, where drugs are poorly regulated and users often lack appropriate information and/or training. While animal productivity and welfare in developing countries like India is compromised by inadequate nutrition, improved nutrition has become a part and parcel of integrated disease management strategies. Efforts are now being made to develop and use nutritional control technologies to be used as adjuncts to chemotherapy, which would not only reduce the use of drugs but also the cost of animal production as a whole. The macronutrient and micronutrient play crucial role in livestock nutrition, so state resource map on macro and micronutrient status is being utilized to enhance production.

However, very little attention is paid on the understanding of the linkages between animal nutrition and animal welfare. Current state of scientific knowledge exists in India and sharing of information on the influence of animal nutrition on animal welfare is the need of the hour. Department of Animal Nutrition, College of Veterinary Science & Animal Husbandry, Anjora, Durg is hosting a two days conference on "The Significance of Veterinary Nutrition for Health & Production of Animals of Agro-ecological Importance" under the aegis of Indian Academy of Veterinary Nutrition and Animal Welfare (IAVNAW) and Indira Gandhi Krishi Vishwavidyalaya (IGKV).

The book "Veterinary Nutrition and Health" is a compilation of working papers of the IAVNAW Symposium which was held during September 24-25, 2011.

Editors

Contents

1

Need of Discovering Traditional Bhartiya Livestock Management Systems for Fruitful Application of Science of Nutrition for Health and Sustained Production

NITYANAND PATHAK
President, Indian Academy of Veterinary Nutrition and Animal Welfare
Izatnagar, (U.P.) - 243 122

Introduction

Bharat is a country of diversity in all aspects of social, cultural, religious, ecological, environmental, agricultural, animal husbandry, veterinary, health management and many other aspects of modern living systems in the world. Animal production is one of the most important subjects of national health maintenance by producing foods of very high nutritive value. In order to maintain and enhance livestock production we were forced to adopt the sciences of animal husbandry and veterinary developed in so called advanced countries of Europe, northern America and Australia because during recurring invasions from west and central Asia and European countries we lost our sciences due to burning of libraries and destruction of ancient literatures.

The veterinary and animal husbandry sciences were fully developed during the Vedic period and could survive for long time during the post Ashokan period. Greater destruction of culture, religion, agriculture, livestock production and health management of animals occurred during the post Gupta period and maximum destruction occurred during different regimes of Mugal period with the exception of short period of Akbar and some of the followers.

Ancient Indian Veterinary Science

1. *The Vedic period*: Probably Ayurveda is the first documented work on health science. This also included Veterinary science with specialization on health and production of important species like cattle, sheep, goats, horses and elephants etc.
2. *Pauranic period*: Although Ayurved is probably a collection of all knowledge developed by different persons who were gathered and given systematic shape by Aswin kumers, the twin son of Surya Deva.

   Aswani Kumars are considered the first teacher of Veterinary science in Bhartiya education system. The development and application of the science of nutrition for health and production, i.e. Veterinary nutrition and dietetics is evident from the statement that "O Aswins you have rejuvenated our emaciated and barren cows with milk". This was possible only when adequate balanced diets were fed for the recuperation of depleted health and revival of fertility and milk production.
3. *The epic period*: Ramayan by Maharishi Valmiki and Mahabharat by Maharishi Vedvyas are the two great epics of India that dealt with culture, politics, economics and different sciences including veterinary and animal husbandry. The cattle remained the principal farm animal for milk and draught but both the epics period was time of great rivalry and war was almost a recurring event in many regions. This favoured the development of horses and elephants.

   Animal sacrifice on establishment of hierarchy was practiced during the Ramayana period as evident from "ashwamedh". Buffalo was tamed during the Ramayana period and evidence of farming for meat is available as Ravan offered buffalo feast to Kumbhakam.
4. *Post epic period*: After epic periods many smaller kingdom rose and Bharat was divided. However, this situation elapsed in short period and with the efforts of Vishnu Gupta (Kautiliya or Chanakiya) Chandragupta was groomed and merger and expansion of Bharat started to take shape by Ashoka the Great. During this period veterinary and animal husbandry again emerged as a state service department and strict rules were framed by Chanakya for the welfare of domesticated and wild animals.

   The system some how contrived during the Mugal period but could not retain academic and national characteristics, and gradually become a family profession. The scientific basis was gradually lost and animal suffering increased to the extent that Rinderpest threatened the survival of cattle and many other species. Other diseases for were also prevalent.

The treatment of sick animals was totally in the hands of quacks and witches. There was no institution for education in Veterinary medicine and animal husbandry upto late eighteenth century British company felt the importance of veterinary services only after the failure of first attempt of equine breeding in 1774 due to outbreak of diseases. In western countries also veterinary education was new and perhaps an organized first veterinary school was established in France at Lyon on 4th August 1761.

5. *Entrance and establishment of western veterinary sciences*: The start of application of European (western) veterinary medicine in India is 1779 when five veterinarians of London Veterinary College came to India for establishing breeding farms for cattle, horse and camel. However, only three of them could continue and two retuned back due to health problems.

East India Company brought William Moorcroft as superintendent of its horse breeding stud at Pusa in 1808. Four important diseases-glanders, farcy (cutaneous glanders), strangles and Barsati in horse were identified. He also identified in Punjab. He could not serve longer and died in 1820.

During this period Major James Lumsdaine started his own camel breeding farm at Hisar in 1809 for supplying draught camel to East India company for transport work This camel breeding farm was later on purchased by the east India company in 1813 but veterinary services were continued by Major Lumsdaine till his death. Afterwards the breeding programme was managed by his brother Major J.T. Hodgson, a veterinarian from London College.

In mean time large number of horses died at Pusa stud due to diseases and Major J.T. Hodgson was brought to Calcutta as a body guard of Governor General in 1821. He was given the responsibility to produce trained "Assistant Apothecaries" as veterinary surgeon for the management of horses in Bengal Army. Only three such trained people were appointed assistant veterinary surgeon in 1923. This programme was discontinued due to lack of even basic facilities for the training of a Veterinarian Hodgson proposed to Governor General for the appointment of a Professor at London veterinary college for training veterinarians for India to carry breeding and management of horses. He also advised for the appointment of Principal Veterinary Officers at Bengal, Bombay and Madras presidencies.

A Group of 12 Veterinary surgeon came to India in 1827. This was followed by another batch of 13 Veterinary surgeons came in 1833. The total number of Veterinary surgeons including Hodgson was 31in three presidencies during 1833. In addition to their specific jobs at studs these veterinary surgeons collected valuable information's regarding farm animals of India. During this period army had its own veterinary staff. In 1881 Griffith Evans of Military veterinary service isolated a flagellate from the blood of horses suffering from surra and the organism was named Trypanosome evinsi.

Start of formal veterinary education in India : On the recommendation of Col. J.H.B: Hallen an Indian civil veterinary department service was formed and establishment of veterinary schools started col. Hallen was appointed by the East India Company in 1850 at Bombay Presidency. Later on he was made Inspecting Veterinary Surgeon of Bombay army in 1862. He established first veterinary school of India at Poona. In 1869 Cal. Hallen was make President of the cattle plague commission in 1869.

Second veterinary school was established at the remount depot (now equine breeding stud) at Babugarh in U.P. during 1874. During same period a third school was opened at Rangoon in Barma (now Mayanmar).

Upgrading of veterinary education in India First Veterinary College, Lahore (Now in Pakistan) : After few years veterinary school at Baubugarh was tranlocated to Lahore to conduct a veterinary diploma course in 1877 and in 1882 it was upgraded to college for awarding Licentiate in Veterinary Practice (LVP). The duration was 2 years and Col. Kettle well was Principal. In 1900 course duration was increased to 3 years and name of college was changed to "*Punjab Veterinary College*". The Course duration was further increased to 4 years and medium of instruction was changed to English from the earlier Urdu medium.

Second veterinary college at Bombay : It was established on 2nd August 1886. In SPCA building donated by Parsi Philanthropist Bai Sakarbai Dinshaw Petit. It was a 3 years degree courses in English medium. J.H. Steel MRCVS was the first Principal of the college at Parel.

Third veterinary college at Calcutta : Although establishment of Veterinary College at Calcutta was recommended in 1971 by the "cattle plague commission" but could be established only in 1891 on donation of 7.5 bigha land and Rs. 30000/- cash by Babu Shoe Buksh Bagla to government for the veterinary college at Belgaechia.

A veterinary school was started in 18 January 1894. Here also Sir Dinshaw Petit offered Rs 25000/- for a veterinary hospital. The school was made college in 1898 to offer a course of 3years duration. Col. F. Raymond was first Principal.

Fourth Veterinary College at Madras : A Veterinary course was conducted in 1882 at The School of Agriculture at Saidapet by James Mills, a Veterinary Surgeon of Madras Presidency. The college was established in 1904 in Madras for 3 years degree in English medium. Major W.D. Cunn was first Principal.

Fifth Veterinary College at Patna : The Bihar and Orissa Veterinary College was started in 1930 in supervision of Mr. D. Quinlean, MRCVS, IVS, Director of Veterinary Services, Bihar and Orissa. This was first college to have an attached Cattle Breeding Farm. Course duration was 3year in English and first principal was Mr. R.T. Davis.

Birth of Imperal Bacteriologist and the Imperial Veterinary Research Institute {Now Indian veterinary research institute, IVRI}

On 9th December, 1889 an Imperial Bacteriologist was appointed and provided space for laboratory at the Science College, Poona. In view of the danger of spillage of wastes from the bacterial laboratory, the site was changed to an isolated place gifted with a natural cold storage (a cave maintaining temperature below 4°C even during summer season. This laboratory gradually grew to Imperial Veterinary Research Institute. In order to improve communication and mobility the major activities were shifted to Izatnagar which became the head quarter. The name was changed to Indian Veterinary Research Institute (IVRI) during 1947.

Birth of Animal Nutrition Research

The dairy animals at the Military Dairy Farms and Equines at some of the equine Breeding Studs suffered from nutritional and metabolic diseases like rickets, spontaneous fracture of bones, night blindness, blindness, reduced fertility etc. In order to solve these problems a Physiological Chemist Dr. F.J. Warth was appointed at the Imperial Agricultural Research Institute at Pusa in Bihar during 1921. Since the investigations involved clinico-pathological investigations, the laboratory was ultimately shifted to IVRI, Mukteswar where it worked upto 10th March 1939 and on 11th March 1939 it was housed in Animal Nutrition Research building inaugurated by his Majesty Lord Linlithigo, Viceroy and Governor General of India. Animal Nutrition Research at IVRI, Izatnagar was organized in laboratories, Viz Animal Nutrition Lab., Nutritional Biochemistry (Minerals) Lab., Nutritional Pathology Lab, Digestion and Metabolism Lab., Toxicology lab, Vitamin lab and Teaching and Training lab. This was a highly balanced set up of animal nutrition research for the prevalent situation of feed resources and health and production status of livestock. However, looking at the historical evolution of animal nutrition research it appears that managers of the division could not translate the idea of laboratory set up in function despite a humble beginning on minerals, vitamins, toxicology and fodder quality improvement research. The method of calcium estimation in feedstuffs by S.K. Talapatra, Ray and K.C. Sen (1940) is still used extensively in many countries.

During this period (around 1926) Dr. P.E. Lander Professor, Animal Husbandry started investigation on nutritional evaluation of common feedstuffs of India with the assistance of Pandit Lalchand Dharmina at the Agricultural College inimical Loyalpur (Now in Pakistan).

New Veterinary Course

Before, 1947 animal husbandry was a neglected subject as a course in agriculture. In Veterinary College, digestion, metabolism and feeding were a neglected aspect of veterinary physiology and received little attention. However, before 1947 an integrated degree course of veterinary science and animal husbandry (B.V.Sc. & A.H) was synthesized and implemented in 1947in all colleges of veterinary education in India.

Status of Research in Animal nutrition

The research on fundamental aspects of nutrition progressed steadily. However, on feeding aspect outcome can be considered only satisfactory little has been done. This happened due to lack of adequate exposer of the research workers about the prevalent feeding systems followed by the livestock owners of this country. In Bhartiya systems of livestock management there is practically no farming system except the seasonal migration and movements of herds from Himalayan Tarai to Bugials of high altitude during the summer and second is the herd movement in dry season from northern Gujrat and greater parts of Rajsthan to bordering areas of Haryana, Uttar Pradesh and Madhya Pradesh, in the search of feed and water.

Animal Feeding research is highly area specific and largely depends on the locally available feed resources, purchase capacity of livestock owners and guidelines available for the feeding of different categories of animals.

Where we lack?

1. The first step was to know the prevalent feeding systems in vogue transferred from one generation to another; and nutritional assessment of such feeding systems for the nutritional adequacy. This was ignored.
2. Most of animal nutritionist came from urban background without any considerable exposure to animal feeding and management system practiced by people for generations.
3. Larger part of our research is still on the lines of research in other countries and many have little relevance for majority of livestock owners.
4. Greater number of scientists is rigid and lacks the flexibility.
5. A tendency of group formation for blind following is increasing. Maneuvering tendency is increasing. To greater extent such tendencies

developed to hide incompetence by persons who acquired a key position in academic and science by non conventional manipulations.

6. A trend of mutualism is increasing and that of critical healthy discussions for the improvement and refinement of scientific approach is vanishing.
7. Young Group and research scholars are not being encouraged for seeking clarifications on doubts and at most of the places they are discouraged.
8. A larger group of senior persons are not tolerating quarries from young group, and generally fearful young group for carrier in the hard competition for appropriate job are avoiding discussions in scientific gathering.

The research works for the development of feed processing and feeding technology in our system of livestock keeping could have started on the basis of systems in vogue in different areas but it could not happen till to date. Hardly any nutritionist is able to enumerate the diversity of even gross composition of rations of a cow or buffalo and the frequency of change in the composition but research is continuing.

The right approach is to know the prevalent feeds used systems of feeding followed, versions of frequent variation in gross composition of daily rations etc.

How a problem can be solved without knowing the problem?

We know that elimination of cattle is not possible in our socio cultural system and we have to feed the huge population of one million. Taking average one third as breedable population, number of animals works out to about 50 million. A feeding strategy on the basis of nutritional knowledge for increasing 500g, 1000g, 1500g or 2000g milk during 240 days lactation may yield additional 6, 12, 18 or 24 million tones milk by feeding 3, 6, 9 or 12 million tones 16-18 medium quality concentrates of 16-18% rude protein and 66-68% TDN.

Western literatures mentioned oats and maize as most common cereal fodder crops. We had more promising fodder crops like sorghum, pearl millet and barley and later two can give several cuts on light irrigations which are secondary in our academic works. There is need of such corrections with experimental evidences.

Wheat and Baja (pearl millet) for fodder and food

Both wheat and bare posse high regeneration ability in favorable conditions. Land under wheat cultivation ranges from 25-27 lakh hectares with grain yield 27-28 quintals per hectare. Assuming 1:1 ratio of grain: straw, the average yield of straw is about 27.80 quintal per hectare. On harvesting wheat crop at 55-60 days of growth with conservative estimates about 27.8 quintal green fodder, 4.17 quintals dry matter (at 15%), 66.2 kg crude protein (at 15%) and 271kg total digestible nutrients of high palatability can be obtained. Thus, total yield of additional nutrients will be around 1.565 million tones CP and 0.6765 million tones of TDN capable of supporting about 13.53 million tone milk production with little protein supplementation.

Other promising dual purpose crops for food and fodder

1. *Bajra or Pearl millet*: Selective harvesting and irrigation stimulates tilering favorable for fodder and food grain production.
2. *Maize*: Consumption of fire roasted young ears at late milk to dough stage is increasing in recent years. Markets of baby corn and sweat corn are also developing in urban areas.

These changes are changing the cropping pattern and providing opportunities for intensive maize production. However, most of the farmers are not utilizing the nutrients in residual green maize stock properly and need education for the conservation of this moderately nutritious residual fodder for livestock feeding.

Need of multidisciplinary approach for solving the livestock production problems encountered by the owners

The relationship of nutrition with health, reproduction and production does not require emphasis. Therefore, for successful livestock production multi disciplinary approach has to be developed in rational manner. This is possible only on breaking the barriers of conservative approach.

Indian Academy of Veterinary Nutrition and Animal Welfare

This organization has no confrontation with any organization of Veterinary Science and Animal Husbandry. The objectives are quite clear as given below:

1. The organization seeks one holiday of each month from the members to organize a free service camp for the livestock and their owners.
2. This needs coordination at institutions through an animal welfare club or similar organization. These services require education and guidance of farmers for increasing income by enhancing production and reducing cost on maintenance.
3. Seasonal farmers awakening exercise for preventive vaccination, treatment and deworming, etc.

4. Guidance for production of value added products for increasing their income.
5. Short duration informal education for persons actually associated with the animal management.
6. To develop liaison with field veterinarians, paravets, extension workers and progressive families with concern for the welfare of each family.
7. Attracting unemployed youth (school dropouts) for earning livelihood through livestock keeping. This may help reduction in migration for search of jobs from rural to urban areas.
8. Maintenance of socio cultural family traditions; large number of young persons are moving away from home in search of job for livelihood. In most of the families aged parents and in some cases grand parents are left behind to live partial starved to starved life with the hope of support from the migrated children.
   (a) Only a small percentage receives continuous support.
   (b) In some cases financial supports continue for few years and then cease gradually.
   (c) Once away from home, many forget family members left behind at rural areas.

   Through this approach attempts are being made to first arose the persons who can contribute in solving these burning problems and then to join hands for infusing confidence in eligible group for earning livelihood through livestock production
9. This approach may contribute some things in poverty alleviation.
10. This may also help food and nutritional security to some extent.

Hope is great. Success depends on awakening of educated group for helping the needy persons.

Only lectures once in a year or two are not going to put impact on livestock owners. Large dairy farmers need little guidance for improving health and production. They are capable of hiring experts from inland and abroad farmers do not care for our recommendations and have more faith in foreign experts.

Let us make this approach a movement for the welfare of animals, their owners, society and nation.

□□□

2

Livestock, Poultry and Fodder Development in Chhattisgarh : Opportunities and Challenges

S.K.PANDEY[1], SUNITA ROY[2] AND GOUTAM ROY[3]
[1]Director Veterinary Services, Chhattisgarh, Raipur, [2] VAS I/C Fodder and Training Section,[3]VAS I/C Assistant Director Statistics.
Directorate of Veterinary Services, Govt. of Chhattisgarh, Raipur - 494001 (C.G.)
1. Director Veterinary Services, Chhattisgarh, Raipur
2. VAS I/C Fodder and Training Section
3. VAS I/C Assistant Director Statistics. Directorate of Veterinary Services
G.E Road, Raipur 494001

Introduction

The state Chhattisgarh, carved out of Madhya Pradesh on 1 November 2000 is a land locked state, sharing borders with seven other states of Indian Union. The geographical area of the State covers over 135,000 Sq. Km and the total population rose from 2.08 Crores in 2001 to 2.55 Crores in 2011. The state is endowed with rich natural resources with basins of great rivers like the Mahanadi, Godavari, and Narmada with a total river length of 1,885 Km. Annual rainfall in the state varies from 1200 to 1600 mm. Nearly 44% of its geographical area is covered with forests.

The present article has four sections. After reviewing the livestock sector of the state in the first section, the departmental initiatives and achievements are discussed in the second section. The third section deals with fodder development situation and finally concluding in the fourth section with the economic aspects, emphasizing the contribution of livestock sector and government investment in past two plan period.

1. Situation Analysis of Livestock and Poultry Sector in Chhattisgarh

1.1 Agroclimatic Situation and Land Use Pattern

The state is broadly classified into three Agroclimatic zones, comprising Northern hills (Koria, Sarguja and Jashpur), Central Plains (Korba, Raigarh, Bilaspur, Janjgir, Raipur, Durg, Mahasamund, Kabirdham, Rajnandgaon and Dhamtari) and Bastar Plateau (Kanker, Bastar, Narayanpur, Bijapur and Dantewada). The Chhattisgarh plains occupy about 54% of the geographical area and share in total cattle population is 55.8%. However, permanent pasture land is only 0.7%, whereas Bastar plateau and Northern hills occupy 46% area with pasture land of 5.7% (Table 1). Permanent pasture land is depleting fast, possibly due to overgrazing, crop encroachment and land acquisitions.

Table 1 : Land use pattern in Chhattisgarh

Agroclimatic Zones	Geo-graphical Area (000 ha)	Land Use (%)						
		Forest	Non Agricultural	Barren / Uncultivable land	Permanent Pastures	Cultivable Waste	Fallows	Net Sown
Chhattisgarh Plains	7,494	33.3	6.3	1.9	0.7	2.0	3.5	44.2
Bastar Plateau	3,263	65.2	2.4	15.2	2.4	5.2	2.1	20.1
Northern Hills	2,847	47.0	4.5	4.4	9.5	0.2	4.5	30.0
Total CG	13,603	43.8	5.0	5.6	6.4	2.4	3.3	35.5

1.2 Animal Distribution Pattern

Agriculture in Chhattisgarh is dominated by the small land holders and the landless (Table2). Of 3.6 million rural households in the state about 18% are landless, 24% are sub-marginal and 19.5% are marginal. These constitute the rural poorest of poor. However, the distribution pattern of animals indicates that 42.8% of small ruminants and 67.9% of backyard poultry are reared by these sections together (Table 2). Small and semi medium farmers account for 50.6% of cattle and 52.4% of buffalo population. This clearly indicates that any poverty alleviation program for rural area in agricultural sector should include Animal Husbandry as a major component. By doing this it is expected to increase productivity and profitability of these poor farming communities bringing them out of the poverty cycle.

Farm mechanization is increasing steadily for large and medium land holders and comparison between 1997 and 2003 livestock census indicates 3.7% and 17.8% decrease in male cattle and buffaloes respectively (Table 3).

Table 2 : Distribution of land holdings in Chhattisgarh

Category	% household 2003	Cattle	Buffalo	Small Ruminants	Rural Poultry	Pig
Landless (0.002ha)	17.6	0.3	0.2	0.7	2.5	11.1
Sub-marginal (0.002-0.5ha)	24.0	14.2	6.7	17.8	14.6	22.1
Marginal (0.5-1ha)	19.5	19.5	15.7	24.3	50.8	24.7
Small (1-2 ha)	19.8	25.0	34.8	23.7	19.6	9.4
Semi medium (2-4 ha)	13.8	25.6	17.6	27.2	8.7	19.2
Medium (4-10 ha)	4.7	12.9	19.6	6.3	3.7	13.3
Large (> 10 ha)	0.5	2.4	5.4	0.0	0.0	0.0
Total	100	100	100	100	100	100

1.3 Livestock and Poultry Population Status

Chhattisgarh is very rich in its livestock wealth with 1.27 crore animals (Table 3-4) against 2.08 crore human population. Cattle population is the highest with 64%, followed by goats (16%), buffaloes (14%) and sheep and pigs being the lowest (6%). Animals in general are smaller in size with poor production potentialities, due to poor genetic potential coupled with inadequate availability of feed and fodder.

Table 3 : Livestock population in Chhattisgarh (in thousands)

Livestock species	Population ('000)					
	1997	2003	% Change	2003	2007	% Change
Total Cattle	8785	8882	1.1	8882	9459	6.50
Male	4643	4469	-3.7	4469	4771	6.76
Female	4142	4413	6.6	4413	4688	6.23
Total Buffalo	1942	1596	-17.8	1596	1599	0.19
Male	1396	1077	-22.9	1077	1007	-6.50
Female	546	519	-04.9	519	592	14.60
Goat	2154	2336	8.4	2336	2761	18.15
Sheep	196	121	-38.1	121	140	15.70
Pig	456	553	21.3	553	412	-25.68
Poultry	6771	8181	20.8	8181	14207	73.66

Source : 16th, 17th and 18th Livestock Census of India

Table 4 : Land and Animal Distribution in three agro-climatic zones

Particulars	Northern Hills	Bastar Plateau	Central Plain	Chhattisgarh
Share in livestock population in %				
Cattle	26.7	17.5	55.8	8462296
Buffalo	28.7	13.9	57.3	1598041
Goat	45.9	22.6	31.5	2335723
Pig	26.6	59.4	14.0	552377
Poultry	24.8	24.9	50.3	8181324
Livestock density (Number/100 ha of net sown area)				
Cattle	178	170	176	175
Buffalo	36	26	34	33
Goat	84	61	27	48
Pig	12	38	3	11
Poultry	160	234	153	170

Livestock is an important source of livelihood for the land constrained poor households especially in the marginal environments. At the state level, the livestock sector contributes about one fourth to the agricultural income, but is subsistence oriented. The livestock in Chhattisgarh, is an integral part of mixed crop-livestock system, where crop production meets most of the feed and fodder requirements of animals and they provide draught power and dung manure for crop production. Such a synergy is considered beneficial for sustainability of crop and livestock production, and household food security. Distribution of livestock holding is more equitable compared to land, indicating that the poor have more opportunities in livestock production compared to crop production.

1.4 Livestock and Livelihood

Livestock are raised as a part of mixed farming systems and are closely associated with socio-economic and cultural ethos of the farming community. In subsistence production systems with underdeveloped markets, the livestock producers are often the consumers of livestock produce and contribute significantly to household nutrition security. Livestock are important assets available to the poor, which can easily be liquidated, compared to land and buildings, into cash during emergency and crisis. This is especially so in drought and dry spell areas. Except cattle and buffalo, the short generation interval and high prolificacy of other livestock species coupled with low initial investment and operational cost make it a viable and suitable enterprise for the poor.

Livestock are important source of manure and draught power, which are vital to preservation of soil fertility and improving soil fertility and improving crop production. In addition, as local transport, draught power is an important energy source saving in petroleum based fuels. Livestock thus contribute to sustainable intensification of farming systems especially of small holders who lack capital to purchase chemical fertilizers and other inputs. Finally, by recycling agricultural residues (straw and stovers) as feed, they save land for food production, which otherwise would have required to produce green fodder and feeds.

1.5 Gender Equity in Livestock Sector

Livestock contribute to women empowerment because there is more ownership and involvement in decision making process regarding livestock related matters than land and other fixed assets of the household. In India, as well as Chhattisgarh, gender equity is more pronounced in livestock sector, as women participants account for about 70% of the labor force while it is only 33% in crop farming. In India, as many as 75 million women are engaged in the sector as against 15 million men. Livestock forms a part of women's daily routine like feeding, watering, calf management, cleaning animals and sheds and in some areas milking and selling of milk. The extent and nature of their involvement however, varies within and between regions.

1.6 Employment Generation

Livestock sector engaged only about 0.5% of the rural workforce in 1999-00 (Table 5) and though latest figures are not available it is estimated to have increased significantly. The reason for low percentage of rural workforce in livestock might be due to the fact that subsistence animal husbandry practices are not labor intensive ventures and livestock in our state's farming community, is not taken up as fulltime economic activity. In India animal husbandry is largely in the domain of women. They comprise over 70% of the total workers in this sector. In Chhattisgarh, women comprise only 29% of the total workers engaged in animal husbandry. However, their share in agriculture is substantial (46%).

Table 5 : Percent of rural workers engaged in agricultural activities.

Agricultural Activities	Chhattisgarh 1993-94	1999-00	India 1993-94	1999-00
Agriculture	90.96	87.88	72.22	70.19
Forestry	0.40	1.05	0.32	0.31
Animal Husbandry	0.26	0.51	5.31	5.49
Fishing	Neg	Neg	0.44	0.31
Non farm	8.65	10.56	21.72	23.70
Total	100	100	100	100

Source : Extracted from NSSO electronic

1.7 Livestock Production and Consumption Pattern

The per capita consumption of food grains declined considerably and that of livestock products increased substantially between 1983 and 1999/00 in India. During this period, milk consumption increased from 43 to 74 Kg per capita pr year, meat from 2.4 to 3.5 Kg and egg from 9.2 to 15.1. Scenario in Chhattisgarh is shown in Table 7. There is considerable disparity in rural urban consumption pattern (Table 6). Sustained economic and income growth and urbanization brought changes in the food basket in India but in Chhattisgarh these trends have not been as robust - annual increase in per capita income was 1.8% and urban population 1.3% both are lower than the country's average.

Compared to staple food, demands for livestock products is more responsive to income changes. If the per capita income and urbanization experience similar trends as at national level, and this is genuinely expected (impact of various employment and/or welfare oriented schemes like SGSY, NREGS, Bharat Nirman, CM Khadyan Suraksha Yojana etc.), then demand for livestock products will increase significantly.

Table 7 : Per capita avilability of major livestock produce in Chhattisgarh

Livestock Produce	2001-02	2010-11	% Change	National Average (2009-10)
Milk in gm / day	104	128	23	300
Egg in No. / year	37	56	51	58
Meat in Kg / year	0.36	1.24	244	3.95

Production of livestock and poultry products is given in Table 8. Meat production is estimated on the basis of records of registered slaughterhouses hence are underestimates, as registered slaughter houses contribute only about 35% of the total meat output in the state. The state contributes 0.9% to the country's milk output, 2% egg output, 0.5% wool and 0.2% meat production. Milk production increased since 2000-01 at an annual growth rate of 6.12% which is much higher compared to 3.8% annual growth at the national level. Growth in egg production is comparable to national average of 3.3%.

Livestock productivity in the state is poor. The average yield of the non descript cow that account for 55% of the total milk output (Figure 1) is less than 1 Kg/Day. This is about one half of the country's average and less than the average yield of a dairy goat in Rajasthan. The average yield of crossbred cow (numbers are increasing with initiatives in AI work by CSLDA) in Chhattisgarh is 3.8 Kg/day, nearly 60% of the national average reflecting poor management practices and feed/fodder shortages.

Table 8 : Production status of livestock products

Year	Milk (Million tonnes)		Eggs (lakh no.)		Meat (000 tonnes)	
	Chhattisgarh	India	Chhattisgarh	India	Chhattisgarh	India
2000-01	0.78	80.6	7326	366323	74.13	1851
2001-02	0.80	84.4	7704	387288	75.42	1922
2002-03	0.80	86.2	7790	398228	83.99	2113
2003-04	0.81	88.1	8091	404031	85.63	2080
2004-05	0.83	92.4	8795	452009	97.78	2211
2005-06	0.84	97.1	8875	472307	107.03	2310
2006-07	0.85	100.8	8967	506630	119.18	2302
2007-08	0.87	104.8	9184	535296	132.66	2571
2008-09	0.91	108.5	9738	558955	204.26	3077
2009-10	0.96	112.4	10529	600696	248.00	4058
2010-11	1.03	*	12446	*	272.23	*
% Annual Growth	3.20%	4.37%	6.99%	7.11%	26.72%	13.25%

* All India Figures not available for 2010-11

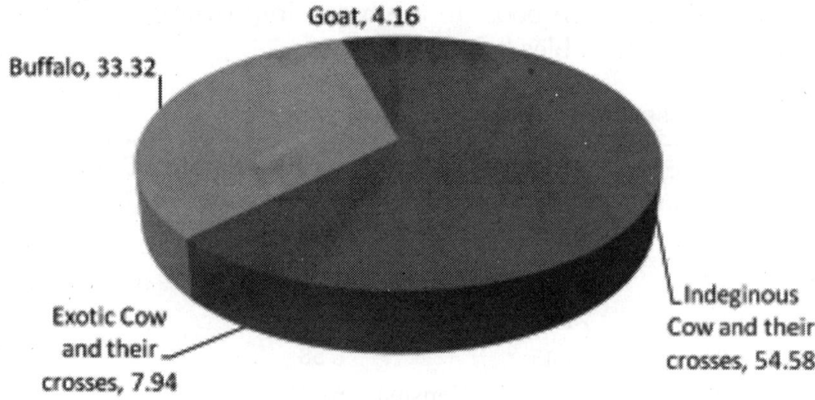

Fig. 1 : Percentage Share of Different Categories of Animals in Milk Production (2010-11)

2. Initiatives and Achievements of the Livestock Development Department

In the year 2009 the name of the department was changed from Animal Husbandry Department to Livestock Development Department wide Chhattisgarh Government Order No. F 1-2/2009/1/1 Dated 14.12.2009.

2.1 Animal Breed Improvement

This sector occupies the top priority among all other activities conducted by the department. The state is not home to any established breeds of domestic animals. However, there are large number of non-descript animals which allows ample scope for breed improvement. Over the past years, the approaches towards this priority sub sector has included the following major shifts –

1. Previous system where only AI Center and AI subscenters were included in AI service delivery was expanded to cover almost all Veterinary Hospitals and Outline Dispensaries.
2. Stationary AI (AI was done largely in Institutions) system has been dispensed with and many of the centers have been provided with small LN container and instructed to perform AI largely at the doorstep of the livestock owners.
3. In order to increase the number of field level inseminators educated unemployed youths were trained and equipped for door step AI services called Private AI Workers (PAIW). They are being given performance linked incentive since 2008-09 under RKVY.
4. Training programs for PAIWs and AVFOs regarding AI at various places on a regular basis has become an integral part of the breed improvement program of the state.

These shifts has given boost to the breed improvement program of the state as reflected in the tables below –

Table 9 : Artificial Insemination and Calf Production

Year	AI Work (In Number Lakhs)	Breedable Animal (Cow and Buffalo) In Number Lakhs	% of Breedable animal under coverage of AI	Calf Production (In Number Lakhs)
2000-01	1.27	29.45(16th Census)	4.31	0.29
2001-02	1.57	29.45	5.33	0.35
2002-03	1.94	29.45	6.58	0.37
2003-04	2.08	30.49 (17th Census)	6.82	0.47
2004-05	2.33	30.49	7.64	0.57
2005-06	3.06	30.49	10.03	0.67
2006-07	5.10	30.49	16.72	0.92
2007-08	5.12	33.62(18th Census)	15.23	1.15
2008-09	4.81	33.62	14.31	1.02
2009-10	5.13	33.62	15.26	1.09
2010-11	4.71	33.62	14.00	1.24

However, in spite of the efforts the the success rate (conception rate and calving rate) may range from 20 to 70% depending on the skill and tools available with the field level inseminator. At present based on figures of 2009-10, the calving rate is 22.66% in the state, which includes Govt. and private inseminators.

Major Achievements in this sector are as below:

Frozen Semen Bull Station – Anjora (Self Sufficiency Attained in XIth Plan)

- Obtained ISO Certification - ISO 9001:2008 Ranked *'Very Good'* by Bureau of Indian Standards overnment of India.
- Increased Semen Prduction from 0.24 Lakhs in first year of production 2005-06 to 5.67 Lakhs in 2010-11
- Collection and Processing of Semen from 9 Improved Breeds.

2.2 Private AI Workers (Unemployed Youth Trained, Equipped and Working)

Since 2005-06 under the Central Sector Scheme - National Program for Cattle and Buffalo Breeding (NPCBB) state unit Chhattisgarh State Livestock Development Agency (CSLDA) Private Artificial Insemination Workers were identified, provided with 1 month theory and 4 month practical training, given AI kit (Liquid Nitrogen Container included) and the department has ensured continual supply of LN2 and semen doses. These PAIWs are rural educated (12th Class pass) unemployed youths who after training are entitled to carry out AI services and minor veterinary activities. Under Rashtriya Krishi Vikas Yojana since 2008-09 the PAIWs are being paid Performance Linked Incentive (Rs. 50 on conducting and registering AI done, Rs. 400 at calf birth and Rs. 200 at the survival of calf upto 6 months). The number of AI done and calves produced by the efforts of PAIWs are on the rise and are given in the Table 10 below-

Table 10 : AI and Calf Production by different classes of Workers

Year	AI Work (In Lakh Number)				Calf Born (In Lakh Number)			
	Department	JK Trust	PAIW	Total	Department	JK Trust	PAIW	Total
2008-09	3.29	1.14	0.38	4.81	0.79	0.21	0.02	1.02
2009-10	3.24	1.44	0.45	5.13	0.81	0.23	0.05	1.09
2010-11	3.14	0.78	0.49	4.71	0.90	0.23	0.11	1.24

3. Cattle Grazers (*Charwaha*)

In our state *Charwaha* (cattle grazers) play important role in traditional management of village livestock. In the past 3-5 years attempts have been made to rope in this community so that they are sufficiently motivated and trained. This may serve to strengthen departmental activities and enhance the social recognition of this hitherto neglected community. About 20,330 charwahas have been identified, enlisted, trained and incentivized by the department. The entire list of identified charwahas, district wise is available in the departmental web site http://ahd.cg.gov.in under the title Livestock Statistics.

4. Bull Distribution for Natural Service in Panchayats of Remote/Tribal Areas

The topography and forested areas of the state coupled with relatively poor connectivity does not permit door to door AI service to be equitable distributed to all livestock owners. It is also realized that in order to increase coverage of breedable animals, as fast as possible, it is important to have as many breeding options made available to livestock owners as possible. Going by this principle breeding bulls are provided to gram panchayats, under a bull custodian, of remote and high demand areas through 100% subsidy. The Table 11 below shows that in the current plan period an average of about 700 bulls were distributed each year.

Table 11 : Bull Distribution in past 2 Plan Periods

Particulars (*Figures in Lakh Numbers*)	**X Plan Period**	**XI Plan Period**	**% Change**
Bulls Distributed - State Plan	1574	2132	36 %
Bulls Distributed - Central Assistance	-	1500	-

Under Rashtriya Krishi Vikas Yojana (RKVY) since 2008-09 a scheme for procurement and distribution of bulls by Govt. Farms is being implemented. Under the scheme AI born graded bull calves from rural livestock owners of the state are purchased by the Govt. Farms, reared till breedable age and distributed to panchayats. The feedback from the field shows that these bulls have better performance and survivability since they are better acclimatized to climatic conditions of Chhattisgarh than the other bulls purchased from outside state. This scheme, operationally implemented by the Cattle Breeding Farms of Anjora, Chandkhuri Raipur and Sarkanda Bilaspur under the department, is currently being expanded.

5. Breed Improvement in Goats

Breed improvement in goats is restricted to natural insemination by distribution of graded Jamunapari goats to rural individual beneficiaries having a sizable goat herd. Table 12 below shows goats distributed in past 5 years averaging about 6700 male goats per year.

Table 12 : Buck Distribution in past 2 plan Period

Particulars (*Figures in Lakh Numbers*)	**X Plan Period**	**XI Plan Period**	**% Change**
Bucks Distributed - State Plan	12,280	20,277	65 %
Buck Distributed - Central Assistance	3,300	13,300	303 %

5.1 Animal Health Sector

The Health Sector puts major emphasis in preventive and control measures for major animal diseases. Earlier, the cold chain infrastructure was very poor causing major hindrance in vaccination measures. At present, state has refrigerators in almost all veterinary institutions, horizontal refrigerators in District HQs, ice lined freezers in 121 block HQs and sufficient numbers of vaccine carriers. This has led to about 116% increase in vaccination in 2010-11 from the base year 2001-02 as shown in Table 13 below.

Table 13 : Vaccinations conducted against Important Animal Diseases

#	Vaccine Category (Figures in lakh numbers)	2000-01	2010-11
1	HS	25.44	48.33
2	BQ	6.47	7.81
3	Anthrax	4.69	1.92
4	FMD	1.34	7.12
5	Swine Fever	0.10	0.23
6	ET	0.94	6.55
7	PPR	0	25.95
8	Rabies	0.04	0.07
9	Poultry vaccines (Fowl Pox and Ranikhet)	22.09	33.52
	Total	**61.11**	**132.05**

State wide PPR Disease Control Program

Peste-des-Petits Ruminants (PPR), a viral disease is popularly known to cause heavy economic loss for the goat and sheep rearers in Chhattisgarh since past decade. The population of sheep and goats together, is 29 lakhs as per 2007 Census. In the open market the cost of goat meat ranges from Rs.200-240 per Kg which makes a 20 Kg adult goat (dressing percentage 56%) to cost Rs.2000-2400 at different places in the state. Thus the total asset value of goats in the state can be projected to around Rs. 640 Crores. Assuming an annual mortality of 5% due to PPR disease (directly due to disease and indirectly due to distress selling), the economic losses due to this disease alone works out to be Rs.32 Crores annually. Thus, it is evident that if PPR disease is controlled effectively it will have direct and significant impact on the producers as well as consumers in the state.

With this background under Rashtriya Krishi Vikas Yojana (RKVY) since 2010-11 State wide PPR Disease Control program, on the lines of Pulse Polio campaign, is being implemented. This has resulted in significant drop in outbreaks of the disease. The Table 14 below attempts to summarize some of the parameters.

Table 14 : State wide PPR Control Program

No.	Parameter	2010-11	2011-12
1	Deworming Phase	12-18 May 2010	23-31 May 2011
2	No. of Deworming done	24.14 Lakhs	27.74 Lakhs
3	Vaccination Phase	10-17 June 2010	13-20 June 2011 5 Districts Sept. 2011 (scheduled) 13 Districts
4	No. of Vaccinations done	19.44 Lakhs	8.45 Lakhs (5 Districts)
5	No. of Village Covered	18,738	Ongoing till Sept. 2011
6	No. of Vaccination Teams	1752	1787
7	No. of Sector In-charges	511	146
8	Expenditure under RKVY	Rs. 137 Lakhs	Rs. 177 Lakhs
9	Base population of Sheep/Goat	29.08 Lakhs (18th Census)	

5.2 Infrastructure Development

The XI Five Year Plan has been a period of rapid infrastructure development for livestock sector as indicated in the table below. Most of the projects with civil works, for which funds have been released to construction agencies, are yet to be finished. This creation of infrastructure, with an investment of Rs. 120 Crores, will contribute immensely towards overall progress of livestock sector in the coming years.

Table 15 : Infrastructure Development in the past 5 years

RKVY (2008-09 to 2010-11)	ASCAD (2007-08 to 2010-11)	Central Assistance for Infrastructure and strengthening of Farms (08-09 to 11-12)	State Plan XI Plan (07-08 to 11-12)
Veterinary Hospital 124 Outline Dispensaries 342 Polyclinic 17 Quarantine Station 11 State Level Vety. Hosp. 1 New Farms 2 Strengthening of Farms 2 Strengthening of Veterinary Hospitals with Equipments and Instruments - 1200	Construction of Disease Investigation Laboratories at all Districts 17 Strengthening of Disease Investigation Laboratories with Equipments and Instruments 17	Vety. Hospital 26 Dispensaries 117 Strengthening of six existing govt. farms	Estab. of 74 Dispensaries Upgradation of 17 Dispensaries into Vety. Hospitals
Total Sanction : Rs. 95.79 Cr.	**Total Sanction: Rs. 4.76 Cr.**	**Total Sanction: Rs. 14.83 Cr.**	**Total Sanction : Rs. 4.52 Cr.**

5.3 Commercial and Cooperative Sector of Livestock and Poultry

The commercial poultry sector has grown at immense pace in the past decade in the state as evident from the 212.5 % increase in number of improved breed poultry population between last two censuses. The egg production in the state rose from 9184 Lakh Numbers to 14624 lakhs in 2010-11 registering a growth of 59% in the past 5 years. This has principally come from the commercial sector with very large poultry farms coming into operation in Raipur, Durg and Rajnandgaon districts.

In commercial dairy sector, the growth has not been to the tune of the commercial poultry sector. Initiatives in livestock products processing sector is yet to be made. In cooperative milk marketing sector the state has started major initiative by bringing all milk unions operated by Raipur Dugdh Sangh (8 Districts of central Chhattisgarh) and Integrated Dairy Development Project area (5 districts) under a Milk Federation. The brand name 'Sanchi' carried forward from erstwhile Madhya Pardesh is being changed to 'deobhog'.

The table below shows the enlisted commercial poultry and dairies of Chhattisgarh with their reported animal holdings according to special survey and enlistment of February 2010 conducted by statistical section of the department.

Table 16 : Status of Commercial Farms in the State

#	Particulars	No. of Units	Total Animal Holdings	Average per Unit animal holding
1	Commercial Dairies (Cow and Buffalo) *Minimum unit size of 5 improved breed animals*	6139	1,15,695	18.84
2	Commercial Broiler Farms *Minimum unit size of 500 birds*	164	31,82,810	19,407
3	Commercial Layer Farms *Minimum unit size of 500 birds*	906	48,81,464	5388

5.4 Integration of Information and Communication Technology in the Department

Since 2010-11 three notable initiatives have been taken. The first one is the creation and updating of the Departmental Website http://ahd.cg.gov.in The second is to put in place online software for monitoring of departmental activities. A link by the icon VETMIS is available in the website through which all major activities conducted by the field staff, once compiled by the district HQ, is entered in the online software and reports are viewable and downloadable by any stakeholder. Efforts are being made to incorporate information regarding government farms, diagnostic laboratories, monthly expenditure reports, beneficiaries' names and other fields. The objective is to make the functioning of department more efficient, transparent and accountable.

The third initiative is under National Animal Disease Reporting System under which all district and block level veterinary institutions has been provided with computer hardware and net connectivity by BSLN. In 2011-12 online software will be made available for by Govt. of India through National Informatics Center so that many parameters concerning animal diseases will be entered by block level institutions in the country and viewed by concerned stakeholder.

5.5 Human Resource Development

Under the preview of the department there are two training centers (Jagdalpur and Mahasaumd) for catering HRD needs of para-veterinary personals. Veterinary professionals undergo regular trainings at reputed institutions like Vety. Collge Anand and Ludhinana, Central Poultry Dev. Organization Bangalore, kerala Livestock Dev. Board. etc. Newly inducted professionals undergo 15 days orientation program.

6. Fodder Development - Situation and Initiatives

Feed and fodder are the most critical inputs in livestock production. Feed cost accounts to almost 60-70% of the total cost of rearing of the animals. According to an estimate made in 2004-05, green fodder available from cultivable land in the state is only 2.3% whereas dry fodder/crop residue accounts for 47.2% of the total feed and fodder available (Table 17). Deficit percentage in concentrates is 68.2% and dry fodder (mainly paddy straw) is 51.3% whereas for green fodder it is a staggering 82.8% deficit (Table 18).

Livestock in Chhattisgarh are raised as a component of mixed farming systems where both the crop and animal production systems are interdependent and contribute to the sustainability of each other. Animals provide dung manure and draught power for crop production and in term derive most of their feed requirement from crop residues and byproducts in addition to grazing on fallows, common lands and forests.

Table 17 : Sources of feed and fodder in Chhattisgarh (2004-05)

	Quantity (Lakh tonnes)	Percent
Dry Fodder	64.59	47.2
Green Fodder	60.53	44.2
Uncultivable land	39.5	28.9
Cultivable land	3.1	2.3
Forest	17.93	13.1
Concentrates	11.75	8.6
Oil cakes	2.21	1.6
Other by products	9.54	7.0
Total	136.87	100.0

Source : Livestock Sector Review: CG AHD,CALPI-CARD 2004-05

Table 18 : Requirement and availability of different feed stuff in Chhattisgarh 2008-09 (lakh tonnes)

	Requirement	Availability	Deficit	Deficit %
Dry fodder	131.0	60.5	70.5	53.8
Green fodder	392.9	64.6	328.3	83.6
Concentrates	39.2	11.8	27.4	69.9

Note : Fodder Requirement Availability - Figures are estimations based on actual survey based figures of 2004-05
Cattle Buffalo Nos. : 2003 Census 104.8 Lakhs, 2007 Census 110.8 Lakhs
Requirement of Fodder calculated on the basis of Stall Feeding Conditions -250 Kg Average Body wt. Cattle.

The livestock in Chhattisgarh however suffers from a shortage of these inputs in terms both quantity and quality. The probable reasons for poor feed status could be

(i) Huge livestock population in relation to available feed resources
(ii) Frequent droughts leading to seasonal feed shortage.
(iii) Poor productivity of common grazing lands due to inappropriate management.
(iv) Dominance of small-holdings mainly used for production of staple crops with almost negligible area allocated to fodder crops.
(v) Low irrigation infrastructure and inadequate natural water bodies.
(vi) Traditional grazing land being converted to cropping area and non agriculture land.
(vii) Inadequate investigation and research on available feed resources.
(viii) Inadequate social consciousness to restrain loitering animals has discouraged innovative farmers from growing off season fodder.
(ix) Inadequate availability of fodder seeds for farmers who are willing to grow fodder in their unutilized land.

In order to mitigate the fodder crisis and after a fair estimation of the constraints the Livestock Development Department of the state is currently implementing several programs and envisages to build up on the strengths to formulate new programs as per the Livestock Development Policy 2008 of the state – discussed briefly below.

1. *Promotion of Urea Treatment of Paddy Straw*: Since past several years' promotion of urea treatment of paddy straw was being implemented under a scheme by which selected beneficiaries received 20 Kg urea,

one bucket, one plastic mug, a polythin sheet of 10'X10' and a token amount Rs. 100 to cover expenses of demonstration and training. The scheme with budgetary framework was operational for two years (2006-07 to 2007-08) following which the promotional scheme continued as an extension activity without budgetary provisions. Encouraging response was obtained in the central plain region of the state. However, in tribal dominated areas of north and south Chhattisgarh the dissemination of technology was at a much slower rate than in central plain areas. This may be due to practice of open grazing in forest and forest buffer area by the farmers in the area and also due to the fact that the practice is labor intensive. No cases of urea toxicity or any other health complications are reported in the state. Under Accelerated Fodder Development Scheme of RKVY in 2011-12 special drive for fodder development has been initiated with a sanctioned outlay of Rs. 469 lakhs. The scheme has 3 components viz, distribution of fodder seed/fertilizer kits, hand/power driven chaff cutters and urea treatment of paddy straw kits.

2. *Promotion of Azola as alternative livestock feed*: Azolla hosts symbiotic blue green algae, *Anabaena azollae*, which is responsible for the fixation and assimilation of atmospheric nitrogen. Azolla, in turn, provides the carbon source and favorable environment for the growth and development of the algae. It is this unique symbiotic relationship that makes azolla, a wonderful plant with high protein content. Azolla is very rich in proteins, essential amino acids, vitamins (vitamin A, vitamin B12 and Beta- Carotene), growth promoter intermediaries and minerals like calcium, phosphorous, potassium, ferrous, copper, magnesium etc. On a dry weight basis, it contains 40 - 60 percent protein, 10 - 15 percent minerals and 7 - 10 percent of amino acids, bio-active substances and bio-polymers. The carbohydrate and fat content of azolla is very low. Its nutrient composition makes it a highly efficient and effective feed for livestock. Livestock easily digest it, owing to its high protein and low lignin content, and they quickly grow accustomed to it. Moreover it is easy and economic to grow.

Table 19 : Comparison of Azolla with different fodder species

Particulars	**Annual Production of Biomass (T/Ha)**	**Dry matter content (%)**	**Protein content (%)**
Hybrid napier	250	50	4
Lucern	80	16	3.2
Cowpea	35	7	1.4
Sorghum	40	3.2	0.6
Azolla	730	56	40

Since 2008-09, all the field functionaries have been trained on the production details of azolla and are instructed to disseminate the technology to appropriate farmers during all veterinary camps, training and other routine field activities. Stock cultures of azolla are maintained at all district and most of the block headquarters.

3. *Azolla demonstration and production unit at all Government Farms*: Under Rashtriya Krishi Vikas Yojana 2009-10, a new scheme is being implemented at all Government Poultry, Pig and Cattle Breeding Farms of the state. Under the scheme all farms will have 10 concrete azolla production tanks of dimension 9 ft (L) x 6 ft (W) x 1ft (D). All the beneficiary oriented schemes where the input supply comes from these farms will have azolla as a mandatory component.

4. *Establishment of seed and fodder production units for demonstration and extension at Departmental Cattle Breeding Farms*: Under RKVY, 2010-11 Fodder Development scheme three cattle breeding farms has 50 Acres of land for fodder seed and/or Hybrid Napier root cuts. Fodder is utilized for the animals kept in the farm reducing the feeding expenditure. Fodder seeds will be made into mini-kits and distributed to farmers in the state to complement the Central Sector Scheme of Fodder Mini Kit Districbution Scheme. The seed and fodder production units for demonstration and extension are proposed to be established at 3 existing farms viz. Chandkhuri (Raipur), Sarkanda (Bilaspur) and Anjora (Durg). The cost for infrastructure and recurring expenditure are required for first year with funds from RKVY and later the recurring expenditures will be met out by state plans.

5. *Central Sector Scheme of Fodder Minikit Distribution*: The state receives fodder minikits from the central allocation. This is much less than what is required. The figures of past few years are given in Table 20. It has been requested to the center regarding increased allocation under this scheme.

6. *Use of Non Conventional Feed Resources*: The state of Chhattisgarh has vast forest resource. Non-traditional or non-conventional materials are available in abundance and can form potential source of feedstuffs for feeding to livestock, if sufficient information on their suitability, nutritive quality, etc. is available. At present these materials are utilized for feeds in small extent. The nutritive quality and economic viability of these resources have to be estimated and demonstrated to farmers to make these acceptable. Adequate resources may be provided to evaluate the utility of NCFR as these are present in abundant quality and underutilized; their use reduce cost of production and dependence on

imports thus saving foreign exchange; and may help in further expansion in components of the animal industries. (See Table 21)

Table 20 : Number of Fodder Minikits Distributed Year Wise

Particulars	04-05	05-06	06-07	07-08	08-09	09-10	2010-11
Kharif							
1 African tall Maize (4 Kg/Pkt)	300	-	700	-		1000	5000
2 MP Chari (3 Kg/Pkt)	2000	-	1000	-			-
3 Jwar Sudex chari (4 Kg/Pkt)	2500	-	1000	-		2000	-
4 Others (Sorghum, Gwarbundel, etc. (3Kg / Pkt)	-	-	-	4700	2000	8000	8000
Rabi							
1 Oat (5 Kg/Pkt)	2500	-	10000	2000	2000	2000	-
2 Berseem (1 Kg/Pkt)	8700	6000	17500	4000	6000	3000	20000
3 Lucerne (1 Kg/Pkt)	2300	6000	-	2000	2000	2000	20000
Total	18300	12000	30200	12700	12000	18000	53000

Table 21 : Non-Conventional Feed Resources

Name	Botanical Name	DCP (%)	TDN (%)
Mahua seed cake	Bassia latifolia	8.0	60.0
Mango seed kernel	Mangifera indica	4.7	70.0
Babul pod chunni	Acacia nilotica	5.8	62.3
Vilayati babul pods	Prosopis juliflora	7.0	75.2
Sal seed meal	shorea robusta	1.6	61.0
Kuvadia seeds	Cassia tora	16.6	59.4
Ambadi cake	Hibiscus cannabinus	5.7	62.4
Kokam cake	Garcinia indica	9.3	70.0
Palas cake	Butea frondosa	6.6	63.5
Niger cake	Guizotia abysbimicacass	10.9	58.7
Kosem cake	Scheilchera oleosa	-	-
Karanj cake	Pongamia globra	25.5	62,0
Neem seed cake	Azadirachta indica	6.5	62,5
Kod husk	Paspalum scorbiculum	-	-

7. *Tree Fodder*: Leaf fodder is another source of feed especially during the lean period (October to June). Its contribution to the animal feed resource is very low but it has a potential for generating extra feed. Farmers have fodder trees and bushes around the homestead and forest either naturally growing or in a few cases transplanted.

In addition to the steps taken by the state to mitigate the fodder crisis some recommendations have been made in the Livestock Development Policy 2008, of the State which are as follows *under Section 3.9* - To Improve feed and fodder resource by capacitating livestock producers and local bodies through provision of information, skills, technologies and management.

1. Promote dual-purpose crops, leguminous fodder crops as intercrops and forage production on rice bunds and multi-utility fodder trees.
2. Improve management of common grazing lands to enhance their productivity and remove encroachments on such lands by promoting users' associations and participation of Panchayati Raj Institutions and civil society organizations. If needed, assist these institutions through financial, technical and legal backstopping.
3. Promote 'community fodder banks' to overcome fodder scarcity in lean seasons.
4. Improve villagers' access to forests for fodder collection. Restrictions on grazing in forests needs clear guidelines. Use of degraded forest land for fodder seed multiplication.
5. Promote private sector and cooperative base manufacturers to produce and market balanced compound cattle and poultry feed.
6. Support and promote higher production of Hybrid maize, soybeans, and oilseed crops etc which are used in compound feed ingredient to meet the market demand.

7. Economic Aspects of Livestock Sector

It has been one decade since the formation of Chhattisgarh State and it has been a decade of rapid development and progress in almost all sectors. The per capita income at current price rose from Rs.12,170 (1999-2000) to Rs. 38,534 (2009-2010) and the state recorded a GSDP growth rate of 11.49% - highest in the country in 2009-10 fiscal year at 2004-05 constant prices. The GSDP at fixed price (1999-2000) in the state during 2001-02 was Rs. 29,250 Crores which has increased to estimated Rs. 60,079.90 Crores in 2009-10. From a revenue deficit stage at Rs. 538.42 Cr. in 2001-02 the state has become revenue surplus, estimated at Rs.888.70 Cr. in 2009-10 and fiscal deficit (as % of GSDP) has fallen from 3.68% to 1.63% during the same period.

In the above scenario the Livestock Sub-sector within Agriculture and Allied Sector has also made significant contribution as evident from the tables below obtained from Economic Survey Report Department of Economics and Statistics 2010-11 GoCG.

Table 22 : Gross State Domestic Products – Chattisgarh (At current prises)

#	Sector	2006-07	2007-08	2008-09	2009-10	% Growth between 08-09 to 09-10	Share of Sectors in Total GSDP
1	Primary Sector *(Agriculture Forest, Fisheries and Mining)*	18368	19801	19111	20501	7.27	26.95
2	Secondary Sector	20693	22376	25429	28776	13.16	37.82
3	Tertiary Sector	19535	21466	23430	26799	14.38	35.22
4	**GSDP at Current Prices**	**58598**	**63643**	**67971**	**76077**	**11.93**	**100.00**
5	Agriculture and Livestock	8738	9743	8313	9203	9.67	12.09
6	Livestock only	N.A					

Rs. In Crores

Value of Livestock for CG state is not available from 2006-07 onwards, it is included in the figures of Agriculture as shown in table above. However, in 2005-06 the value of Livestock at current prices was Rs. 5362 Cr. and Livestock GDP as % of Agricultural GDP for Chhattisgarh state was 34% current prices and ranked 6th in India. The table below shows the budgetary provisions and utilizations in past 2 plan period indicating overall growth of 66.94% in plan budget which is lower than proportional growth of 128.56% in non-plan. Hence, in 12th plan period it is expected that there will be rise in plan budget and the department is set to take-up the challenge and meet the expectation of general public and particularly the livestock owners of the state.

Table 23 : Allocation and Utilization of Budgets in 10th and 11th Plan Period

#	Particulars	X Plan(02-03 to 06-07) Allocation	X Plan(02-03 to 06-07) Utilized	XI Plan (07-08 to 11-12) Allocation	XI Plan (07-08 to 11-12) Utilized	% Change in Utilization
A	**Plan**	**232.70**	**165.62**	**373.26**	**276.49**	**66.94**
1	State	195.00	148.38	189.95	142.59	
2	Centrally Sponsored Schemes	16.31	10.13	32.39	23.39	
3	Central Sector Schemes	21.39	7.11	25.07	5.99	
4	RKVY	Nil	Nil	125.85	104.52	
B	**Non Plan**	**243.57**	**233.51**	**567.69**	**533.73**	**128.56**

Rs. In Crores

The prospects for livestock production are generally very good. Demand for, and production of, livestock and livestock products in less developed countries (LDCs) is expected to double over the next 20 years. Livestock production has been growing faster than any other agricultural sub-sector, and it is predicted that by 2020 livestock will account for more than half of total global agricultural output in financial terms. (This process has been termed the *'livestock revolution'*.)

With the above discussion there are two major goals of the department in the recent future. Firstly, to increase the overall growth of livestock sector by improving the efficiency in productivity / profitability, service delivery system, marketing and processes to build a self sustained livestock economy that enhances income and employment opportunities and food and nutritional security of the large masses and absorb the risks of crop failure.

Secondly to utilize livestock as a tool to reduce poverty, economic and social inequalities by enabling the underprivileged and resource poor rural households to participate in the livestock development processes and help them improve their competitiveness to face challenges of market liberalization and globalization.

❑❑❑

3

Evolution of Poultry Sector in India through Policy & Planning

P.K.SHUKLA * AND SUJIT NAYAK **
* Joint Commissioner and **Livestock Officer
Government of India, Ministry of Agriculture, Department of Animal Husbandry, Dairying & Fisheries, Krishi Bhawan, New Delhi

Introduction

Poultry production is highly dynamic in terms of structural and management changes. In today's business environment, faster the ability to adapt to the changing system requirement, faster is the growth. However sustainability often requires dependence on other sectors like feed/ingredient inputs and processing facilities.

In India, poultry sector growth may be attributed to many factors like rising incomes and a rapidly expanding middle class, together with the emergence of vertically integrated poultry producers that have reduced consumer prices by lowering production and marketing costs. Integrated production, market transition from live birds to chilled and frozen products, and policies that ensure supplies of competitively priced corn and soyabeans are keys to future poultry industry growth in India. Further, disease surveillance, monitoring and control will also decide the fate of this sector. Concurrently, India's unorganised and backyard poultry sector is also one of the potent tool for subsidiary income generation for many landless/ marginal farmers and also provides nutritional security to the rural poor.

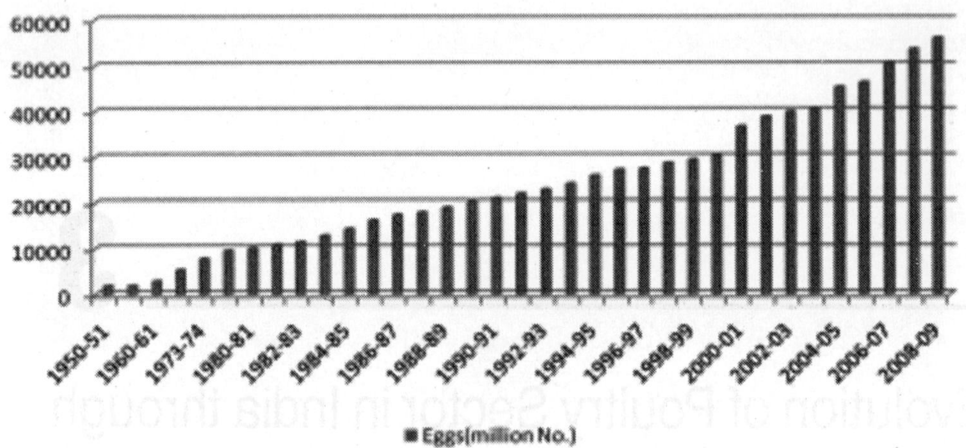

Fig: Estimates of Egg Production in India

Poultry is one of the fastest growing subsectors of Animal Husbandry. Annual egg growth rates in IX Plan, X Plan were 7.3%, 5.6% respectively and XI Plan (so far) is also around 5 percent. Similarly for poultry meat also the growth rate has been around 6 percent.

The per capita egg availability has increased from 29 at the end of VIII Plan (1996-97) to 51 before the end of XI Plan, again a 5% increase over last three Plan periods.

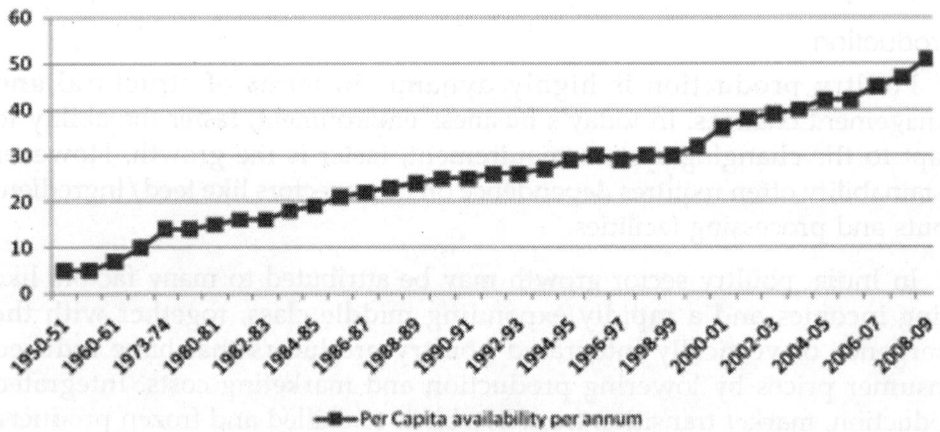

Fig: Per capita availability per annum

Exports of poultry products also increased from Rs. 88.84 crore at the start of IX Plan period (1997-98) to 156.47 crore at the start of X Plan (2002-03) which comes to nearly 15% per annum. This further increased to Rs. 441 crore at the start of XI Plan. This was again a 13% increase per annum.

However, while comparing allocation to poultry in DADF , the amounts are miniscule with Rs. 46.20 crore in IX Plan (2.1% of total allocation to DADF), Rs. 65 crore in X Plan(2.6% of total allocation to DADF) and Rs. 325 crore in XI Plan (4% of total allocation to DADF). If we compare with total allocation to Ministry of Agriculture, the allocation for Poultry schemes in DADF will come to less than 0.5 percent. Whereas the share of value of output is 10% of total livestock sector and nearly 2.5% of the agriculture and allied sector, the fund allocation for the poultry subsector is far from commensurate.

The value of output at the start of IX Plan period (1997-98) was 10,335 crore at current prices and at the start of XI Plan it was Rs. 23,443 crores (2007-08) i.e. it has gone more than twice as much as it was at the start of IX Plan.

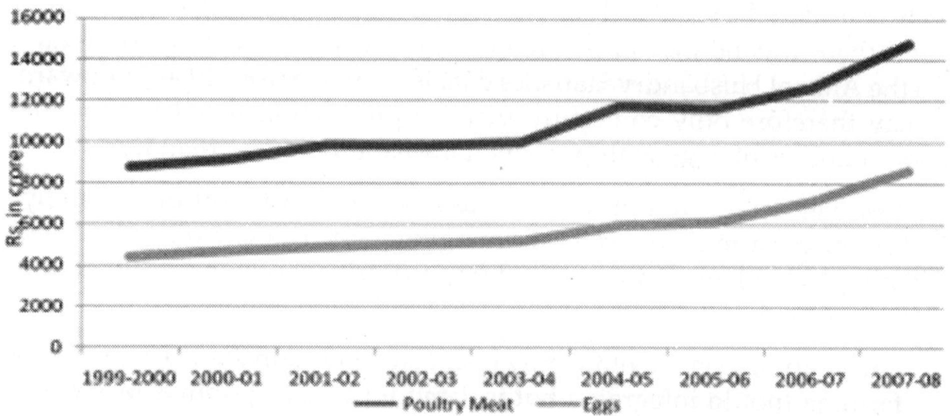

Fig: Increasing trend of Value of Output from Poultry Meat and Eggs (At Current Prices

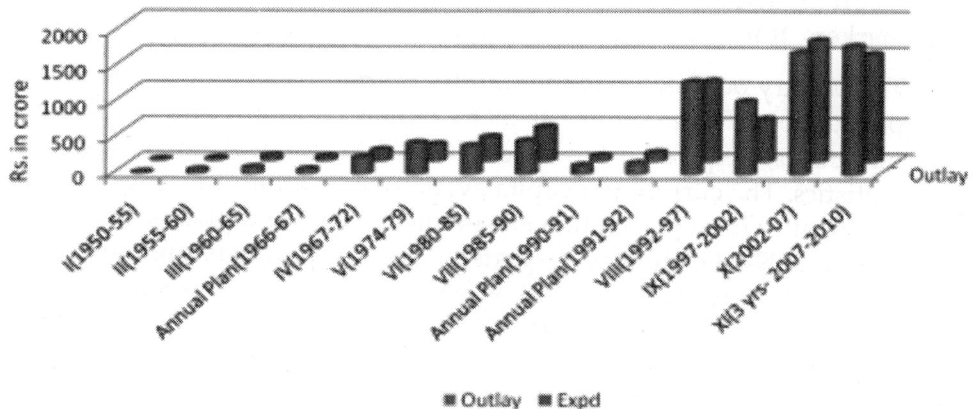

Fig: Outlay and expenditure of centraland centrally sopnsored schemes under animal husbandry and dairying sector from first plan - All India

These achievements and growth rates are still being sustained despite the ingress of avian influenza which was a severe setback for the industry, showing the resilience of the subsector, perseverance of the private sector and timely intervention by the Government.

To assess the future trends we have to review the past planning and present scenario to extrapolate the future. The externalities and variables are often unprecedented and sudden. Both empirical and statistical methods need to be accounted for while making any predictive assumptions. The 'Livestock Revolution 2020' study by Delgado *et. al.* gained such acceptability and popularity because variables and factors like economic crises and increase in consumption of meat products etc. were integrated in the study.

Pre-Independence Scenario : Poultry was not a recognized sector and was merely considered a backyard activity. The concept of farming had not caught up and there was no investment made with the aim of having any returns. Even the Animal Husbandry Statistics data is available from 1950-51 onwards. We may therefore only conjecture that the production was less than 1800 million numbers of eggs with per capita availability of less than five.

However scientific applications led to a near revolution whereby a scientific modern industry started emerging. Government played a role in facilitating technology induction and import; private sector readily adopted and extrapolated and replicated the successful interventions.

- Layer farming on scientific principles commenced in the 1970s and broiler farming (not in integrated but isolated form) was popular in 1980s.
- Scientific breeding & genetics came a long way from mass selection, trapnesting, cross / pedigree breeding of neo-independent period to recurrent selection, use of Osborne and selection indices, BLUP, DNA markers, transgenics, genome mapping etc. of the more modern period
- The poultry population in the country is around 648 million and the egg production of the country is 59.84 billion (2009-10) and 61.45 billion numbers anticipated achievement in 2010-11 as per Animal Husbandry Statistics. The current per capita availability is around 51 eggs per year. The poultry meat production is estimated to be 2.03 million metric tonnes as per 2009-10 estimates. Exports of poultry products are currently at around 372 crores in 2009-10 as per available data from Agricultural and Processed Food Products Export Development Authority (APEDA).

Development of Poultry Sector through Plan periods

First Five Year Plan (FYP) : Poultry keeping recognised as an important subsidiary industry of the poorer classes in the rural areas.

- Breeds like white Leghorn, Rhode Island Red, and Black Minorca considered for improving both the number and the size of the eggs.
- Selective breeding and proper development of poultry have also been included as a part of the key village scheme
- The Indian Veterinary Research Institute by a process of selective breeding has evolved an Indian strain which would substantially step up the yield
- Effective vaccine against Ranikhet disease brought out

Second FYP : proposed to set up five regional farms;

- Problems of cold storage facilities and other diseases recognised
- Up-gradation / breeding with RIR, WLH

Third FYP : expansion & strengthening infrastructure of State poultry farms, regional poultry farms and extension-cum-development centres.

Fourth FYP : Favourable atmosphere created for the growth of ancillary industries such as organised poultry feed, poultry equipment, and sales organisations for eggs and dressed birds.

- Propagation of stock with high feed conversion efficiency
- proposed to take up a coordinated poultry breeding programme at Central and State farms to evolve superior lines and explot hybrid vigour.

Fifth FYP : Particular emphasis will be laid on scientific poultry breeding programme.

Sixth FYP : NAFED continue its efforts to take a commanding share of marketing of eggs and poultry at regional and national levels and in exports;

- An aggressive consumer education programme will form a major component of market promotion activity.
- Market surveys within the country and abroad will be conducted from time to time.
- Duck development will be intensified in potential areas, particularly in the north eastern states.

Seventh FYP : At the Central Poultry Breeding Farms, poultry layer strains like HH-260 and BH-78 were evolved and released to the commercial farms.

- I.C.A.R. also evolved high egg-laying strains like ILI-80 and fast growing broiler strains such as IBL-80 and IBB-80 for release.

- For the marketing of eggs, 111 egg and poultry production-cum-marketing centres were established during the Plan period.
- A National Hatchery Registration Programme was also introduced during the Plan period to enforce production and supply of quality chicks of both layer and broiler types.

Eighth FYP : High yield layers/broilers will be developed and private entrepreneurship encouraged;

- Poultry rearing activities by private units or on cooperative basis was decided to be promoted. Incentives given to these organisations in terms of finances, appropriate training and guidance.
- Quail, duck and guinea fowl rearing farms established at State Poultry Centres.
- Additional cold storage facilities for storing eggs and broiler at selected districts will be created to overcome variation in production and demand.

IX FYP : poultry sub- sector has also made significant progress due to research and development activities. The egg production which was at the level of 22 billion nos. during 1991-92 increased to 28.2 billion nos. during 1996-97. The per-capita availability of eggs increased from 25 to 30 per annum, for the same period.

- Established a pyramid-programme for low-input technology bird dissemination through propagating ICAR, State Universities, GOI organizations stocks by multiplication of GP/Parent stock in Central Poultry Development Organisations;
- Multiplication of parents into commercial stock through strengthening of infrastructure of State farms.

X Plan : System of production of commercial hybrid broilers and layers has become highly successful.

- Give a boost to export of poultry products, measures undertaken for the development of infrastructure like cold storage, pressured air cargo capacity and reference laboratory for certification of health and products.
- The venture capital fund scheme for poultry components ushered in private entrepreneurship development.

XI FYP : In case of poultry the emphasis would be on development of rural poultry.

- Scheme of Poultry Venture Capital Fund supported 632 units since 2005-06 till 2010-11
- Rural Backyard Poultry Development Project launched alongwith Poultry estates (pilot basis) under Centrally sponsored scheme, "Poultry Development'

Present day capabilities

High yielding breeding stocks : India has the technical know-how in maintaining the high-yielding stocks and some companies have entered into franchisee agreement with pureline/ Grandparent stock providers. Commercial birds with laying capacity of around 315+ in case of layers and with Feed Conversion Ratio of less than 1.7 in 4-5 weeks of age are now common in this segment. Some of the stocks available are as follows:

Layers

Purelines: Babcock, CARI Gold layer

Grandparents: Bovans, Hyline, Lohmann

Broilers

Purelines: Cobb, Hubchicks, CARIbro, Indbro, Marshall

Grandparents: Ross, Hybro, Hubbard, Lohmann broiler

Most of the GP stocks are imported eg. Ross(UK), Hybro, Bovans(Netherlands), Hubbard, Hyline (USA/ Germany) etc. Market share is approximately 65% by Babcock in layer segment and 40% by Cobb alone in broiler segment, both of Venkateshwara Hatcheries (VH) Group.

Low-input technology breeding stock: This segment of poultry gained its importance due to its role in rural poultry development, as village-hardy birds that can serve at the farmers' doorstep were needed. Private sector was initially least interested due to lack of commercial gain and the onus was entirely on the public sector and suitable stocks were developed & tested in the Government R&D institutes like Central Poultry Development Organizations - CPDOs located at Chandigarh (Northern Region), Bhubaneswar (Eastern Region), Mumbai (Western Region) and Hessarghatta (Southern Region) , Central Avian Research Institute, PDP Hyderabad, many veterinary colleges/ universities like and a few private sector players like Keggfarms, Kalyani, Deejay etc. Some of the stocks developed for the purpose are Chabro, Kalinga Brown, Vanaraja, Giriraja, Girirani, Krishna-J, Kalyani DK, Kuroiler, Deejay Dekalb etc.

Poultry equipment: The demand for modern poultry equipment in India is fuelled by an increase in the size of the poultry farms. Previously poultry farms had production of only a few hundred birds (200-500 chickens) per cycle. However presently, poultry units with fewer than 5,000 birds are an exception with the majority of the farms breeding more than 500,000 birds. Similar is the case with layer poultry farms.

The Indian poultry equipment market is estimated at approximately $500 million and estimated to grow at 10 percent annually. Another factor that provides substantial stimulus to the poultry machinery industry is the rapid growth of the poultry processing industry. With increasing demand for quality poultry products, the adoption of better machinery to ensure quality has become very important to the Indian poultry units.

Barring a few items like egg graders, poultry processing equipment etc. most of the equipment are available/ produced in the country. India is almost self-sufficient in indigenous production of most of the basic equipment like hatchers/ incubators, feeders, poultry houses, even environmentally controlled & pre-fabricated houses etc.

Poultry feed & feed supplements: The total feed requirement of organized poultry sector is nearly 14 MMTs and nearly the whole of it is in compounded form. Most of the feed ingredients are available in the country but the rate of growth of maize production is not commensurate with the rate of growth of poultry; eventually shortages are felt. Recently tariff rate quota was removed and imports allowed for one year at nil duty. Feed supplements like antibiotics, probiotics, vitamins, minerals, amino acids, mold inhibitors, enzymes, preservatives, coccidiostats, antioxidants etc. are mostly imported.

Poultry vaccines and biologicals: This sector depends almost equally on indigenous and imported products. Technical know-how for the vaccines and biological production are mostly present in the country against the prevalent diseases. Further, the VH group are also having facilities to produce SPF for production of vaccines among other uses. Vaccine and biological centers are present in both public and private centers. Alongwith the production centers there are quality control centers at the apex level at Standardization Division of Indian Veterinary Research Institute (IVRI) and at National Institute for Animal Health, Baghpat.

Disease diagnostic labs: There are numerous disease diagnostic labs for poultry exclusively, across the country and some of the large integrator firms have their own sophisticated labs. At the apex level, Regional Diagnostic Labs, IVRI, High-Security Animal Disease Lab (mandated for exotic disease diagnosis only) are present besides the various State Government networks.

Poultry processing: This is still at a very nascent stage but both the quantity and value of the exported processed poultry products have increased during the last few years. The wet market dominates with processed products accounting for only about 5 percent. In case of eggs the processing is even lesser. Further, value-addition is miniscule.

Export of poultry and poultry products: Major items exported are table eggs, egg powder, hatching eggs, SPF eggs, live birds, and poultry meat. The value of exports has increased marvelously from a mere Rs. 11 crore in 1993-94 to present annual target of more than Rs. 422 crore in 2008-09. The strength of exports mainly lies in the competitive cost of production, proximity to international markets and successful regaining of freedom from Highly Pathogenic Avian Influenza (HPAI).

Research and HRD infrastructure: The research and training are quite well established in the organized sector. At the public sector, most of the veterinary institutions are having poultry departments and training is also undertaken by various State Governments as well as Central Organizations like CPDOs especially for rural poultry. At the private sector also research is more oriented towards breeding and poultry health.

Major Policy interventions

There are many major and minor policy interventions by the Government during the last few decades that has resulted in the metamorphosis this sector. Some of the major ones are enumerated below:

- R&D focus was strengthened and poultry research especially in the field of breeding & genetics was given a major boost. Productivity increased from 210 to 310+ over the years and as correlated responses, the egg mass, weight, feed efficiency, albumin quality, fertility & hatchability have also increase. CARI naked neck was the first commercial broiler developed in the country.
- The Central Poultry Development Organizations (the erstwhile Central Poultry Breeding Farms, Regional Feed Analytical Laboratories, Central Duck Breeding Farm, Central Poultry Training Institute and Random Sample Poultry Performance Testing Centers) were established and they not only helped in breed development like HH260 but popularizing the scientific farming of poultry. Diversification with other species like duck, turkey, guinea fowl, Japanese quails etc. was also a major initiative taken by this organizations.
- GP imports were put in the OGL category and imports commenced from 1995, increasing broiler production manifold. The FCR presently is well below 2 from an earlier as high as 4.0.

- Government has been liberal in allowing vaccines and medicines against the prevalent diseases and which were available adequately indigenously.
- Feed additives were put under chapter 23.09 of ITC-HS and imports were facilitated under OGL.
- A recent policy initiative has been to identify the role of backyard poultry as mentioned above in rural development and accordingly State Government farms have been assisted by the Central Government to strengthen their infrastructure for producing stocks suitable for backyard rearing.
- The CPDOs were accordingly reorganized and their mandate revised to give thrust to the area. As a next step, a scheme on Rural Backyard Poultry is being envisaged to directly aid the farmers through mother unit & cluster approach.
- Containment and control of the damage done by the avian influenza is another area where a series of policy initiatives has not only helped India reclaim freedom from HPAI but has also put a surveillance and monitoring system in place to prevent further ingress of the disease.
- Assess the risk to domestic industry in post-WTO era and placing in place TRQ regime; also increased bound rate tariff to 100% on cut up chicken parts to dissuade dumping
- Acts: Livestock Importation Act 1898, amended (2001) in light of bird flu to prevent ingress of the disease and 'The Prevention and Control of Infectious and Contagious Diseases in Animals Act, 2009' further strengthens the reporting and surveillance
- Veterinary services were strengthened and support through diagnostic and prophylactic facilities enhanced by way of BSL lab upgradations
- Risk analysis undertaken for various livestock products
- Recommended States for treating Poultry at par with agriculture and promote eggs in mid-day meal scheme
- Extended relief under debt-waiver relief announced in 2008
- National Poultry and Meat Processing Board set up
- Food Safety and Standards Authority set up
- National Biosecurity Network Proposed
- National Institute of Animal Health set up for veterinary Biological Products Quality Control

- Scheme launched to strengthen surveillance - National Animal Disease Reporting System
- National Livestock Policy in the pipeline and proposes a holistic approach for the sector's development
- There have been other policy and fiscal initiatives of the Government :
    - facilitating exports through initiatives of Department of Animal Husbandry, Dairying & Fisheries, EIC of India, APEDA, Ministry of Food Processing etc.
    - boost to hygienic production of poultry meat by setting standards
    - With the view to review & revise the specifications for commercial broilers, layers, parent stock and other avian species, poultry feed standards were framed in 2004-05 by DADF in consultation with experts in the field from both public & private sector.
    - Took up issues of dioxin, nitrofurazone contamination
    - exemption of processed & branded chicken meat preparations from duties & levies
    - freight subsidy for exports, reduction of customs duty on raw material for animal health products
    - reduction of custom duty on capital equipment for processing
    - packaging, washing, grading and stamping etc.
    - to boost exports the Government is aiding by negotiating one to one with prospective importing countries
    - putting in place the annual Residue Monitoring Plan to facilitate exports
    - Proposals of compartmentalization examined
    - Continual meetings with DG Sanco, European Union Food Inspectors and other countries/ trade blocs to assess their requirement sort out differences
- On the private sector side organizations like NECC, Bromark, Suguna Broilers by declaring egg and broiler prices have bought some stability to this highly sensitive products market.
- Economic and other relief measures to the poultry sector
    - To bail out the affected farmers from bird flu outbreaks in the country during 2006 and again in 2008, a number of economic relief measures like conversion of unpaid principal & interest on working capital into term loans and reschedulement etc. have been announced.

Subsidized grains unfit for human consumption were allocated specially for poultry industry in 2006.

- An interest subvention of 4% was given in 2006 for the whole country and recently again a 4% interest subvention on the outstanding non-overdue loan amount as on 01.01.2008 to the Poultry units of West Bengal for the period from 01.01.2008 to 31.03.2009 has been agreed to by the Government. The guidelines are being issued for the same.
- The Reserve Bank of India has already issued guidelines for the 'Agricultural Debt Waiver and Debt Relief Scheme, 2008' announced during the Union Budget 2008-09 wherein allied activities includes poultry among others.
- To control the increasing prices and reduced availability of maize, the exports were banned for some period during 2008 to enable the poultry sector to benefit from domestic production.

Some Challenges and negative impact of Livestock production in general

Competition with human food

It is implicated that each year livestock consume 77 million tonnes of protein from feed that is potentially suitable for human consumption, whereas only 58 million tonnes of protein are contained in food products supplied by livestock. In terms of dietary energy, the proportionate loss is much greater. This loss is a result of the recent trend towards more concentrate-based diets for livestock.

We are not factoring into this the fact that proteins contained in animal products are of higher quality for human nutrition than those in the feed provided to the animals. It is also amply demonstrated that from an economic perspective, hunger and food insecurity are mostly a demand problem, due to lack of purchasing power.

Livestock and their feed also make a contribution to food security objectives by providing a buffer in national and international markets that can be drawn upon in case of food shortages. This has been demonstrated in the previous world food crises of 1974/75 and 1981/82, and in the most recent food crisis in 2007 and 2008 where livestock sector provided an important buffer function by contracting or switching to alternative feed supplies, thus contributing to lowering demand for grains.

Industrialization

The majority of the recent growth in the production of meat, milk and eggs comes from intensive industrial systems. Globally, intensification involves a switch from no-input or low-input-low-output animal keeping (pastoral or mixed farming) to high-input-high-output animal production. Intensive farming is characterized by increasing productivity and yield through indoor or feedlot housing, concentrate feeding, high density in farms, selective breeding and/or a switch to commercial high input breeds. Though these yield higher production, it is implicated that they externalize many of their costs/ impacts like subsidizing feed cost and energy, health and environmental impacts etc.

Land use

Livestock production is one of the activities having largest human use of land which is implicated at the cost of forests etc. Grazing systems alone cover the largest land area and are currently estimated to occupy some 26 percent of the earth's ice-free land surface. As stated previously a large area of arable land is used to produce feed for animals that are increasingly reared in intensive systems.

However, alternatively we also have examples where intensive livestock production is tried as an alternative to tropical deforestation. The model developed in Colombia employs perennial crops with high biomass production potential (sugarcane with forage trees for pigs, poultry and sheep).

Environment and climate

Livestock production is implicated for seven billion tonnes of greenhouse gas emissions globally each year (9 per cent of all carbon dioxide, 37 per cent of all methane and 64 per cent of all nitrous oxide); it is also implicated as one of the largest polluting sectors-including phosphorus, nitrogen and pesticide contamination of water.

Biodiversity

Livestock production has both favourable and unfavourable impacts on biodiversity - it may maintain biodiverse rich grasslands but also causes deforestation for pasture and the growing of feeds. Of the 35 global 'hotspots' where biodiversity is most threatened, livestock production is a contributing factor in 23 cases. A total of 7 616 breeds are recorded in the Global Databank, comprising 6536 local breeds and 1080 transboundary breeds. Of these, 1491 are classified as being "at risk"

Water

It is estimated that 8% of global water is used primarily for irrigation of feed crop. it is estimated that 990 litres of water to produce one litre of milk. The growth of industrial livestock systems is increasing the need for water to be poured into feed crop production.

Public health

About 75% of the new diseases that have affected humans over the past 10 years have been caused by pathogens originating from an animal or from products of animal origin. Many of these diseases have the potential to spread through various means over long distances and to become global problems. This is strongly affected by how farmed animals are treated - the use of industrialized systems can increase risks.

Sustainable Production Model

Since 2009, a new component under Centrally Sponsored Scheme of Government of India, 'Poultry Development' has been introduced viz: "Rural Backyard Poultry Development". The basic rationale behind culmination of the concept into the scheme component had been the recommendations of the workshops, studies earlier held, studying of different models, discussions with State Governments, various experts, consultants, technical personnel / agencies, financial institution experts etc.

Central idea of this scheme component revolves around providing higher potential birds to nearly 3.85 lakh beneficiaries to help increase their income from their enterprise similar to small agriculture farmers being provided with improved seeds to increase productivity & their income from same land holding. Further, the scheme component has created an intermediate step - 'mother units' for rearing chicks upto 4 weeks of age prior to distribution to avoid high mortality when introduced as day-old chicks in the field directly.

At the time of project preparation, there have been an estimated 23.82 crore desi birds as per Animal Husbandry Statistics. Through this scheme it has been envisaged to replace nearly 10% of desi fowls (the non-descript type and not the indigenous defined varieties) through distribution of 4-week old chicks to target beneficiaries and assist rural backyard poultry farmers/ families in terms of chick cost for 3 cycles in tapering numbers. Beneficiary receives 4-6 week old birds & sells them at 14-16 weeks. Therefore farmer will realize cash returns in a lumpsum every 10 weeks. It was decided that target beneficiaries should comprise of below Poverty Line families.

The major items of assistance are as follows:

i. The SHGs/ NGOs, entrepreneurs may take up mother unit activity wherein they qualify for maximum Rs. 20,000 fixed capital subsidy and Rs. 36,000 interest-free loan to meet out their recurring expenditure. A provision for upto Rs. 1 lakh is also kept for mother unit demonstration centres at State Poultry Farms which have earlier been strengthened under the scheme component Assistance to State Poultry Farms. These mother units will procure the day old chicks either from the State Poultry

Farms or from the private hatchery and will rear the birds upto 4 weeks of age.

ii. This scheme component aims at supporting BPL beneficiary families with tapering assistance, wherein 4-week old chicks, suitable for rearing in the backyard, reared at the 'mother units' are further distributed to them in three batches of 20, 15 and 10 birds.

iii. Further, to raise the birds in a bio-secure manner, a provision of Rs. 750/- per beneficiary for night-shelter etc. is made in the scheme.

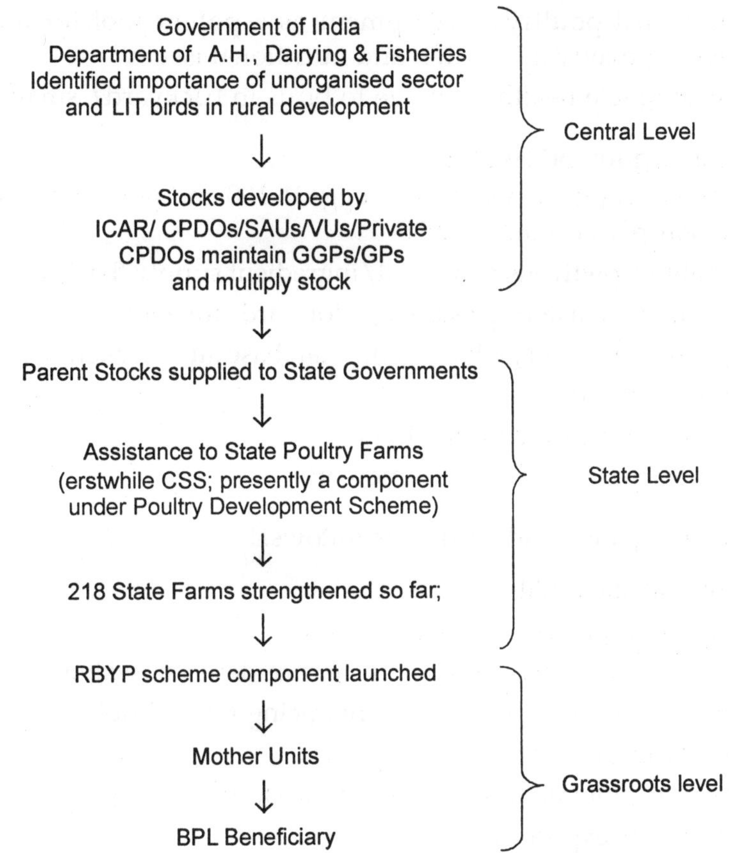

In addition to the chicken, there are other avian species like Quail, Ducks, Pheasants and Guinea Fowl, which are special avian species and have not been seriously exploited commercially because of the preoccupation of the urban poultry producers with layer and broiler chicken. These species, if introduced in the rural areas and raised like the layer and broiler chicken through farmers cooperatives and marketed by them directly can help in increasing rural poultry production and thus better employment, incomes and food for the rural people.

Strategic Planning for Future

A strategic planning for the programs of the Department of Animal Husbandry, Dairying and Fisheries was undertaken to set the roadmap for future development of the sector and representatives for the private sector also participated. The following major issues emerged:

The aspirations of the sector were clearly demarcated in case of private and public sector as follows:

Backyard/ Unorganised sector

1. Use backyard poultry development as a potent tool for addressing livelihood, poverty alleviation and nutritional issues
2. Ensure complete health coverage to birds in backyard/ small sector

Commercial/ Organised Sector

1. Increase per capita availability of eggs to 100 and poultry meat to 5 Kgs per person per annum by 2030
2. Sustainable growth ensuring feed/ingredient supply (backward linkage)
3. Substantial increase in processing (forward linkage)
4. Realistic national and global poultry database and marketing intelligence
5. Upgrade technology
6. Epidemic / Pandemic mitigation
7. Standards implementation framework

The major gaps were identified as follows:

- Lack of realistic database
- Inadequate improved stocks(LIT birds)
- Lacking effective door-step health service delivery system
- Absence of corpus/ institutional financing for technology upgradation
- Standards implementation framework
- Pandemic/epidemic risk mitigation measures missing
- Incentives for exports wanting
- Inadequate HRD for specialized poultry operations
- Non-recognition of poultry as agriculture activity in many States

Milestones have also been set to commensurate with existing programs. This will help shape the Results Framework Document which will address the issues on quantifiable terms.

□□□

4

Agro-Ecological Approach of Veterinary Nutrition for Sustainable Livestock Production

P.K.SHUKLA* AND SUJIT NAYAK**
*Joint Commissioner and **Livestock Officer
Government of India, Ministry of Agriculture, Department of Animal Husbandry, Dairying & Fisheries, Krishi Bhawan, New Delhi

Introduction

One of the great challenges currently posing us is how to feed an estimated nine billion people by the year 2050, 40% more than presently inhabit the planet , even more formidable is the challenge to achieve this without damaging the environment. The challenge is how to increase the food supply, particularly food of animal origin, in light of increasing global demand from predominantly urban populations with increased purchasing capacity. (FAO, 2009)

There is a need for urgent action in the global food system as a plethora of factors converge to impact demand, production and distribution of food over the next 4 decades. These drivers for change are the expected growth in the world human population; increase in incomes globally; urbanization, competition for land, water and energy resources; the need to reduce greenhouse gas emissions; and adaptation to a changing climate. (Foresight, 2011).

Livestock contribute 40 percent of the global value of agricultural output. It also supports livelihoods and plays an important role in food security of almost a 1.3 billion people. Major objective of livestock production is to provide safe and healthy animal food/ protein for the growing population. However there are many serious challenges cropping up on its sustainability.

Therefore, the significance of sustainability and agro-ecological approaches are highly significant not for current situation only but to plan for the long-term future as well. Further these approaches are pluri- and inter-disciplinary in nature and cross over many specialized domains. Therefore a integrated approach is also necessary.

Alleged Negative Contributions of Livestock

Competition with human food

It is implicated that each year livestock consume 77 million tonnes of protein from feed that is potentially suitable for human consumption, whereas only 58 million tonnes of protein are contained in food products supplied by livestock (Steinfeld *et. al.*, 2006). In terms of dietary energy, the proportionate loss is much greater. This loss is a result of the recent trend towards more concentrate-based diets for livestock.

It is also often deduced from this that food for the poor and hungry could be made available by reducing demand for feed. Actually the relationship between feed demand and food security is far complex, involving many agro-ecological considerations.

We are not factoring into this the fact that proteins contained in animal products are of higher quality for human nutrition than those in the feed provided to the animals. It is also amply demonstrated that from an economic perspective, hunger and food insecurity are mostly a demand problem, due to lack of purchasing power.

Actually it is conjectured that if there is no competition between human food and animal feed, there is actually no increase in availability of food for humans. Further they are particularly useful in converting vast renewable resources from rangeland, pasture, and crop residues or other by-products into food edible for humans. Besides, nutrients in by-products are utilized and do not become a waste-disposal problem. Analysis of the costs/returns of edible energy and protein for humans are dependent on the production system used. The efficiency with which livestock and poultry convert edible energy and protein for humans into meat or milk is highly dependent on on regional production practices.

However, it is also acknowledged that while livestock may not directly take food from the deprived, but they instigate in raising overall demand, and thus prices, for crops and agricultural inputs. Besides, livestock and their feed also make a contribution to food security objectives by providing a buffer in national and international markets that can be drawn upon in case of food shortages. This has been demonstrated in the previous world food crises of 1974/75 and 1981/82, and in the most recent food crisis in 2007 and 2008 where livestock sector provided an important buffer function by contracting or switching to alternative feed supplies, thus contributing to lowering demand for grains.

Industrialization

The majority of the recent growth in the production of meat, milk and eggs comes from intensive industrial systems. Globally, intensification involves a switch from no-input or low-input-low-output animal keeping (pastoral or mixed farming) to high-input-high-output animal production. Intensive farming is characterized by increasing productivity and yield through indoor or feedlot housing, concentrate feeding, high density in farms, selective breeding and/or a switch to commercial high input breeds. Though these yield higher production, it is implicated that they externalize many of their costs/ impacts like subsidizing feed cost and energy, health and environmental impacts etc.

Land use

Livestock production is one of the activities having largest human use of land which is implicated at the cost of forests etc. Grazing systems alone cover the largest land area and are currently estimated to occupy some 26 percent of the earth's ice-free land surface. As stated previously a large area of arable land is used to produce feed for animals that are increasingly reared in intensive systems.

However, alternatively we also have examples where intensive livestock production is tried as an alternative to tropical deforestation (Murgueitio 1990). The model developed in Colombia employs perennial crops with high biomass production potential (sugarcane with forage trees for pigs, poultry and sheep).

Environment and climate

Livestock production is implicated for seven billion tonnes of greenhouse gas emissions globally each year (9 per cent of all carbon dioxide, 37 per cent of all methane and 64 per cent of all nitrous oxide) (FAO, 2006); it is also implicated as one of the largest polluting sectors - including phosphorus, nitrogen and pesticide contamination of water (WPSA, 2011).

Biodiversity

Livestock production has both favourable and unfavourable impacts on biodiversity - it may maintain biodiverse rich grasslands but also causes deforestation for pasture and the growing of feeds. Of the 35 global 'hotspots' where biodiversity is most threatened, livestock production is a contributing factor in 23 cases (Mittermeier, 2004). A total of 7 616 breeds are recorded in the Global Databank, comprising 6 536 local breeds and 1 080 transboundary breeds. Of these, 1491 are classified as being "at risk".

Water

It is estimated that 8% of global water is used primarily for irrigation of feed crop. it is estimated that 990 litres of water to produce one litre of milk. The growth of industrial livestock systems is increasing the need for water to be poured into feed crop production (FAO, 2009).

Public health

About 75% of the new diseases that have affected humans over the past 10 years have been caused by pathogens originating from an animal or from products of animal origin. Many of these diseases have the potential to spread through various means over long distances and to become global problems. (WHO, 2011). This is strongly affected by how farmed animals are treated – the use of industrialized systems can increase risks (WPSA, 2008).

Consumption and Production of major animal Food

Table 1 : Consumption – Meat, Milk and Eggs – India and World

Region	kg/capita/year					
	MEAT		MILK		EGGS	
	1980	2005	1980	2005	1980	2005
India	3.7	5.1	38.5	65.2	0.7	1.8
World	30	41.2	75.7	82.1	5.5	9

(*Source :* FAO, 2009)

Table 2 : Production – Meat, Milk and Eggs – India and World

Region	Million Tonnes					
	MEAT		MILK		EGGS	
	1980	2007	1980	2007	1980	2007
India	2.6	6.3	31.6	102.9	0.6	2.7
World	136.7	285.7	465.5	671.3	27.4	67.8

(*Source :* FAO, 2009)

Therefore it is evident that compared to world figures, India is close only in terms of milk consumption and lagging behind in others.

Sustainability

According to FAO (FAO, 1988), sustainable development is "The management and conservation of the natural resource base, and the orientation of technological and institutional change in such a manner as to ensure the attainment of continued satisfaction of human needs for present and future generations. Such sustainable development conserves (land,) water, plants and (animal) genetic resources, is environmentally non-degrading, technologically appropriate, economically viable and socially acceptable".

Some define sustainability in terms of resource availability where it is emphasized accounting for the rates at which resources are produced and depleted. Principles are framed in light of strategies for conservation, regeneration and substitution for increasingly scarce resources. Some define sustainability in terms of functional integrity emphasizing dynamic system models of complex ecological and social processes of reproduction, and frame sustainability principles on basis of system vulnerability to anthropogenic stress.

More stress and greater research capacity is available for analyzing issues under a resource availability paradigm, but functional integrity approaches are more likely to yield social and ethical consensus over the goals and purposes of livestock production. Some opine that functional integrity paradigm is better for understanding the importance of biodiversity, and the relationship between society and ecology. (Thompson and Nardone, 1999)

It is argued that identification of livestock-specific criteria is impossible because of the large heterogeneity of livestock production systems and the non-linear relation between livestock-specific criteria and agroecological criteria. Therefore, a system specific analysis is needed to assess the overall effect of livestock inclusion in an agricultural system on each of the proposed general criteria for sustainability. These are: demand and supply of consumable livestock products; potential human population supporting capacity; land area utilized for agriculture; degree of equity in food distribution; variability of production; net annual soil losses; nutrient balances and losses; water availability and utilization; soil organic matter; fossil energy and drug utilization. (WiP *et al.,* 1995).

Criteria for Sustainability

Livestock production system

To assess the sustainability it is indispensible that the LPS should be classified carefully. The variables proposed as criteria for sustainability are influenced by various factors related to the size and nature of LPS, their relation to other production activities, and local ecological conditions. Livestock One possible system classification distinguishes pastoral/ grazing- intensive or extensive, mixed- irrigated or rain-fed and intensive/ industrial LPS. Lately there have been major transformations in LPS from small-holder mixed systems to large-scale commodity-specific systems, from roughages to concentrated feeds, from fragmented/ dispersed to concentrated production etc.

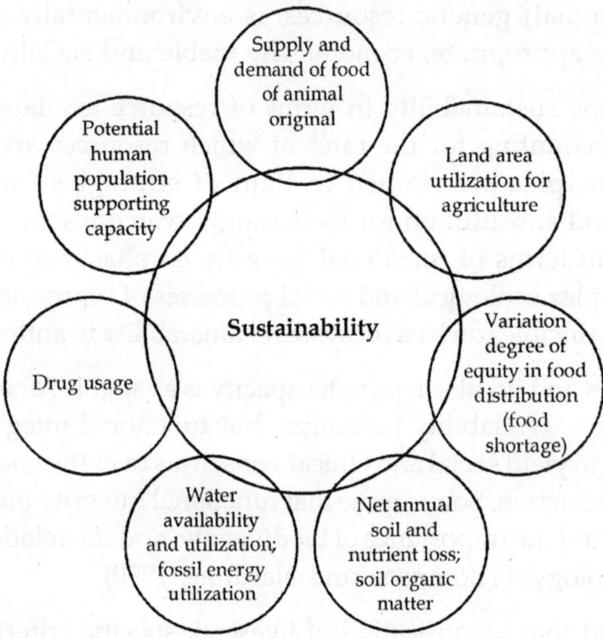

Fig. 1 : Model for various criteria for measuring sustainability of livestock systems (adapted from De Wit. 1993)

Table 3 : Use of feed concentrate – India and World

Region	1980 Million Tonnes	2005 Million Tonnes
India	15.5	37.1
World	908.4	1250.1

(*Source :* FAO, 2009)

As an example, China has seen an enormous increase in production of poultry meat and eggs through a combination of a growing number of birds and increasing productivity per bird. Today, the commercial broiler market is dominated by large, integrated companies that control the entire production and marketing chain: feed, breeding, fattening and processing. One large, integrated operation in Fujian Province, produces around 50 million broilers a year and employs 4 000 employees – one job for every 12,500 birds produced annually (FAO, 2009).

Another good example of transformation is dairy sector in India and Kenya. Less than 5 percent of animals in the Indian dairy herd were crossbred In 1982. By 2003, this proportion had nearly trebled. It has been estimated that 56 percent of production growth can be attributed to increased number of milch animals and 37 percent to higher productivity of the crossbred animals. Smallholder dairy production received an important impetus from the active support of government sponsored programmes, such as Operation Flood, and a major effort to market milk in urban areas (Staal *et al.*, 2008).

Agro-ecology

Agro-ecology is the "application of ecological science to the study, design and management of sustainable agro-ecosystems"(Altieri, 2007). As a set of agricultural practices, agro-ecology seeks ways to enhance agricultural systems by mimicking natural processes, thus creating beneficial biological interactions and synergies among the components of the agro-ecosystem. Contribution of agro-ecology is tremendous in ascertaining various objectives of defeating hunger by increasing availability through improvement in productivity at field level, by reducing poverty through increasing accessibility, adequacy by improvement in nutrition, farmers' participation enabling dissemination of best practices and by contributing to sustainability e.g. through adaptability to climate change etc. Some examples are enumerated below.

- Integration of livestock into farming systems, such as dairy cattle, pigs and poultry, provides a source of protein to the family, as well as a means of fertilizing soils; so does the incorporation of fish, shrimps and other aquatic resources into farm systems, such as irrigated rice fields and fish ponds.
- Agro-ecology helps to support incomes in rural areas through promotion of on-farm fertility generation. Instead of mineral fertilizers many are applying livestock manure or by growing green manures.
- Dairy-goat development project in Ethiopia, which significantly increases poor households' access to foods of animal origin.
- Use of Low-Input Technology birds as a potent tool for poverty alleviation, gender empowerment and in some places community development has been a very remarkable example of agro-ecological approach to sustainability.
- Green Revolution approaches have focused primarily on boosting cereal crops. However, rice, wheat and maize are mainly sources of

carbohydrates with relatively little protein and some other nutrients essential for adequate diets. The shift from diversified cropping systems to simplified cereal-based systems thus contributed to micronutrient malnutrition in many developing countries (Demment *et. al.* 2003). Therefore agro-ecological approaches help increase nutritional diversity by enabling increased diversity in the field, in turn proving very helpful for children and women mostly.

- Livestock genetic diversity is key to global food security; The "Global Plan of Action for Animal Genetic Resources" adopted by all FAO member countries in 2007, has become a key instrument for the conservation and sustainable use of animal genetic resources at global, regional and national level.

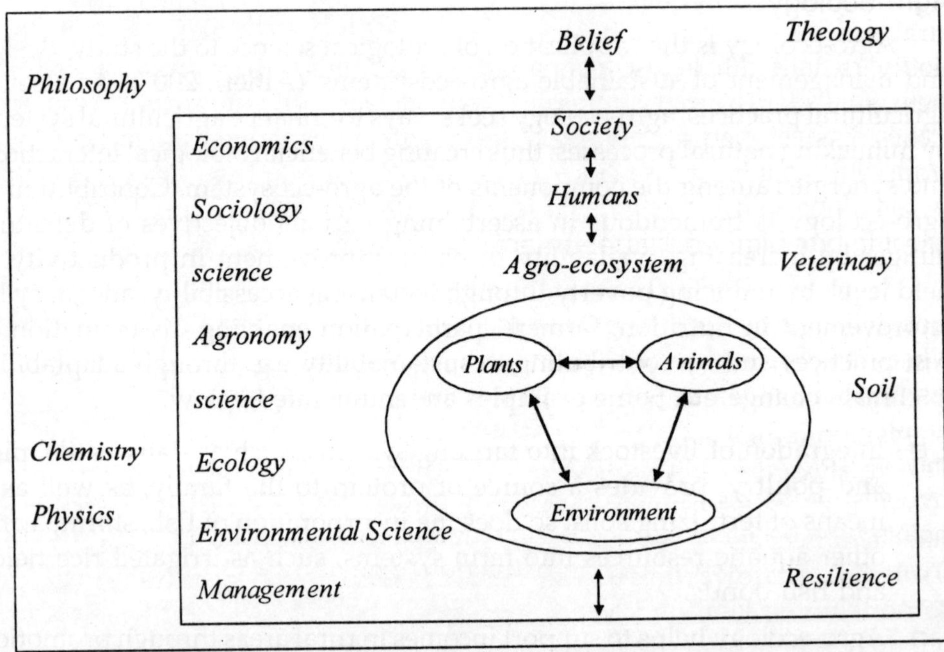

Fig 2: Agro-system concept (adopted and modified from Checkland, 1999)

- Agro-ecology improves resilience to climate change. Besides it helps increase diversity of species and also of farm activities which are ways to mitigate risks from extreme weather events, as well as from the invasion of new pests, weeds and diseases, that will result from global warming. Agro-ecological modes of farming are better equipped to support shocks of natural disasters. Agro-ecology also puts agriculture on the path of sustainability by delinking food production from the reliance on fossil energy (oil, gas etc.). However in case of livestock production in intensive system it is very difficult.

- The participation of farmers is vital for the success of agro-ecological practices. Agro-ecology has mostly been spread through farmer field schools and farmers' movements. Farmer field schools have been shown to significantly reduce the amounts of pesticides use, as inputs are being replaced by knowledge. Studies recorded 34 to 66 per cent reduction in pesticide use, combined with 4 to 14 per cent better yields recorded in cotton production in China, India and Pakistan (Van den Berg and Jiggins, 2007).

Welfare

Welfare of animals is also an integral part of a sustainable, agro-ecological approach for livestock farming. The rearing and use of animals has a major impact on the global environment and on society, particularly in terms of rural livelihoods, public health, greenhouse gas emissions, land use and biodiversity. Animals also play a vital role in our lives, whether we rely on them for food, revenue, transport, companionship, or to help balance our ecosystems. Therefore it is felt necessary to integrate welfare issues in the production system.

Need for Resilience Management

Approaches to natural resource management are often based on a probabilistic responses to management and external drivers such as climate. Where the objectives include long-term sustainability, linked social-ecological systems behave as complex adaptive systems, with the management specialist as integral components of the system. Further, uncertainties are big and it may be difficult to reduce them as fast as the system changes. Sustainability involves maintaining the functionality of a system when it is disturbed, or maintaining the elements needed to renew or reorganize if a large perturbation drastically alters structure and function. The ability to do this is termed "resilience." (Walker, 2002).

Role of Veterinary Nutrition towards Agro-ecologically Compliant Sustainability

Feed & fodder deficit & measures

India suffers from serious deficiency of feed and fodder to fully exploit the production potential of our livestock. As the area under fodder production is almost constant, the increasing fodder requirement has to be met through development of high yielding fodder varieties with better nutritive value. It is important to note that presently only 4 per cent of the cropping area is under fodder cultivation and over 55 per cent of the fodder for livestock is met from crop residues and agricultural by-products. Therefore, new dual purpose, high-yielding, disease resistant hybrid varieties of forages should be developed and their nutritive value for different categories of livestock assessed. (Planning Commission, GOI, 2010)

Fodder seed production and availability is a major constraint in fodder production. Production of quality seed of high yielding varieties of fodder crops and pasture grasses/ legumes needs to be ensured.

Although an impressive growth in rice and wheat production has increased to some extent the availability of crop residues as well. However, it is felt that due to use of more dwarf high yielding varieties of other crops, the stock/ residues have actually depleted. The availability of straw from coarse cereals is stagnant due to a decline in area, resulting in higher prices. Dry matter availability from grazing lands and common property resources has declined due to encroachment, overgrazing, and lack of management. Though the availability of concentrate feed has improved, its use is limited to large landholders and commercial peri-urban systems. Improved animal nutrition technologies such as urea treatment of straws, urea molasses mineral blocks, and bypass protein have not gained wide acceptance.

A huge livestock population not commensurate with available feed resources is an impediment to improving productivity. Options such as optimizing livestock numbers to match available feed resources and/or improving feed availability through breeding of dual-purpose crop varieties with better digestibility coefficient, improving the cost-effectiveness of existing nutrition technologies, and bringing more land under fodder crops need to be explored (Birthal and Rao, 2002). The Systemwide Livestock Program (SLP) has played a major role in fostering partnerships for key staple crops eg. sorghum, millet and groundnut in India. Successful forage species testing by International Centre for Tropical Agriculture (CIAT) and use of para grass grown in wastewater by International Water Management Institute (IWMI) & ILRI are some of the noteworthy actions taken towards this direction (Birthal *et. al.*, 2006).Some of the major initiatives suggested to be promoted are (Planning Commission, GOI, 2010) :

- Development of high yielding forage varieties and popularisation of food crops / varieties having high straw yield;
- Establishment of fodder banks to collect and store surplus crop residues in fodder surplus areas, under public-private partnership for distribution in fodder scarcity areas;
- Technologies to harvest and pack the straws & strovers from major food crops, like wheat, rice, maize and pulses which are otherwise burnt
- Production and distribution of good quality seeds of outstanding varieties by establishing supply-chain networking relevant agencies and farmers;

- Promotion of fodder production on degraded and wastelands and community pasture lands and under different farming systems;
- Promotion of post-harvest technologies for storage of fodder and improving nutritive value of roughages;
- Popularisation of complete feed, feed with by-pass protein, microbial protein, azola, spirulina and non-traditional feed ingredients;
- Decentralised production of complete feed through community initiatives, using locally available biomass.

The availability and cost of maize and soybean meal generally determine the cost of compounded feed. Average increase in corn availability is far below the growth rate of egg or meat production. Therefore, only two options are left with either to increase maize production markedly by increasing yield or area under production or to utilize other cereals as alternate to maize.

Animal scientists are already working on ways to produce meat with less feed. One possible solution may be using DDGS, or dried distillers grain solubles which is left over after corn is turned into ethanol. Growing use of cereals and oilseeds to produce fossil fuel substitutes – ethanol and biodiesel – represents a significant challenge for the livestock sector in terms of competition for resources.

Current trends

The world protein shortage is acute as demand of protein has increased manifold. The following table illustrates the trend in various regions (Table 4).

Table 4: Daily protein supply from livestock and from all sources in 1980 and 2002 *in grams per capita*

Region	Total Protein from Livestock		Total Protein	
	1980	2002	1980	2002
Sub Saharan Africa	10.4	9.3	53.9	55.1
Near East	18.2	18.1	76.3	80.5
Latin America	27.5	34.1	69.8	77.0
Developing Asia	7.0	16.2	53.4	68.9
Industrialized Countries	50.8	56.1	95.8	106.4
World	20.0	24.3	66.9	75.3

Source: Steinfeld *et. al.* (2006)

- Single-cell protein products such as algae, bacteria and yeasts are now showing promise to meet the demand.

- The synbiotics (probiotics and prebiotics) have been considered as suitable substitute of antibiotics, which are slowly being phased out, especially the gut-acting ones.
- The production of enzymes, singly or in combination, for enhancing utilization of feeds with high fibre or with anti-nutritional non-starch polysaccharides (feed enzymes) and phytate (phytase), has been priority area for research lately.
- Technology has made it feasible to produce transgenic feeds with high protein and amino acid contents (quality protein maize with high lysine & tryptophan), low anti-nutritional factors (Canola meals with low erucic acid, tannins, and glycosinolates) and with high vitamin activity (yellow sorghum with high beta-carotene activity), etc.
- Micro-organism have been selected and optimized by classical biotechnological methods to produce amino acids in fermentation process to produce the limiting amino acids in particular in large quantities for the feed industry. Production of trace mineral proteinates (organic minerals) utilizing yeast (*Saccharomyces cerevisae*) has become feasible in augmenting availability of various trace minerals including zinc, manganese, chromium, selenium, copper, etc.
- Impaired nutrition has been shown to be associated with reduced capacity of host to form specific antibodies; decrease in the phagocytic activity; interference with production of non-specific protective substances; reduced non-specific resistance to bacterial toxins; altered tissue integrity; diminished inflammatory response, collagen formation and wound healing, decreased antibody affinity and complement system; and variable endocrine activity. Hence the present strategy towards control of diseases have been a joint approach including vaccination programmes, selective breeding for augmenting disease resistance capacity of birds, improved management to curtail environmental stresses to a minimum level, and nutritional management (Sasidhar, 2006).
- Safety of feed also determines the food safety as is epitomized by the Bovine Spongiform Encephalopathy (BSE) or Mad Cow Disease associated with feeding of meat & bone meal (MBM). There is also concern on use of GM crops and concerns of contaminations with unintentional Persistent Organic Pollutants (uPOPs) like dioxins. Hence not only there is a dire need for high-end equipment like High-Resolution Mass Spectrophotometer etc. & skilled personnel but also adoption of principles of GMP & HACCP as well as addressing of issues of traceability in the feed industry urgently.

To sum up

Animal husbandry is at a crossroads with health, biosecurity, climate change and sustainability implications. For last more than thirty years, since the early 1980s, neither the private sector nor governments were interested in investing in agriculture. This is now changing. The reinvestment in agriculture, triggered especially by the 2008 food price crisis, is essential to the substantive realization of the right to food.

The increase of human population and its consumption of food of animal is driving the Livestock Production systems (LPS) both complex and intensive use of both anthropogenic and environmental resources. The threat to various livestock production systems is understood due to depleting resources or fragility of systems interactions. The pressures of sustainable production is thus increasing day by day.

There is a need for further research into Livestock Production systems (LPS). This sort of research involves strong interaction with a wide range of disciplines outside animal science to provide an improved understanding of the potential for the integrated development of LPS.

Veterinary nutrition approaches should assimilate the multi-disciplinary agro-ecological information and pay attention to resilience management to have a sustainable future for the livestock sector.

References

Altieri M.A. (1995). Agroecology: The Science of Sustainable Agriculture, 2nd ed., Boulder, Colorado, Westview Press.

Birthal P.S., Taneja V.K. and Thorpe W. (eds). (2006). *Smallholder Livestock Production in India: Opportunities and Challenges. Proceedings of an ICAR-ILRI international Workshopheld at National Agricultural Science Complex, DPS Marg, Pusa, New Delhi 110 012, India, 31 January-1 February, 2006.* NCAP (National Center for Agricultural Economics and Policy Research)- ICAR (Indian Council of Agricultural Research), New Delhi, India, and ILRI (International Livestock Research Institute), Nairobi, Kenya. 126 pp.

Birthal, P. and Parthasarathy Rao, P. (eds). (2002). Technology options for sustainable livestock production in India: proceedings of the Workshop on Documentation, Adoption, and Impact of Livestock Technologies in India, 18–19 Jan 2001, ICRISAT-Patancheru, India. New Delhi 110 012, India and Patancheru 502 324, Andhra Pradesh, India: National Center for Agricultural Economics and Policy Research and International Crops Research Institute for the Semi-Arid Tropics. 220 pp.

Checkland, P. (1999). *Systems Thinking, Systems Practice* Chichester: John Wiley & Sons, Ltd. In: Dalgaard T, Hutchings N.J., Porter J.R. Agroecology, scaling and interdisciplinarity http://basecologica.blogspot.com/2007/08/texto-4-agroecology-part-1.html accessed on 31July 2011.

De Wit, J., Oldenbroek J.K., van Keulen H., Zwarff D. (1995). Criteria for sustainable livestock production: a proposal for Implementation. *Agriculture. Ecosystems and Environment* 53 (1995) 219-229.

De Wit, J. (1993). Criteria for measuring sustainability of livestock production systems, IVG-Ropon B-394, Zeist, The Netherlands.

Demment M.W., Young M. and Sensenig R.L. (2003). Providing micronutrients through food based solutions: a key to human and national development," *Journal of Nutrition*, 133, pp. 3879-3885.

FAO 1988. Document CL 94/6 94th Session of the FAO Council, (1988). In: *FAO (1994)* Development and Education Exchange Papers (DEEP): Sustainable Agriculture and Rural Development: Part 1: Latin America and Asia, *Rome.*

FAO, (2006). Livestock's Long Shadow: environmental issues and options. Food and Agriculture Organization of the United Nations, Rome.

FAO, (2009). State of Food and Agriculture. Food and Agriculture Organization of the United Nations, Rome.

FAO, (2009). The State of Food and Agriculture. Food and Agriculture Organization of the United Nations, Rome, http://www.fao.org/docrep/012/i0680e/i0680e.pdf accessed on 28 July 2011

Foresight, (2011). The future of food and farming. Final project report The Government Office for Science, London. http://webarchive.nationalarchives.gov.uk/+/http://www.bis.gov.uk/foresight/our-work/projects/current-projects/global-food-and-farming-futures/reports-and-publications accessed on 29 July 2011.

Mittermeier, R.A., Robles Gil, P., Hoffmann, M., Pilgrim, J., Brooks, T., Mittermeier, C.G., Lamoreux, J., and da Fonseca, G.A.B. (2004). Hotspots Revisited. Mexico: CEMEX, quoted in FAO 2006.

Murgueitio, E. Intensive sustainable livestock production: an alternative to tropical deforestation. Ambio, (1990). Vol. 19 No. 8 pp. 397-400 http://www.cabdirect.org/abstracts/19910653089.html;jsessionid=6202EFBCF09C7717D218356B2C5E4009 accessed on 24 July 2011.

Planning Commission, Government of India, (2010). Report of the Advisory Committee on Animal Husbandry & Dairying, Government of India, Yojana Bhawan, New Delhi.

Sasidhar PVK (Ed.) (2006). Poultry Research Priorities to 2020. Proceedings of National Seminar (November 2-3). Central Avian Research Institute, Izatnagar-243 122 (India).

Staal, S.J., Pratt, A.N. & Jabbar, M., eds. (2008). Dairy development for the resource poor. Part 1: Pakistan and India dairy development case studies. Nairobi, International Livestock Research Institute.

Steinfeld, H., Gerber, P., Wassenaar, T., Castel, V, Rosales, M. & de Haan, C. (2006). Livestock's long shadow. Environmental issues and options. Rome, FAO.

Thompson P.B. and Nardone A. (1999). Sustainable livestock production: methodological and ethical Challenges. *Livestock Production Science* 61 (1999) 111–119.

Van den Berg H. and Jiggins J. (2007). Investing in Farmers. The Impacts of Farmer Field Schools in Relation to Integrated Pest Management," World Development, 35:4, pp. 663-686.

Walker, B., Carpenter S., Anderies J., Abel N., Cumming G., Janssen M., Lebel L., Norberg J., Peterson G.D., and Pritchard R. (2002). Resilience management in social-ecological systems: a working hypothesis for a participatory approach. Conservation Ecology 6 (1): 14. [online] URL: http://www.consecol.org/vol6/iss1/art14.

WHO, (2011). World Health Organization: Zoonoses and veterinary public health http://www.who.int/zoonoses/vph/en/ accessed on 25 July 2011.

WSPA, (2011). Why livestock and humane, sustainable agriculture matter at Rio+20. INTERNATIONAL (World Society for Protection of Animals). United Kingdom. http://www.wspa-international.org/Images/Policy%20doc%20-%20Why%20livestock-Final-sm_tcm25-21763.pdf accessed on 27 July 2011.

□□□

5

Applications Abuses and Alternatives to Antibiotics

S.S. SIKKA
Senior Nutritionist cum Head, Department of Animal Nutrition
Guru Angad Dev Veterinary and Animal Sciences University, Ludhiana

"LET FOOD BE THY MEDICINE AND MEDICINE BY THY FOOD"

It was proclaimed some 2500 years ago by Hippocrates. An Antibiotic is produced by a microorganism that inhibits or kills other microorganisms. The word 'antimicrobials' is often used to encompass any substance of natural or of synthetic origin (chemotherapeuticals). A century ago first antimicrobial (Salvarsan) was used for treating syphilis in 1910. Use of antimicrobials was expanded in 1930's with the use of sulphanomides (first chemotherapeutical) in human medicines. Penicillin though discovered in 1929 by Alexander Fleming was introduced for therapeutic use in 1941 for curing various bacterial diseases. Antimicrobials are the single most important discovery in the history of medicine being considered as miracle drugs because of saving millions of human and animal lives. Table 1 depicts the history of treatment of ailments.

Antimicrobials As Growth Promoters (AGP's)

Growth promoting properties of antimicrobials in poultry was first reported by Moore *et al.* (1946) and in pigs by Jukes *et al* (1950). Feeding of sub-therapeutic doses of antimicrobials to the farm animals was readily adopted. Various antimicrobials used in animal/ poultry production are given in the table 2.

Table 1 : Use of medicines for treating ailments

Year	Prevailing Medical advice
2000 BC	Here eat this root
1200 AD	This root is heathen, say this prayer
1500 AD	Prayer are superstitious, drink this potion
1900 AD	This potion is snake oil, Swallo this pill
1950 AD	This pill is ineffective, take this antibiotic
2000 AD	This antibiotic is synthetic, eat this root.

Table 2 : Antimicrobial agents approved for use in broiler production

Sulfonamides	Ionophores	Others
Sulfachloropyrazine	Lasalocid	Amprolium Arsanilate
Sulfamethazine	Maduramycin	(arsenical) Buquinolate
Sulfadimethoxine Sulfamyxin	Monensin Narasin	Clopindol Dequinate
Sulfanitran Sulfaquinoxaline	Salinomycin	Nequinate Robenidine Zoalene
Antibiotics and arsenicals		

Aminocyclitols (spectinomycin); Aminoglycosides (streptomycin, neomycin, gentamycin); Arsenicals (roxarsone, arsanilic acid); Bacitracin* Decapeptides (bacitracin); Bambermycin; B-Lactams (penicillins); Carbadox;; Erythromycin*; Fluoroquinolones (enrofloxacin, sarafloxacin); Laidomycin; Lasalocid; Lincomycin*; Lincosamides (lincomycin); Macrolides (erythromycin, tylosin); Monensin; Novobiocin Oleandomycin Roxarsone; Streptogramins (virginiamycin); Tiamulin; Tetracyclines (chlortetracycline, oxytetracycline, tetracycline);

* Identical to human-drugs

[a]Adapted from NRC, 1999 and USDA, 2001. [b]Labeled as growth promoter [c]The most commonly used arsenical compound in poultry feed. SOURCE: Hancock TC, Miller CV, Denver JM, Riedel GF. Fate and transport of arsenical fee amendments in Chesapeake Bay watersheds. Society of Environmental Toxicology and Chemistry 21st Annual Meeting; 2000 Nov 12–16; Nashville, TN.

As growth promoters, antibiotics are fed to healthy animals at concentrations below 200 grams per ton of feed for more than 14 days (FDA, 2000). The therapeutic doses are very high. Small doses result in conditions which are particularly conducive to selection for resistance in bacteria. Antimicrobials for therapeutic purposes are available only on prescription, but as growth promoters, these products are freely accessible and sold over the counter.

The overall outcome of use of AGPs is the availability of more nutrients for growth and production of the farm animals and poultry. Improvement of growth rate and feed conversion ratio (feed: gain) has been 16% and 9% in piglets, 9% and 5.5% in growing pigs, 3-10% and 3-5% in broiler chickens, 2% and 1% in layers, 7-10% and 4-5% in veal calves (Avcare, 2003). Effects of uses of AGP's on broad issues are depicted in table 1.

Exact mechanism as to how AGP's promote growth is not entirely clear. It is widely assumed that AGP's act mainly through their effect on intestinal flora. With less than 10 % of intestinal micro-flora identified, there has been little chance of fully understanding AGP's mode of action.

It is postulated that AGP's allow the animal to express their natural potential for growth, which is achieved through their direct influence on (Bedford 2005) i.e. reducing the total number of intestinal microorganisms, creating a more favourable balance between beneficial and non-beneficial ones, proportionally sparing of nutrients for absorption and weight gain. Intestinal bacteria inactivate pancreatic enzymes and metabolize dietary protein with the production of ammonia and biogenic amines. Antibiotics help in inhibiting these activities and increase the digestibility of dietary proteins. Experimental results obtained with some antibiotics commonly used as growth promoters (chlortetracycline, penicillin and sulfamethazine) have shown that treated pigs have higher serum levels of a growth factor similar to insulin.

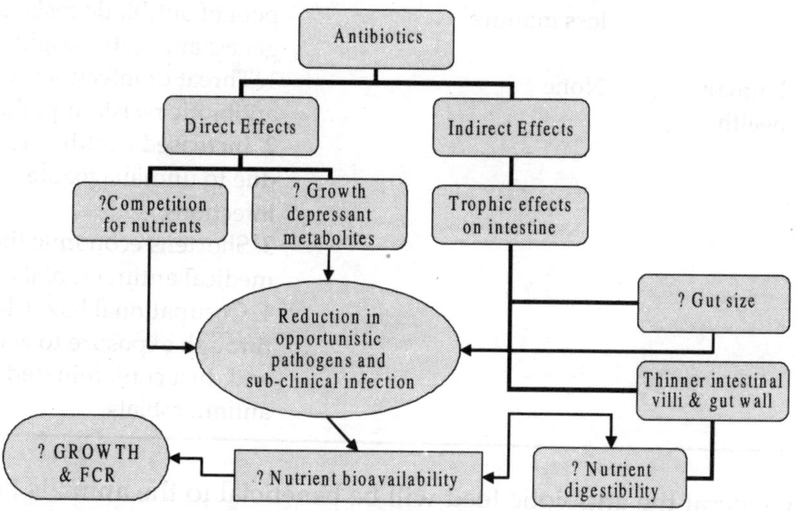

Fig. 1 : Schematic diagram showing possible mechanism of action of antiobiotics for growth promotion

Table 1 : Effects of AGP in Relation to Some Broad Issues of animal production.

S No.	Broad issue	Positive effect	Negative effect
1	Health	Control of certain diseases (primarily enteric) to some extent	1. Development of antimicrobial resistance 2. Masks sub-clinical disease and infection 3. Limits incentives for hygienic improvements
2.	Welfare	Alleviates and dampens disease signs	1.Camouflages stress associated with sub-clinical disease 2. Allows higher stocking rates
3	Husbandry	Increased 1.Production & 2. Productivity	Stimulates, increase and intensify animal production
4	Feed	Enhance shelf life.	1. Camouflages bad feed quality. 2. Hampers improvements in feed formulation 3. Development of alternatives
5	Production system	Lower labour demand due to more intense production methods. Better crop security.	Hampers the development of animal-friendly production systems. Development of antibiotic resistance even for pathogens of crop animals.
6.	Environment	Better utilization of feed; less manure.	Increases the environmental pool of antibiotic resistance genes; antibiotic residues.
7.	Human health	None	1. Threat of infection by antibiotic resistant pathogens. 2. Increased health care cost due to unmanageable infections. 3. Shortens economic life of medical antimicrobials. 4. Occupational hazards through exposure to aerosol and dust contaminated with antimicrobials.

In general the antibiotic feed will be beneficial to the animals because of inhibition of sub clinical infections, reduced gut motility, reduced mucin secretion, reduced toxin (eg. ammonia and biogenic amine from protein formulation) production, bile salts modification, thinning intestinal wall, increase in digestive enzyme output, improve the digestibility, increase the uptake of nutrients along the alimentary canal, reduce the opportunity for harmful bacteria to establish in the gut, activation of the intestinal immune system and reduction in microbial use of nutrients thus sparing the nutrients for the host (Sikka, 2008).

The ultimate impacts of use of antimicrobials as growth promoters in farm animal/aquaculture production systems are increased growth rate of animals/fish/shell fish, better feed conversion, improved egg production in laying hens, increased litter size in sows, un physiological early weaning of piglets, increased milk yield in dairy cows, economize the animal production systems, reduced incidence of disease, allow high stocking rates which raise questions on animal ethics and welfare and provides some protection against certain diseases

In spite of tremendous beneficial effects in improving feed efficiency and live-stock productivity, antibiotics were soon found loosing ground as additives in animal feed because of their effect on development of resistance in some deadly bacteria in the animal gut and in the terrestrial environment. Today, there is considerable controversy and a growing concern over the use of antibiotics to promote growth in animals raised for food.

The continued feeding of antibiotics containing feed not only produce resistant bacteria in the body of the animal but also introduce low levels of antibiotics in the soil and water through the animal excreta, in turn producing antibiotic resistance in soil bacteria, which may contain pathogens too. In recent years, public has become increasingly more alarmed by the emergence and spread of antibiotic-resistant bacteria. It is true that microbial resistance to antibiotics is on the rise, and is even becoming something of a crisis in some countries' health care programmes. Overuse of prescribed drugs in human and veterinary medicine, as well as their use as growth promoters in animal in live-stock feeds has all been blamed as the cause of growing antibiotic resistance.

Dose of Antibiotics

The recommended inclusion levels in diets of poultry and pig were 4 ppm for the narrow-spectrum and 10 ppm for the broad-spectrum antibiotics in 1950's, but these levels have increased 10 to 20 folds since then. In case of fish and fishery products certain antibiotics are permitted to as high a level as up to 100 ppm, with the result, the development of antibiotic resistance by several infective bacteria has become a serious problem as some of these bacterial infections which could normally be treated by specific antibiotics have turned out to be untreatable by these antibiotics. To manage such resistant bacterial infections, health authorities are forced to search for newer and more effective antibiotics. If this trend continues, the day will come when some infectious pathogens may emerge which have developed resistance to all the known existing antibiotics currently in use. In short, it is some thing like unknowingly creating a pathogen similar to AIDS, resistant to all treatment methods- a man made threat to mankind. World over health authorities are seriously pondering on this issue.

Therapeutic use of Antibiotics in Livestock Production

Therapeutic use of antibiotics is a significant issue in livestock, aquaculture and poultry industry. Farm animals and birds suffering from infectious diseases are benefited from the use of antibiotics. However, food safety and quality assurance aspects of food products such as injection site lesions, antibiotic residues, and antibiotic resistance of bacteria must be considered. The injection site lesions are the visible tissue damage due to mechanical and chemical irritation caused by the injection as well as inflammatory response to the irritation. Lesions may occur when any drug, vaccine or even saline water is injected. Injection site lesions may be detected in tissues for years after the injection.

The term 'antibiotic residue' is the small amount of an antibiotic or its breakdown product(s) that remains in or on an agricultural product following treatment with that antibiotic. Every antibiotic approved for use in livestock production has a maximum residue limit or tolerance level that is established based on consideration of the potential risks to human beings exposed to the drug residue in food. These health risks (Callan,2003) include allergic reactions (penicillin), bone marrow suppression (chloramphenicol, sulfonamides), nephrotoxicity (gentamycin), carcinogenicity (sulfonamides), or the potential for developing antibiotic resistant bacteria (all antibiotics). Moreover, antibiotic residues in milk can also affect starter cultures used in cheese and yogurt manufacture.

Antibiotics in Soil Environment and Food Chain

Antibiotics are not fully used by the animals. A major portion i.e.30- 80 percent of antibiotic dose may be excreted as waste because of poor adsorption. When manure is used to fertilize croplands, antibiotics in the manure may get into the soil and eventually end up in streams, lakes or rivers. Antibiotic residues in the excreta have potential impact on the environment as compared to industrial chemicals; the exposure routes of veterinary medicinal products to the environment are depicted in figure 1. Antibiotics used as veterinary medicines enter the environment by two ways:

(i) Directly when using the drugs i.e. the unabsorbed as waste and

(ii) Subsequent excretion of absorbed antibiotic residues and their metabolites through urine and faeces of the animal.

The dominating pathways of environmental release in the terrestrial compartment are: application of FYM in arable soil, and in fish farms, an unknown part of food-pellets containing the medical compound (most often an antibacterial drug) will not be eaten hence reach the sediment directly without any change. Antibiotics after consumption may be excreted partly as unchanged compound or as metabolites, which finally reaches the sediment. The group of antibiotics used as non-therapeutics is to be used as growth permoters especially in pigs and also in cattle and poultry. Coccidiostat is only used as growth promoters in poultry production. The medicinal mixtures with antibiotics sold as "premixed" drugs are used for therapeutic treatment of pigs, cattle, poultry, fish and shellfish.

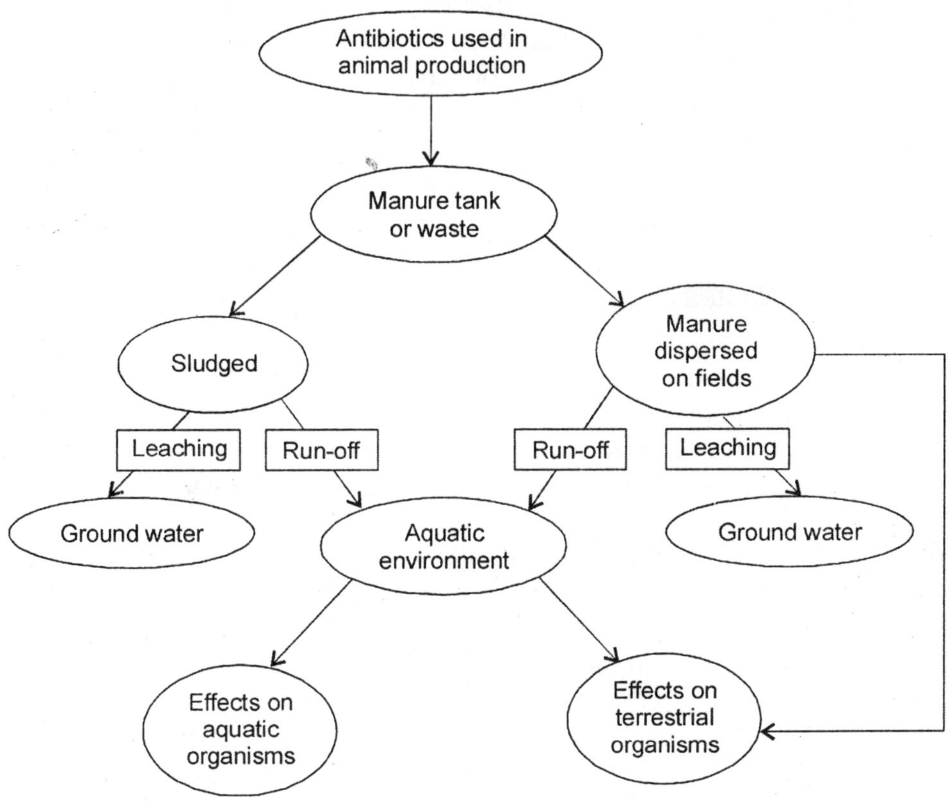

Schematic diagram showing anticipated exposure pathways for veterinary antibiotics in the environment (Sarmah *et al.*, 2006)

No information is available on the fate of veterinary medicinal products with antibiotics during storage of manure/cow dung slurry. There are two types of substances, (i) hydrophilic and (ii) hydrophobic, available in the manure /slurry. Hydrophilic substances dissolve in the aqueous fraction of the manure/slurry while hydrophobic substances get adsorbed on the particulate matter. The antibiotics residues present in dung depending on its chemical properties either undergo degradation or leach to the soil in cases of rain. In grazing animals drugs released in urine immediately reach the soil and if water soluble, leach further down to groundwater or adjacent water systems. Most drugs excreted through the urine are by nature relatively water soluble, whereas drugs excreted via faeces in general is less soluble.

Livestock population in the country is bound to increase in future. This will result in increase in livestock population in the country suggesting that in future still higher amounts of antibiotics will find their way into terrestrial environment. There is a tremendous growth in poultry production for meeting increased demand for meat and eggs in the country. Continuous use of antibiotic laden poultry meat, fish & manure can ultimately lead to severe environmental problems in terms of various toxic effects from residual antibiotics and their metabolites on soil micro-flora and fauna as well as development of antibiotic resistance in some pathogenic bacteria, whose control in case of an infection may become impossible with the available antibiotics- a man made unmanageable infection similar to ***AIDS***.

Antibiotics in Wastes

Spreading of manure/slurry and dropping of excreta by field animals may lead to a run-off of especially hydrophilic substances in case of subsequent rains. Microorganisms are essential to life on earth as they are responsible for nutrient re-cycling, organic matter decomposition and a variety of other functions. Antibiotics, which are designed to kill disease causing bacteria especially broad spectrum antibiotics could work havoc on natural microbial communities in the soil. Antibiotics might disrupt essential biological activity in the soil. One major consequence of this phenomenon is the emergence of antibiotic-resistant bacteria that could infect humans, livestock, fish & shellfish and wildlife. After consumption of antibiotic laced feed to the animals, unused antibiotics will eventually enter the environment. In fish and shellfish farming, antibiotics are given as feed additives, and are directly released into the aquatic environment (Thurman *et al.*, 2002). Approximately 70 to 80 % of antibiotics administered to fish & shellfish enter the environment. Antibiotic residues with significant antibacterial activity have been reported in the sediments from fish and prawn hatcheries and farms (Samuelsen *et al.*, 1992) in this country.

Of the total drugs administered 40 to 90 % are excreted as parent compounds by the animals after medication (Halling-Sorensen *et al.*, 2001; Winckler and Grafe, 2001). The most common antibiotics present in swine, beef, and poultry/turkey manures are tetracyclines (oxytetracycline and chlortetracycline), tylosin, sulfamethazine, amprolium, monensin, virginiamycin, penicillin, and nicarbazine (Webb and Fontenot, 1975; De Liguoro *et al.*, 2003; Kumar *et al.*, 2004, 2005). The concentration of these antibiotics varies from traces to as high as 216 (mg L^{-1}) of manure slurry (Kumar *et al.*, 2005). Concentration of antibiotics in manure excreted from treated animals can be as high as several hundred of mg kg^{-1} (Migliore *et al.*, 1997; De Liguoro *et al.*, 2003). Soil and water contamination from manure fertilization and at concentrated animal operations has been frequently reported (Rabolle and Spliid, 2000; Hamscher *et al.*, 2002; Boxall *et al.*, 2002). There is concern that residual concentrations of antibiotics in agricultural soil can easily reach levels similar to pesticides if the manure loading for fertilization increases to the kilograms per hectare level (Thiele-Bruhn, 2003). These antibiotics generally remain stable during manure storage and end up in agricultural fields on manure applications (Boehm, 1996 and Migliore *et al.*, 1995). Widespread contamination of veterinary antibiotics exposes humans and animals to a constant low concentration of antibiotics. This threatens the human and animal health by diminishing the success of antibiotic treatment. Evidence has been presented that antibiotic resistant genes from microorganisms in the environment can be transferred directly to humans. Leaching and runoff of antibiotics from manure-fertilized lands is threatening the quality of drinking water. Though the effects of long-term exposure to low concentrations of antibiotics are not yet clear, the potential danger resulting from veterinary antibiotic contamination to human and animal health cannot be neglected.

Persistence of Antibiotics in Soil

There are very few studies on reaction of antibiotics in soil. Photolysis, hydrolysis, bio-degradation and binding on to soil particles through adsorption process are some of the reactions of these antibiotics and their products that can take place in soil and influence their persistence in soil. They may form complexes with soluble organic materials in the soil and may become more mobile and contaminate even groundwater while still in its parent form. Soil pH plays important role in ionization of most of the antibiotics reacting soil. Tetracycline group of antibiotics behaves as amphoteric compounds in soil. They are stable under low pH conditions but not under basic soil conditions. These compounds can form chelate-complexes with divalent metal ions like Ca^{2+}, Mg^{2+}, Fe^{2+}, Mn^{2+}, Zn^{2+}, and Cu^{2+} etc. Sulfonamides, on the other hand, have two pKa values, they behave as weak acids and form salts both under acid and basic conditions. Some of the strongly bound antibiotics absorbed antibiotics in the soil can contaminate the surface waters when these move with the soil and sediments move along with the run-off water. Aminoglycosides are polar compounds, they are highly water soluble. They can easily move with the percolating water and can contaminate the ground water resources, but they are photodegradable, therefore, easily decompose when subjected to sun-light. Penicillin belongs to â-lactam class of antibiotics is stable under a wide range of pH values from strong acid to strong alkali conditions. Fluoroquinolones, also resist break down through hydrolysis and therefore are highly stable in soil.

European Agency for the Evaluation of Medicinal Products has recommended a more intensive environmental safety evaluation of veterinary medicinal products if any ingredient or metabolite is present in manure in concentrations > 0.1 mg/kg. WHO of UN in the year 2000, recommended ban on antibiotics as growth promoters in animal feed if these antibiotics are also used in human therapy and in absence of risk-based evaluation. In 2006, EU completely banned the use of antibiotic–growth promoters in animal agriculture and aquaculture. *There is need to collect precise data on antibiotic use in animal farming, aquaculture and agriculture and the potential reservoir for residual antibiotics in the terrestrial environment in the country. Besides, research work is needed to understand kinetics of biodegradation and potencies of degraded products of various antibiotics in different soils, manures and waste water.* Antibiotics can influence the biological processes in the soil and can affect the organic matter transformation, biological N fixation, degradation of herbicides/pesticides in the soil.

Numerous studies have suggested that aerobic conditions were always beneficial for the degradation of antibiotics in manure and water. *It has been suggested that there is need to develop technologies to enhance the degradation of antibiotics in soil and to prevent them from contaminating surface and ground water, a more effective and practical way to reduce contamination from veterinary antibiotics, would be eliminating the antibiotics in the manure before its application to agricultural land as fertilizer.* There is considerable need for further research into environmental effects such as sorption, mobility, and microbiological changes. This is also the case for other substances that have not undergone valid environmental risk assessment.

Degradation of Antibiotics

Antibiotics like ciprofloxacin, ofloxacin, and virginiamycin degrade very slowly and may persist in soil in its original form up to 30-80 days while bambermycin, tylosin, and erythromycin completely degrade in a period of one month at temperatures ranging from 20-30°C. Most of the antibiotic residues in manure generally remain stable during manure storage until its application to agriculture fields. On repeated application of antibiotic-laden manure to the soil result in significant concentration in the soil making them potential source to contaminate the terrestrial environment. Persistence of antibiotics in soil is determined by a number of soil and environmental factors. Properties of antibiotics which influence their persistence in soil are photo-stability, binding with soil particles, adsorption on soil colloids through surface reactions, water solubility, biodegradation, making complexes with organic matter and may become more mobile, move faster and contaminate ground waters while still retaining its original structure.

Factors like adsorption reactions, effect of type of Soil, type of clay minerals and soil temperature are also responsible for the persistence of antibiotics in the soil.

Eco-toxicological Impacts

Antibiotics when enter the soil, its environment is affected in several ways:

(i) Alter the composition and diversity of indigenous soil microbial communities, which are of fundamental importance for ecosystem.

(ii) Change function in nutrient cycling,

(iii) Change decomposition, and

(iv) Changes in energy flow (McCracken and Foster, 1993; Schmitt *et al.*, 2004).

(v) Cause the formation of resistance (even cross and multiple), in organisms in the soil environment (Al-Ahmad *et al.*, 1999; Sengelov *et al.*, 2003).

Organic matter in antibiotic exposed soil is not decomposed resulting in reduced release of nutrients for plants affecting crop growth and crop yield. *How antibiotics affect soil fauna and flora, enzymatic activity and nutrient cycling needs greater emphasis for investigation.* These impacts could be direct such as antibiotic toxicity to soil microbes and indirect effect such as nutrient availability due to changed microbiological activity in soil. Decomposition of organic matter in the form of manures and crop residue depends on various microbial processes, which, in turn depend on type and population of microorganisms in soil. Repeated application of antibiotics in soil through manures may adversely affect decomposition process by curtailing the microbial population and also by allowing only the antibiotic-resistant microbes to flourish. Oxytetracycline or chlortetracycline residues in manure which when applied to the soil result in more evolution of due to higher proportions of easily decomposable/degradable C compounds. Ionophore antibiotics such as monensin favours growth of Gram-negative bacteria in animal gut, which, inturn changes the fermentation dynamics, improves dietary protein efficiency, and results in less methane production by as much as 25%. The effect of monensin in decreasing feed intake by animals and reduced excretion of nitrogenous compounds such as ammonia and also methane are environmentally beneficial. Similarly tylosin addition in pig feeds can result in reduced N excretion by as much as 10%. This means if we ban the use of antibiotics in the animal husbandry, there could be 7-10% increased loading of environmental N (NAAS, 2010).

Impact on Non-target Microorganisms

Antibiotics like streptomycin-laden manure has been found to decrease bacterial count in soil upto 50-75% over several months. The effect will depend upon the nature of bacterial population; a more resilient population shows effect only for a limited period as compared to non-resilient population. Streptomycin has been specifically found to adversely affect the nitrifying bacteria as NO_3-N concentration in the soil decreased. Gram-negative bacteria like *nitrosomonas spp* are responsible for nitrification in soil. Therefore, broad-spectrum antibiotics like tetracyclines, aminoglycocides, and sulfonamides in manure and soil are expected to inhibit the nitrification process in soil, however, narrow spectrum antibiotics such as sefdiazine, oxolinic acid, and tylosin simulated the nitrification process. Veterinary antibiotics may also inhibit SO_4 reduction as well as OM decomposition. Build up of tylosin in soil can cause selective pressure on soil bacterial population, shifting bacterial communities from Gram-positive to a Gram-negative; the consequences of such a selective change in population are well known (Pasricha, 2008).

Emergence of Antibiotic Resistance

Microbial resistance to antibiotics is on the rise, and is even becoming something of a crisis in some countries' health care. For bacteria to develop resistance to antibiotics, they must first receive exposure to them. Overuse of prescribed drugs in human and veterinary medicine, as well as their use as growth promoters in animals has all been blamed. Widespread use of antibiotics and their subsequent release into the environment may lead to the selection of antibiotic-resistant bacteria. There has been a frequent observation on shortening of the time between introduction of a new antibiotic and development of resistance of the targeted microbial species. If spontaneous mutations were the only cause of antibiotic resistance, it would have been restricted to only a few bacterial species. A higher degree of vancomycin resistance (60%) in various enterococci isolates from the broiler droppings has been reported. Similarly, a high level of resistance among Gram-positive and Gram-negative isolates from various meat products have been observed for such antibiotics as penicillin, erythromycin, sulfamethoxine, tetracycline, ceftibiotics, and gentamycin. Therefore, animal manure containing such antibiotics can cause elevation of resistance in soil bacteria after manure application year after year. The studies have shown that development of resistance is quite rapid, it has been found that within 3 weeks of antibiotic feeding; more than 70% of faecal bacteria were resistant to penicillin and tetracycline. All these studies show that antibiotic feeding of animals provides an environment that permits selection of resistant strains and perhaps also encourages the transfer of genetic information from even unrelated bacterial species.

Every time some drug becomes ineffective against resistant bacteria, it adds to the cost of treatment. Research takes place for 10-15 years, costing more than one $ billion, with about 5,000 early testing trials and only one will get regulatory approval. Doctors need to wait for more than 8 to 10 years for evolving a new antibiotic. It is thus important we should look for safer growth promoters and use antibiotics to a bare minimum especially those antibiotics that are used by both animals and humans. *If possible antibiotics used for managing human infections shall be totally banned for use as growth promoters.*

Antibiotics as routine feed additives are used at low concentrations, which appear to prevent some infectious diseases. The antibiotic dose depends on the type and size of the animal and the type of antibiotic. These low quantities of antibiotics encourage the selection of antibiotic resistant bacteria in the environment. Overuse of antimicrobials may diminish their effectiveness and the strains of resistant bacteria would arise. Of the 1,415 microorganisms known to cause diseases in humans, 60% are *zoonotic*. Many bacterial species multiply rapidly enough to double their numbers every 20–30 minutes, and their ability to adapt to changes in the environment and survive unfavourable conditions often results in the development of mutations that protect them.

Resistance

Microorganisms exist on the classical concept *"SURVIVAL OF THE FITTEST."* Microbes produce certain compounds to kill other microorganisms for their own survival and propagation. In our language these compounds are called the Antimicrobials. Antibiotic resistance means the ability of bacteria to loose their susceptibility to specific antibiotic drugs. Bacterial capacity to adapt to external changes using these mechanisms is called resistance development and this allows the resistant organisms to proliferate in the prevailing conditions. Resistance takes in two forms.

(i) *Inherent or intrinsic resistance*: The species is not normally susceptible to a particular drug. This may be due to the inability of the antibacterial agent to enter the bacteria cell and reach its target site, or lack of affinity between the antibacterial and its target (site of action), or absence of the target in the cell.

(ii) *Acquired resistance*: The species is normally susceptible to a particular drug but certain strains express drug resistance, which may be mediated through a number of mechanisms. When resistance develops, the antibiotic is no longer capable of curing or treating the disease caused by the infective agent. A low level of resistance may be detected by a slight increase in the minimal inhibitory concentration (MIC) for the antibiotic from the usual value, which is not necessarily of clinical significance. A higher degree of resistance is characterized by an MIC that exceeds, sometimes by several orders of magnitude, the concentrations of drug safely attainable in the patient's tissues. There are two types of resistances which occur.

Vertical Transmission: Resistance through mutation in existing genes that is the resistant trait would be confined to the mutant clone and spread of resistance is confined to that clone only. *Horizontal transmission*: Resistance developed through the uptake of existing genes. In this case, the resistance trait through mobile genetic elements can also spread to other bacterial clones, species and even to other genera.

Transfer of resistance

Resistant genes are flowing freely between animal and human bacteria through the food chain, which makes the situation more alarming. Of great concern was the possibility that resistance generated on the farm could lead to a loss of effectiveness of key antibiotics in human medicine.

Risks of resistance transfer: Generally two risks are considered independently.

Risk associated with the transmission of resistant bacteria from aquaculture environments to humans, i.e. the increase of resistance in human bacterial pathogens as a direct consequence of the use of antibiotics in aquaculture; and

Risk associated with the introduction in the human environment of nonpathogenic bacteria containing antimicrobial resistance genes and the subsequent transfer of such genes to human pathogens.

Mechanism of Resistance

Different mechanisms exist in bacteria that make them resistant to a specific antibiotic of a common chemical group. Antibiotic resistance is conferred by variations in the genetic makeup of bacteria. The genes that confer antibiotic resistance are carried on the bacterial chromosome or on separate plasmids that can be transferred between different bacteria. Thus, one bacterium can transfer antibiotic resistance to another bacterium. In addition, genes that confer resistance to antibiotics tend to group together such that resistance to multiple antibiotics is transferred by a single plasmid. These properties of antibiotic resistant genes complicate the control of antibiotic resistance and contribute to the concern over the use of antibiotics in livestock and public health. Antibiotics can promote the establishment of an antibiotic resistant population of bacteria by killing the susceptible bacteria leaving behind the resistant bacteria. Antibiotics do not induce the genetic changes that confer resistance, rather, they select for the bacteria that already have the genetic changes responsible for resistance. Indiscriminate or inappropriate use of antibiotics can promote the selection of antibiotic resistant bacteria. It is extremely important that antibiotics are used appropriately and according to the manufacturer's recommendations unless otherwise specified by the animal nutritionist/veterinarian.

Resistance in food-borne pathogens

Development of resistance in in the food-borne pathogens is a real problem, because these infections can become difficult to treat with traditional antibiotics, thus threatening human and animal life. The reports of several incidences of infection by multidrug-resistant *Salmonella typhimurium DT 104* in the past decade is the result of such a possibility. Out of 120 isolates of *E.coli* from animal food showed that around 20% were resistant to multi-antibiotic drugs. Similarly, a wide range of tetracycline-resistant genes of *E.coli* have been observed as isolated from human and animal sources. A recent study showed that not only Gram-negative enterobacteria but also Gram-positive bacteria are the major source of antibiotic-resistant integrons in animal litters. Selection of tetracycline-resistance occurs in the animal gut and these resistant bacteria are released into the environment when the wastes from these animals are used as manure.

Antibiotics and Plant Uptake

Until recently, research on antibiotics use has been mainly directed toward their beneficial and adverse effects on the end user, humans and animals. Consumers may unknowingly be ingesting some of these antibiotics when they eat vegetables grown on manure-applied lands. Some adverse impacts of consuming antibiotics in vegetables (sweet corn) and fruits are speculated.

- *Allergic or toxic reactions* - Some of the antibiotics when ingested by humans, especially children, may cause serious allergies or toxicity (Patterson *et al.*, 1995). There may be some interaction effects from simultaneous ingestion of two different antibiotics. It has been shown that some of the macrolide antibiotics present in animal feed have interacted with other antibiotics like monensin and have resulted in toxicity of monensin and the death of affected cattle (Basaraba *et al.*, 1999).

- *Antibiotic resistance*- Antibiotics present in plant materials ingested by humans may provide resistance to human pathogens thus resulting in illnesses that may be difficult to cure with presently available antibiotics. It has been shown that resistance of gut bacteria to antibiotics increased when fed with increasing concentrations of penicillin in contaminated waste milk (Selim and Cullor, 1997; Langford *et al.*, 2003). Small amounts of tetracycline can act as a catalyst in triggering the horizontal gene transfer between different bacteria (Shoemaker *et al.*, 2001).

Increasing resistance may be of concern both for human and animal health if antibiotics are present in food crops. Our knowledge regarding the implications of manure based antibiotics on the terrestrial environment and human health is limited. There is an urgent need to study

(i) Fate of different antibiotics present in manure,

(ii) Which antibiotics and their degradation products may be taken up by plants grown on antibiotic-laden manure amended soils,

(iii) Whether or not antibiotics present in food degrade when cooked, and

(iv) Whether or not antibiotics or their degradation products are still bioactive to impart antibiotic resistance to gut and soil bacteria or cause adverse immunological reactions in humans.

Thus, the use of antibiotics anywhere in the world can increase antibiotic resistance somewhere else, following the simple ecological principle that "*Every thing is connected to everything else*". The transfer of resistant bacteria is not restricted to a particular country or a continent as animal products are traded world-wide. This suggests that prevention of further spread of resistance from the bacterial communities via animal products required global regulations. Lest the day microbes developing resistance to all existing antibiotics and infecting human beings with out any management option similar to AIDS cannot be ruled out.

Warnings on the Use of Antibiotic Growth Promoters

Worldwide legislation to control use of antibiotics has eventually fuelled the reduction of antibiotic use, at least their non-therapeutic use. Doctors may still prescribe antibiotic treatment to patients where it can be ineffective, but consumers in many advanced countries are no longer keen to eat meat / livestock products from the animals raised on feeds containing antibiotics. As per WTO proclamation, sanitary and phyto-sanitary measures are to be used to an extent required to protect animals and plants by following scientific methods. The chance for residual effects can be reduced by adopting package of practices through which the farmers are advised to follow a standard operating procedure for antibiotic use and withdraw antibiotic feed additives seven to ten days or a suitable period to permit metabolism and excretion of residues prior to sacrifice/ harvest for use as food. This strategy may prevent unwanted antibiotic residue directly reaching human body at the same time it may not affect the pattern of antibiotic residues from animals and fish reaching the soil and water and inducing antibiotic resistance in the microbes there. Moreover, of late there is societal transition from cheap food to "safe" food. Animal welfare activists demand for natural products. The net result has been world over rejection of antibiotics.

Use of ionophore antibiotics (monensin, lasolacid, etc.) has been extensive in the animal husbandry. Efforts are being made to ban in many countries, but the experience has not been satisfactory, as the disease incidence has been increased resulting much more use of therapeutic antibiotics. However, the antibiotics are classified as (i) Feed Antibiotics and (ii) Therapeutic Antibiotics to curb the use of therapeutic antibiotics at sub-therapeutic levels as feed additives for animal production.

The WHO, American Medical Association, and the American Public Health Association have urged a ban on use of antibiotics as growth promoting additives (GPAs), arguing that their use leads to increased antibiotic-resistant infections in humans. In contrast, commercial interests have argued that their removal will have a significant impact on the cost of production in farm animals (Smith *et al*,2002; Casewell *et al*, 2003). Studies have shown that the use of growth promoting antibiotics contributes to contamination of flocks and food products by antibiotic- resistant pathogens, including *Campylobacter, Salmonella* and pathogenic *Enterococcus* and *Escherichia coli* and thereby increasing risks of human infections untreatable by certain antibiotics (Fienman, 1979; Cohen and Tauxe, 1986). In 2004 the U.S. Food and Drug Administration banned the non-therapeutic use of *Eenrofloxacin* (a *fluoroquinolone* applied for therapeutic uses) for growth promotion in food animals on the grounds that its use has contributed to fluoroquinolone-resistance in human pathogens. In recent years, concerns about the use of antimicrobial products in food-producing animals have focused on human food safety because foods of animal origin are identified as vehicles of food borne disease in humans, than any other group of food. As a result of treating animals with antibiotics, food borne bacteria may also become resistant to the antibiotics used to treat human disease.

By the early 1950s the problem of antimicrobial resistance was well acknowledged. Table 2 depicts some of the warnings and actions for the use of antimicrobials.

Table 2 : Warnings/Actions against the use of antibiotics as animal feed additives.

S. No	Year	Warnings / action
1	1945	Alexander Flemming warns against misuse of penicillin as 'microbes are educated to resist'
2.	1950s	Antibiotic resistance widely recognised – vertical transmission.
3.	1950	Tuberculosis bacteria resistant to Streptomycin.
4.	1953	Certain strains of dysentery bacillus was found resistant to Chloromphenicol, Tetracycline, Streptomycin, and Sulphanilamides
5	1958-59	Tetracycline resistant to poultry.
6	1960s	Horizontal transmission recognized.
7	1969	Swann Committee recommends severe restrictions on antimicrobials supplementations in animal feeds.
8	1970s	Swann committee recommendations implemented in the UK and EU
9	1975	Swann committee recommendations relaxed: tolysin and spiramycin still permitted as growth promoters; vancomycin comes into use.
10	1977	Swedish Agriculture Board considers potential risk of antibiotic resistance, but concludes it is negligible
11	1984	Swedish farmers ask for government ban on antimicrobials in animal feed because of health and consumer concerns.
12	1985	Swedish ban on grounds of antibiotic resistance in animals and it's 'uncertain' long-term effects
13	1995	Avoparcin and Vancomycin resistant Enterococci in pigs and poultry.
14	1995	Norway banned Avoparcin
15	1996	German government banned Avoparcin
16	1997	EU banned Avoparcin
17	1997	Swedish report concludes that risk of antibiotic resistance in humans is 'far from negligible'
18	1997	WHO scientific meeting concludes that it is 'essential to replace growth promoting antimicrobials'
19	1998	Danish government banned Virginiamycin due to Streptococcus resistance.
20	1998	EU bans five antimcirobials in animal feed as 'precautionary' measure, such as Avoparcin, Bacitracin Zn, Spiramycin, Virginiamycin and Tylosin in animal feedstuffs.

21	1999	EU Scientific Steering Committee recommends phase-out of antimicrobials that may be used in human/animal therapy
22	1999	Pharmaceutical industry opposes EU bans and takes EU to the European Court; judgement expected end 2001
23	2000	WHO recommends ban on antimicrobials as growth promoters if used in human therapy and in absence of risk-based evaluation.
24	2006	European Commission authorized use of Flavophospholipol, Monensis Na, Salinomycin Na and Avilamycin in the diets of poultry, beef cattle, pigs, rabbits and calves, as these are not used in human medicine. The act is ADUFA- Animal Drug user Fee Act, STAAR- Strategies to address antimicrobial drug resistance and PAMTA- Preservation of Antibiotics for Medical Treatment Act.
25	August, 2008	US congress passed a legislation regarding AGP's
26	November, 2008	Brain storming session was held at NAASC, New Delhi.
27	May, 2010	Policy paper no 43 " Antibiotics in manure and soil- A grave threat to human and livestock health" NAAS (2010)

These issues were discussed at different levels in different countries.

Spectinomycin and Enrofloxacin in USA,

Cloramphenicol and Nitrofurans in Argentina, Canada, EU, Japan, USA andIndia and

Rifampin Not labelled in USA or Canada have banned for use as growth promoters in animal husbandry. Govt. of India also banned Chloranphenicol, Nitrofurans including Furaldone, Furazolidone, Furylfuramide, Nifuratel, Nifuroxime, Nifuraprazine, Nitrofurantrin, Nitrofurazone, Neomycin, Nalidixic acid, Sulphamethoxazole, Aristolochia spp. And preparations thereof, Chloroform, Chlorpromazine, Colchicine, Depsona , Dimetridazole, Metronidazole, Ronidazole, Ipromidazole, Other nitroimidazoles, Clenbuterol, Diethylstilbestrol (DES), Sulfonamide drugs (except approved Sulfonamethixine, Sulfabromomethazine and Sulfaethoxy pyridazine), Fluroquinolones and Glycopeptides in aquaculture

Worldwide, there are great differences in the regulatory control of antimicrobials for therapy, prophylaxis and growth promoting purposes. In US, low doses of Tetracycline and Penicillin are still used as feed additives for prophylaxis and growth promotion without veterinary prescription, while therapeutic antimicrobials are often used based on prescription.

Alternatives to Antibiotic Growth Promoters (AGPs)

Resistant genes are flowing freely between animal and human bacteria through the food chain, which makes the situation more alarming. Of great concern was the possibility that resistance generated on the farm could lead to a loss of effectiveness of key antibiotics in human medicine. Continuous use of antimicrobials in feed is one of the major sources of overuse and misuse of antimicrobials in animal production. The usage of antimicrobial agents as feed additives is a complex issue with implications for human and animal health, animal welfare, food safety, environmental aspects, development of production systems, feeding practices and management of the animals.

Ban on use of AGP's has created the need to explore the alternatives that can improve the general health status and enhance the immunity to fight against disease. This increased the interest of nutritionists toward natural substances like botanicals, herbs, nutraceuticals, enzymes etc. Some of the potential alternatives tried in the past are zinc oxide, copper sulphate, plasma proteins, egg yolk antibodies, organic acids, probiotics, prebiotics, enzymes, bioactive peptides, botanicals (herbs/spices), essential oils and fermented liquids feeds (Sikka,2008)

Several foods besides containing nutrients also contain certain compounds that enhance the production by providing either the nutritional balance, improving the metabolism or preventing the disease. Moreover at the same time there is increased interest over the food safety, environmental contamination and the general health risks that have made *natural* the norm, promoting the trend towards alternative strategies to manage and feed the animals and birds without reliance on antibiotics. Such types of foods are labeled as adaptogens, dietetics, nutracines, nutraceuticals or multifunctional additives.

Acid Barrier- Central and Hind Gut

Acidic conditions prevailing in the stomach due to the secretion of hydrochloric acid acts as a powerful antimicrobial barrier. This mechanism is inadequately developed in the newly weaned piglets. Lactic acid originating from the fermentation of lactose by lactic acid bacteria (naturally occurring and probiotic additives) is helpful but limited by relatively small amount of bacterial activity in the stomach and proximal small intestine. Anything that increases acid production post weaning (Prebiotics, SCFA, Probiotics, Lactic Acid) can enhance antimicrobial competence and improve the barrier to orally acquired pathogens.

Bacterial Metabolism

End products of bacterial carbohydrate metabolism are acids, short chain fatty acids (SCFA) mainly acetic, propionic and butyric acids. SCFA are weak organic acids with bacteriostatic properties in common with the organic acids used as preservatives. SCFA play an important role in the prevention of potentially harmful bacteria escaping the stomach and migrating forward through the small intestine, but more important is the reverse flux of harmful bacteria from hind gut to small intestine. Higher butyrate concentrations contribute to a healthier intestine because butyric acid is a strong stimulator of the gastrointestinal cell growth, not only for the colonocytes, but also for the enterocytes of the small intestine (Pouillard P, 2003). Immune cells form part of the intestinal epithelial lining whose function is to monitor, react and coordinate a response to the components of the intestinal microflora. Prebiotics and probiotics increase the chances of a favourable response to the monitoring process, minimising immune activation with its highly beneficial impact on appetite and nutrient partitioning to growth. Growth responses to pre and probiotics achieve statistical significance during the first 14 days after weaning in piglets that confirms they can be fast acting in their influences (Corrent, 2002).

The gastrointestinal (GI) tract of vertebrates contains a species-diverse group of microflora. Bacteria, particularly gram-positive, predominate (Savage, 1977; Mackie *et al.*, 1999). As many as 500 bacterial species exist in the GI microflora, with numbers up to 10^{10} to 10^{12} bacterial cells/g of colonic content or faeces (Moore and Holdeman, 1974; Savage, 1977; Lee, 1984; Jensen, 2001). These numbers are consistent with the estimation that bacterial cells out number the host cells by 10:1 (Gaskins, 2001). The bacterial population influences a variety of immunological, physiological, nutritional, and protective processes of the GI tract and exerts profound effects on the overall health, development, and performance of monogastrics. Indeed, experiments comparing conventionally reared versus sterile (germ-free) animals have demonstrated that commensal bacteria play important role in organ, tissue, and immune system development, as well as providing a variety of nutritional compounds (Gaskins, 2001; Snel *et al.*, 2002). The commensal bacteria compete with the host for nutrients, secrete toxic compounds, and induce an ongoing immune/inflammatory response in the GI tract. All of these costs negatively impact animal health and performance. Two important areas for future research are

1) To determine the optimal microflora for animal health and performance under commercial growth conditions in other words, to discover the microflora that maximize the benefits while minimizing the costs and

2) To develop dietary and other interventions to foster development of this microflora.

Balance of Gut Microflora

A delicate balance between the beneficial bacteria (Lactobacilli, Bifidobacteria and Eubacteria) and the potential pathogenic bacteria (E Coli, Salmonella, Staphylococci, Listeria, Shigella, Veillonella, Brachyspiro (Serpulina), Clostridia and Coliforms) exists in the gut. A ratio of 9:1 between beneficial and pathogenic bacteria is considered to be ideal. But the factors like drug administration, stress, environmental and managemental changes, spoiled feed or change in gastric pH can alter this ratio. The pig monitors what bacteria are within its gut and reacts to what is there. Pigs grow faster or slower according to what it 'sees' in its gut!

The digestion efficiency in poultry and pigs depend upon the micro organisms which live naturally in its digestive tract. The microbial population present in the intestine of chicken comprises more than 90% of all the living cells in the bird. The intestinal microflora have important and differing effects, including regulation of epithelial cell turnover, competition for ingested nutrients, modification of digestion, competitive exclusion of pathogens, metabolism of mucus secretions and modulation of mucosal immunity (Hooper *et al,* 2002). To make the environment conducive for the beneficial bacteria pre and probiotics are added in the feed. These are beneficial nutritional modifiers for monogastrics.

Veterinary Nutraceuticals

The term nutraceuticals is a combination of nutrients and pharmaceutical. Their use is not a newer concept, but it is an example of history that is repeating itself (Dzanis 1999). Word 'Nutraceutical' was first coined by Stephen Defelice, the founder Chairman of "Foundation for Innovation in Medicine (FIM)". Sarah (2003) reported that nutraceuticals must improve the performance effectively & economically, with little therapeutic use, without causing cross resistance to other antibiotic at actual use level, without involving with transferable drug resistance, without causing any deleterious disturbance to the normal gut flora and should not create environmental pollution. Moreover these must be non toxic to the animals and its handlers. A non-drug substance that is produced in purified or extracted form and administered orally to provide agents required for normal body structure and function with the intent of improving health and well being of animals.

Dietary Supplements

Any substance that contain a vitamin, a mineral, herb or other botanicals, an amino acid, a dietary substance for use to supplement the diet by increasing the total dietary intake, or a concentrate metabolite, constituent extract or combination of any of the previously mentioned ingredients. A new concept i.e. Nutrition Based health, according to this concept feed and feeding programmes must be designed to reduce stress and to assist the animals in resisting disease challenges (Adams, 2005). Judicious use of various nutrients and bioactive feed components like acidifiers, antioxidants, bacterial inhibitors, enzymes, flavours etc. to support animal health is the right approach of Nbh. A term *'pronutrient'* i.e. a micro ingredient included in the formulation of animal feed in relatively small amounts with specific physiological and microbiological functions different from any other nutrient is included in the feed additive list. Many active ingredients from plants must be considered pronutrients due to their effects against the colonization of different pathogenic organism and stimulation of beneficial bacteria eg zinger for the treatment of dysentery.

Broadly nutraceuticals / natural therapy is classified as Herbs & Botanicals, Antioxidants (Vitamins C, A, beta carotene), Enzymes and Prebiotics and Probiotics or Direct Fed Mcrobials (DFM).

Herbs/Botanicals

Vegetative parts of the plants (leaves, bark, fruit, roots, seed and their extract) containing a variety of chemical compounds that are used as body restoratives are called herbs. While drugs are made from any part of plant (root, leaves, bark etc), essential oils or any of a class of volatile oils obtained from plants, possessing the odour and other characteristic properties of the plant, used chiefly in manufacture of perfumes, flavours and pharmaceutical, is extracted after hydro distillation (Webster Dictionary of English, 1989).

These chemical compounds are active in altering the physiological and biochemical processes in the body. Herbs and spices have compounds with antibacterial effects for example garlic contain allicin and ajoene which exhibits broad spectrum anti microbial properties (Naganawa *et al*, 1996) and is effective in reducing cholesterol of liver, breast and thigh muscle (Kopnjufca *et al*, 1997). Another example is Yucca Schidiger which improve growth & FCR (Headon et al 1991).

Recently, Sikka and Singh (2010) elaborated the use of herbs and botanicals. These help in improving the performance by reducing the stress associated with handling, transport and poor health by providing nutrients and or active principles which act as anti stress agents. Being adaptogenic manage stress and improve egg production in birds. Increase the feed consumption due to the flavours present. Ensure the normal gut functioning. Improve the digestion by activating digestive secretions. Improve the feed conversion efficiency there by growth and production. Improve the liver functioning. Act as toxin binder and reduce the risk of mycotoxicosis. Normalize the kidney functioning. Improve the immunity as an immune modulater, act as antioxidant, coccidiostat and anti helminthic. Stimulate endocrine system. Stimulate intermediate nutrient metabolism. Stabilize gut environment. Ameliorate the effect of ANF's present in the feed. Used for the treatment of bacterial (Yuan *et al,* 1993), viral (Yu & Zhu, 2000) and parasitic diseases (Pang *et al* 2000). Reduce ammonia and other noxious gases in the GI tract through their binding to the saponins and excreted in the excreta and reduce the ascitic mortality in broilers (Menocal, 1995).

These properties of various herbs are due to the active secondary metabolites that belong to class of isoprene derivatives, flavonoides and glucosinolates. Intercation between different active components within and between extract may have either cummulative or antagonistic effect. Use of herbs in poultry and pig feeds are now gaining momentum as it claim to have no side effect, safe and eco friendly. A term botanical / natural broiler/pig can be used when only botanical / natural materials are used for enhancing performance and prevention of disease. Sikka and Singh, (2007).

The desired activity of herbs varies due to variability of the composition of plant secondary metabolites, environmental conditions, different harvesting time, stage of maturity, method of extraction and conservation, anti nutritional factor and nature of diet in which it is supplemented because it have to compete with nutrients present in the feed.

Prebiotics

Prebiotics are short chain non-digestible oligosaccharides with 2-10 units of monosaccharide present in feed ingredients. These are commonly found in soybean and rapeseed meal. Legumes, cereals and yeast cell walls contain respectively á-galactooligosaccharides (GOS), fructooligosaccharides (FOS) and mannanoligosaccharides (MOS). Lactobacilli, Bifidobacteria and Eubacteria selectively ferment some prebiotics. Prebiotics modify the gut microbial population balance by promoting the growth of beneficial flora in the intestines (Gibson *et al,* 1996,2004, Flickinger & Fahey 2002) thereby providing a healthier intestinal environment. These are not easily digestible and provide competitive advantage to favourable bacteria, inhibiting the colonization of harmful microbes and promoting the beneficial ones.

It is generally accepted that high *Villi : Crypt* depth ratios are indicators of a healthier and more efficient intestinal mucosa. Prebiotics have a beneficial effect on the gut integrity especially in the distal end of small intestine, the area with the greatest levels of fermentation. In a recent experiment, it was observed that ratios were enhanced in distal area, with enhanced fermentation along the entire small intestine (Decuypere, 2003). Through a variety of mechanisms prebiotics are thought to increase resistance to infection. Prebiotics enhance the physical barrier (modulation of paracellular permeability, mucosal trophic action), improved functional barrier (mucosal immunity), have competitive adhesion to epithelial receptors, increased SCFA production along the gastro-intestinal tract, inducing a shift to a more saccharolytic (carbohydrate fermenting) flora, lowers intestinal pH, reduce the colonization of harmful bacteria excreting harmful bacteria. They also have competitive exclusion (colonisation resistance).

Galacto-oligosaccherides (GOS), Mannanoligosaccharides (MOS), Fructo-oligosaccharides (FOS) are frequently used in poultry diets (Ishihara et al 2000, Zhang *et al,* 2003). Harmful bacteria attach themselves to both the FOS and MOS and are excreted. Fructo- oligosaccharides (FOS), derivative of inulin, stimulate the growth of Bifido bacteria, improve the mucosal morphology of the colon (Howard et al 1995) and inhibit the growth of pathogenic microorganism such as clostridia and salmonella. Wang & Gibson (1993) revealed the increase in egg production and feed efficiency of layer with the use of dietary oligofructose and inulin. The inulin is required for the growth of Lactobacilli (Gibson, 1999). FOS has been reported to improve growth in the weaned pigs by 5.1 % and feed efficiency by 2.0% (Mul & Perry, 1994) On the other hand MOS found to improve daily weight gain by 7.4% and feed utilization by 5.2 % in nursery pigs (Vender beke, 1997) by improving the structural integrity of G-I-tract. Spring and Privulescu (1998) revealed that oligosaccharides stimulate the secretion of cytokine and there by enhance the immune system of the pig to resist pathogenic bacterial challenge.

Probiotics

The live microbial food supplement which when fed improve the intestinal microbial balance of the host are called probiotics or Direct Fed Microbials (DFM's). Probiotics improve the survival with better growth, better-feed conversion and inhibition of diarrhea in piglets (Jin et al 1996). Lactobacilli, Streptococci, Bi-fido bacteria, *Bacillus, Bacteriods, Pediococcus, leuconostoc, Propionibacterium,* and some yeast (*Saccharomyces cerevesiae*) and fungi (*Asperzillus oryzae*) are commonly used DFM's. B *Subtilis* and B *licheniformis* are used in nursery pig rations as they are spore forming and are able to resist the environmental conditions of high temperature and moisture occurring during the pelleting process.

Probiotics are administered through drinking water and by mixing in the feed. Probiotics should be given once or twice daily, after which the bacteria should establish itself in the alimentary canal and replace disease-promoting microorganisms. Furthermore, it is practically impossible that probiotic bacteria could establish themselves in a stable alimentary canal system. Therefore these must be added to the feed on regular basis. Use of probiotic bacterial cultures have greater effect during the early stages of growth, when, the gut is sterile and when the alimentary flora are unstable, viz after weaning and subsequent to an extended period of treatment with antibiotics. Probiotics, improve health and growth by modifying intestinal microbial balance by competitive exclusion, adhering to intestinal mucosa (Jonsson and Conway, 1992), preventing attachment of pathogens, (Green & Sainbury, 2001), production of antimicrobial compounds (Hentges, 1992) such as bacteriocins and organic acids, competition with pathogens for nutrients (Freter,1992), stimulation of intestinal immune responses (Perdigon and Alvarez,1992), affect the gut permeability, increase nutrients uptake (Stavric *et al*, 1995; Mulder *et al*, 1997; Lee *et al*, 1999).

Some bacterial cultures when fed in single or multiple (few) doses to newly hatched birds establish an intestinal flora quickly and it prevents colonization by pathogenic bacteria. For example lactobacilli acidophilus produces lactocidin which has antibacterial effects on E coli. Lactobacilli modify gut pH, competition for nutrients and absorption sites, boost cell immune response, inhibition of bacterial growth by hydrogen peroxide production and cell signaling to turn off pathogenic function (Fuller,1999). Competitive Exclusion(CE) preparations are not always pure cultures of bacteria and their microbial composition may not be completely known. Few CE cultures have proven effective in protecting chicks from *Salmonella* infections.

Interest in the use of probiotics in poultry and pig diets is to curtail sub-therapeutic doses of antibiotics in feed. Like antibiotics, probiotics appear to have a more pronounced effect on farms where housing and hygiene are not optimal (Mulder *et al*, 1997; Thomke and Elwinger, 1998). Supplementation of probiotics containing *Lactobaccilus acidophilus, Streptococcus faecium* and yeasac @ 0.025% in the diets of broilers were found to be beneficial in early stage of growth. In broilers supplementation of yeast culture at 0.1 % level increased the body weight and performance (Tollaba *et al* 2004) due to quantitative and qualitative alteration in the digestive tract flora with better nutrient utilization (Sara *et al* 2003).Use of combination of several strains at a time improved the weight gain and feed efficiency in broilers (Mazurkiewicz *et al* 1992) and in chicks (Nguyen *et al*,1998). Feeding of mixture of S. *cerevisae*, L.*bulgaricus* and S. *thermophilus* did not show any effect on the production of layers (Svetic *et al* 1996).

Dietary supplementation of probiotics results in no effects on growth (Bold *et al*, 1993; Yadav *et al*, 1994) or have better growth performance (Couch, 1978, Arendz 1981), with improvement in feed efficiency and low mortality during finishing (Bhatt *et al*, 1993), increased immunity and carcass characteristics (Panda *et al*, 2005) and can also replace the anti microbial compounds in the broiler chicks (Ramarao *et al*, 2004). In layers improvemnet in egg production and feed efficiency have been reported by Nahashon et al (1993), Mohan et al (1996). In pigs the intestinal microflora is capable of resisting the establishment of certain intestinal pathogens (Lopez & Marquez 1994). Bera & Samanta (2005) fed probiotics (alone or in combination) to the piglets and reported superior growth performance in the pre and post weaning periods with yeast +MOS(YMOS), followed by Yeast + lactobacillus (YL) and control (C) with higher profit. Better FCR in pigs with yeast+ lactobacillus and yeast + MOS was observed (Bera & Samanta ,2005; Siuta 2000; Tardani and Terreni 1996). However, Charles and Duke (1978) observed no effects Incosistent resuts observed with the supplementation of probiotics were due to the variations in bacterial cultures used, age and species of animals, feed composition and feed form, feeding management practices adopted, dose levels and Different strains of organism used, interaction with other dietary feed additives (Chesson 1994).

Organic acids/acidifiers

Organic acids (C1-C-7) are widely distributed in nature as normal constituents of plants or animal tissues. Organic acids posses both the antibacterial and anti mould activities and therefore have long been used as preservative to prevent spoilage by checking microbial growth and are also used to maintain the proper gut health. Organic acids are very efficacious when their use is adapted to the physiology and anatomy of poultry birds.

Types of Acidifiers

Generally two types of acidifiers are used in the feed industry.

1. *Feed Acidifiers*: These lower the pH of the feed and inhibit the growth of pathogenic microflora. This inhibition reduces the micro flora competing for the host nutrients and prevent the occurrence of diseases which results in better growth and performance.
2. *Gut Acidifiers*: Gut acidifiers (organic acid) acidify the intestinal tract and modulate the intestine bacterial population in a positive and natural way. Since many harmful bacterial species have pH optimum for their growth around 7 where as useful bacterial species such as *Lactobacillus* and *Enterococcus* have their best growth pH around 6. Maintenance of healthy gut for proper productivity is of utmost importance. Amongst various options available to poultry and pig feed industry, short chain fatty acids have shown tremendous promise in maintaining gut health through their varied modes of action.

Selection of Organic Acids : The antimicrobial activity of organic acids is related to reduction in pH and its ability to dissociate, which is determined by the pKa value of the respective acid and the pH of the surrounding environment. The selection of organic acid is very critical in determining the efficacy of the product.

Functions of Acidifiers : Acidifiers help in maintaining an optimum pH in stomach, stimulate feed consumption, improve growth rates, improve feed conversion ratio, inhibit the growth and colonization of pathogenic bacteria, prevents damage to epithelial cells of intestines, reduce microbial competition with host for nutrients, reduce endogenous nitrogen losses, lower the incidence of sub clinical infections, reduce the production of ammonia and other growth depressing microbial metabolites, increase pancreatic secretions, increase protein and amino acid digestibility by correcting activation and function of proteolytic enzymes, improve energy digestibility, increase mineral digestibility as acid ion complex with minerals, serve as substrates in intermediary metabolism and have energy content, check problem of Salmonella, E. coli, entritis and diarrhoea in pigs, check entritis and mortality syndrome.

Supplementation of organic acids improve the weight gain, feed consumption and feed utilization (Denli *et al,* 2003) reducing the production of toxic components by pathogenic bacteria and reduces the colonization of pathogens on the intestinal wall, thus preventing the damage of the epithelial cells (Langhout, 2000). In poultry diets organic acids are mainly used in order to sanitize the feed to avoid the problems releated with salmonella (Berchieri & Barrow,1996). However Waldroup *et al* (1995) reported the inability of citric acid at the dietary concentration up to 1 % to prevent the salmonella colonization in caeca. In poultry nutrition organic acids have not gained as much attention as in swine nutrition (Langhout, 2000). Edwin (2000) reported that addition of 2% lactic acid to the diet without growth promoters increased the weight gain by 2.6 % with improved FCR. Propionic acid based products were found effective in alleviating the enteritis and mortality syndrome in turkey poults (Roy et al 2002). Several organic acids like citric acid, fumaric acid, formic acid, propionic acid were tried on pig for their impact on the growth performance (Partanen & Mroz, 1999). Their supplementation in weaning pig diets give most pronounced impact on the growth performance (Roth & Kirchgessner, 1998). Blank *et al* (1999) reported that the incorporation of organic acids into nursery pig rations has been shown to reduce bacterial load and increase the digestibility of energy and amino acid in the ileum, resulting in improvement in feed efficiency and reduction in the incidence of diarrhea. These pigs often suffer from digestive problems due to infection of *E coli.* An insufficient production of HCl, digestive enzymes and feeding of high protein pre starter diets are another reasons for the digestive upset at this stage. Supplementation of organic acid increases the gastric proteolysis, protein and amino acid digestibility. The acid anion has been shown to complex with Ca, P, Mg, and Zn which results in an improved digestibility of these minerals. Kirchgessner and Roth (1988) also revealed the role of organic acid as substrates in the intermediary metabolism. Supplementation of 1.5% citric acid to control diets did not significantly effect the pH, concentration of VFA's / non VFA or microflora (total anarobes, *Lactobacilli, Clostridia, E. coli*) in the contents from the stomach, jejunum, caecum or lower colon of weanling pigs (Risley *et al,* 1992,). Similar results were reported for the Fumaric acid (Risley *et al,* 1992). Sodium fumarate when added to a control pig diet at a level of 0.3%, no significant effect on the concentration of SCFA and the density of lactobacilli or E coli along the GI tract was observed (Sutton *et al,* 1991). Supplementation of 1 % lactic acid lowers the gastric pH (Thomlinson & Lawrence, 1981) and reduced the level of *E coli* in the duodenum and jeunum of 8-week-old piglets (Cole *et al* 1968). Addition of formic acid or potassium diformate reduces the pH, (Fevrier et al 2001) and number of coliform bacteria in stomach, duodenum, jejunum and rectum of growing pigs (Overland *et al,* 2000). Waldroup *et al* (1995) reported the reduction of caecal pH with the addition of a formic acid/ propionic acid blend in a concentration of 1% in the broiler chicken. It seems that these short chain fatty acids can nearly compensate for the effects of antibiotic growth promoters in pigs, although these effects are less consistent (Partanen and Mroz, 1999).

Feeding of Excess of Organic acids : Excess level of strong dietary acid can reduce the pH too quickly after feed ingestion but the stomach may not develop its parietal secretary cells that produce HCl. This inhibits the normal gut development. Therefore use of organic acids must be done judiciously.

Mode of action : Over the years, it was thought that a pH reduction of the gastrointestinal tract (GIT content was the mode of action. Research in the food preservation field has brought clear explanations on the mode of action of organic acids on bacteria and numerous trials have shown that the concept works both in pigs and poultry. More likely, the organic acids in poultry might play a direct role on the GIT bacteria population, reducing the level of some pathogenic bacteria (*C. perfringens*) and mainly controlling the population of certain types of bacteria that compete with the birds for nutrients. Animal has the capacity to maintain its GIT environment homeostasis in order to warrant the normal functioning of all digestive functions. Also, the strong buffering capacity of the feed prevents any significant GIT pH modification. Logically, organic acids added to feeds should be protected to avoid their dissociation in the crop and in the intestine (high pH segments) and reach far into the GIT, where the bulk of the bacterial population is located.

State of the organic acids whether undissociated or dissociated is extremely important to define their capacity to inhibit the growth of bacteria. As a general rule, more than ten to twenty times the level of dissociated acids to reach the same inhibition of bacteria are required as compared to undissociated acids. The antibacterial capacity of organic acids at pH below 3.0-3.5 is very high and almost all organic acids are very efficacious in controlling bacteria growth.

The sequence of mode of action of organic acids on bacteria is as: Undissociated organic acids enters the bacterial cell. Bacterial membrane disrupts (leakage, transport mechanisms). Essential metabolic reactions (ex. glycolysis) are inhibited. Stress on intracellular pH homeostasis. Toxic anions are accumulated in the cell. Energy stress response to restore homeostasis. Chelation as permeabilizing agent of outer membrane and zinc binding.

The key basic principle on the mode of action of organic acids on bacteria is that non-dissociated (non-ionized) organic acids can penetrate the cell wall and disrupt the normal physiology of certain bacteria E. coli, Salmonella spp., C. perfringens, Listeria monocytogenes, Campylobacter spp. This is called "pH-sensitive," meaning that they cannot tolerate a wide internal and external pH gradient.

The dual mode of action of organic acids make them more attractive as at low pH they do not disassociate where as at higher pH, the acid disassociates .The un dissociated form of organic acid prevents the cell membranes. In the alkaline environment of bacterial cytoplasm, the organic acids disassociate and release H+ ions and acidifies the cell contents., Microbial enzyme working is inhibited due to low pH in the cell and the distressed cell start pumping out the H+ ion in order to return to equilibrium. The energy required to eject the H+ ion is thought to weaken the already distressed cell, there by slowing both the growth and reproduction. Anions of organic acids deactivate RNA transferase enzyme, which damage the nucleic acid multiplication process and eventually result in death of the organism.

Pumped out H+ ion acidify the intestinal contents which favours the acid producing bacteria (Lactobacilli, bifidobacteria) and inhibits the acid hating bacteria (Salmonella, E Coli, Campylobacter sp). All acids have different dissociation constant (pKa values), low pKa values indicates strong acidification power. Some acids have multiple pKa value and these acids can dissociate at different parts of the GI tract. Acids can be used singly or in combinations. By combining several organic acids, which disassociate at different pH levels, it is possible to exploit the effects of both modes of action over a larger proportion of the range of pH found in the intestines.

Problems of feeding Organic acids: The unprotected acids can cause a fast drop in pH and by dissociating quickly in the stomach or upper small intestine may not be effective. Without protection, organic acids are readily dissociated in the first part of the gastrointestinal tract and rendered useless. Acids can also be used in protected form by using the encapsulation technology for their slow release in the GI tract.

Antioxidants

Nutrients in the body on oxidation release energy for various metabolic processes physiological activities and to transform dietary nutrients into body tissue along with generation of heat. Auto oxidation results in the production of free radicals which damage the cellular tissue and cause many disorders (Lerson & Summer, 2002). To prevent auto oxidation antioxidants are frequently used. Nutritional antioxidants are very helpful in reducing physiological stress both at an organ and cellular level due to free radical formation.

Feed antioxidants help by protecting the feed nutrients during storage, helping the absorption of the oxidation sensible substances in the GIT, reducing aging by keeping the membrane intac, enabling the system for better exploitation of genetic potential

In poultry diets mostly vitamins A, beta- carotene, E, C and its calcium and sodium salts, ethoxyquin, lecithin, butylated hydroxytoulene (BHT), propyl gallate, chelated metal ions are commonly used as an antioxidants. The beneficial effects of antioxidants are due to their scavenging nature for free radicals (Bulger & Hilton, 1998), maintaing the potency of dietary vitamins and stimulating bird's immuno- responsiveness to infections. Antioxidant defence system includes the enzyme superoxide dismutase, catalase, and glutathione peroxidase. During stress free radicals in the body increase while the level of these enzymes decrease. Ascorbic acid also plays a role in collagen synthesis, carnitine synthesis along with its primary function of antioxidants (Gross *et al,* 2000). It scavenges neutrophill oxidants, hydroxyl radicals, hydrogen peroxide and hypochlorous acid (Bulger & Helton, 1998). Raju et al (2005) revealed that herbal Vit C (0.025%) improve the performance of bird by alleviating the effect of aflatoxicosis. Similarly the primary physiological role of Vitamin E is to act as antioxidant (Matthai, 1996). Many studies have shown that supplementation of Vitamin A, C & E can attenuate the side effects of extreme environmental stress (Kafri & Cherry, 1984, Njoku, 1986). Brahma Rasayana a polyherbal antioxidant was found useful in ameliorating the effects of free redicals generated due to heat stress (Ramnath *et al,* 2007). Herbs like garlic, green tea, amla also posses antioxidant properties.

Essential Oils

Essential oils are highly concentrated extracts produced by refinement of botanicals by hydro-distillation. Essential oils are standardised products, often based on a blend of plant metabolites such as allylisothiocyanates, thymol, carvacrol, capsaicin, cinnamaldehyde, piperin etc. Any class of volatile oils obtained from plants, possessing the odor and other characteristic properties of the plant are used chiefly in the manufacture of perfumes, flavors and pharmaceuticals (extracts after hydro distillation).

Plants contain hundreds of substances with different properties but essential oils are composed mainly of nine groups (and many sub-groups) of molecules that are of interest to us. There are many chemical constituents but no two oils are alike in their structure and effect. One must distinguish between non-purified plant extracts containing numerous different molecules interacting and pure active compounds, either extracted from plants or synthesized (nature identical). According to the plant chosen, one or more active compounds are dominant and the quantity found will differ according to factors like plant variety, soil, moisture, climate, time of harvest and other factors

Functions of Essential Oils : Nutritionally, metabolically and toxicologically, we have a clear interest in using as low levels of essential oils as possible in animal nutrition. Essential oils are extremely potent substances, which are rapidly absorbed in the duodenum and can not interact with the microflora. Essential oils are used as flavouring agents to increase their attractiveness of the feeds, to reduce feed intake, manipulate/disturb GIT microflora, antimicrobial, antioxidant, coccidiostat, antiviral properties, to increase the digestive enzyme secretions, increase the appetite, improve the immune function, improves the performance and accumulation in animal tissues and products

There are reports of synergy between organic acids and essential oils. The synergy is thought to come from the ability of the essential oils to weaken bacterial cell walls, increasing its permeability to the organic acids.

Mode of Action : It is extremely difficult to generalize on the mode of action of essential oils (EO) on bacteria and yeasts because each has different properties and each type of microorganism has a different sensitivity. Generally, Gram+ve bacteria are considered more sensitive to essential oils than Gram-ve bacteria because of their less complex membrane structure.

Essential oils work by inhibiting the growth of the bacteria. These compounds influence the biological membranes of bacteria. The cytoplasmic membrane of bacteria has two principal functions 1. Barrier and energy transduction which allow the membrane to form ion gradients that can be used to drive various processes and 2. Formation of matrix for membrane-embedded proteins influencing the ATP-synthase complex, sharply reducing intracellular ATP pool through a reduction of ATP synthesis and increased hydrolysis; education of the membrane potential, which is the driving force for ATP synthesis; the membrane becoming more permeable to protons; and reduction of the internal pH.

Judicious use of Essential oils : Most essential oils are generally recognized as safe (GRAS) but they must be used properly and cautiously because they can be toxic (allergens), potent sensitizers and their odor and/or taste may contribute to feed refusal. They are also very volatile and will evaporate rapidly, leading to large variation in concentration in the finished products. Essential oils are very rapidly absorbed in the duodenum and cannot interact with the microflora.

Enzymes

Non starch polysaccharides or NSP (cellulose, glucans and xylans etc)) of the cereal grains (Henry, 1985) like wheat, rye, oats possess antinutritive activity (Annison & Choct, 1991) which leads to the formation of viscous gel in the gut that intrferes the proper absorption of nutrients (Choct & Annion, 1992) and also produces sticky droppings in poultry. Similarly phytic acid and its salts as phytates present in the feedstuffs also binds minerals, carbohydrates, proteins and form insoluble complexes which make these nutrients especially minerals like phosphorus unavaiable to the monogastrics and are excreted in faeces. Supplementation of exogenous enzymes in the diets decrease gut viscosity and improve the availability of nutrients from feed, lower the feed cost and help in reducing the environmental pollution by minimizing the waste excretion. Exogenous enzymes in the diets of young animal complement the endogenous enzymes. Their use in the poultry and pig feed industry has become a routine (Bedford, 1997, Sikka, 2003, Sikka and Singh, 2009).

The enzymes in pig and poultry feeds are added to achieve the following goals viz. to supplement the endogenous enzymes especially to young birds and pigs due to immature digestive system, to counter ANF's present in feed, to increase the availability of dietary nutrients, to improve the AME level of the feeds, to release the bound nutrients and pre treatment of certain feeds / ingredients such as feathers and offals.

Phytase enzyme was found to improve the performance and availability of phytate phosphorus as well as other organic nutrients (Singh & Sikka 2006). Similarly supplementation glycosidase has been found to increase the energy utilization in birds. Higher body weight gain and better feed efficiency in Japanese Quails with supplementing of 0.05%, non starch polysaccharidase (Edwin *et al,* 2004) and in broiler (Srivastava *et al,* 2005) with enzymes mixture of amylase, cellulose, lipase and protease and in weaner pigs (Owsley et al 1986) with diminsihing digestive disturbance (Kitchen 1997, Partridge &

Hazzledine, 1997). Reports indicate the improvement in young pigs was more than older one (Bohme *et al,* 1990). The use of beta glucanase and xylanase are beneficial with high fiber grains like wheat, barley and their by products (Chesson, 1987, Sikka & Chawla 2002). Thomke *et al.* (1980) also reported that b-glucanases could improve performance in barley fed pigs. Alpha galactosiadse is used to breakdown the galactose units in raffinose and stachyose found in soyabean. The efficacy of enzyme supplementation depends upon types of diet, enzyme supplementation (Singh *et al,* 2010), animals, chemical linkage in the substrate that need to be cleaved etc.

Immuno-modulators

Nutrition and disease have close connection as the nutritional status of animal influence immunological function and resistance to disease. Health status of the organism is influencing the animal's nutritional requirements. Many nutrients like protein & energy (Praharaj *et al,* 1999), methionine (Tsiagbe *et al,* 1987, Swain & Johri 2000), Vitamin A (Friedman & Sklan 1997), Vitamin E &Se (Swan *et al,* 2000, Areceli & Saavedra, 2003, Hooda *et al,* 2005, Singh *et al,* 2006), Vitamin C (Amakya anim *et al,* 2005) and trace element like Zn, Fe, Cu & Mn (Dardenne 2002) have the immuno modulating ability. In pigs nucleotides (Tibbetts 2000), β glucans (Diluzio & Jacques 1985), vitamins, PUFA, antibodies from products such as blood derivatives (eg, plasma protein), freeze dried eggs containing pig related antibodies and possibly some whey protein products have been reported to improve the immune response. Reduced immune activity promotes growth by increasing appetite and partitioning nutrients to growth.

Idea concept

Immuno modulation through nutrition gave birth to a new concept the ***'IDEA'***, which stands for Impulse, Digestibility, Economics and Advance. The IDEA concept seeks to enhance immunity development, giving opportunity for better nutritional management, reduce feed costs, reduce intestinal challenges by coccidia and bacteria without the use of drugs and conditioning the gut for better coccidiosis management especially in broilers. The IDEA concept is simple and an innovative approach to feed management which redefines the birds nutritional and management needs during critical phases.

Supportive Dietary Modifications

Bacteriostatic approach is supported by alteration in the diet to reduce the amount of substrate available to the intestinal microflora. Diets must be modified to reduce "By-Pass Nutrients"! This is best achieved through increased digestibility of ingredients by the addition of enzymes, herbs, probiotics, acidifiers etc. The aim is to reduce the protein and carbohydrate fraction of the diet, which can escape digestion and absorption and remain available as a nutrient source for microbial fermentation by intestinal microflora. Bacterial fermentation of indigestible protein produces ammonia and biogenic amines, which are toxic and increase the risk of diarrhoea. Piglet starter diets must be highly digestible and must encourage a shift to protein fermentation in the hindgut by being 'carbohydrate' deficient. The addition of fermentable carbohydrates (prebiotics) to pig diets reduces protein fermentation through increased carbohydrate fermentation in the hindgut. The reduced efficiency of bile salts can be countered by adding emulsifying agents (lecithin) directly to the diet and by improving the saturated to unsaturated fatty acid ratio in the diet to aid absorption. Alterations such as switching from DL-Methionine to Liquid MHA-FA, an organic acid, are another small change that can increase the antimicrobial status of a pig diet. The efficiency of the intestinal epithelium structure and function can be upgraded with the use of Betaine.

Recommendation for Future Research

Until new alternatives are finalized for AGPs, withdrawal of antibiotics all of a sudden from feed will lead to significant reduction in aquaculture, poultry and live stock production. This can raise issues of food security. A workable strategy in this context will be to classify the available antibiotics into two groups. One group consisting of chloramphenicol, nitrofurans including: furaltadone, furazolidone, furylfuramide, nifuratel, nifuroxime, nifurprazine, nitrofurantoin, nitrofurazone, neomycin, nalidixic acid, sulphamethoxazole, chlorpromazine, colchicines, dapsone, dimetridazole, metronidazole, ronidazole, ipronidazole, other nitroimidazoles, clenbuterol, sulfonamide drugs (except approved sulfadimethoxine, sulfabromomethazine and sulfaethoxypyridazine) and fluroquinolones should be exclusively used as therapeutic antibiotics, for treating human and animals. All other antibiotics including tetracyclines are to be listed in a second group of antibiotics, which can be permitted as AGPs indicating maximum permissible concentration in feed, withdrawal time as well as method of disposal of solid and liquid based metabolic waste. Implementation of such a practice will drastically reduce the chances of developing resistance to therapeutic antibiotics, thereby sparing the therapeutic antibiotics for long-term use in disease management. Once suitable alternatives to AGPs are developed use of antibiotics as AGP can be completely banned.

There is urgent need to gather precise information on the use of antibiotics in the animal husbandry in the country and its potential reservoir in soil and water. The most important of all is the need to perfect our capability in developing precise mechanism for identification and response to dangerous resistance trends in bacteria responsible for causing deadly infections in human and animals. There should be a blanket ban on the use of those antibiotics in animal feeds which are commonly used in controlling bacterial infection in humans.

Alternative nutritional strategies should be developed for enhanced digestion and absorption of the feed stuffs. The challenge for live-stock productivity is to find suitable, reliable and cost effective management routines and feed additives for a sustainable and successful production. There could not be a better time to agree or review a health plan for pig and poultry units. Cleaning and disinfection routines should also be reviewed and upgraded. Until alternatives to AGPs are developed it is better to restrict the therapeutic antibiotics only for disease management and to set apart a set of other antibiotics for meeting AGP needs. There is need for constant monitoring by compound livestock feed manufacturers association (CLFMA), ICAR, Drug controlling agencies for production and distribution of antibiotics for non-therapeutic uses.

References

Adam C A (2005). *Feed International* 26: 25-27.

Al Ahmed, A *et al.* (1999). *Arch. Env. Contamination and Tox*. 16: 462

Amakye- Anim J, Lin TL, Hester PY, Thiagarajan D, Watkins BA and Wu CC (2000). *Poult Sci* 79:680-688.

Annison G & Choct M (1991). *World poultry Sci. J.* 47:232-42.

Araceli Pinelli-Saavedra (2003). *Reprod. Nutr. Dev.* 43 397-408

Arends L J (1981). *Poult. Sci.* 60:1619.

Avcare Ltd. (2003). The role of enteric antibiotics in livestock production - a review of published literature, May 2003, Australia.

Basaraba, R.J., F.W. Oehme, M.W. Vorhies, and G.L. Stokka. (1999). *J. Vet. Diag. Invest.* 11:79–86.

Bates, J., Jordens, J. Z. and Griffiths, D. T. (1994). *Journal of Antimicrobial Chemotherapy.* 34: 507–516.

Bedford M R (1997). Farmers Poultry Forum, London

Bedford, M. (2005). *Horizon.* p 49.

Bera J & Samanta G (2005). *Indian J Anim Nutr* 22(3): 156-159.

BERCHIERI, A JR. and BARROW P. A. (1996). *Poult. Sci.*75:339

Bhatt R S, Katoch B S, Dogra K K, Gupta R, Sharma K S and Sharma C R (1995). *Indian J. Poult. Sci.* 30:117-121.

Boehm, R. (1996). Dtsch. Tieraerztl. *Wochenschr.* 103:264–268.

Bolder N M, VanLith L A J T, Putirulan F F and Mulder R W A W (1993) In. Proc 12,probiotics and pathogenicity (J fjensen, M H Hinton and RWAW Mulder Eds.) CONP_DLO, Beekbergen, Netherlands, pp115-122.

Boxall, A.B.A., D.W. Kolpin, B. Halling-Sørensen, and J. Tolls. (2002). *Environ. Sci. Technol.* 37:287A–294A.

Brchieri A, Jr and Barrow PA (1996). *Poult. Sci.* 75:339-341.

Bulger and Hilton (1998). Gastroenterol Clin. *North Am.* 27:403-419.

Callan, R. J. (2003). H. M. Colorado State Univ. www.cvmbs.colostate.edu/ilm/proinfo/cdn/2003/CDNmay03insert.).

Casewell, M., Friis, C., Marco, E., McMullin, P., Phillips, I. (2003). *J Antimicrob Chemother* 52:159-161.

Charles O W and Duke S (1978). *Poult Sci* 57:1125 (abstract).

Chesson A (1994). In principles of pig science (Ed DJA Cole, J wisemann and MA varley) pp197-214. Nottingham University Press. Nottingham.

Choct M & Annison G (1992). *Br. Poult. Sci.* 33:821.

Cohen, M.L. and Tauxe, R.V. (1986). *Science*, 234:964-969.

Cole DJA, R Beal, M & Luscombe JR (1968). *Veterinary Record* 459-464.

Corrent, S. (2002). Nutreco trial report, p 172.

Couch, J R (1978). *Feedstuffs*. 50:6

De Liguoro, M., V. Cibin, F. Capolongo, B. Halling-Sorensen, and C. Montesissa. (2003). *Chemosphere* 52:203–212.

Decuypere, J. (2003). Western Nutrition Conference. Canada.

Denli M, Ferda Okan, & kemal Celik (2003). *Pakistan J. of Nutrition* 2(2);89_91.

Derdane M (2002). *European Journal of clinical Nutrition* 3 :20-23.

Diluzio NR and Jacques P (1985). In advances in immunopharmacology. Ed L Chedid, JW hadden F Spreadico, P Dukor, and Willoughby. Pub Permagon Press. NY. P-369-375.

Edvin S C, Viswanathan K, Mohan B, & Purushothaman M R (2004). *Indian J. Poult Sci* 39:241-245.

Edwin MR (2000). *Feed Mix* 8 :15-17.

Food and Drug Administration. New animal drugs for use in animal feeds [cited 2005 Mar]. 21CFR558.3; 2000.

Fedral Food, Drug and Cosmetic (FFDC) ACT (1998) title 21,united states Code, US, Govt. printing office,Washington DC.

Feinman, S.E. (1979). CRC handbook series in zoonoses: antibiotics, sulfonamides, and public health. Boca Raton: CRC Press; 151-71.

Fevrier C, Gotterbarm G, Jaghelin- Peyraud Y, Lebreton Y, Legouevec F and Aumaitre A (2001). In digestive physiology of pigs. Ed By Lindberg JE, Ogle B, CABI Publishing. Pp-136-138.

Fleming, A. (1929). *British Journal of Experimental Pathology*, 10: 226–236.

Flikinger,E A and Fahay G C (2002). *Br. J. Nutr.* 2: 297-300.

Freter, R (1992). In: Probiotics. Thescientific basis (R Fuller, Ed.), Chapman Hall, London, UK. 111-144

Friedman A and Sklan D (1997). *World Poultry Sci J* 48;101-11.

Gaskins, H.R., C.T. Collier and D.B. Anderson, (2002). *Anim. Biotechnol.* 13:29-42.

Gibson G R (1999). *J. Ani. Sci.* 73 (1):82.

Gibson GR, William A, Reading S and Cllins MD (1996). *Proc Nutr. Soc* 55:899-992.

Gibson, G R, William B A, Icwakkel, R P, Li H S, Li, X P, Luo J Y, Li W K and Verstegen M W (2004). *Poult Sci* 83:175-182.

Green A A & DWB Sainsbury (2001). XV European Symposium on the quality of poultry meat. 9-12. Sep-2001. Kusadasi/Turkey 245-251.

Gross K I, Wedekind K J, Cowell C S et al (2000). Ms, Thatcher CD, remillard RL, et al (eds) Small Animal Clinical Nutrition ed 4 Topeka, KS Mark, Morris institute. pp 21-107.

Hamscher *et al.* (2002). *Anal. Chem.* 74: 1590

Halling-Sørensen, B., S.N. Nielsen, P.F. Lanzky, F. Ingerslev, H.C. Holten Lutzheft, and S.E. Jørgensen. (1998). *Chemosphere* 36:357–393.

Halling-Sørensen, B *et al.* (2001). *Arch. Environ. Cont. Toxicology.* 42: 263

Headon, D R., Buggle K A., Nelson A B and Killeen G F (1991). In Biotech in feed industry Ed. TP lyons, Alltech tech Publication, KY .pp 95-108.

Henry R J (1985). *J. Fd. Sci & Agric.* 36:1243-1253.

Hentges D J (1992). (R Fuller ed) Champman and Hall London UK. pp 87-110.

Hooda S, Tyagi Praveen, Tyagi Pramod and Sharma D (2005). *Indian J. of Poult Sci.*40:33

Hooper LV *et al.* (2002). *Annu Rev Nutr* 22:283-307.

Howard Md, DT Gordon, LW Pace,KA Garleb and MS kerley (1995). *J.of Pediatr. Gastroenterology Nutr.* 21:293-303.

Ishihara N, Chu D C, Akachi S and Juneja L R (2000). *Poult Sci.* 79:689-697.

Jin LZ, Ho YW Abdullah, N jalaludin S (1996). *World Poult Science J* 53:351-369.

Jonsson E and Conway P (1992). In Probiotics, the scientific basis (R Fuller Ed) Champman and Hall London UK .pp 260-316.

Kafri I and Cherry J A (1984). *Poult Sci* 63(1), 125-126.

Kirchgessner M and Roth FX (1988). Ergotype Effekte durch organische sauren in der ferkalautzucht und schweinemast. *Ubersichten Zur Tierernahrung* 16 :93-108.

Kitchen DI (1997). In proceeding of Alltech 13th Annual symposium (ED TP Lyons and KA Jacques) pp-101-113. Nottingham University Press. Nottingham.

Kopnjufca V H. Pesti G M and Bakali R I (1997). *Poult Sci.* 76: 1264-1271.

Kumar, K., A. Thompson, A.K. Singh, Y. Chander, and S.C. Gupta. (2004). *J. Environ. Qual.* 33:250

Kumar, K., S.C. Gupta, Y. Chander, and A.K. Singh. (2005). *Adv. Agron.* 87.

Langford, F.M., D.M. Weary, and L. Fisher. (2003). *J. Dairy Sci.* 86:3963–3966.

Lee Y K, Nomoto K, Salminen S, Gorbach S (1999). Handbook of probiotics, NY, John Wiley and Sons Inc. 1999.

Lopez DC & Marquez GPC (1994). Proceedings of the 13th International Pig Veterinary Society Congress. Bangkok, Thiland. Pp 293.

Matthai J (1996). *Indian J. Pediatr.* 63:242-253.

Mazurkiewicz M, Jamroz D, Gawel A, Wieliczko A, Klimentowski S and Madej J A (1992). *Medcyna Wet* 48:369-371.

Menocal J A (1995). In Biotechnology in the feed industry (TP Lyons & KA Jacques eds.) Nottingham University Press, Loughborough.

Migliore, L., C. Civitareale, G. Brambilla, and G.D.D. Delupis. (1995). *Water Res.* 31:1801-1806

Mohan B, Kadirvel R, Natarajan A and Bhaskaran M (1996). *Br. J.Poult.Sci.* 37:395-401.

Moore, PRA Everson TK. Luckey E.McCoy, E.A.Elvehjem and E.B.Hart (1946). Use of sulphasuccidine, Streptothricin and streptomycin in nutrition studies with the chick. *J. Bio. Chem.* 165:437-441.

Morales, R *et al.* (2005). *Horizon.* p102.

Mul AJ & perry FG (1994). In recent advances in animal Nutrition. Ed PC Garnsworthyand DJA Cole) pp57-79. Nottingham University press. Nottingham.

NAAS, (2010). "Antibiotics in manure and soil-A grave threat to Human and Animal Health" Policy paper No. 43. National Academy of Agricultural Sciences, New Delhi pp20.

Naganawa R, Iwata, N., Ishikawa, K., Fukude, M., Fujino, T and Suzuki, A. (1996). *Appl. Environ Microbiol.* 62:4238-4242.

Nahashon S N, Nakave H S and Mirosh LW (1993). *Poult Sci.* 72:87 (abstract).

Njoku P C (1986). *Anim. Feed Sci. Technol.* 16:17-24.

Oswley WF, Orr DE & Tribble LF (1986). *J. Anim Sci.* 63:497-504.

Overland M, Granli T. Kjos NP, Fjetland O, Steien SH, Stokstad M (2000). *J Anim Sci* 78 (7): 1875-1884.

Pang F H, Xie M Q and Ling H H (2000). *Chinese J. Vet med.* 8:1-3.

Partanen KH and Mroz Z (1999). *Nutr Res Rev.* 12 (1):117-145.

Partridge G & Hazzledine M (1997). Proceeding of American Society of SWINE Practitioner. Pp 183-193.

Pasricha, N S (2008). Paper presented in Brain Storming session held at NASC New Delhi.

Patterson, R., R. DeSwarte, P. Greenberger, L. Grammer, J. Brown, and C.A. Choy. (1995). Ocean Side Publ., Providence, RI.

Perdigon G and Alvarez S (1992). In. probiotics the scientific basis (R Fuller ed) Champan and Hall, London UK pp-146-180.

Pouillard, P. (2003). *International Forum Agrosante* 2003, 1-2 April.

Praharaj NK, Reddy VR and Rama Rao SV, Shyam Sunder G and Reddy BLN (1999). *Archiv Fur Geflugelkunde* 63:1-8.

Ramarao S V, Reddy M R, Raju MVLN and Panda A K (2004). *Indian J. Poult Sci,* 39:125.

Risley *et al.* (1992). Cited from " An overview of the effect of organic acids on gut flora and gut health. By Nuria canibe, Ricarda M Engberg and Bent B.Jensen, Danish Institute of Agricultural Sciences. Research Centre Foulum, Denmark

Roth FX and Kirchgessner m (1998). *Journal of Animal Feed science* (7) 25-33.

Roy RD, Eidens FW, Parkhurst, CR Quereshi MA & Havenstein GB (2002). *Poult. Sci* 81: 951-957.

Sarah H. (2003). Poultry Industry, Alternative to antibiotics. www.engromix.com

Sarmah, A. K., Meyer, M.T. and Boxall, A.B.A. (2006). *Chemosphere,* 65 725–759.

Sebastian S, Touchburn S P and Chavez E R (1998). *World Poultry Sci J.* 54: 24-27.

Selim, S.A., and J.S. Cullor. (1997). *J. Am. Vet. Med. Assoc.* 211:1029–1035

Shoemaker, N.B., H. Vlamakis, K. Hayes, and A.A. Salyers. (2001). *Appl. Environ. Microbiol.* 67:561–568.

Sikka S S (2003). In Compendium "Tech Adv. In Livestock & Poultry Production and Management- Specific Reference to Rural Development".

Sikka S S (2009). Paper presented in Brain Storming session held at NASC New Delhi.

Sikka SS and Cawla JS (2002). *Ani. Nut. & Feed Tech* 2:11-18.

Sikka SS and Singh J (2007). In Proceeding of XXIV annual conference of Indian Poultry Science Association and National Symposium on poultry production for rural employment and nutritional security.25-27th April. 2007.Punjab, India..pp-62-67.

Sikka SS and Singh J (2010). In procd. ANA world Coference, NASC New delhi.

Singh Jaswinder & Sikka S S (2006). *Indian J. Poult Sci* 41;171-175.

Siuta A (2000). The influence of polish robotics on rearing performance of piglets. *Roczniki-Naukowe- Zootechniki* 6 :213-217.

Smith, K L, J E Hillerton and R J Harmon (2001). National Mastitis Council guidelines on normal and abnormal raw milk based on somatic cell counts and signs of clinical mastitis. http://nmconline.org/docs/abmilk.pdf.

SOU, (1997). 'Antimicrobial feed additives', Swedish Government Official Reports, p. 132.

Srivastava S P, Singh S and Saraswat BL (2005). *Indian J Anim Nutrition* 22: 13-15.

Stavric S, Kornegay E T, Wallace R J (ed) Chesson A (1995). Weinheim Germany:VCH Verlagegesellschaft mbH. Pp 205-231.

Sutton *et al.* (1991) cited from " An overview of the effect of organic acids on gut flora and gut health. By Nuria canibe, Ricarda M Engberg and Bent B.Jensen, Danish Institute of Agricultural Sciences. Research Centre Foulum, Denmark.

Svetic M, Dumanovski F, Kekej M, Ivekovi CD and Prpic B (1996). *Nutr Abstr Rev* 66:121.

Swain BK and Johri TS (2000). *Br Poult Sci.* 41:83-88.

Swain BK, Johri TS and MAajumdar S (2000). *Br. Poult. Sci* 41:287-92.

Tardani, A., and M. Terreni. (1996). *Bacillus cereus* in diets for pigs. *Riv. Suinicol.* 37:27.

Thomke S, Elwinger K (1998). *Ann Zootech.* 4: 245-271.

Thomke S, Rundgren M and Hesselman K (1980). In proc. Of the 31st European Association of Animal Production Germany. P-5.

Thomlinson and Lawrence (1981). cited from "An overview of the effect of organic acids on gut flora and gut health. By Nuria canibe, Ricarda M Engberg and Bent B.Jensen, Danish Institute of Agricultural Sciences. Research Centre Foulum, Denmark.

Tsiagbe VK, Cook ME, Harper AE and Sunde ML (1987). *Poult. Sci* 66:1138-42.

Vander Beke N (1997). Thesis high scholl gent. Belgium.

Waldroup *et al* (1995). cited from " An overview of the effect of organic acids on gut flora and gut health. By Nuria canibe, Ricarda M Engberg and Bent B.Jensen, Danish Institute of Agricultural Sciences. Research Centre Foulum, Denmark.

Wang X and GR Gibson (1993). *J. Appl Bact* . 75:373-380.

Webb, K.E., Jr., and J.P. Fontenot. (1975). *J. Anim. Sci.* 41:1212–1217.

Webster's Encyclopedic Cambridge Dictionary of English Language (1989). Gramercy Books, New York.

WHO, (2000). http://www.who.int/emcdocuments/zoonoses/hocdscsraph20004c.html.

Yadav B S, Srivastava R K and Sjukla P K (1994). *Indian J. Anim Nur.* 11: 225-227.

Yu, J G & Zhu LY (2000). *J. Tradi Chi. Vet. Med.* 6:3-4.

Yuan Y L, Fan Bt & Zhang Y X (1993). *J. Tradi Chi. Vet. Med.*, 3:6-10

Zhang W F, Li D F, Lu WQ & Y, GF (2003). *Poult Sci*, 82 :657-663.

□□□

6

Recent Development in Microbial Degradation of Tannins in Rumen and thier Effect on Animal and Human Health

S.N. RAI
Principal Scientist
National Dairy Research Institute, Karnal-132001, India

ABSTRACT

Quantitative biodegradation of tannins in terms of different monomers in rumen have been achieved using babul (Acacia nilotica) pods as a source of tannins. Under in vitro studies six total mixed rations (TMR) containing 0, 40, 60, 80,100,120 g tannin/kg substrate, were assessed for nutrient digestibility and gas production and degraded products of tannins with rumen fluid of crossbred cattle, buffaloes and goats using HPLC. The digestibility of dry matter, organic matter and crude protein decreased ($P<0.05$) with increased levels of tannins beyond a certain a level. Similarly, gas production was also reduced ($P<0.05$) with increased levels of tannins in the TMR. Gallic acid, phloroglucinol, resorcinol and catechin were identified. Phloroglucinol and resorcinol were the major end products of tannin degradation while catechin and gallate was produced in traces. The in vivo results also depicted the presence of similar degraded products of tannins in different biological samples of cows. The use of various degradation products of tannins are documented for its therapeutic value which may be used as protective measures against several ailments such as cancer, cardio vascular diseases, diabeties and enhances the immunity status in the body and reproductive efficiency. The details of different aspects of human health have been discussed in this article.

Introduction

In tropical region like India, there is large deficit of conventional feeds. Due to shortage of conventional feeds especially grains and their milling by-products as well as oil cakes, alternative approach to substitute this gap through use of new unconventional feed resources as animal feed has been coming up gradually. However, their use as animal feeds is limited because of the presence of anti-nutritional factors like tannins. Tannins are classified into hydrolysable and condensed tannin. Hydrolysable tannin contains carbohydrate core in which hydroxyl groups are esterified to gallic acid (gallotannin) or ellagic acid (ellagitannin). Condensed tannin contains phenol of flavon group and yield anthocyanidin on acid hydrolysis as it also known as proanthocyanidin. Tannins are reported to have a negative effect on digestibility of nutrients and thus lower the production performance and also cause toxicity to the vital organs if provided in excess amount.

Babul pod (*Acacia nilotica*) is one of such tannin containing nutritionally potential unconventional feed resource seasonally available in huge quantities in many tropical countries. About 60 x 10^3 tonnes of *Acacia nilotica* pods are available annually in India as per the rough estimate. It is essential to find out the non-toxic level of *Acacia nilotica* tannin in diet of ruminant to avoid possible harmful effect on nutrient digestion. HPLC has been used to evaluate tannin present in unconventional feeds in last few decades. HPLC was also used to estimate tannins metabolites in different biological samples of rat. Mass spectrometry was also used to study the chemical nature of vegetable tannins. Scanty literatures on nutritional potentiality of *Acacia nilotica* pods and its tannin metabolites in ruminant tempted us to find the factual influence on animal productivity and nutraceutical effects. Hence, during last decade, attempts were made to assess the microbial degradation of tannins in the rumen of cattle, buffalo and goats (using a series of *in vitro* and *in vivo experiments)* and a novel methodology was developed for their identification and quantification of degradation products in the different biological fluids using different levels of *Acacia nilotica* pods in total mixed ration (TMR) as substrate.

Nutrient Digestibility and Gas Production

Nutrients digestibility was decreased ($P<0.05$) with increased level of tannins from 0 to 120g tannin/kg TMR. It is clear from the study that digestibility of DM, OM and CP is reduced with increased level of tannin in the TMRs. Crude protein digestibility was greatly affected by tannin contents. The pronounced reduction in protein in this case, might be due high ratio of soluble to insoluble tannins in *Acacia nilotica* pods. As high ratio of soluble to insoluble tannins affect the protein digestibility more than that of carbohydrate.

In contrary to this, it was reported that enzymatic hydrolysis of casein, pea meal and soybean meal protein increased in presence of tannic acid (1 to 5 % w/w). However, natures of tannins of Acacia nilotica pods were different from that tannic acid as it contains epigallocatechin gallate. Decreased in digestibility of other nutrients was observed with increased level of tannin which was reflected through decreased in IVGP.

There is a great geographical variation in *Acacia nilotica* pods for the content of tannin in it. It was reported that goat of Tanzania and Zimbabwe consumed less (< 40g DM/day) *Acacia nilotica* pods and showed negative nitrogen balance. However, in India, feeding of *Acacia nilotica* pods which contained > 180 g tannins/kg, did not affect dry matter intake and N balance in crossbred calves fed on diet containing 61 % *Acacia* pods in the concentrate mixture. Similarly, intake and N balance did not affect at 40 % level of inclusion in the concentrate mixture of cows.. Babul seed chuni a byproduct of *Acacia nilotica* did not affect nutrient utilization by cows even at higher level of inclusion namely 0, 30 and 45 % in the concentrate mixture. However, inclusion of similar levels of babul seed chuni in the concentrate mixture of calves diet significantly reduced (P<0.05) the CP digestibility, but not other nutrients. Lesser or no effect of babul seed chunni on nutrient utilization is due its low tannin content.

Determination of Tannin Degraded Products using HPLC

Tannin metabolites using HPLC such as Phloroglucinol, Gallic acid, Resorcinol and (+) Catechin were first time identified and quantified (patented) at NDRI, Karnal in TMR containing 4, 8 and 12 per cent tannin.

A. nilotica leaves contain the relatively uncommon catechin gallate tannin (Self *et al.*, 1986), while *A. nilotica* pods and bark contain (-) epigallocatechin gallates (Ayoub, 1985). *A. nilotica* pods also contain catechin gallates as the degradation products revealed (+) catechin but not the (-) epicatechin, gallocatechin or epigallocatechin. Tanner *et al.* (1990) also reported detecting catechin gallates in *A. nilotica* pods. These flavanol gallate tannin give positive colour reactions for condensed and hydrolysable tannin when in fact neither of these tannin classes is present (Self *et al.*, 1986) which has led to some confusion in the literature (Ngwa *et al.*, 2001).

Identification of Tannin Degraded Products

Incubation with rumen liquor from buffalo, cattle and goat yielded phloroglucinol, resorcinol, (+) catechin and gallic acid as degradation products from the *A. nilotica* tannin in addition to two unidentified compounds. The (+) catechin concentrations were broadly similar between the animal species (0 to 12 mg/g tannin). However, large differences occurred in phloroglucinol concentrations between animals and with time (0 to 491 mg/g tannin). Resorcinol showed much smaller differences (0 to 63 mg/g tannin).

Phloroglucinol was rapidly degraded in cattle rumen liquor, but accumulated in higher concentrations in buffalo and goat rumen liquor especially at the 8 and 12 per cent tannin levels. It would appear that there was a time delay between the phloroglucinol and the resorcinol peaks, which occurred at 18 or 30h and 30 or 42h, respectively. Gallic acid and (+) catechin can both be degraded by bacteria to phloroglucinol and resorcinol (Murdiati *et al.*, 1992; Lowry *et al.*, 1996; Hopper and Mahadevan, 1997; Arunachalam *et al.*, 2003). Pyrogallol is a known metabolite of gallic acid. Absence of pyrogallol and presence of very little gallic acid were detected after 18h incubation, suggested that these were rapidly metabolized to phloroglucinol (Zhu *et al.*, 1995; Tor *et al.*, 1996). The absence of pyrogallol is in contrast to the results of others who found it in cattle and goat rumen liquor after 24h incubation with tannic acid (Odenyo and Osuji, 1998; Nelson *et al.*, 1995). Tannic acid consists largely of pentagalloyl glucose (Self *et al.*, 1986) and, therefore, appears to give rise to a slightly different degradation pathway than the catechin gallates. Pyrogallol was either not produced from the catechin gallates of *A. nilotica* or metabolised to phloroglucinol in less than 18h. (Fig.1).

The time course of the appearance and disappearance of these metabolites seemed to vary between the three animal species, which suggests that the microbial populations produced slightly different effects. Goat microbes appeared to degrade most of the tannin to (+) catechin and phloroglucinol. Buffalo microbes also produced high levels of phloroglucinol. In contrast, cattle rumen liquor degraded phloroglucinol rapidly and accumulated much more resorcinol.

Interestingly, the gas production from cattle and goat microbes showed a lag phase, which suggests that the microbes were adapting during the first 12h. Long lag phases as a result of *A. nilotica* tannin have also been reported by Mueller-Harvey *et al.* (1988). However, there was no lag phase in buffalo rumen liquor. As buffalo microbes, at 12 per cent tannin, resulted in the lowest total gas volume and the largest decrease of gas production due to tannin between 6 to 18h incubation, it is suggested that the buffalo microbial populations were least adapted to these tannin. Microbes in goat rumen liquor may be most capable to cope with this tannin, as they produced a big response from 5 ml at 6h to 20 ml after 12h and only small differences between the 0, 4, 6, 8 and 10 per cent tannin TMRs.

Decarboxylation and reductive dehydroxylation of phenolics occurs principally in the rumen. The resulting gallic acid is less toxic than tannic

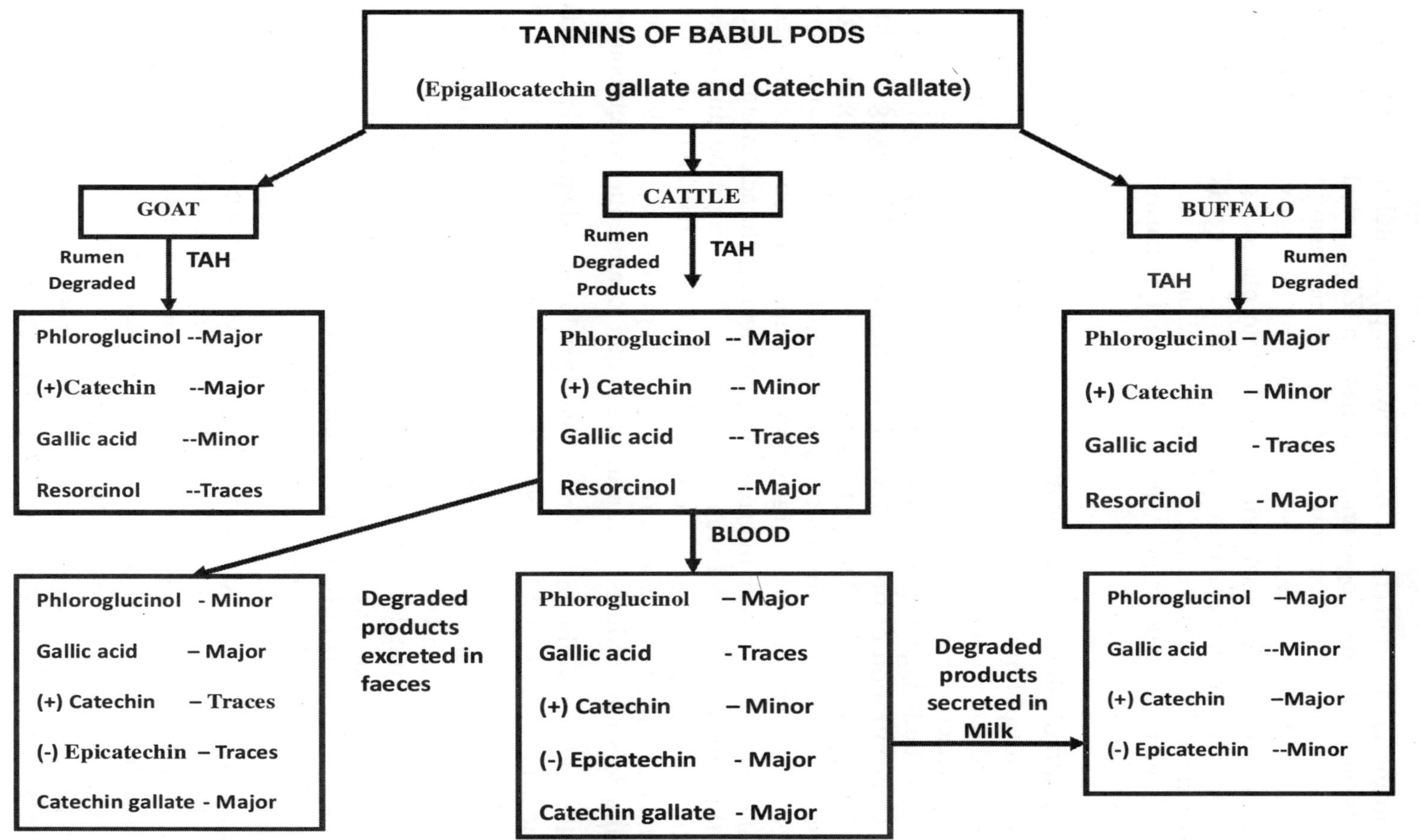

Fig. 1 : Identification of degraded products of tannins from Babul Pods in different biological samples in ruminants (TAH = Tannin Acyl Hydrolase)

acid according to Murdiati *et al.* (1992). However, pyrogallol is considered to be responsible for methaemoglobinaemia in sheep (Zhu *et al.*, 1995; Tor *et al.*, 1996). Lowry *et al.* (1996) also concluded that an increasing fraction of the ingested *A. nilotica* tannin was being degraded as the recovery of urinary metabolites in sheep decreased with time. Certain phenolics, such as gallic acid and (+) catechin, can apparently act as source of energy (Tsai and Jones, 1975; Tsai *et al.*, 1976; Patel *et al.*, 1981; Krumholz and Bryant, 1986; Lowry *et al.*, 1996; Bhat *et al.*, 1998) and, therefore, may not be harmful at moderate levels.

Quantification of Tannin Metabolites

Gallic acid, phloroglucinol, resorcinol and Catechin were appeared as degraded products of *Acacia nilotica* tannin. In addition, one unidentified peaks had been detected. Presence of catechin but not epicatechin as a metabolite of *Acacia nilotica* tannin, gave an indication that *Acacia nilotica* contained catechin gallate. Concentration of phloroglucinol was highest (8-135 mg/g tannin) followed by resorcinol (15-63 mg/g tannin) and catechin (3 – 10 mg/g tannin). Gallic acid was produced in traces. Gallic acid and catechin both can be degraded to phloroglucinol and resorcinol by rumen microbes. Sometimes, pyrogallol may produce as an intermediary product in gallic acid metabolism. But in this study pyrogallol was not detected. This might be due rapid degradation of pyrogallol to phloroglucinol. Uncommon nature of tannin of *Acacia nilotica* might follow different way of degradation in which either pyrogallol does not produced or rapidly degraded to subsequent metabolites.

Gallic acid, pyrogallol and resorcinol were produced as degraded products of tannic acid in urine and faecal sample of rats. Gallic acid, resorcinol and catechin were detected in urine and faecal samples as metabolites of *Acacia nilotica* tannins. *Selenomonas ruminantium* and *Streptococcus caprinus* are two major bacteria, which involves in tannin degradation in the rumen has been isolated from the ruminal content of feral goat browsing on tannin rich *Acacia* species. A *Selenomonas* species capable of tannin degradation was isolated from the enrichment culture of rumen microflora of sheep and goat. Hydrolysable tannin degraded to gallic acid, pyrogallol, phloroglucinol and resorcinol by the enzyme tannin acyl hydrolase (Tannase) produced by rumen bacteria. Such degraded products of hydrolysable tannin can be used as energy source after their conversion into acetate and butyrate through HOHN (3-Hydroxy-5-Oxohexanoate) pathways by a numbers of rumen bacteria. Hydrolysable tannins content of TMR ranged from 38.1 to 112.1 g/kgDM. Resorcinol, a degraded product of hydrolysable tannin anaerobically converted to acetyl CoA by reduction and then to a six-carbon keto acid through hydrolysis. The resultant six-carbon keto acid however, not degraded further by rumen bacteria and excreted as urinary phenolic conjugate. The catechin and epicatechin, degraded products of condensed tannin further degraded first to diaryl propanol which then converted to acetic acid and phenylvalarolactone through ring scission can also be used as source of energy.

Acacia nilotica tannin reduced the *in vitro* digestibility of dry matter, organic matter and crude protein. Degraded products of tannins from *Acacia nilotica* pods in rumen fluid of cattle were phloroglucinol, gallic acid, resorcinol and catechin. Phloroglucinol. Resorcinol was the major degraded products while gallate was produced in traces. From this study it becomes clear that, cattle harbour the tannin degrading bacteria in the rumen microflora without a pre exposure to tannin containing diet.

Degraded Products of Tannin Secreted in Milk of Cows

Phloroglucinol, gallic acid, (+) catechin and (-) epicatechin were identified and quantified by developing a novel method using HPLC. At low level of pods (20 % in diet) all the tannin monomers were secreted in milk where phloroglucinol and resorcinol were the major components of metabolites and other two were produced in traces. At 20 per cent level, there was no gallic acid detected in serum, however, it was found in milk, indicated that there was some inter conversion of monomers occurred in mammary gland. The concentration of phloroglucinol, gallic acid, (+) catechin and (-) epicatechin per 100 ml of milk were estimated as 268.26, 2.89, 29.82 and 2.14 mg respectively at 20 per cent level of babul pods in the diet.

Degraded Products of Tannin Excreted in Urine of Cows

Phloroglucinol, gallic acid, resorcinol, (+) catechin, (-)epicatechin and catechin gallate were identified and quantified by developing a novel method using HPLC across all levels of inclusion of babul pods. Phloroglucinol and catechin gallate were the major end products of babul pods tannin in the urine of cows at both 20 (2.68±1.12, 13.11±11.75 mg/g tannin) and 40 (2.06±0.84, 1.30±0.67 mg/d tannin) per cent level of babul pods. Total excretion was similar at both levels (5.50±1.61, 14.85±12.02 mg/g tannin), although excretion at higher level (40 %) was found higher in comparison to low level (20 %) of babul pods. It is apparent that, when the level of tannin increased in the diet of cows, excrete more tannin through urine than at low level where excretion was more through faeces.

Reviewing the recent information suggested that research work in the field of tannin metabolism with respect to known threshold level of dietary tannin in dairy animals, changes in quantity and quality of milk produced from tanniniferous feed containing diet and role of tannin metabolites secreted into milk as a nutraceutical value demands high priority. Therefore, a number of experiments were planned to establish the nutraceutical effects of different degradation products of tannin through feed to milk and milk products on laboratory animals in order to evaluate for their value addition as well as efficacy of preventing against various human ailments.

Therapeutic Value of Tannin Metabolites

Tannins, being bioactive compound, have both positive (antioxidants) and negative (anti-nutrient) effects on biological system depending on their concentration and nature. Tannins monomers, due to their valuable biological properties as a antioxidant and putative role in reducing oxidative damage associated with many diseases including cancer, cardiovascular diseases, cataracts, atherosclerosis, diabetes, asthma, liver injury, arthritis, immune deficiency diseases and aging, have been raising a high interest among human and animal nutritionist.

Gallic acid, a bioactive compound of tannins inhibits nitrozation and thus the formation of carcinogenic nitrosamine. Catechins have various functions in biological system like inhibit lipid peroxidation and oxidation of low density lipoproteins, up regulate the synthesis of some hepatic phase II enzymes that are involved in the detoxification of some xenobiotics, including chemical carcinogens, have antithrombotic activity and may aid in lowering total cholesterol and LDL-cholesterol levels, stimulate the secretion of bile salts and fecal excretion of cholesterol. Catechins have also been found to promote thermo genesis.

Value addition of milk and milk products through natural sources is the major concern in present era to improve immune status of animals as well as humans through animal products. Tannins at relatively high concentrations usually inhibit the activity of enzymes, but at low concentrations they often stimulate enzyme activity (Maxson *et al.*, 1973).

The binding of tannins with proteins participates in the anti-diarrhoeic activity of tannins by protecting the digestive organs from injurious attack. It also participates in the antihaemorrhagic effects of tannin rich drugs. The detoxification of snake venoms and bacterial toxins by persimmon tannin is another activity most probably based on the strong binding activity of this tannin (Asquith and Butler, 1986: Murdiati and McSweeney, 1987). The natural occurrence of tannins, in pasture species, in addition to its potential of controlling bloat, could have a direct nutritional benefit by protecting leaf protein from degradation in the rumen of animals (Mangan, 1988). The inhibition of mutagen city of several carcinogens by tannins has been partly attributed to the binding of tannins with these compounds. Mechanism of inhibition rather depends on the type of the mutagen. Strong inhibition of tumor promotion is exhibited by several tannins and has been demonstrated experimentally on two stage carcinogenesis. Several oligomeric hydrolysable tannins and related compounds revealed strong host mediated antitumor activity which may be due to the enhancement of immune response of the host animals through the actions on tumor cells and some immunocytes (Okuda *et al.*, 1991).

Acacia Tannins as Ayurvedic medicine

Acacia tannins contain different polyphenolic compounds that have shown a potential medicinal value in different diseases. Significant and positive linear correlation was found between total antioxidant capacities and phenolic contents, indicating that phenolic compounds were the dominant antioxidant constituents in the plants. It contains of two types namely hydrolysable and condensed tannins.

Approaches to increase bioavailability

Mixing tea flavan-3-ols with 50% bovine, soy, and rice milk, respectively increased total flavan-3-ol (EC, EGC, EGCG, ECG) recovery to 52, 55, and 69% after digestion. The recovery of flavan-3-ols after the addition of 30 mg of ascorbic acid showed differential effects on EGC, EGCG, EC, and ECG (74, 54, 82, and 45%) (Green, *et al.*, 2007). The addition of up to 50% of fruit juice (grapefruit, orange, lemon, or lime) also improved the recovery of EGC (81–98%), EGCG (56–76%), EC (86–95%), and ECG (30–55%).

Drug Potential of these Tannin metabolites

Percival *et al* (2002) reported that the mice consumed wine rich in phenolic components as catechin, epicatechin, gallic acid, ellagic acid showed increased antioxidant activity. Gallic acid (GA) also showed strong antioxidant activity by preventing lipid per oxidation. GA is a strong antioxidant that possesses antimutagenic and anticarcinogenic activities

Green tea contain (+) - gallocatechin (GC), (-)- epicatechin (EC), (-)-epigallocatechin (EGC), (-)- epicatechingallate (ECG), (-)- epigallocatechingallate (EGCG) which show numerous biological activities including antibacterial, antioxidant, antitumor and cancer preventive activities. Catechin serve as powerful antioxidant against lipid peroxidation when phospholipid bi-layers are exposed to aqueous oxygen radicals. When the superoxide dismutase (SOD) - like activity of natural antioxidants was evaluated by measuring the inhibition of pyragallol autoxidation that is catalyzed by the superoxide radical, (+) - catechin and (-) - epicatechin showed effective SOD-like activity (Kim *et al.*, 1995). Jasmine green tea, which contain (-) – epicatechin (EC), (-) epicatechingallate (ECG), (-) epigallocatechin (EGC) and (-)

epigallocatechingallate (EGCG) showed a strong protection for RBC membrane to hemolysis induced by an azo free radical initiator.

Administration of 5 mg of procyanidin B-2 3, 3ⁱ-di-o-gallate also led to a significant increase in renal functional parameters (Yokozawa *et al.*, 1993).

(+) Catechin prevents cancer (liver, lung, breast and colon cancer) in at least one of three ways. First, they can prevent the formation of carcinogens, second, they tone up the body's natural detoxification defenses, and finally, they suppress cancer promotion. In the laboratory, animal studies have shown that (+) catechin has other promising qualities: acting as an antibacterial and antiviral agent, regulating cholesterol and blood pressure, and reducing blood clotting tendencies that may cause heart attacks or strokes. (+) Catechin and (-) epicatechin have strong antimicrobial activity and can be used for the treatment of periodontal (mouth) disease. They also showed insulin enhancing activity.

Cardiovascular Diseases and Catechins

Cardiovascular disease (CVD), principally heart disease and stroke, are the leading cause of mortality in both men and women in all racial and ethnic groups. The risk of atherosclerosis is increased by high blood pressure, hypertension, kidney disorders, obesity, diabetes, smoking, excessive alcohol consumption, stress, thyroid and adrenal gland problems, and lipid disorders (Crespy and Williamson 2004). Tea contains many compounds, especially poly-phenols and epidemiologically studies show that polyphenolic compounds present in tea reduces the risk of a variety of diseases. Catechins are the main compounds in green tea; they consist of (-)-epicatechin, (-)-epicatechin-3-gallate (ECg), (-)-epigallocatechin, (-)-epigallocatechin-3-gallate (EGCg) etc. (Graham, 1992).

Out of these 30 studies, 17 studies indicated the statistically significant beneficial effects of green tea. These results suggest a plausible mechanism for the beneficial effects of green tea.

Effect on antioxidant markers and oxidative stress

Antioxidants are compounds that protect cells against the damaging effects of reactive oxygen species, such as singlet oxygen, superoxide, peroxyl radicals, hydroxyl radicals, and peroxynitrite. An imbalance between antioxidants and reactive oxygen species results in oxidative stress, leading to cellular damage. Catechins are hypothesized to help protect against these diseases by contributing, along with antioxidant vitamins (i.e. Vit. C and E) and enzymes (i.e. superoxide dismutase (SOD), and catalase), to the total antioxidant defense system.

Duthie, *et al.*, (2006) reported that short-term supplementation (two weeks) with cranberry juice (contained significant levels of vitamin C, total phenols, catechins and anthocyanins with associated antioxidant activity measured as FRAP) did not influence several biomarkers of blood lipid status and had no cytoprotective effect on either basal or induced oxidative DNA damage in a group of young, healthy volunteers.

Tannin monomers and Antioxidant activity

The use of alkylgallates as antioxidants of fatty oil and the use of gallic acid as a preservative of fresh fish are examples of practical applications of this effect. The long lasting inhibitory effects of tannins may be due to the presence of many phenolic hydroxyl groups which produce stable free radicals one after another. The formation and solublization of precipitates with several metal ions is accompanied by reduction of the metal ions. This property of tannins may induce a reduction in the toxicity of several metallic ions under mild conditions..

Catechin serve as powerful antioxidant against lipid peroxidation when phospholipid bilayers are exposed to aqueous oxygen radicals.

When the superoxide dismutase (SOD)-like activity of natural antioxidants was evaluated by measuring the inhibition of pyragallol autoxidation that is catalyzed by the superoxide radical, (+) – catechin and (-) – epicatechin showed effective SOD-like activity .

The glomerular filteration rate, renal plasma flow and renal blood flow were significantly increased in rats given (-)– epicatechin 3-o gallate at a dose of 5 or 10 mg/ kg body weight/day for 24 days. Administration of 5 mg of procyanidin B-2 3, 3[i] -di-o-gallate also led to a significant increase in renal functional parameters (Yokozawa *et al.*, 1993). Gallic acid also showed strong antioxidant activity by preventing lipid per oxidation (Dufour *et al.*, 2002).

Percival *et al* (2002) reported that the mice consumed wine rich in phenolic components as catechin, epicatechin, gallic acid, ellagic acid showed increased antioxidant activity and did not result in lower T lymphocytes and natural killer cells in the blood when the injection of lipopolysaccharides (LPS), a compound derived from bacteria, was given to mice.

Effects on lipid profiles

Green tea catechins affect lipid metabolism by different pathways and prevent the appearance of atherosclerotic plaque. Green Tea Extract (GTE) intake decrease the absorption of tri-glycerides and cholesterol (Raederstorff, *et. al.* 2003 and Loest, *et. al.* 2002) and these findings are in accordance with the fact that faecal fat excretion increases (Raederstorff, *et. al.* 2003). Some studies report that green tea catechins decreases plasma total cholesterol and blood triglyceride levels, but the effects differ among studies (Miura, *et. al.* 2001, Murase, *et. al.* 2002 and Tijburg, *et. al.* 1997). This difference could be due to the different animal models used. Moreover, regarding the green tea catechins intake levels, plasma cholesterol apparently decreases only when green tea intake is >0.5% of the diet. Green tea catechin ingestion also decreases LDL cholesterol. Concurrently, HDL cholesterol increases, showing that green tea polyphenols exert an anti-atherosclerotic effect. These results demonstrate that long term feeding of tea catechins can be beneficial in the suppression of high-fat-diet-induced obesity by modulating lipid metabolism. By this mechanism, green tea could possibly reduce the risk of associated diseases, including diabetes and coronary disease.

Effect on carbohydrate metabolism

Diabetes, especially type 2 is a heterogeneous disorder that involves resistance of glucose and lipid metabolism in peripheral tissues to the biological activity of insulin and inadequate insulin secretion by pancreatic â cells.. Catechins also reduced plasma triglyceride levels in an oral glucose tolerance test in normal rats. These results suggest that green tea catechins could act as preventive agents and could have a beneficial effect against lipid and glucose metabolism.

Epigallocatechin gallate (EGCG) enhances oral glucose tolerance in severely diabetic mice and in moderately diabetic rats. The *in vivo* and *in vitro* findings suggested that the reduction of Effective glucose production (EGP) and increase in glucose-induced insulin secretion contributed to the antidiabetic effects of EGCG. EGP is main determinant of fasting glucose levels. EGCG supplementation causes a pronounced decrease of glucose levels in food-deprived animals, which exceeds the decrease of glucose levels in animals not deprived of food. The increase in insulin concentration in fed mice supplemented with EGCG could either be caused by direct stimulation of insulin secretion in response to feeding or by a positive effect of EGCG on the pancreas.

Conclusion

The available data on biodegradation of tannins from babul pods depicted similarity of degradation products in various biological samples and thereby releases in the milk of cows to a significant extent. Hence, it is suggestive of having better therapeutic value of milk which may be used as protective measures against several human ailments such as cancer, cardiac problems, diabetes, renal impairment and enhances the immunity status in the body of the animal.

References

Arunachalam, M., Mohan, N., Sugadev, R., Chellappan, P. and Mahadevan, A. (2003). Degradation of (+) catechin by *Acinetobacter calcoaceticus* MTC 127. *Biochim. Biophys. Acta* 1621: 261-265.

Ayoub, S.M.H., (1985). Flavanol molluscicides from the Sudan *Acacias. Int. J. Crude Drug Res.* 23: 87-90.

Bhat T.K, Singh, B. and Sharma, O.P. (1998). Microbial degradation of tannin – a current perspective. *Biodegradation* 9:343-357.

Hopper, W. and Mahadevan, A. (1997). Degradation of catechin by *Bradyrhizobium japonicum. Biodegradation.* 8: 159-165.

Krumholz, L.R. and Bryant, M.P. (1986). *Eubacterium oxidoreducens* sp. Nov. requiring H_2 or formate to degrade gallate, Pyrogallol, Phloroglucinol and auercetin. *Arch. Microbiol.*, 144 : 8-14.

Lowry, B.J., McSweeney, C.S. and Palmer, B. (1996). Changing perceptions of the effect of plant phenolics on nutrient supply in the ruminant. *Aust. J. Agric. Res.* 47: 829-842.

Mueller-Harvey, I., McAllan, A.B., Theodorou, M.K., Beever, D.E. (1988). Phenolics in fibrous crop residues and plants and their effects on the digestion kinetics in ruminants. In: Reed, J.D., Capper, B.S. and Neate, P.J.H. (Eds.) Plant breeding and the nutritive value of crops. Proceedings of a workshop held at ILCA, Addis Ababa, Ethiopia, 7-10 December 1987. ILCA, Addis Ababa. p. 97-132.

Murdiati, T.B., Mcsweeney, C.S. and Lowry, J.B. (1992) . Metabolism in sheep of gallic acid, tannic acid and hydrolysable tannins from *Terminalia oblongata, Aust. J. Agric. Res.*, 43 : 1307-1319.

Nelson, K.E., Pell, A.N., Shofield, P. and Zinder, S. (1995). Isolation and characterisation of an anaerobic ruminal bacteria capable of degrading hydrolysable tannins. *Appl. Env. Microbiol.* 61: 3293-3298.

Ngwa, A.T., Nsahlai, I.V., and Bonsi, M.L.K. (2001). The rumen digestion of dry matter, nitrogen and cell wall constituents of the pods of *Leucaena leucocephala* and some *Acacia* species. *J. Sci. Food Agric.* 82: 98-106.

Odenyo, A. A. and Osuji, P.O. (1998). Tannin-tolerant ruminal bacteria from East African ruminants. *Can. J. Microbiol.*, 44,905-909.

Patel, T.R., Jure, K.G. and Jones, G.A. (1981). Catabolism of phloroglucinol by rumen microbes *Coprococcus. Appl. Environ. Microbiol.* 42:1010-1017.

Self, R., Eagles, J., Galletti, G.C., Mueller-Harvey, I., Hartley, R.D., Lea, A.G., Magnolata, D., Richli, U., Gujer, R. and Haslam, E., (1986). Fast atom bombardment mass spectrometry of polyphenols (syn. vegetable tannins). *Biomed. Mass Spectrom.*, 13: 449-468.

Tanner, J.C., Reed, J.D. and Owen, E. (1990). The nutritive value of fruits (pods and seeds) from four *Acacia* sp. compared with extracted noug (*Guizotia abyssinica*) meal as supplements to maize stover for Ethiopian highland sheep. *Anim. Production,* 51: 127-133.

Tor, E.R., Francis, T.M., Holstege, D.M., Galey, F.D. (1996). GC/MS determination of pyrogallol and gallic acid in biological matrices as diagnostic indicators of oak exposure. *J. Agric. Food Chem.*, 44: 1275-1279.

Tsai, C.G. and Jones, G.A. (1975). Isolation and identificaiton of rumen bacteria capable of anaerobic phloroglucinol degradation. *Can J. Microbiol.*, 21 : 794-801.

Tsai, C.G., Gates, D.M. Ingledew W.M. and Jones G.A. (1976). Products of anaerobic phloroglucinol degradation by *Coprococcus* Sp. Pe.15. *Canadian J. Microbiol.*, 22 : 159-164.

Zhu, J., Filippich, L.J. and Ng, J. (1995). Rumen involvement in sheep tannic acid metabolism. *Vet. Hum. Toxicol.*, 37:436-440.

□□□

7

Influence of Nutrition on Bovine Reproduction

ANKITA KILLEDAR
Reproductive Biology Research Unit, College of Veterinary Science & Animal Husbandry
Anand Agricultural University, Anand-388110,Gujarat

The reproductive performance of dairy animals in this article is covered under two topics :

1. Achievement of early Puberty and
2. Postpartum reproductive perfomance

Nutrition is a critical factor that affects reproduction. Successful reproduction is based on the same necessary nutrients as those needed for maintenance, growth and lactation. These nutrients include energy, protein, vitamins and minerals. Nutrient deficiencies or excesses can lead to reduced reproductive performance. Pubertal heifers require feed for their growth and development. Primiparous heifers require feed in addition for foetal development. In post partum cows during early lactation, the demand for nutrients to support maintenance and milk production is given the highest priority. Thus, reproduction takes a "back seat" until these demands for nutrients are met.

Effect of Nutrition on Pubertal Development

The achievement of puberty i.e., expression of estrus and the age at first conception in heifers are two main benchmarks which are used to assess the reproductive performance of heifers. The age at first calving is the result of these two events. The effect of feeding heifers adequately, underfeeding and overfeeding are discussed below. Heifers that are not fed adequate amounts of energy reach sexual maturity later. Dairy heifers reach sexual maturity when they are 70% of their adult weight. Heifers raised on quality hay or grazed on late summer pastures often are energy-deficient.

Overfeeding energy to heifers before they reach puberty also is very harmful. Heifers which are overfed will reach adequate weight at an early age but will lack sufficient bone growth, especially in the pelvic area, which increases calving difficulty. Excessive weight gain is more harmful to heifers before they reach puberty than after they are bred. Overfeeding heifers before puberty (before nine months of age) can cause heifers to store excessive fat tissue in the developing udder and decrease the amount of milk-producing tissue.

Poor nutrition delays puberty, reduces conception rate and increases pregnancy losses in heifers (Fleck *et al., 1980*). Maintaining dairy heifers on only 62% of their energy requirements delays puberty until 20 months of age (Gerloff and Morrow, 1986). Young growing animals needs specific attention from this point of view, as it determine the achievement of required body weight for attaining puberty and sexual maturity whereas in adults it will lead to the loss of sexual desire, irregular estrus or anoestrus and reduced conception rate (Kaur, 1994).

Generally both the under and over feeding is detrimental to the reproductive status of animals. The effect of dietary intake on the time of onset of puberty was clearly demonstrated by Asdell (1955), who found that when he fed Friesian heifers on high, medium and low planes of nutrition, puberty occurred at 9, 11 and 15 months of age, respectively. The heifers required 1.89, 1.64 and 1.33 services per conception, respectively.

First calf heifers may be more sensitive to protein deficiencies than mature cows. Heifers that are raised on a protein deficient diet lack the skeletal growth in relation to their size, especially in the pelvic area. These heifers are older when they start cycling, have more difficulty in calving, and may not milk as well once they enter the milking herd.

Leaver (1977) fed Friesian heifers from 6 weeks before, to 6 weeks after, artificial insemination on three different levels of nutrition. These gave growth rates of 0.68 (high), 0.50 (medium) and 0.34 (low) kg/day, respectively, producing a wide range of body condition score at the time of mating. Pregnancy rates were 42, 72, 70 and 63% for poor, moderate, good and very bodily condition, respectively. Thus, heifers that are in poor or moderate condition achieve improved pregnancy rates when dietary intake is increased but those in good condition show no response. This study also suggests that heifers that are overfed and fat have impaired fertility.

Reid *et al.* (1964) also found that heifers reared on a very high level of nutrition had more breeding problems subsequently than those fed moderately. As the feeding level increases, the age at puberty decreases.

Additional feeding after insemination improved conception rates only in those heifers growing at less than 750 g/day before insemination (Rochet, 1973). It was therefore recommended that Holstein-Friesian dairy heifers should be growing at a rate of 0.7 kg/day to achieve optimum fertility. As a guide, target weights are that Friesian-Holstein heifers should be at least 330 kg and Jersey heifers 280 kg, a month before mating commences (Fielden *et al.*, 1977). In Gujarat under field conditions the crossbred heifers weighing 270 kg start showing regular estrus irrespective of age(Personal communications).

Olivares *et al.* (1981) studied effect of prepartum and postpartum supplementation on the reproductive performance of Brahman heifers. They studied the effect of feeding as below:

Parameters	I	II	III	IV
Prepartum weight loss (g/day)	770	737	1362	1366
Postpartum weight loss upto 120 days (g/day)	41	81	163	162
% cows cycling	67	58	25	8
% cows conceiving	50	25	8	8
Calf weight at birth (kg)	27	29	28	29
Calf weight at 120 days (kg)	104	102	119	108

I = Fed 2 kg concentrates for 22-25 days prepartum and 90 days postpartum
II = Fed 2 kg concentrates prepartum, only for 22-25 days prepartum
III = Fed concentrates postpartum only 90 days postpartum
IV = Received no concentrates (control)

Patel *et al.* (2009) studied the estrus induction response and circulatory profiles of calcium, inorganic phosphorus and trace elements (Co, Cu, Fe, Zn) in prepubertal (15-20 months old) HF heifer without (n=7) and with (n=7) mineral supplementation @ 50g/day for 75 days. The concentration of phosphorus, cobalt, calcium and iron were significantly higher in treatment group, so also the growth rate. In treatment and control groups, 5 (71.43%) and 2 (28.57%) heifers, exhibited estrus within 105 days from the beginning of feeding trial and all of them conceive with first AI only, suggesting beneficial role of mineral supplementation in including fertile in prepubertal exotic heifer.

Postpartum Reproductive Performance

The post partum reproductive performance criteria are ;

1. Interval from calving to first Post partum estrus and first AI
2. Interval from calving to conception (Service Period)

Interval of these two criteria will result in prolonged or shorter calving interval. Feeding and management of cows and buffaloes not just after calving but before calving also affects the postpartum fertility.After parturition, cows should be fed balanced rations to maximize dry matter intake so that body weight losses are minimized. This allows the cow to attain a positive energy balance in a shorter period of time (Harris, 2009).

Roche (2006) has defined the effect of infertility on dairy farm profitability as:

i) Prolonged calving interval with fewer calves and less milk per cow;
ii) Increased replacements costs; Increased labor, semen and veterinary bills; and
iii) An extended low production or dry period which increases BCS (body condition score) at calving and also reduces fertility at the subsequent breeding season.

Management problems in feeding : Cows too thin at calving take longer to recover and to start cycling for rebreeding. These cows will have lower conception rates that cow in moderate-to-good condition at calving. It is important to bring thin cows into condition now, to improve the odds of success at the start of the breeding season. All cows that are offered the same ration after calving will not be able to maintain uniform condition. Competition at the feed bunk, social rank and efficiency of nutrient use for maintenance and milk production influences a cow's ability to maintain weight. Even when a high plane of nutrition is being offered after the calving, some cows will lose weight. Timid, young or smaller animals may not have adequate access to the feed buck and will not be able to obtain their full daily ration. Nutrient intake of these cows will be reduced followed by problems with rebreeding. Management tools such as dividing the cow herd into two groups according to nutritional needs and feeding them accordingly will not drastically increase feeding cost and could have significant impact on rebreeding success (Lori, 2007).

In terms of the effect of inadequate nutrition, the most severe effect of inadequate nutrition is the cessation of cyclical activity, although other less severe manifestations are silent oestrus, ovulatory effects, conception failure and fetal and embryonic death. In particular, inadequate nutrition will increase the time interval to the first ovulation, which should normally occur 17-42 days postpartum. The time interval to the first insemination is thereby delayed. If the period of postpartum acyclicity extends beyond the earliest service date (Butler and Smith, 1989).

Nutrition plays a major role in the reproductive performance of buffalo, as with other farm animals. However there is a strong possibility that the consequences of poor nutrition are often interpreted as seasonality of breeding in buffalo. Under feeding, over feeding or unbalanced feeding, as well as deficiencies in minerals, vitamins or trace elements score at calving affects fertility, characterized by prolonged post-partum intervals, reduced conception rates, and more services per conception. A very low protein diet can cause cessation of estrus (Agrawal, 2003).

Body Condition Score (BCS) and Reproductive Performance

Because of the strong relationship between body condition loss in early lactation and reproductive performance, body condition scoring is a useful tool for predicting reproductive performance. In the United State, most people score body condition on a scale of 1 to 5 as proposed by Wildman,1982. The recommended body condition score on the 1 to 5 scale at calving is 3.5 to 4.0 with acceptable body condition score loss after calving not to exceed 1 score. Therefore, animals calving with a score of 3.5 should not be less than a 2.5, five to seven weeks postpartum..

Steenkamp *et al.* (1975) compared the conception rates of cows of similar weight that differed in condition score and found that condition at mating was more important than weight. A condition score is based on the amount of fat and muscle tissue covering the skeletal frame and is indicative of the animal's nutritional status (van Niekerk, 1982).

Moran (2005) described those changes in partitioning of nutrients over a lactation period towards body condition and utilization for other purpose as follows:

Period	Utilization of nutrients
Dry Period	1. Intake goes to body condition. 2. No milk. 3. Body condition increasing.
Early Lactation	1. Intake and body condition go to milk. 2. Milk production high. 3. Body condition high but decreasing.
Mid Lactation	1. Intake goes to milk. 2. No Body condition to milk. 3. Milk is less than peak. 4. Body condition low but steady.
Late Lactation	1. Intake goes to body condition and milk. 2. Milk decreasing. 3. Condition increasing.

Effect of Nutrition on Resumption of Postpartum Cyclicity and Fertility

General : Resumption of ovarian activity in high producing dairy cows is determined by energy status of the animal. Therefore, feeding management that minimizes loss of body condition during the early postpartum period and incidence of metabolic disorders during early lactation should increase the number of cows experiencing a first ovulation during the first 4 to 6 week postpartum.

Energy deprivation reduces the frequency of pulses of luteinizing hormone (LH); Thereby impairing follicle maturation and ovulation. Furthermore, under nutrition inhibits estrous behavior by reducing responsiveness of the central nervous system to estadiol by reducing the estrogen receptor in the brain (Hileman *et al.*, 1999).

Generally, the first postpartum ovulation in dairy cattle occurs 10 to 14 d after the nadir of NEB (Butler, 2003). The anovular cows not only have reduced estrous detection and conception rates, but also have compromised embryo survival (Santos *et al.*, 2004). Severe weight and BCS losses caused by inadequate feeding are more likely to be anovular; which compromises reproductive performance at first postpartum insemination. Prolonged postpartum an ovulation or anestrous extends the period from calving to first AI and reduces fertility during the first postpartum service (Santos *et al.*, 2008).

Morris (1976) considered that, if the weight loss between calving and 60 days postpartum is = 5% there should be concern; if it exceeds 10%, there is likely to be poor fertility. Hence, Morris advised that positive action needs to be taken before such problems occur; this means regular weighing, accurate body scoring or the use of a girth band measure regularly after calving.

The percentage change in the cow's bodyweight during the first 2 weeks after calving is inversely related to the number of days to first ovulation (Stevenson and Britt, 1980; Butler *et al.*, 1981). Cows should be fed well for 22-25 days before parturition and, if possible, for 90 days after parturition (Olivares *et al.*, 1981).

Patil and Deshpande (1981) found that Gir cows that gained weight in the first three months after parturition showed heat during that period, while those that lost weight remained anoestrous. Cows that lost weight had lower blood glucose and serum protein concentration than cows that gained weight, it could be used as an indicator.

1. *Influence of Nutrition on endocrine mechanisms :* The mechanisms through which nutrition controls reproduction in postpartum cows are of great interest. The energy required to ovulate a follicle, form a corpus luteum, and maintain an early pregnancy is miniscule compared with the other

energy demands of lactating cows. Therefore it is necessary to establish pregnancy early in lactation.

2. *Figure* : Endocrine Mechanisms through Which Nutrition Affects Reproduction In postpartum cows

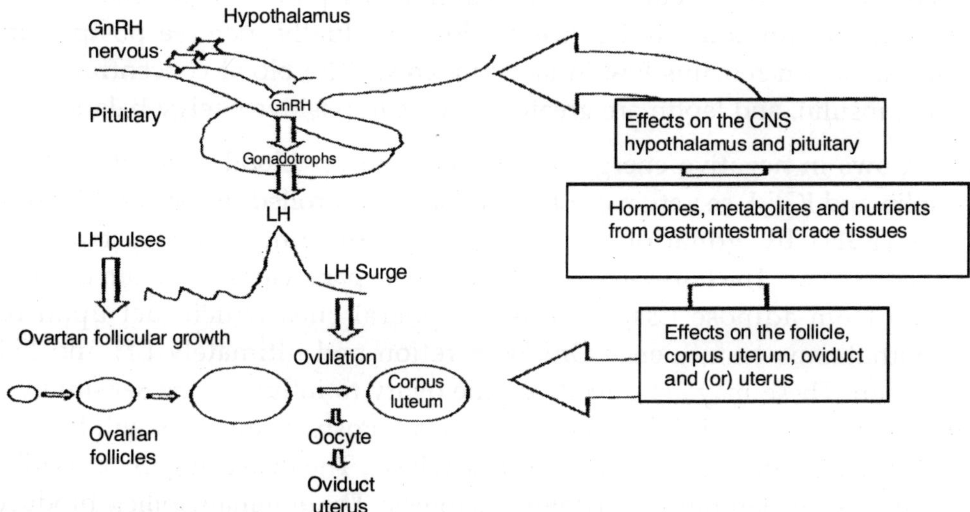

Conceptual model shows the mechanisms through which nutrition affects reproduction in postpartum cows. Hormones, metabolites, and nutrients from the gastrointestinal tract and nutrient-responsive tissues affect GnRH and LH secretion through their actions on the central nervous system (CNS) and hypothalamus and same hormones and metabolites may have direct effects on ovarian function (both follicles and corpora lutea) as well as the oocyte, oviduct and uterus. The combined effects of each axis determine postpartum fertility (Lucy, 2000).

Follicular growth continues during pregnancy but diameters of dominant follicles decrease, perhaps because of a decrease in LH pulsatility in late pregnant cattle (associated with high steroid concentrations during late pregnancy). Follicular development begins shortly after calving with a transient increase in FSH, a follicular wave and the development of a dominant follicle. The first postpartum dominant follicle undergoes one of three fates 1) ovulation; 2) atresia and turnover; or 3) cyst formation. A principal component of the process is the secretion of LH during the early postpartum period. Low LH pulsatility is associated with follicular turnover and anestrus; moderate LH pulsatility is associated with ovulation; and extreme LH pulsatility and lack of an LH surge is associated with the development of cystic ovaries. (Beam and Butler, 1999):

Metabolic cues or indicators which signal GnRH secretion and ovarian cyclicity

Changes in metabolic hormones are dynamic in postpartum cows and reflect the shifting metabolic status of the animal. Blood concentrations of insulin like growth factor (IGF)-I, insulin, and leptin decrease shortly after calving. Insulin and IGF-I concentrations gradually increase postpartum, whereas leptin remains low in lactating cows. The blood concentrations of IGF-I, insulin, and leptin are greater in cows in positive energy balance.

Cows in negative energy balance have lower blood concentrations of insulin and IGF-I. secretion of LH and FSH is controlled primarily (LH) or in part (FSH) by gonadotropin releasing hormone (GnRH) from the hypothalamus. The hormones insulin from the pancreas; IGF-I from the liver; leptin from adipose tissue act as peripheral cues which act upon the hypothalamus to influence GnRH secretion and ultimately LH and FSH secretion. These may act directly on the ovary to influence the sensitivity of the ovary to LH and FSH. (Lucy *et al.*, 2000). Postpartum cows will begin to cycle once LH pulsatility reaches a critical level. The increasing LH pulsatility stimulates the maturation of a dominant follicle. The dominant follicle produces estradiol, that reaches a threshold level to trigger an LH surge. The cow will have an LH surge and ovulate as long as the LH surge mechanism (positive feedback of estradiol) is established. In addition to this blood insulin and IGF-I concentration increase as well. Thus there is a coordinated series of events that act to promote follicular development and eventually ovulation.

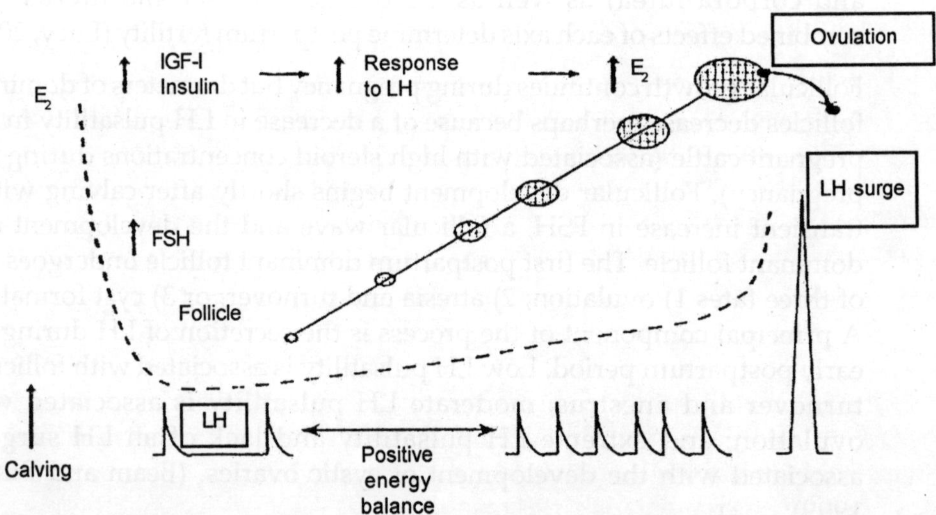

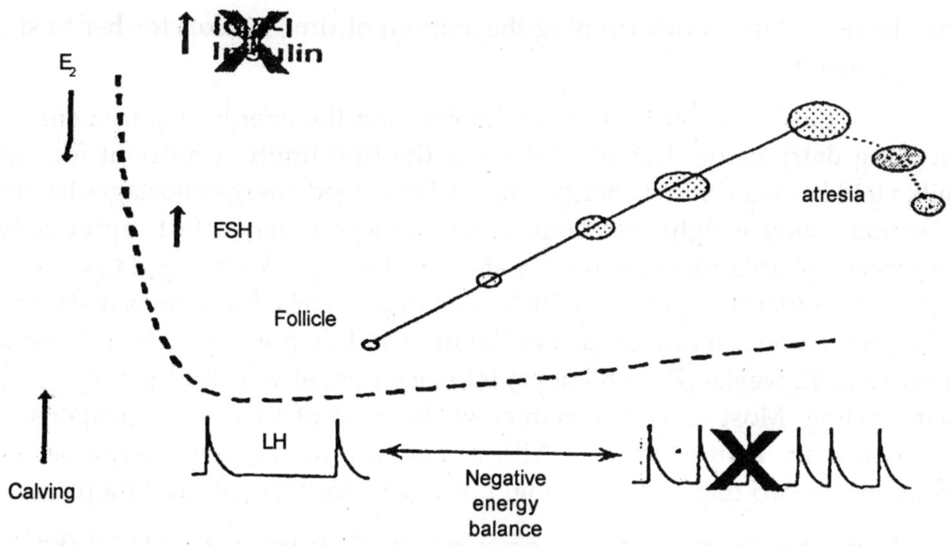

Energy balance reflect the difference between energy consumed and that expended for maintenance and milk production. Interval to first ovulation after calving has been reported to increase with increasing negative energy balance (Butler *et al.*, 1981. It is not possible to measure energy balance accurately in practice , *hence physiological indicators of metabolic status may better reflect the signals controlling resumption of ovulation*. In cows that have been selected for increased or decreased milk yields, a significantly longer interval to first ovulation after calving was observed in animals producing more milk, which was associated with higher circulating concentration of growth hormone and ß-hydroxy butyrate, and lower concentrations of insulin and glucose (Gong *et al.*, 2002). Other studies have demonstrated significant relationship between PPAI (postpartum anoestrus interval) and the ratio of insulin to growth hormone in plasma (Beam and Butler, 1997).

Physiological basis for this association has been cited as: a reduced LH pulse frequency; reduced circulating concentration of insulin and IGF-1; reduced production of oestradiol by ovarian follicles during NEB; and possible deleterious effects of the metabolites NEFA and BHB (beta hydroxybutyrate), together with low circulating glucose concentrations on oocyte development (Leroy *et al.*, 2006).

Role of Energy

Improvement in a cow's energy may be an important signal to the ovaries to start cycling. Cows may start cycling when they are still in negative energy balance but are starting to return to a positive value. When a cow is returning to a positive energy balance, the magnitude of the negative energy balance may be important in determining the amount of time it takes for her to start cycling again.

Most nutritionist use TDN for determining the energy requirements for lactating dairy cattle. Usually energy is the first limiting nutrient for high milk yield because of low energy forages. Prolonged energy shortages leading to serious body weight and body condition losses may affect reproductive efficiency. Maintaining energy balance in the early lactating dairy cow is extremely difficult, especially with low energy forages. Most cows reach peak milk production around 35 days in lactation and do not reach energy balance until 10 to 12 weeks (70 to 85 days) into lactation, at which time they would start cycling. Most early lactation cows, because of their slow response to increasing dry matter intake (DMI), usually are in negative energy balance from one or two days after calving, until 70 to 85 days into lactation.

To meet their energy needs, cows rely on their body store of fat (known as body condition). For every pound of body fat mobilized, enough energy can be supplied to support the production of 7 lbs of milk. Cows gaining weight during early lactation have higher conception rate and need less service per conception compared to those losing weight.

It is now widely accepted that negative energy balance (NEB) in early lactation is associated with reduced fertility performance (Roche *et al.*, 2002).

It is absolutely essential to optimize feed intake in early lactation to avoid excessive NEB and maintain acceptable fertility. Mayne *et al.* (2002) demonstrated this by showing that herds with higher intakes of metabolisable energy and dry matter in the first 100 days after calving had better fertility.

Diskin *et al.*, (2006), reported that feeding higher levels of concentrate in early lactation did not improve conception rate to first service, but did improve conception rate to second service for dairy cows. This is an important finding when one considers that 50 to 70% of cows on most dairy farms will be presented for a second service.

Ahlawat and Derasari (2009) studied 22 cows of a panjarapole to know the variation in metabolic profile due to physio-pathological status of the cow. The cows were divided in to two groups, viz. cyclic (n=12) and anoestrus (n=12) group. Blood sample were collected at 11 days interval over 2 months period from all animals. They found that the blood glucose (93.67±3.78 vs. 49.15±2.14 mg%) and plasma cholesterol (165.43 ± 4.65 vs. 109.80 ± 4.52 mg%) levels were significantly higher in cyclic as compared to anestrous cows.

Role of Protein

Protein is a basic requirement for dairy cows recuperating after calving, required for milk production and maintainance and resumption of cyclicity.

Whether the use of total crude protein for ration balancing is adequate for replacement and lactating cows remain unresolved. However, increasing amounts of data indicate that animal performance (growth, gain, milk production and reproduction) may be enhanced and optimized by properly formulating diets for rumen undegradable intake protein (UIP) and rumen degradable intake protein (DIP) and total crude protein (CP).

Tamminga (2006) clearly state that feeding high levels of RDP delays the first ovulation or oestrus reduces the conception rate to first insemination, increases the number of days open and lowers the overall conception rate.

Protein defiencies in lactating cows may increase the incidence of silent heats,cow releases the egg but she is not seen in heat and lower conception rates while at the same time decreasing feed intake and milk production. Cows which are deficient in protein increase milk production within a couple of days when additional protein is added to the diet.

It is generally recommended that for a dairy cows producing more than 30 kg of milk per day, 16% crude protein per dry matter is the optimum. In a study involving high yielding Friesian cows (Treacher *et al*.,. 1976), it was found that if cows were fed 75% of the recommended CP intake, the mean calving to first oestrus interval was extended to 46 days compared with 35 days for the control group on a normal intake; however, the calving interval was shorter in the low protein group. First lactation cows had better conception rates (65 vs. 36%) when fed diets of 16% crude protein per dry matter (CPDM) that contained more rumen degradable protein.

Gerloff and Morrow (1986) concluded that a marginal depression of conception rate occurred at CP levels of 16-18%, but the reduction was significant at =19% CP. The 20% dietary CP increased the incidence of RFM, dystopia and postpartum metritis compared with a 13% level. It had been suggested that there was also impaired intrauterine leukocyte function in cows receiving the higher level of protein (Anderson and Bartone, 1987).

Many authors consider that the toxicity of high levels of CP occurs as a consequence of excess RDP, leading to increased circulating concentrations of ammonia and urea. In consequence, abnormal high concentration of urea and ammonia are present in the uterus (Jorden *et al*., 1983), where they may be toxic to spermatozoa (Hossain, 1993), oocytes or embryos (Robinson And McEvoy, 1996), or adversely affect aspects of uterine function (Elrod, 1992).

Excesses of protein ,crude protein in the total diet greater than 17-20% results in lowering conception rates with increases seen in the number of services per conception and days open. These observations have not been consistent and may depend more on the amount and type of protein and amount of energy supplied in the diet than the amount of crude protein. Some studies have indicated that blood urea nitrogen (BUN) above 20 mg/ 100 ml may decrease the chances of pregnancy.

Role of Fat

There are several potential mechanisms by which polyunsaturated fatty acid (PUFA) supplements may improve fertility in dairy cattle (Staples *et al.*, 1998). These include:

i) a glucose sparing effect at the mammary gland which may improve circulating concentrations of glucose, with a positive effect on LH release pattern;

ii) increased circulating concentrations of cholesterol, a precursor of progesterone; and

iii) inhibiton of PGF 2α and oestradiol 17ß in order to improve the lifespan of the corpus luteum and potentially improve the survival of the embryo.

The potential effect of PUFAs in reducing embryonic mortality is interesting because Diskin *et al. (2006)* indicated that the main reason for reduced fertility in modern-day dairy cattle is increased early embryonic mortality. In support of this hypothesis, Petit and Twagiramungu (2006) have demonstrated that supplementation with flax seed (a rich source of linolenic acid, an omega-3 PUFA) significantly reduced embryonic mortality in comparison to other fat supplemented groups. Fatty acids from the omega-3 family reduce ovarian and endometrial synthesis of PGF2 á and may result in reduced embryonic mortality (Mattos *et al.*, 2004).

Omega-6 (linoleic acid) and omega-3 (linolenic acid) fatty acid are classified as essential fatty acids (EFA) for dairy cows. Actually, the rumen microbes' biohydrogenate both of these EFA to stearic acid. To restrict it EFA can be fed as long chain calcium salts.

Polyunsaturated fatty acids (PUFA) are precursors to cholesterol, which is an antecedent to steroid hormones. The corpus luteum (CL) uses cholesterol to make progesterone and estradiol (Staples *et al.*, 1998); thereby reducing PGF?Ü secretion and decreasing the sensitivity of the CL to PGF?Ü. This helps prolong the life and functionality of the CL and allows it to increase P4 concentrations. Higher pre-breeding concentrations of P4 have a positive impact on conception rates.

Jones *et al.* *(2008)* describe the potential chain of endocrine events if amounts of PUFA are insufficient due to: (1) Insufficient dietary supplementation. (2) Insufficient absorption in the small intestine due to microbial biohydrogenation in the rumen.

Pregnancy recognition in the bovine occurs between d 15 and 18 post estrus with the concepts maintaining the CL of pregnancy. Not unexpectedly, then, it is estimated that 40% of embryonic death loss occurs during d 8-17 post estrus and could largely be a result of inability to maintain the CL. This is accomplished through the production of interferon-tau (INF) which inhibits the ability of the uterine endomentrium to produce pulsatile PGF?Ü which is responsible for the degradation of luteal tissue (Thatcher *et al.*, 2001).

Role of Minerals and Vitamins

Adequate trace mineral intake and absorption is required for a variety of metabolic function including immune response to pathogenic challenge, reproduction and growth. Mineral supplementation strategies quickly become complex because differences in trace mineral status of all livestock and avian species in critical in order to obtain optimum production in modern animal production systems

Reproductive performance of cattle may be compromised if zinc, copper, or manganese status is in the marginal to deficient range. Inadequate zinc levels have been associated with decreases fertility, abnormal estrus, abortion, and altered myometrial contractibility with prolonged labor (Maas, 1987). Common copper deficiency symptoms in cattle include delayed or suppressed estrus, decreases conception, infertility and embryo death. Manganese deficiency in cows results in suppression of conception rates.

Feeding complex trace minerals to dairy cows enhances reproductive performance early in the breeding season. Research result in cattle indicate that first calf heifers have confirmed pregnancies 10 day earlier (Swenson, 1998), a 17 to 35% improvement in AI conception rates, a 15 day reduction in open days and a 8 day reduction in days to first service. Strategic complex trace mineral supplementation in cattle targets 60 days pre calving through 80 day post calving. Dairy producers can benefit from year round complexed trace mineral supplementation due to additional effects such as improved claw integrity, enhanced milk production and reduced somatic cell counts. Improving reproductive performance of beef and dairy cows by achieving confirmed conception rates early in the breeding period can have economic returns to the producer. In a study on 700 postpsrtum cows and buffaloes, 125 animals came into estrus just by regular feeding of mineral mixture. (Ankita Killedar, 2010, DBT Project).

Butani *et al.* (2009) studied 12 normal cyclic/fertile buffaloes, and found that the buffaloes conceive having high zinc and iron than buffaloes that do not conceive (1.15±0.02 ppm vs. 0.91±0.08 ppm; 4.57±0.36 ppm vs. 3.78±0.22 ppm). Whereas there is no much difference in copper (0.74±0.04 ppm vs. 0.78±0.03 ppm).

The primary vitamins A, D and E play major role in bovine reproduction. The vitamin requirements of dairy cows are met by a combination of rumen and tissue synthesis , natural feeds and feed supplementation. Most commercial concentrates contain supplemental vitamins so the probability of infertility due to a vitamin deficiency is greatly reduced. When commercial concentrates are not fed, vitamin supplements should be provided. Proper vitamin and mineral balance must be provided in dry cows rations when feed intake is restricted and (or) low quality forage is fed to control or reduce body condition. To ensure adequate intake, vitamins and minerals should be fed in small amounts of low energy concentrates or mixed in a complete dry cow ration. Byers (1994) proposed the adequate levels of vitamins are provided to cattle are vitamin A @ 100,000 IU/d, vitamin E @ 1000 IU/d, vitamin D @ 15,000 IU/d.

Conclusion

1. Nutrient deficiencies, excesses or imbalances have been shown to be capable of altering reproduction.
2. During early postpartum period, the dairy animals gaining body weight conceive easily at an earlier stage than either maintaining or reducing body weight.
3. Negative energy balance results into impairment of postpartum reproductive function, viz., ovarian rebound, oestrus signs, conception etc..
4. Nutrition influences ruminant fertility directly by the supply of specific nutrients required for the processes of oocyte development, ovulation, fertilization, embryo survival and establishment of pregnancy.
5. Optimal cow nutrition starts with feeding during the dry period. This will promote better body condition score, fewer calving problems, flatter lactations, better cow health and improve fertility, all of which make significant contributions to farm profitability.
6. The function of trace minerals and vitamins in reproduction and overall animal performance is of considerable economic concern. Supplemental vitamin and trace minerals improve immune function of dairy cattle, especially during the peripartum period.

References

Agrawal, K. P. (2003). Augmentation of reproduction in buffaloes. Proceedings of b4th Asian Buffalo Congress, New Delhi, India: 121

Ahlawat, A. and Derashi H. J (2009). *Ind. J. Field Vet.*, 4(4):13-16.

Ankita Killedar, (2010). DBT Project. socio economic development of rural women through reproductive bio technology in cattle and buffaloes.

Beam, S. W., and W. R. Butler. (1999). J. Reprod. Fertil. Suppl.54:411-424.

Butani, M.G., Kumar, R., Dhami, A. J., Kavani, F. S. and Killedar, A. (2009). *Ind. J. Field Vet.*, 4(2): 1-4.

Butler, W.R., and Smith, R.D. (1989). *J. Dairy Sci.*, 72:767-783.

Fleck, A.T., Schalles, R.R. and Kiracofe, G.H. (1980). *J. Anim. Sci*, 51:86.

Fielden, E.D., Macmillan. K.L. and Moller, K. (1997). Pregnancy, parturition and the postpartum period Bovine Practitioner, Advances in bovine theriogenology in New Zealand, 11:10.

Ganguli, N. C. (1981). Buffalo as a candidate for milk production. International Dairy Federation Bulletin, 137.

Gerloff, B.J. and Morrow, D.A. (1986). In current Therapy in Theriogenology and edn, ed. D.A. Morrow.

Gong, J. G., W. J. Lee and R. Webb (2002). Reproduction 123:419-427.

Grainger, C., G. D Wilhelms, and A. A. McGowan (1982). Effect of body condition at calving and level of feeding in early lactation on milk production of dairy cows.

Gerloff, B.J. and Morrow, D.A. (1986). In: Current Therapy in Theriogenology, 2nd edn, ed. D.A. Morrow.

Harris, B. (2009). Feeding for maximum milk production and reproductive performance. U.S.Department of Agriculture, Cooperative extension Service, University of Florida.

Hegazy, M.A., Essawi, S.A. and Youssef, A.H. (1997). *Vet. Med. J. Giza*, 45:147.

Huzzey, J.M., Veira, D.M., Weary D.M. and von Keyserlingk, M.A.G (2007). *J. Dairyn Sci.*, 90: 3220-3223.

Jones, B., Bowen, A., Martin, M. and Ax. R. (2008). Dietary Essential Fatty Acids and Reproduction in Dairy Cows. High Plains Dairy Conference. Department of Animal Sciences, University of Arizona.

Kaur, H. (1994). Influence of nutrient deficiency on reproduction. In proceedings of ICAR summer school on " Recent advances in animal reproduction and gynecology".Held at PAU, Ludhiana (25th july to 13th Aug.). pp. 99-102.

Larry, D.G. and Joe, W. (1994). Nutrition and Reproduction Interactions in Dairy cattle. The University of Georgia, College of Agriculture And Environmental Sciences. Bulletin 1111.

Leaver J. D. (1997). *Anim. Prod.*, 25:219.

Lori, W. S. (2007). Vet. Clin. N. Amer. *Food Anim. Pract.* 3:633-646.

Lucy M. C. (2000). J. Dairy Sci. 83:1635-1647.

Mc Dougall, S. (2001). N.Z. Vet. 49:187-194.

Morris, R. S. (1976). Diagnosis of infertility in Larger Dairy Herds, Proc No. 28. Refresher Course for Veterinarians, Sydney.

Mattos, R., Staples, C.R., Arteche, A., Wiltbank, M.C., Diaz, F.J., Jenkins, T.C and Thatcher, W.W. (2004). *J. Dairy Sci.*, 87:921-932.

Morrow, D.A. (1969). Phosphorus deficiency and infertility in dairy heifers. *J.Am. Vet. Med. Assoc.* 154:761-768.

Olivares, R., Chicco, C., Redrigvez, C. F., Hernandez, R. and Verde, O. (1981). Prepartum and postpartum supplements for Brahman heifers. Memoria Associational Latinoamericana de Production Animal, 16:48 (Animal Breedings Abstracts, 52:6521).

Opsomer, G, Y. T. Grohnm, J. Hertl and A. deKruif. (2000a). *Therigenelogy* 53:841-857.

Pathak, N. N. (1992). Buffalo production, World Animal Science C6. (Ed. N. M. Tulloh and J. H. G. Holmes). Elsevier Science Publishers, Amsterdam, Netherlands.

Patil, J. S. and Deshpande, B.R. (1981). Ind. Vet J., 58:376-379.

Patel, B.B., Pate, J.A., Dhami, A.J. And Patel, D.M (2009). *J.Field Vet.*, 4(3):1-4.

Reid, J. T., Loosli, J. K., Trimberger, G. W., Turk, K. L., Asdell. S. A. and Smith, S.E. (1964). Cornell University Agricultural Experiment Station Bulletin (87. Ithaca, New York, USA.

Roche, J. F. (2006). The effect of nutritional management of the dairy cow on reproductive efficiency. *Anim. Repro. Sci.*, 96:282-296.

Rochet, M. (1973). Physical constraints on voluntary intake of forages by ruminants. Ann. Zootech., 22:227.

Rubio, M. Corro, E. Castillo, C. S. Galina and C. Murcia. Rev. Fac:Argen (Luz) (1999). 16: 637-650.

Randhawa, S.S. and Randhawa, C.S. (1994). Ludhiana (25th July to 13th Aug.) pp. 103-121.

Robinson, J.J. and McEvoy, T.G. (1996). *J. Vet. Res.*, 44(3):139-51.

Staples, C.R., Burke, J.M. and Thatcher, W.W. (1998). *J.Dairy Sci.*, 81:856.

Steenkamp, J.D.G., van der Horst, C. and Andrew, M.J.A (1975). *J. Anim. Sci.*, 5:103-110.

Staples, C. R., Burke, J. M. and Thatcher, W. W. (1998). *J. Dairy Sci.*,81:856.

Tamminga, S. (2006). *Amin. Repro. Sci.*, 96:227-239.

Thatcher, W.W., Guzeloglu, A., Mattos, R., Bineli,. *Theriogenology*, 56:1435-1450.

Vasconcelos, J.L.M., Sangsritavong, S., Tsai, S.J. and Wiltbank, M.C. (2003). *Theriogrenology*, 60:795-807.

□□□

8

Nutritional Aspect of Fertility in Peripartum Dairy Cows

R.P. TIWARI, BIPIN P. SONAR AND NIRMAL KEDIA
Department of Veterinary Gynaecolgy & Obstetrics
College of Veterinary Science & A.H., Anjora, Dug 491001 (Chhattisgarh)

Introduction

Nutrition has an important impact on the reproductive performance of cattle. Energy is the major nutrient required by adult cattle and inadequate energy intake has a detrimental impact on reproductive activity of the female bovine. Immediately after parturition, rate of milk production increases dramatically. Intake of energy is not sufficient to meet requirements for maintenance and milk production. Consequently, virtually all dairy cows will experience negative energy balance during early lactation. Negative energy balance may occur prior to parturition if dry matter intake declines appreciably prior to calving. Nutritional status of early lactation dairy cows is related in many ways to reproductive performance, however, energy status is probably the most important nutritional parameter affecting reproduction. Cows under negative energy balance have extended periods of anovulation. Postpartum anestrus, as well as infertility, is magnified by losses of body condition during the early postpartum period. Resumption of ovulatory cycles is associated with energy balance, and the underlying mechanisms seem to be associated with metabolic signals and regulatory hormones primarily insulin and insulin-like growth factor (IGF). Feeding diets that promote increases in plasma glucose and insulin may improve the metabolic and endocrine status of cows in early lactation (Santos, 2009). Shifts in blood metabolites and hormones might compromise ovarian function and fertility. It has also been reported that energy balance and dry matter intake (DMI) might affect plasma concentrations of progesterone (Villa-Godoy *et al.*, 1988), which may interfere with follicle development and maintenance of pregnancy. Deficiencies of most nutrients can be avoided by appropriate modifications in diet formulation, i.e., increase nutrient density. However, if a cow is not consuming enough dry matter to provide sufficient energy to support maintenance, milk production, and reproduction, energy density of the diet can only be increased so far without compromising animal health. Excessive feeding of concentrates may initiate acidosis and off-feed problems. Excess of dietary protein has been suggested as detrimental to fertility, although the evidence is weak. When protein is fed in excess of requirements, the result is elevated blood urea nitrogen levels, which have been linked to decreased fertility in most (Blanchard *et al.*, 1990; Butler *et al.*, 1996; Canfield *et al.*, 1990; Ferguson *et al.*, 1993; Jordan and Swanson, 1979a; Kaim *et al.*, 1983), but not all (Barton *et al.*, 1996; Carroll *et al.*, 1988; Howard *et al.*, 1987) studies dealing with feeding high protein diets to dairy cattle. Addition of moderate amounts of supplemental fat to the diet improves energy intake, modulates PGF2á secretion by the uterus, affects ovarian dynamics, enhances luteal function and embryo quality, and has moderately positive effects on fertility. More specifically, some fatty acids (FA) might impact fertilization rate and embryo quality in dairy cows. The amount of fat that can be included in the diet must be restricted to $\leq$ 5% of ration dry matter to ensure maximum dry matter intake and to avoid depression in fiber digestion.

Transition Period

The occurrence of health problems during the transition period is clearly a major complicating factor for subsequent reproductive performance (Ferguson, 2001), resulting in additional economic losses. The transition period for a dairy cow is from 3 to 2 wk prepartum until 2 to 3 wk postpartum. A number of profound physiologic changes occur in the transition cow that modifies her metabolism drastically.

It was recognized that many of the metabolic disorders afflicting cows during the periparturient period are interrelated in their occurrence and are related to the diet fed during the prepartum period (Curtis *et al.*, 1985). They determined that increased energy content of the diet fed during the prepartum period was associated with decreased incidence of displaced abomasum and that increased protein content of this diet was associated with decreased incidences of retained placenta and ketosis (Curtis *et al.*, 1985).

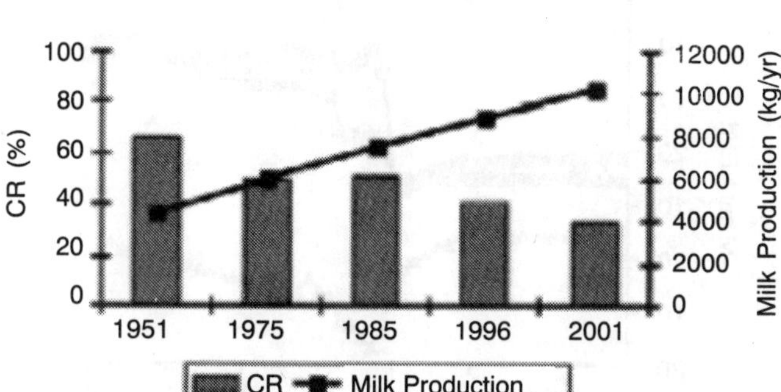

Fig. 1 : The inverse relationship between conception rate (CR%) and annual milk production of Holstein dairy cows. (Butler, 2003)

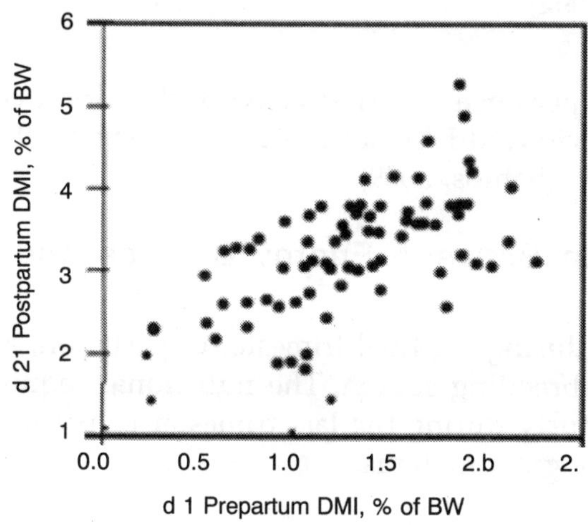

Fig. 2 : Relationship between DMI at 1 d prepartum and 26 d postpartum

Energy Balance of Periparturient Cows

Energy balance has been positively related to reproductive performance in dairy cattle (Butler and Smith, 1989). Energy balance is equal to energy consumed minus the energy required for maintenance and the conceptus or milk production. Energy consumed is a function of dry matter intake and the energy density of the diet. A typical profile for energy requirement, intake, and balance of peripartureint dairy cattle is shown in figure below. The most severe negative energy balance occurs shortly after calving. The magnitude and duration of negative energy balance can vary greatly. Figure shows cows reaching zero energy balance at 3 weeks postpartum, but the duration may be much longer for cows that do not receive adequate diets postpartum.

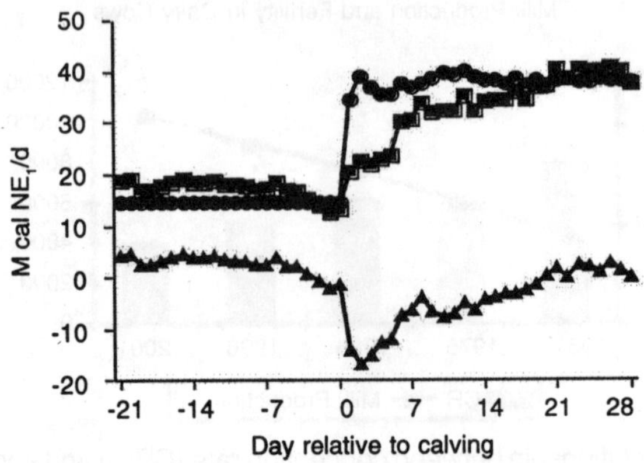

Fig. 3 : Energy requirement (squares), intake (circles), and balance (triangles) of transition cows (Bertics *et al.*, 1992).

When cows experience a period of NEB, the blood concentrations of nonesterified fatty acids (NEFA) increase, at the same time that IGF-I, glucose, and insulin are low. (Santos, 2009).

The Relationship Between Energy Balance and Reproductive Performance

Energy intake during the final trimester of gestation, affects pregnancy rate the following breeding season. The nutritional requirement of a cow increases tremendously during the last trimester of pregnancy to meet the needs of the rapidly growing fetus.

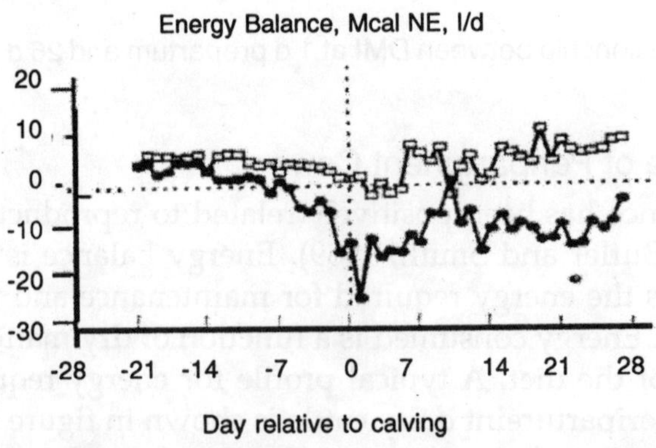

Fig. 4 : Estimated NE, and CP balance of a transition cow which experienced severe DMI depression prepartum (circles) or a cow which experienced virtually no DMI depression prepartum (squares).

Negative energy balance can affect cow reproductive performances through some biological mechanisms:

- Metabolic hormonal modifications regulated by pituitary-hypothalamic axis (as LH, FSH, GH, insulin, leptin, IGF-1, oestrogen and progesterone
- Interactions between blood metabolites and ovarian activity (glucose, NEFA, BOHB)
- Relationship between uterine functionality and immune response during pregnancy and transition period. (Rossi *et al*, 2008)

The lipomobilization that distinguishes this disease, due to the low plasmatic level of insulin and to the high concentration of GH (growth hormone), is the basis of the increase of non-esterified fatty acids (NEFA) in blood. These metabolites have a direct toxic effect on the follicles with induction of cumulus cells apoptosis, necrosis and follicular development arrest (Jorritsma *et al.*, 2004; Friggens, 2003). A probable negative effect is also supported by ketone bodies.

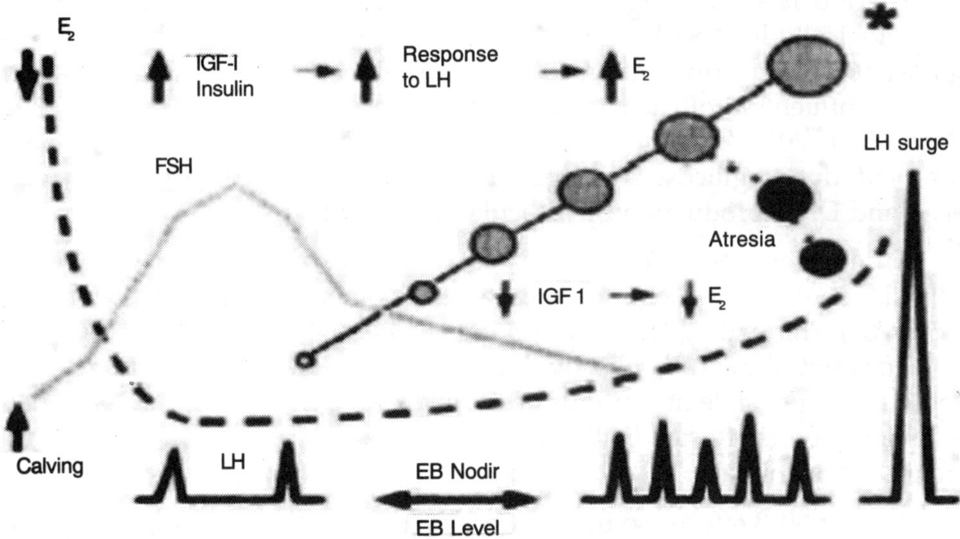

Fig. 5 : A schematic model describing dominant follicle development (circles) and function in relation to changing metabolic and reproductive hormones, and energy balance during the first follicular wave postpartum in dairy cows. The first follicle ovulates (*) or undergoes atresia (Beam and Butler, 1999).

NEB is able to negatively change ovarian activity also through other metabolic pathways. The plasmatic insulin, IGF-1 (Insulin-Like Growth Factor 1) and leptin decrease has direct effects (lower ovarian sensibility to pituitary gonadotropins) and indirect effects on follicular development, such as on lower pulse secretion frequency of pituitary LH. Insulin has a positive effect on ovarian sensibility to gonadotropins, resulting in best recruitment of small follicles and development of the dominant follicle.

During post-calving, follicle capacity to produce required oestrogens for next ovulation is directly influenced by insulin and IGF-1 plasmatic concentration (Butler, 2003); in particular the latter can result in 40-50% lower levels during negative energy balance in the first two weeks post-calving, and can reflect the same molecular concentration in follicular fluid (Fenwick *et al.,* 2008; Fitzpatrick *et al.,* 2007). Therefore, there is an high decrease of IGF-1 plasmatic levels in the first post-calving week and this fall directly influences several reproductive parameters (calving to first ovulation and to conception intervals). IGF-1 is essential to improve gonadotropins activity on ovariahatsn structures and to stimulate cell proliferation and follicular steroidogenesis (Wathes *et al.,* 2007). Unlike IGF-1, lower insulin plasmatic levels have not shown a strong influence on follicular cell proliferation, but can participate to the regulation of oestrogen production in case of serious energy decrease (Wathes *et al.,* 2007). Glucose concentration in blood during NEB period is significantly reduced. However, cow hematic glucose is physiologically low because of reduced ruminal absorption of glucose after almost complete fermentation to propionic acid (47.2 - 55.8 mg/dl) and it directly influences follicular fluid glucose concentration (Lopez *et al.,* 2003; Martin *et al.,* 2008). During NEB and ketosis, a delayed oocyte development is observed, due to glucose shortage, fundamental molecule for energy (ATP), RNA and DNA production by follicular and oocyte cells.

Another consequence of the post-calving lower energy is a lack of follicular ovulation, which continues its development to follicular cyst (Boland *et al.,* 2001). This pathogenesis is supported by the lack of pituitary LH secretion that does not allow follicular ovulation and a major oestrogen production. These are responsible of continue cysts development and of the characteristic behavior of cows affected by this pathology, (increase of walking activity and mount other animals).

Among NEB effects, some authors (Van Knegsel *et al.,* 2007) mention the effect on progesterone (P4) plasmatic concentration; during the first post-calving days, NEB impacts corpus luteum activity (lower energy availability for lutheal cells), and consequently progesterone production, especially during second and third oestrus cycles. This condition does not allow changes in endometrial morpho-functional characteristics at the time of post-calving first service, and negatively affects intrauterine environment, necessary for embryo implantation. The uterine effects of negative energy balance are identified as a delayed uterine involution after post-calving (30-40 days) and a major incidence of herd endometritis. These facts, responsible for strong delay in resume of normal reproductive functions after calving, are due to alteration of some genes expression connected with NEB, that regulate the immune response of the reproductive tract (IL 1â and IL 8 encoding) and the recondition of normal uterine size (Boland *et al.*, 2001). The latter problem derived from alteration that regulate protein change and collagen catabolism of uterine wall (matrix metalloproteinases MMPs-1), that result poorly tonic, unable to expel the fetal membranes and virtually defenseless towards pathogens because of lack of mononuclear cells (Wathes *et al.*, 2007). Retained placenta, is a serious disease connected with the two previous illnesses, resulting from problem in separation of placental cotyledons from endometrial caruncles and hence lack expulsion of fetal membranes within 24 hours after calving.

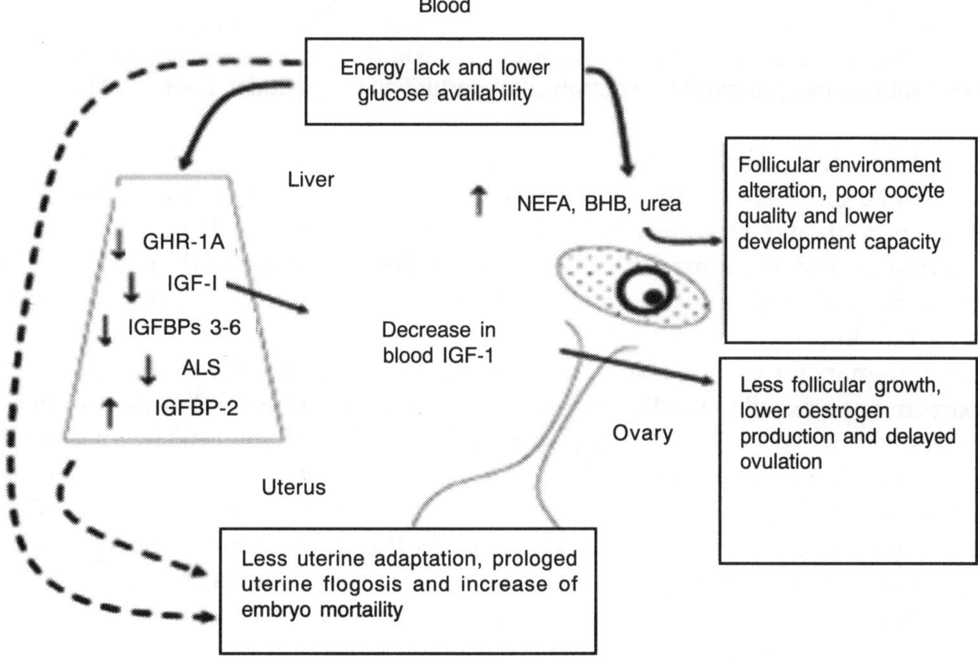

Fig. 6 : Summary diagram of negative energy balance direct and indirect effects on the reproductive apparatus function, mediated by metabolic-hormonal change that involve bloodstream and liver: decrease of GH receptors (GHR-1A) and IGF-1, IGF binding protein (IGF-BP) and acid-labile subunits (ALS) (Wathes *et al.*, 2007 modified).

In several studies (Butler, 2006; Schneider, 2004; Wathes *et al.*, 2007) it was concluded that the decrease of one point BCS at the moment of post-calving first insemination, can reduce cow reproductive efficiency by 17-38%. Consequently interval from calving to conception can increases over 120-130 days (usually if cow exceed 180-200 days after calving, becomes to high culling risk).

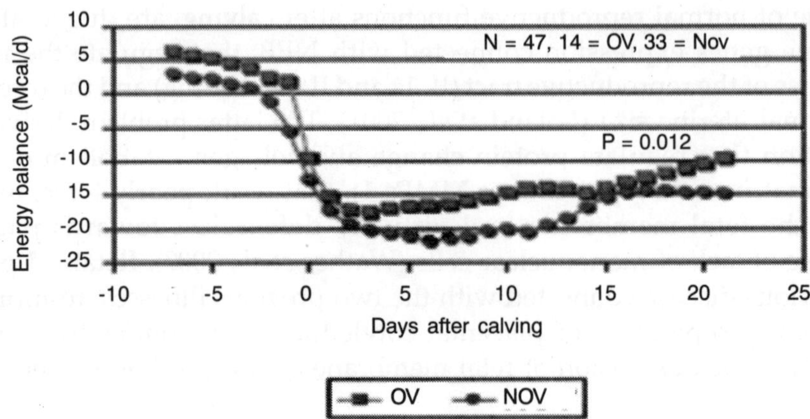

Fig. 7 : Energy balance becomes negative a few hours before calving and remains on very negative values in cows with delayed ovulation (NOV) while tend to rebalance in cows with normal pre-ovulatory activity after parturition (OV) (Butler, 2006 modified).

It has been demonstrated (Roche *et al.*, 2007) that with optimal or high BCS during the steaming-up and immediately after calving (BCS 2,75-3,25), there is a greater tendency to correctly express a oestrus during voluntary waiting period, compared with cows that exhibiting poor body condition in the same period. Besides the strong influence of BCS on duration of anoestrus after calving, lower body condition during transition period can influence also pregnancy rate (PR). The loss of a point BCS during the first week post-partum is an excellent indicator of cow reproductive potential at the moment of first service after calving. According to Montiel et Ahuja (2003), cows with 0,5-1 BCS losses show a 53% potential conception rate, While a loss higher than one point BCS may reduce to 17% the potential conception rate, which consequently affects PR. These data express the fundamental importance to assess BCS of dry and transition dairy cows, for indirectly estimate reproductive capacity at the moment of first service.

Butler and Canfield (1989) monitored early lactation dairy cows and cows that were dried off immediately after calving to study the relationship between negative energy balance and time to first ovulation. They clearly demonstrated a positive relationship (R^2=.72) between the days to negative energy balance nadir (most extreme negative energy balance) and days to first ovulation. Early resumption of estrous cycles is important because pregnancy rate (services per pregnancy) is decreased as the number of heats experienced by a cow prior to 60 days postpartum is increased.

The mode of action by which energy balance affects reproductive performance has not been established. Energy requirements of ovarian tissue are minor relative to total energy requirements for maintenance plus milk production. Therefore, negative energy balance probably does not directly effect ovarian function through a caloric deficiency. It is more likely that negative energy balance influences endocrine status of the animal which in turn regulates ovarian function. Butler et al. (1981) estimated that ovulation resumes approximately 10 d following the point of greatest negative energy balance. Negative energy balance may prohibit the development of pulsatile GnRH and LH patterns required for the reestablishment of ovulatory cycles (Butler and Canfield, 1989). In dairy cows, as energy balance on day 15 postpartum was increased, plasma LH concentration and size of the largest follicle on the ovary was increased (Lucy *et al.*, 1991). Insulin was suggested as a metabolic signal that may influence LH secretion (Butler and Canfield, 1989). Plasma insulin concentration is low immediately postpartum and is positively correlated to energy balance. Insulin-like growth factor (IGF)-I, a potent stimulator of granulosa and luteal cell steroidogenesis was lowest in cows with the greatest negative energy balance (Spicer *et al.*, 1990). Beam and Butler (1997) conducted a study in which cows were grouped into those that ovulated during the first follicular wave postpartum and those that did not ovulate during the first follicular wave. Cows that failed to ovulate had a longer interval until negative energy balance nadir, smaller maximum follicular diameter, lower peak estradiol, and lower plasma IGF-I. Prolonged postpartum anovulation or anestrus extends the period from calving to first A1 and reduces fertility during the first postpartum service (Santos *et al.*, 2009). In fact, anovular cows not only have reduced estrus detection and conception rates, but also have compromised embryo survival (Santos *et al.*, 2004).

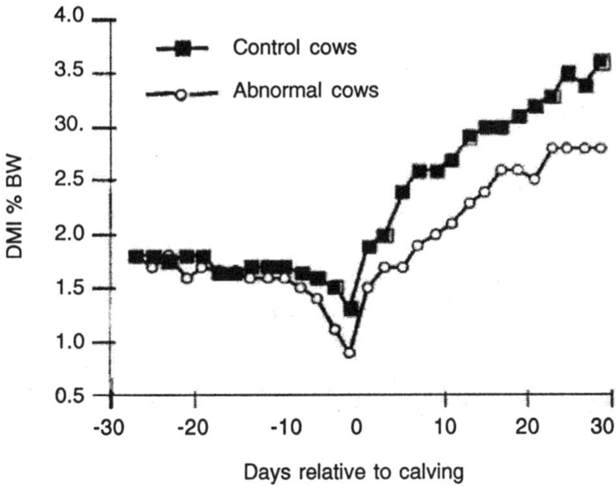

Fig. 8 : Dry matter intake of cows that did (abnormal) or did not (control) develop postpartum disorders. (Zamet et al, 1979)

High producing dairy cows may return to positive energy balance by 6 to 8 weeks postpartum but still not conceive for another 60 days. Britt (1992) speculated that this may reflect the lag time between initial development and maturation of a follicle. Follicles destined to ovulate between 50 and 90 days postpartum are in the initial stages of development between 2 weeks prepartum and 4 weeks postpartum. It is clear that the period of most severe negative energy balance is during the time that follicles due to ovulate during the desirable breeding period are just beginning to develop. According to Britt (1992), the developing follicles may become "imprinted" by the adverse metabolic environment associated with negative energy balance and eventually produce eggs that are less fertile and corpora lutea that secrete less progesterone. Energy balance, particularly during the first 3 wk postpartum was correlated negatively with interval to first ovulation (Butler *et al.*, 1981; Ducker *et al.*, 1985; Berghorn *et al.*, 1988; Staples *et al.*, 1990). Because conception rates improve as the number of estrous cycles postpartum increases (Britt, 1992), it is reasonable to assume that feeding strategies that hasten the initiation of postpartum ovulatory cycles may improve reproductive performance. Luteal function may influence fertility by affecting conception and embryo survival. Villa-Godoy et al. (1988) indicated that energy balance within 9 d postpartum was correlated positively with milk progesterone concentrations during the second and third estrous cycle postpartum.

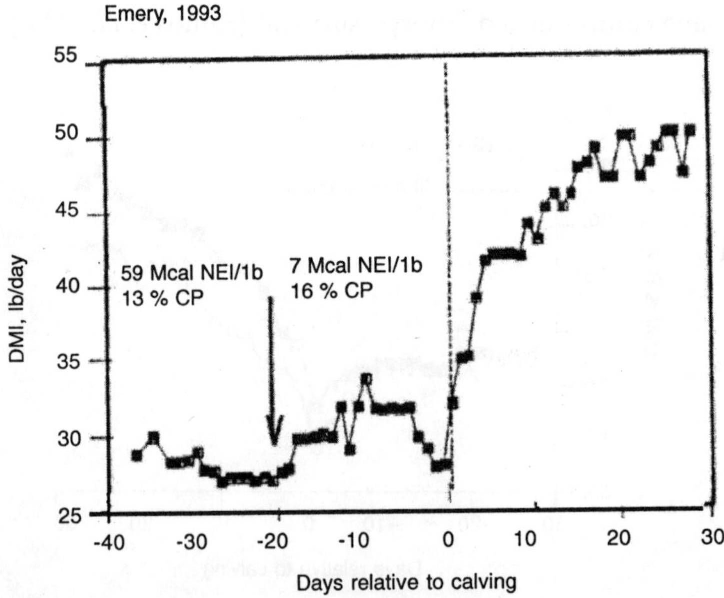

Fig. 9 : Effect of increasing nutrient density of the prepartum diet on DMI.

Nutritional Strategies to Improve Energy Balance and Reproduction

To improve energy balance, milk production must be reduced or energy intake must be increased, or both. Clearly, reducing milk production in not a desirable strategy. Consequently, energy intake must be increased. This can be achieved by increasing dry matter intake, increasing energy density of the diet, or both. Dry matter intake following calving is positively related to dry matter intake prior to calving (Grummer, 1995).

Increasing energy density of diets fed to early lactation cows can be difficult. Energy density can be increased by substituting high energy concentrates such as cereal grains for forage or by supplementing fat. Insulin and/or IGF-I concentrations are greater in cows whose first dominant follicle ovulated (Beam and Butler, 1997), are positively related to CL development and progesterone concentrations (Spicer *et al.*, 1990; Thatcher et al, 1996), and are positively related to energy status and follicular growth rate (Lucy *et al.*, 1992a). Miyoshi *et al.* (1995) drenched cows with 500 ml PG/day from day 7 to 42 postpartum and observed increased energy balance and blood glucose and insulin. Days to first ovulation was decreased (32 vs 44), duration of luteal phase during the first estrus was increased (6 vs 13 days), and although not statistically significant, conception rate at first breeding was increased from 25 to 57%. Formigoni et al. (1996) fed 300 ml PG(Propylene glycol) /day for the final 20 days of the dry period and then drenched the same amount of PG on days 0, 3, 6, 9, and 12 postpartum. Although they did not detect an increase in blood insulin, plasma nonesterified fatty acids were decreased and IGF-I and IGF binding protein were increased. Percentage of cows remaining acyclic was reduced with PG as time postpartum increased.

Fat and Fatty Acids

Because of the limitations associated with feeding high levels of concentrates, supplemental fat has become common in dairy diets and considerable research has been conducted to examine the effects on reproduction. Feeding calcium salts of long chain fatty acids (Ca-LCFA) of palm oil improved pregnancy of dairy cows (Schneider *et al.*, 1988), although the authors did not report statistical significance. Several theories have been suggested for why supplemental fat may improve reproductive performance of dairy cattle; not all of them involve improved energy balance. The three major theories are:

1. Feeding fat improves energy balance so that the cow returns to estrus sooner and conceives earlier.
2. Cows fed fat have higher plasma progesterone concentrations; progesterone is positively related to fertility because it enhances implantation and embryo survival.

3. Specific long chain fatty acids inhibit prostaglandin synthesis by the uterus and, therefore, prevent regression of the corpus luteum and increases the chances of embryo survival.

Energy Balance. It is unlikely that improvements in energy balance explain improvements in reproductive performance of cows fed supplemental fat. Several studies have reported improved conception or pregnancy rates when energy balance or body weight or body condition score changes (i.e., indicators of energy balance) were not improved by feeding fat (Staples and Thatcher, 2000). It is common for energy status to not be enhanced when feeding fat because milk yield increases, feed intake decreases, or both occur. Therefore, it is likely that fat improves reproduction independent of energy balance.

Higher Plasma Progesterone. Improved fertility in cattle has been associated with high circulating concentrations of progesterone during the luteal phase prior to and following insemination (Grummer and Carroll, 1991). Cholesterol is a precursor for luteal cell progesterone synthesis and can be derived from cellular de novo synthesis or uptake of plasma lipoprotein cholesterol; most species are dependent on the provision of lipoprotein cholesterol (Grummer and Carroll, 1988). Feeding fat to dairy cattle almost always increases plasma cholesterol and the increase is independent of the type of fat supplement. Consequently, it has been postulated that feeding fat may improve reproductive performance by increasing conversion of cholesterol to progesterone. Feeding fat commonly increases plasma progesterone (Grummer and Carroll, 1988, Staples and Thatcher, 2000). Grummer and Carroll in1991 concluded that greater plasma progesterone is probably not a result of greater production from cholesterol. Maximum rates of progesterone synthesis are obtained when lipoprotein cholesterol is added to luteal cell cultures at concentrations below those in plasma of unsupplemented cows (Carroll *et al.*, 1992). Fat feeding does not alter lipoprotein composition, therefore, binding and uptake of lipoprotein cholesterol by luteal cells is probably not enhanced when feeding fat (Carroll *et al.*, 1992). Therefore, it would seem unlikely that increases in plasma progesterone concentrations during fat feeding are due to increases in plasma lipoprotein concentrations.

A summary indicated that size of the dominant follicle is frequently increased when feeding supplemental fat and the average increase was from 12.9 to 16.4 mm (Staples and Thatcher, 2000). It is possible that larger dominant follicles result in larger CL and higher concentrations of progesterone in blood. (Vasconcelos *et al.*, 1998; Garcia-Bojalil *et al.*, 1998).

Table 1 : Effects of fat on diameter of the dominant follicle (Staples, 2000)

Reference	Fat Source	Experimental Diet Control	Fat
		----mm----	
Lucy *et al.*, 1991	Calcium salt	12.4	18.2
Lucy *et al.*, 1990	Soybean oil	7.0	10.2
Lucy *et al.*, 1993	Calcium salt	16.0	18.6
	Yellow grease	16.9	20.9
Beam and Butler, 1997	Tallow/yellow grease	11.0	13.5
Staples *et al.*, 2000	Soybean oil/fish oil	14.3	17.1
Average		12.9	16.4

Inhibition of Prostaglandin Synthesis: PGF2á plays an important role in reestablishing estrous cycles after parturition and thereafter until conception. The uterus produces it when conception does not occur and it causes regression of the CL and initiation of a new estrous cycle. Research indicates that certain fatty acids such as linoleic acid (C18:2) cause inhibition of PGF2á production. Therefore, following conception, if C18:2 can "help" suppress prostaglandin production, there is a greater likelihood that the CL and progesterone production will be maintained and the embryo will survive . Linoleic acid may also inhibit estradiol prodcution. Estradiol stimulates PGF2á production by the uterus and sensitizes the CL to PGF2á. Studies have indicated lower estradiol concentrations in cows fed fat or lower estradiol prodcution from granulosa cells harvested from cows fed fat (CLCFA).

Linoleic acid is a polyunsaturated fatty acid that is extensively hydrogenated by microbes in the rumen. The amount of C18:2 that must "bypass" the rumen to elicit an effect on prostaglandin synthesis is not known. If the amount required is relatively small, then feeding oils high in C18:2 or feeding C18:2 in a form that reduces hydrogenation in the rumen (for example, as a calcium salt) may provide enough C18:2 to the bloodstream to elicit an effect.

Dietary Protein

Lactating animal ration containing crude protein (CP) between 16 and 18 % of its total dry matter is typical. Diets with limited CP can compromise microbial growth and rumen fermentation reflected in declines in feed intake and milk production. On the other hand, feeding protein in excess of what is needed by the cows has been implicated in increased ammonia and urea concentrations in blood and milk, which have been used as markers for reduced fertility (Butler, 1998). The suggested decline in fertility of cattle fed excess protein is caused by alterations in uterine physiology with a decline in uterine pH during the early luteal phase of the estrous cycle (Butler, 1998). A more acidic uterine environment is less conducive with maintenance of pregnancy in cattle (Ocon and Hansen, 2003).

Additional undegradable protein fed during late gestation improved body condition at calving in dairy heifers and beef cattle (Curtis et al, 1985). Mature Holstein cows fed higher amounts of undegradable protein prepartum had significantly reduced incidence of clinical ketosis and reduced days open compared to cows receiving a similar diet containing lesser protein amount (Van Saun *et al*, 1995). Increasing prepartum dietary undegradable protein content improved glucose status in cows and tended to decrease NEFA concentrations, suggesting a possible effect on ketosis incidence (Putnam *et al*, 1996). Cows fed a higher protein prepartum diet, independent of energy content, had lower serum NEFA concentration, NEFA to cholesterol ratio, and fatty liver score (Holtenius *et al*, 1990). Cows afflicted with either ketosis or LDA were found to have lower serum apoproteins associated with very low density lipoprotein (VLDL) structures, suggesting an inability of the liver to export triglycerides (Oikawa et al, 1997). These studies emphasize the critical role of amino acids in maintaining glucose homeostasis and fat metabolism during the transition period. Clinical responses to supplemental protein circumstantially suggest current recommendations for dietary protein during pregnancy are being underestimated.

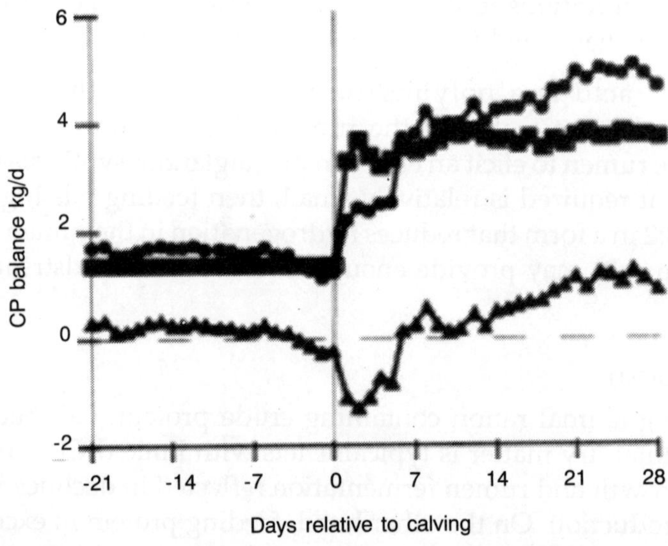

Fig. 10 : Crude protein requirement (squares), intake (circles), and balance (triangles) of transition cows. (Bertics et al, 1992)

Prepartum protein deficiency may then result in depletion of the labile protein pool to support gestation rather than early lactation when gluconeogenesis is critically needed. Prepartum protein depletion adversely affects periparturient metabolic status, resulting in greater incidence of ketosis, hepatic lipidosis and other metabolic diseases. Subsequent lactation and reproductive performance may also be impaired either directly as a result of limited amino acid availability or indirectly as a result of metabolic disease. concentrations to pregnant cows, As discussed above relative to DMI declines during the close-up dry period, dietary protein content will need to be appropriately adjusted. However, excessive dietary protein content (>16% CP) should not be generally recommended as its negative impact on energy balance in excreting excess urea. One study feeding higher levels of protein (15%), all from rumen degradable sources, reported a 66% incidence of downer cow syndrome with high death loss compared to a lower protein (8%) diet (Julien et al, 1977). Cows fed diets for the entire dry period low in dietary crude protein (8 percent) had a higher incidence (50 percent) of retained placenta compared with cows fed 15 percent crude protein (20 percent incidence) (Julien *et al.*, 1976).Another issue to be addressed is distribution of dietary crude protein into soluble, degradable and undegradable fractions. Most studies with improved animal performance from increased prepartal dietary protein have used additional undegradable protein sources. Deficient crude protein or excess degradable protein intake may lead to repeat breeding problem in dairy animals.

Macrominerals

Cows diagnosed with clinical hypocalcemia were 3.2 times more likely to experience retained placenta (RP) than cows that did not have clinical hypocalcemia (Curtis *et al.*, 1983).Whiteford and Sheldon (2005) also found thathypocalcemia was associated with occurrence ofuterine disease in lactating dairy cows.

A periparturient disease most frequently associated with macromineral nutrition is parturient hypocalcemia or milk fever. Milk fever is a rather nasty periparturient disease problem as a result of its association with 8 other periparturient disease processes and its negative effect on postpartum DMI (Curtis et al, 1983). Following decades of milk fever research, the underlying pathogenesis has been related to a failure of the calcium homeostatic system to maintain blood calcium concentrations with the onset of lactation. Kidney and bone are the target organs of concern which are unresponsive to parathormone stimulation. A number of prepartum dietary factors have been identified as influencing this target organ responsiveness; however, there is no consensus on predisposing factor(s) and mode of prevention. Prepartum dietary amounts of calcium and phosphorus and their ratio were first considered as primary determinants of milk fever (Boda and Cole, 1954). Subsequent research showed that extremely low dietary calcium (<20 gm/ day) could eliminate the problem, but these diets were not practical with available feedstuffs (Goings *et al*, 1974; Wiggers *et al*, 1975). Further work has shown a role for magnesium in calcium homeostasis and subsequently, milk fever problems (Van de Braak *et al*, 1986;). Practitioners have recognized a transition from classic "textbook" milk fever cases responsive to calcium gluconate infusion alone, to milk fever cases requiring both calcium and magnesium supplementation for a Reinhardt *et al*, 1988positive response. Another study had suggested that dietary sulfur content was a primary determinant of milk fever incidence (Oetzel, 1991). More recently, dietary potassium and sodium rather than (Goff and Horst, 1997). calcium content has been implicated as a primary inducer of milk fever (Dishington and Bjornstad 1982). High dietary potassium not only interferes with magnesium availability, but contributes to metabolic alkalosis which hinders target organ response to the calcium homeostatic system (Reinhardt et al, 1988; Goff and Horst, 1997). Dietary cation-anion difference (DCAD) as it relates to metabolic acidity or alkalinity has been a more recent area of active milk fever research relative to inciting factors and possible prevention.(Reinhardt et al, 1988; Dishington and Bjornstad 1982; Block, 1984 and Goff et al 1991). In spite of a tremendous increase in knowledge about calcium homeostasis, there is no tremendous gains in minimizing incidence of milk fever in aged dairy cows. Beyond the initial attempts at reducing calcium and phosphorus intakes to various modes of supplementing vitamin D metabolites or their analogs; manipulating prepartum DCAD shows the greatest promise for a practical method of milk fever prevention (Oetzel, 1993 and Wang et al, 1994) Rising forage potassium content places a serious strain on magnesium status and DCAD in many prepartum diets, leading to increased milk fever problems in a herd. This is a critical issue to be addressed by the practitioner. Although anionic salt programs are seen as a practical method of dealing with milk fever problems using available feed ingredients; they do not come without risk. Most anionic salts are unpalatable and their use generally results in reduced DMI during this critical period just prior to calving. Other issues include costs; safe time frame for feeding; and required dietary calcium, phosphorus and magnesium content for appropriate clinical response. Problems associated with attempted anionic salt programs stem mostly from use of partial anionic salt programs and inaccurate assessment of DCAD as a result of incomplete forage analysis data. Many herd "outbreaks" of milk fever can be directed back to a change in forage without consideration to changes in macromineral content and its effect on DCAD. Practitioners can provide a tremendous service to their dairy clients by routine monitoring of dry cow forages and diet for changes in macromineral content and subsequent alterations in DCAD. If not using anionic salt programs, similar monitoring would be critical to maintaining moderate calcium and phosphorus intake and appropriate magnesium content relative to dietary potassium concentration.

The rate of retained placenta was associated with imbalances in calcium and phosphorus metabolism (Noorsdsy *et al.*, 1973; Pelissier, 1976). Hypocalcemia results in loss of muscle tone in the uterus, which may contribute to the increased incidence of retained placenta (Goff and Horst,1997) Low levels of calcium may contribute to retained placenta, which may develop into uterine infection. Imbalance of calcium and phosphorus lead to repeat breeding problem. Wide Ca:P ratio or over-supplementation with calcium is a remote cause of cysic ovaries. Phosphorus deficiency, especially in heifers or excess phosphorus lead to anoestrus condition. (www.das.psu.edu/teamdairy).

Microminerals and Vitamins

Although microminerals and fat-soluble vitamins are not directly associated with periparturient metabolic disease problems, they do play a role in transition cow and neonate performance. Trace minerals are lost during gestation to the fetus where they are concentrated in the liver to be used as a postnatal mineral reserve (Abdelrahman and Kincaid, 1993; Graham *et al*, 1994 and Van Saun et al, 1994) Fetal hepatic micromineral reserves are also augmented by consumption of colostrum, a highly concentrated source of most essential nutrients. Therefore, available neonatal nutrient reserves are the sum of placental transport and colostrum consumption, both of which are highly influenced by maternal nutrient status. In contrast to the microminerals, fat-soluble vitamins like vitamins A and E do not appreciably cross the placenta resulting in no gestational liver reserve (Van Saun *et al*, 1989 and Van Saun, 1991). The neonate's primary source of vitamins A and E comes via colostrum ingestion supplied from an adequately supplemented dam (Mechor *et al*, 1992 and Van Saun, 1991). Nutrient concentrating ability of the fetal liver can only partiallycompensate for maternal nutrient deficiencies. A greater decline in nursing beef calf's selenium (Se) status was observed in calves from Se-deficient compared to Se-adequate dams (Koller *et al*, 1984). Adequacy of neonatal nutrient reserves might explain differences in time frame and severity of specific nutrient deficiency disease occurrence. From the dam's perspective, gestational micromineral and vitamin losses may significantly affect her reserves and their metabolic function. All too often mineral and vitamin supplementation is reduced or interrupted during the dry period. Deficiencies of microminerals and fat-soluble vitamins have been related to retained placenta and compromised immune function problems (Van Saun, 1991, Weiss et al 1990 and Ferguson, 1991) A compromised immune system may lead to increased incidence of metritis, mastitis or other infectious disease process. In short, it is absolutely essential that the pregnant cow receive an adequate amount of all minerals to support both maternal maintenance and conceptus development throughout the duration of gestation to minimize deficiency disease problems of either the dam or neonate.

In cows selenium deficient diets (0.05 to 0.07 mg/kg), supplemental selenium substantially reduced the incidence of retained placenta (Julien *et al.*, 1976 b,c)Administration of selenium and vitamin E in combination was more effective in reducing retained placenta than either antioxidant alone. Avitaminosis was shown to increase the incidence of retained placenta (Ronning *et al.*, 1953; Roberts, 1961; Nicholson and Cunningham, 1965). Ronning *et al.*, (1953) demonstrated a decrease in the incidence of retained placenta with increased intake of carotene. Selenium and vitamins A or E deficiencies may lead to uterine infection. For preventing this condition to occur it is adviced to Administer injectable selenium-vitamin E preparation at least 21 days prior to expected calving. Selenium and vitamin E deficiency may also lead to abortion cases. vitamins A, D, and E and carotene deficiency lead to repeat breeding problem. lack of fat-soluble vitamins iron, selenium or vitamin E. , plant hormones and antihormones lead to anoestrus condition in dairy animals. For avoiding this problem one can provide cows with adequate amounts of fresh forage for at least four to six weeks each year. Inadequate intake of vitamins A and E, carotene or selenium lead to cystic ovaries problem. For avoiding these problems to arise Submit forage samples for standard and mineral tests and submit feeding program for evaluation. This feeding program to be implemented in farm by dairy manager. (www.das.psu.edu/teamdairy).

References

Abdelrahman, M. M. and R. L. Kincaid, (1993). Deposition of copper, manganese, zinc, and selenium in bovine fetal tissue at different stages of gestation. *J. Dairy Sci.* 76: 3588.

Barton, B. A., H. A. Rosario, G. W. Anderson, B. P. Grindle, and D. J. Carroll, (1996). Effects of dietary crude protein, breed, parity, and health status on the fertility of dairy cows. *J. Dairy Sci.* 79: 2225-2236.

Beam, S. W., and W. R. Butler, (1997). Energy balance, metabolic hormones, and early postpartum development in dairy cows fed prilled lipid. *J. Dairy Sci.* 81:121-131.

Berghorn, K. A., R. D. Allrich and C, H, Noller, (1988). Energy balance and reproductive traits of post partum dairy cattle. *J. Dairy Sci.* 71(Suppl. 1):171 (Abstr.)

Bertics, S. J., R. R. Grummer, C. Cadorniga-Valino, D. W. LaCount, and E. E. Stoddard. (1992). Effect of prepartum dry matter intake and liver triglyceride concentration and early postpartum lactation. *J. Dairy Sci.* 75:1914.

Blanchard, T. *et al.* (1990). Effect of dietary crude-protein type on fertilization and embryo quality in dairy cattle. *Am J Vet Res* 51: 905-908.

Block, E. (1984). Manipulating dietary anions and cations for prepartum dairy cows to reduce incidence of milk fever. *J Dairy Sci* 67:2939-2948.

Boda J M. and H.H. Cole, (1954). The influence of dietary calcium and phosphorus on the incidence of milk fever. *J Dairy Sci* 37:360.

Boland M.P. Lonegan P., O'Callaghan D. (2001) "Effect of nutrition and endocrine parameters, ovarian physiology and oocyte and embryo development" *Theriogenology*. 55: 1323-1340.

Britt, J. H. (1992). Reproductive efficiency in dairy cattle as related to nutrition and environment. Page 30 in Proc. Adv. Nutr. Sem. for Feed Prof. University of Wisconsin, Madison.

Butler W.R. (2003). Energy balance relationships with follicular development,ovulation and fertility in postpartum dairy cows. Livestock Production Science. 83: 211-218.

Butler W.R. (2006). Relationships of negative energy balance with fertility. Penn State Dairy Cattle Nutrition Workshop pp. 51-60.

Butler, W. R. and R. D. Smith. (1989). Interrelationships between energy balance and postpartum reproductive function in dairy cattle. *J. Dairy Sci.* 72:767.

Butler, W. R. and R. W. Canfield, (1989). Interrelationships between energy balance and postpartum reproduction. In Proc. Cornell Nutrition Conference for Feed Manufacturers, October 24-26, 1989, Cornell University, Ithaca.

Butler, W. R., J. J. Calaman, and S. W. Beam, (1996). Plasma and milk urea nitrogen inrelation to pregnancy rate in lactating dairy cattle. *J Anim Sci* 74: 858-865.

Butler, W.R. (1998). Review: effect of protein nutrition on ovarían endotcrine physiology in dairy catlle. *J. Dairy Sci.* 81:2533-2539.

Butler, W. R., R. W. Everett and C. E. Coppock, (1981). The relationship between energy balance, milk production and ovulation in postpartum Holstein cows. *J. Anim. Sci.* 53:742.

Canfield, R. W., C. J. Sniffen, and W. R. Butler, (1990). Effects of excess degradable protein on postpartum reproduction and energy balance in dairy cattle. *J Dairy Sci* 73: 2342-2349.

Carroll, D. J., B. A. Barton, G. W. Anderson, and R. D. Smith, (1988). Influence of protein intake and feeding strategy on reproductive performance of dairy cows. *J Dairy Sci* 71: 3470-3481.

Carroll, D. J., R. R. Grummer, and F. C. Mao, (1992). Progesterone production by cultured luteal cells in the presence of bovine low and high density lipoproteins purified by heparin affinity chromatography. *J. Anim. Sci.* 70:2516.

Carroll, D. J., R. R. Grummer, and M. K. Clayton, (1992). Stimulation of luteal cell progesterone production by lipoproteins from cows fed control or fat supplemented diets. *J. Dairy Sci.* 75:2205.

Curtis, C.R., H.N. Erb, C.J. Sniffen, R.D. Smith and D.S. Kronfeld, (1985). Path analysis of dry period nutrition, postpartum metabolic and reproductive disorders and mastitis in Holstein cows. *J Dairy Sci* 68:2347.

Curtis, C.R., H.N. Erb, C.J. Sniffen, R.D. Smith, and D.S. Kronfeld, (1985). Path analysis of dry period nutrition, postpartum disease, reproductive performance and mastitis in Holstein cows. *J. Dairy Sci.* 68:2347-2360.

Curtis, C.R., H.N. Erh, C.J. Sniffcn, R.D. Smith, P.A. Powcrs, M.C. Smith, M.W. White, R.B. Hillman, andE.J. Pcarson, (1983). Association of parturient hypocalccmia with cight poriparturient disordois in Holstoin cows. *JAVMA*. 183:559-561.

Dishington, I.W. and J. Bjornstad, (1982). Prevention of milk fever by dietary means, the effect of a concentrate fortified with mineral salts. *Acta Vet Scand* 23:336-343.

Ducker, M. J., R. A. Haggett, W. J. Fisher, S. V. Morant and G. A. Bloomfield, (1985). The effect of level of feeding in late pregnancy and around the time of insemination on the reproductive performance of first lactation dairy heifers. *Anim. Prod.* 41:1.

Dyk, P., and R. Emery, (1996). Reducing the incidence of peripartum health problems. Proc. Tri-State Dairy Nutr. Conf., M.L. Eastridge, ed.

Emery, R.S. (1993). Energy needs of dry cows. In: Proc. Tri-State Dairy Nutr. Conf. Ohio State Univ., Michigan State Univ., and Purdue Univ., Ft. Wayne, IN. pp 35.

Fenwick M.A., Fitzpatrick R., Kenny D.A., Diskin M.G., Patton J., Murphy J.J., Wathes D.C. (2008). Interrelationships between negative energy balance (NEB) and IGF regulation in liver of lactating dairy cows. *Domestic Animal Endocrinology*. 34: 31-44

Ferguson, J.D. (2001). Nutrition and reproduction in dairy herds. *In:* Proc. 2001 Intermountain Nutr. Conf., Salt Lake City, UT, pages 65-82.

Ferguson, J. D., D. T. Galligan, T. Blanchard, and M. Reeves, (1993). Serum urea nitrogen and conception rate: The usefulness of test information. *J Dairy Sci* 76: 3742-3746.

Ferguson, J.D., (1991). Nutrition and reproduction in dairy cows. *Vet Clinic NA: Food Anim Pract* 7(2):483-507.

Fitzpatrick R., Llewellyn S., Kenny D.A., Murphy J.J., Scaramuzzi R.J., Wathes D.C. (2007). Effect of negative energy balance on the insulin-like growth factor system in pre-recruitment ovarian follicles of post partum dairy cows. *Reproduction*. 133: 627-639.

Formigoni, A., M. C. Cornil, A. Prandi, A. Mordenti, A. Rossi, D. Portetelle, and R. Renaville. (1996). Effect of propylene glycol supplementation around parturition on milk yield, reproduction performance, and some hormonal and metabolic characteristics in dairy cows. *J. Dairy Res.* 63:11.

Friggens N.C. (2003). Body lipid reserves and the reproductive cycle: towards a better understanding. *Livestock Production Science*. 83: 219-236.

Garcia-Bojalil, C. M., C. R. Staples, C. A. Risco, J. D. Savio, and W. W. Thatcher, (1998). Protein degradability and calcium salts of long-chain fatty acids in the diets of lactating dairy cows: reproductive responses. *J. Dairy Sci.* 81:1385.

Goff, J.P. and R.L. Horst, (1997). Effects of the addition of potassium or sodium, but not calcium, to prepartum rations on milk fever in dairy cows. *J Dairy Sci* 80:176-186.

Goff, J.P., R.L. Horst, F.J. Mueller, J.K. Miller, G.A. Kiess and H.H. Dowlen, (1991). Addition of chloride to a prepartal diet high in cations increases 1,25-dihydroxyvitamin D response to hypocalcemia preventing milk fever. *J Dairy Sci* 74:3863.

Goff, J. P., and R. L. Horst, (1997). Physiological changes at parturition and their relationship to metabolic disorders. *J. Dairy Sci.* 80:1260– 1268.

Goings, R.L., N.L. Jacobson, D.C. Beitz, E.T. Littledike and K.D. Wiggers, (1974). Prevention of parturient paresis by a prepartum, calcium-deficient diet. *J. Dairy Sci.* 57:1184.

Graham, T. W., M. C. Thurmond, F. C. Mohr, C. A. Holmberg, M. L. Anderson, and C. L.Keen, (1994). Relationships between maternal and fetal liver copper, iron, manganese, and zinc concentrations and fetal development in California Holstein dairy cows. *J Vet Diag Invest* 6:77.

Grummer, R. R, and D. J Carroll, (1991). Effects of dietary fat on metabolic disorders and reproductive performance of dairy cattle. *J. Anim. Sci.* 69:3838.

Grummer, R. R. (1995). Impact of changes in organic nutrient metabolism on developing feeding strategies to minimize stress during the transition from late pregnancy to early lactation. *J. Anim. Sci.* 73:2820.

Grummer, R. R., and D. J. Carroll, (1988). Review of lipoprotein cholesterol metabolism: importance to ovarian function. *J. Anim. Sci.* 66:3160.

Holtenius, P. and M. Hjort, (1990). Studies on the pathogenesis of fatty liver in cows. *Bovine Practitioner* 25:91.

homeostasis in ruminant. *Vet Clinic NA: Food Anim Pract* 4(2):331-350.

Howard, H. J. *et al.* (1987). Influence of dietary protein on reproductive performance of dairy cows. *J Dairy Sci* 70: 1563-1571.

Jordan, E. R., and L. V. Swanson, (1979a). Effect of crude protein on reproductive efficiency, serum total protein, and albumin in the high-producing dairy cow. *J Dairy Sci* 62: 58-63.

Jorritsma R., Cesar M.L., Hermans J.T., Kruitwagen C.L.J.J., Vos P.L.A.M., Kruip T.A.M. (2004). "Effects of non-esterified fatty acids on bovine granulose cells and developmental potential of oocytes in vitro" *Animal Reproduction Science.* 81: 225-235.

Julien, W. E., H. R. Conrad, and D. R. Redman, (1976). Influence of dietary protein on susceptibility to alert downer syndrome. *J. Dairy Sci.* 60:210– 215.

Julien, W. E., H. R. Conrad, J. E. Jones, and A. L. Moxon, (1976). Selenium and vitaminEand incidence of retained placenta in parturient dairy cows. *J. Dairy Sci.* 59:1954– 1959.

Julien, W. E.,H. R.Conrad, J. E. Jones, and A. L. Moxon, (1976). Selenium and vitamin E and incidence of retained placenta in parturient dairy cows. II. Prevention in commercial herds with prepartum treatment. *J. Dairy Sci.* 59:1960– 1962.

Julien, W.E., H.R. Conrad and D.R. Redman, (1977). Influence of dietary protein on susceptibility to alert downer syndrome. *J Dairy Sci* 60:210.

Kaim, M., Y. Folman, and H. Neumark, (1983). The effect of protein intake and lactation number on post-partum body weight loss and reproductive performance of dairy cows. *Anim Prod* 37: 229-235.

Koller, L.D., G.A. Whitbeck and P.J. South, (1984). Transplacental transfer and colostral concentrations of selenium in beef cattle. *Am J Vet Res* 45:2507.

Lopez Gautius F., Yaniz J., Madriles-Helm D. (2003). "Effects of body condition score and score change on the reproductive performance of dairy cows: a metaanalysis" *Theriogenology*. 59: 801-812

Lucy, M. C., C. R. Staples, F. M. Michel, and W. W. Thatcher, (1991). Effect of feeding calcium soaps to early postpartum dairy cows on plasma prostaglandin F2a, luteinizing hormone, and follicular growth. *J. Dairy Sci.* 74:483.

Lucy, M. C., C. R. Staples, W. W. Thatcher, P. S. Erickson, R. M. Cleale, J. L. Firkens, M. R. Murphy, J. H. Clark, and B. O. Brodie, (1992b). Influence of diet composition, dry matter intake, milk production, and energy balance, on time of postpartum ovulation and fertility in dairy cows. *Anim. Prod.* 54:323.

Lucy, M. C., J. Beck, C. R. Staples, H. H. Head, R. L. de la Sota, and W. W. Thatcher, (1992a). Follicular dynamics, plasma metabolites, hormones and insulin-like growth factor-I (IGF-I) in lactating cows with positive or negative energy balance during the preovulatory period. *Reprod. Nut. Dev.* 32:331-341.

Lucy, M. C., R. L. de la Sota, C. R. Staples, and W. W. Thatcher, (1993). Ovarian folicular populations in lactating dairy cows treated with recombinant bovine somatotropin (Semetribove) or saline and fed diets differing in fat content and energy. *J. Dairy Sci.* 76:1014.

Lucy, M. C., T. S. Gross, and W. W. Thatcher, (1990). Effect of intravenous infusion of soybean oil emulsion on plasma concentration of 15-keto-13,14-dihydro-prostaglandin F2? and ovarian function in cycling Holstein heifers. Livestock Repro. Latin Amer., Internat. Atomic Energy Agency, Vienna, p119.

Lucy, M. C., W. W. Thatcher, and C. R. Staples, (1992c). Postpartum Function: Nutritional and Physiological Interactions. Page 135 in Large Dairy Herd Management. H. H. Van Horn and C. J. Wilcox, eds. American Dairy Science Association, Champaign, IL.

Martin B., Golden E., Carlson O.D., Egan J.M., Mattson M.P., Maudsley S. (2008). Caloric restriction: Impact upon pituitary function and reproduction. *Ageing Research Reviews*. 7: 209-224.

Mechor G.D., Y.T. Gröhn, L.R. McDowell and R.J. Van Saun, (1992). Specific gravitymeasurement of bovine colostrum immunoglobulin concentration as affected by temperature and colostral components. *J Dairy Sci* 75:3131-3135.

Miyoshi, S., J. L. Pate, and D. L. Palmquist, (1995). Productive, reproductive, and metabolic responses to daily administration of propylene glycol in early lactation. *J. Dairy Sci.* 78(Suppl. 1):306 (Abstr.).

Montiel F., Ahuja C. (2005). Body condition and suckling as factors influencing the duration of postpartum anestrus in cattle: a review" *Animal Reproduction Science.* 85: 1-26.

Nicholson, J. W. G., and H. M. Cunningham, (1965). Retained placenta, abortion, and abnormal calves from beef cows fed all barley rations. *Can. Vet. J.* 6:275- 281.

Noorsdsy, J. L.,H.W. Leipold, D. L. Carmahan, R. A. Frey, J. Vestweber, M. G. Robl, G. Kennedy, J. R. Dunham, T. E. Chapin, and W. E. Moore, (1973). Metabolic disturbances in the dairy cow influenced by managerial practices: Case reports and epidemiological studies. Rumen Function Conf., Chicago, IL.

Ocon, O.M., and P.J. Hansen, (2003). Disruption ofbovine oocytcs and preimplantation cmbryos by urea and acidic pH. *J. Dairy Sci.* 861 194-1200.

Oetzel, G.A., (1991). Meta-analysis of nutritional risk factors for milk fever in dairy cattle. *J Dairy Sci* 74:3900.

Oetzel, G.R., (1993). Use of anionic salts for prevention of milk fever in dairy cattle. *Comp Cont Ed* 15:1138-1146.

Oikawa, S., N. Katoh, F. Kawawa and Y. Ono, (1997). Decreased serum apolipoprotein B-100 and A-1 concentrations in cows with ketosis and left displacement of the abomasum, *AJVR* 58:121-125.

Pelissier, C.L. (1976). Dairy cattle breeding problems and their consequences. *Theriogenology.* 6:575- 583.

Putnum, D.E., G.A. Varga, T.W. Cassidy and J.E. Vallimont, (1996). Increasing dietary protein density increases N balance in late gestation Holstein cows. *J Dairy Sci* 79(Suppl. 1):207, Abstract.

Roberts, S. J. (1961). Page 225 *in* Veterinary obstetrics and genital diseases. Edwards Bros., Ann Arbor, MI.

Roche J.R., Macdonald K.A., Burke C.R., Lee J.M., Berry D.P. (2007). Associations among body condition score, body weight and reproductive performance in seasonal-calving dairy cattle. *Journal of Dairy Science.* 90: 376-391.

Ronning, M., E. R. Berousek, A. H. Kuhman, and W. D. Gallap, (1953). The carotene requirements for reproduction in Guernsey cattle. *J. Dairy Sci.* 36:52- 56.

Rossi F., Righi F., Romanelli S., Quarantelli A. (2008). Reproductive efficiency of dairy cows under negative energy balance conditions. *Ann. Fac. Medic. Vet. di Parma.* XXVIII: 173–180.

Santos, J.R.P. (2009). Nutrition and Reproduction in Dairy Cattle. Dairy Caltle Reproduction Conforcnce. Minneapolis, MN. Boise, ID.

Santos, J.E.P., H.M. Rutigliano, and M.F. SA Filho, (2009). Risk factors for resumption of postpartum cyclicity and embryonic survival in lactating dairy cows. *Anim. Reprod. Sci.* 110:207-221.

Santos, J.E.P., W.W. Thatcher, R.C. Chcbol, R.L.A. Ceni, and K.N. GalviXo. (2004). Thc cffect of embryonic death rates iu cattlo an the efficacy of eshous synchronization programs. *Anim. Rcprod. Sci.* 82-83C:513-535.

Schneider J.E. (2004). Energy balance and reproduction" *Physiology and Behaviour*. 81: 289-317.

Spicer, L. J., W. B. Tucker, and G. D. Adams, (1990). Insulin-like growth factor-I in dairy cows: relationships among energy balance, body condition, ovarian activity, and estrous behavior. *J. Dairy Sci.* 73:929.

Schneider, P., D. Sklan, W. Chalupa, and D.S. Kronfcld, (1988). Feeding calcium salts of fatty acids to lactating cows. *J. Daily Sci.* 71:2143-2150.

Staples, C. R., and W. W. Thatcher, (2000). Nutrition and reproduction: feeding for breeding. Pages 1-16 in 4-State Professional Management Seminar. Midwest Plan Service, Ames, IA.

Staples, C. R., M. C. Wiltbank, R. R. Grummer, J. Guenther, R. Satori, F. J. Diaz, S. Bertics, R. Mattos, and W. W. Thatcher, (2000). Effect of long chain fatty acids on lactation performance and reproductive tissues of Holstein cows. *J. Dairy Sci.* 83(Suppl. 1): 278. (Abstr.)

Staples, C. R., W. W. Thatcher, and J. H. Clark, (1990). Relationship between ovarian activity and energy status during the early postpartum period of the high producing dairy cow. *J. Dairy Sci.* 73:938.

Thatcher, W. W., L. de la Sota, E. J-P. Schmitt, T. C. Diaz, L. Badinga, F. A. Simmen, C. R. Staples, and M. Drost, (1996). Control and management of ovarian follicles in cattle to optimize fertility. *Reprod. Feril. Dev.* 8:203-217.

Van de Braak, A.E., A.Th. Van't Klooster and A. Malestein, (1986). Influence of a deficient supply of magnesium during the dry period on the rate of calcium mobilisation by dairy cows at parturition. *Res Vet Sci* 42:101-108.

Van Knegsel A.T.M., Van Den Brand H., Dijkstra J., Kemp B. (2007). Effects of dietary energy source on energy balance, metabolites and reproduction variables in dairy cows in early lactation. *Theriogenology*. 68s: 274-280.

Van Saun, R.J. and C.J. Sniffen, (1995). Effects of undegradable protein fed prepartum onlactation, reproduction, and health in dairy cattle. II. Postpartum diets and performance. *Journal of Dairy Science* 78(Supplement 1):265, Abstract #P341.

Van Saun, R.J., (1991). Dry cow nutrition: The key to improving fresh cow performance. *Vet Clinics NA: Food Anim Pract* 7(2):599-620.

Van Saun, R.J., T.H. Herdt, and H.D. Stowe, (1989). Maternal and fetal selenium concentrations and their interrelationships in dairy cattle. *J Nutr* 119:1128.

Van Saun, R.J., T.H. Herdt, and H.D. Stowe, (1989). Maternal and fetal vitamin E concentrations and selenium-vitamin E interrelationships in dairy cattle. *J Nutr* 119:1156.

Vasconcelos, J. L. M., R. Satori, H. N. Oliveira, J. N. Guenther, and M. C. Wiltbank, (1998). Reduction in size of the ovulatory follicle reduces subsequent luteal size and pregnancy rate. *J. Dairy Sci.* 81:(Suppl. 1):224. (Abstr.).

Wang, C., J.S. Velez, C.A. Risco, G.A. Donovan, A.M. Merritt and D.K. Beede, (1994). Recent advances in prevention of parturient paresis in dairy cows. *Comp Cont Ed* 16: 1373-1381.

Wathes D.C., Fenwick M., Cheng Z., Bourne N., Llewellyn S., Morris D.G., Kenny D., Murphy J., Fitzpatrick R. (2007). Influence of negative energy balance on cyclicity and fertility in the high producing dairy cow. *Theriogenology*. 68s: 232-241.

Weiss, W.P., D.A. Todhunter, J.S. Hogan and K.L. Smith, (1990). Effect and duration of supplementation of selenium and vitamin E on periparturient dairy cows. *J Dairy Sci* 73:3187.

Wiggers K.D., D.K. Nelson and N.L. Jacobson, (1975). Prevention of parturient paresis by a low calcium diet prepartum: A field study. *J Dairy Sci* 58:430.

www.das.psu.edu/teamdairy- O'Connor, M., Griswold, D., Adams, R. and Hutchinson, L. Trouble-shooting infertility problems in cattle. DAS 00-10 and VSE 00-01: 1-6.

Zamet, C.N., V.F. Colenbrander, C.J. Callahan, B.P. Chew, R.E. Erb and N.J. Moeller, (1979). *Theriogenology* 11:229.

□□□

9

Meat Production, Export Potential, Policy and Quality Concerns

M.K. AGNIHOTRI
Principal Scientist & COE (Edn.), Education Division, ICAR, KAB-II, Pusa, Delhi-12
Ex –Joint Commissioner (Meat and Meat Products) DADF, Ministry of Agriculture
Government of India, New Delhi

Introduction

Livestock sector plays an important role in the national economy and socioeconomic development of the country as it provides not only rural employment and economic security but also essential nutrition through various products and also raw material base for the leather and allied sector industry. India, with about 11 % of the world livestock population, occupies a significant place numerically in respect of livestock wealth. With 2.3% of the land area of the world, it maintains nearly 17% of world's human population and about 11% of the livestock.

The cattle, buffalo, sheep, goat and pigs population which was 185.20, 97.90, 61.50, 124.4, 13.50 millions in 2003 reached to 199.10, 105.30, 71.60, 140.5, 11.1 millions, respectively in 2007 (18th Live stock census, DADF, M/o Agriculture). The average annual growth rate in population of these species during the corresponding period was 1.83,1.84,3.87,3.10,(-)4.74 percent. Buffalo has surpassed the cattle population growth rate for various reasons viz., use for milk, meat and draft purposes as well as PFA standards for %fat and SNF favoring buffalo milk rather than cow milk production. Country possesses about 57% of buffaloes, 14 % of cattle, 16 % of goat, 6 % of sheep and 1.5 % of world pig population. With such large population of livestock, on meat production front, it contributes meager 2.42 percent to the world total meat production of 269 million tones (FAO, 2007).

In general, productivity of our livestock is very low, in comparison to the world average. The average milk production in cattle is about 1200 kg/ lactation as against 2100 kg being the world average. Average carcass yield from sheep, goat and pigs is 12, 10, 35 kg as against the world average of 16, 12 and 79 kg, respectively (Table-1). Due to shrinkage in pasture and grazing land, dwindling feed and fodder resources, use of course grains (which are generally used as feed ingredients) for ethanol production (for bio-energy), emerging new diseases, indiscriminate use of pesticides/insecticides in various crops and their presence at higher level in various crop residues and agro industrial by-products, biotic and abiotic stress due to various other factors and climatic changes, livestock sector faces many challenges to attain the optimum growth rate and increase the livestock products production.

Table 1: Meat yield from various Livestock in India

S.No.	Species	Average carcass weight/ per animal (kg)		
		India (FAO)	India (DAHD)	World
1	Cattle	103	89	202
2	Buffalo	138	110	140
3	Sheep	12	12.6	16
4	Goat	10	9.6	12
5	Pig	35	32.2	79

Current Status

Meat industry in India has great economic potential but received limited attention for its growth and development. Yet the value of output from meat group as per estimates of Central Statistical Office (CSO) at current prices in 2009-10 was Rs.64,073 crore(Rs.3,40,473 crore for total livestock sector). It is envisaged to achieve 10% growth rate in meat sector during 11th Five Year Plan period.

Slaughterhouses have been under the control of municipal authorities/ local bodies and no systematic efforts have been made to make meat production an economic activity. Barring a few export-oriented abattoirs, it has been in the hands of those who have no knowledge of slaughterhouse hygiene, sanitation, meat quality and animal rights. The hygienic conditions in most of the slaughterhouses are appalling and animal by-products are not properly handled and processed.

As per FAO (2007) estimates, 12.45 million cattle, 10.86 million buffaloes, 19.54 million sheep, 54.30 million goats and 14.20 million pigs were slaughtered for meat production.

Production and supply of meat for local consumption is one of the most neglected and poorly organized sectors in the country. Meat is sold in open places attracting contamination from dirt, dust, flies, water etc. Though the consumption of meat and meat products is on rise, hygiene, safety and quality aspects have not changed much. Except poultry (20%), less than 1% of meat produced from cattle, small ruminants and pigs is under organized sector.

With the introduction of National Food Safety and Standard Authority under the provision of the Food Safety and Standards Act 2006, production, packaging, transportation, supply, marketing and storage of meat and meat products under strict hygienic condition has become essential to safe guard human health.

Meat Demand

Presently the animal protein supply per caput per day is only 10 g as against the world average of 29 g.

The per capita consumption of meat in the country, as per FAO (2007) estimates is 13.70 g /day whereas the world average is 106.85 g. In USA, it is 337g, the highest followed by 331 g in Spain, 323 g in Australia. In China, it is about 148g/caput/day.

This is due to not enough production of livestock products. The poor productivity in livestock is not only due to poor genetic makeup but also because of lack of adequate feeding and nutrition. Growing population and incomes, along with fast changing food preferences, are rapidly increasing demand for livestock products in the country while globalization is boosting trade in livestock inputs and their products.

It is estimated that by 2020 country would require about 147million tones of milk and 14 million tones of meat (Dastagiri, 2004), which could be possible only through improving the productivity rather than number of livestock. Increasing productivity per unit time rather than their numbers is also important from environmental view point as livestock is considered as one of the important contributors of greenhouse gases (Agnihotri and Rajkumar, 2008).

Export and export potential

There is a preference for meat exported from India because of certain inherent merits such as its lean character, relative freedom from toxic feed additive residues and near organic meat production. Currently India has been exporting meat to more than 60 countries. Buffalo meat is exported in frozen bone less and de-glanded form and is free from FMD virus due to its ageing for minimum of 24 hrs at 2°C to bring down the meat pH below 6.0. Meat is available at very competitive prices. The Indian buffalo and lamb meat has established itself in the markets' of South-East Asia, Middle East and African countries.

Out of total meat production of 6.50 million tones, buffalo alone contributed about 1.50 million tones. With this much production of buffalo meat, India ranks first followed by Pakistan (0.68 million tones) and China (0.31 million tones).The world total buffalo meat production was 3.32 million tones in 2007.

India is the 5th largest producer of meat. The top five meat producing countries are as under:

S No	Name of the country	Quantity (in million tones)	% of world total meat production
1.	China	70.46	26.19
2.	USA	42.02	15.62
3.	Brazil	18.89	6.94
4.	Germany	7.41	2.75
5.	India	6.50	2.42
	World total	269.00	-

Source: FAO Stat (2007).

Country is 5th largest exporter of bovine (buffalo) meat in the world.

The top five bovine meat exporting countries are as under

S.No	Name of the country	Quantity of bovine meat exported (in million tones)	% of total bovine meat export
1.	Brazil	1.96	20.74
2.	Australia	1.28	13.54
3.	USA	0.60	6.34
4.	Ireland	0.53	5.61
5.	India	0.48	5.10
	World total	**9.45**	-

Source: FAO-Stat (2007).

Buffalo meat is one of the major commodities, among livestock products, exported from the country. Among the animal products exported from India, meat and meat products account for more than 90% of the total exports volume. Remaining 10% are dairy products and honey.

On private sector, there are about 16 modern integrated abattoirs cum processing units where quality meat is produced adopting OIE guidelines and international quality standards.

The major meat production centers in the country for exports are- Aurangabad, Nanded, Mumbai and Satara in Maharashtra; Goa; Zaherabad and Medak in Andhra Pradesh; Derabassi in Punjab; Barabanki, Unnao, Aligarh, Meerut, Saharanpur, Noida and Ghaziabad. in UP; Mourigram in West Bengal and Gurgaon in Haryana.

The Malaysia, Philippines, Saudi Arabia, Angola, Jordan, UAE, Kuwait are major destinations for buffalo meat. Though there is no religious biasness for buffalo meat, its demand in domestic market is very limited due to limited liking .Therefore, buffalo meat with production of 1.47 million tones offers great potential for exports especially from male buffalo calves.

The EU is expected to import large volume of bovine meat over the next few years as abolition of subsidies might lead to rapid decrease in production of livestock products .The Central America and the Caribbean, Russia, Middle East, East Asia and most of the African countries are the bovine meat deficit regions. The major demand for bovine meat is expected to come from these areas and also from the EU. South America, Oceania (Australia and New Zealand) and India are emerging as the major bovine and buffalo meat surplus countries. The continuous drought has been affecting Australia's herd building during the last few years and BSE issue limits the potential of North America. There are also serious concerns that Brazilian bovine meat supply may not be able to keep pace with sharply increased export projections for bovine meat. This offers a great opportunity for India, to grow its international trade in meat.

Salvaging Male Buffalo Calves for Meat Production

As per 18th Livestock Census (2007), India's buffalo population is 105.3 million and country ranks 1st in world in buffalo population. Buffalo population trends over the years, reveal positive growth in buffalo population. Presently, primary importance of buffalo in the country is largely for purposes of milk and to a small extent for production of meat and draft purposes.

It is estimated that about 8 million male buffalo calves are removed from buffalo production system in the country due to due to inadequate feeding by farmers with a view to save on mother's milk and other feed resources leading to parasitism, stunted growth and untimely deaths. Livestock farmers do not consider raising male animals to be remunerative; as a result, the country suffers a loss of about Rs.750 million per annum.

High mortality of buffalo calves has been reported in a study conducted by Central Leather Research Institute (CLRI), Chennai, which indicated mortality ranging from 42-88% in different parts of the country (Table 2). These calves could otherwise be salvaged for meat production and recovery of hides, skins, bones etc. thereby improving economic condition of farmers and providing quality meat for export market and domestic consumption. Raising these male buffalo calves will also generate additional employment in rural areas. In most of the states only culled old and unproductive animals are permitted to be slaughtered. It requires change in the state's policy so that such male calves when reared for meat purposes are allowed to be slaughtered.

Table 2 : Percentage of young stock to total deaths in bovines

S. No.	State	Cattle			Buffalo		
		Total death (Nos.)	Calf mortality (Nos.)	% of calf death to total deaths	Total death (Nos.)	Calf mortality (Nos.)	% of calf death to total deaths
1.	2.	3.	4.	5.	6.	7.	8.
1.	Andhra Pradesh	146	89	61	213	171	80
2.	Bihar	251	88	35	168	91	54
3.	Chhattisgarh	254	82	32	67	28	42
4.	Jharkhand	128	38	30	25	12	48
5.	Kerala	191	89	47	7	6	86
6.	Madhya Pradesh	197	66	34	173	101	58
7.	Maharashtra	304	84	28	149	92	62
8.	Punjab	195	146	75	887	778	88
9.	Rajasthan	747	234	31	143	68	48
10.	Tamil Nadu	153	61	40	42	25	60
11.	Uttar Pradesh	276	95	34	467	275	59
12.	Uttarakhand	281	77	27	240	129	54
13.	West Bengal	410	179	44	19	10	53
	Total	**3533**	**1328**	**38**	**2600**	**1786**	**69**

Source : Report of All India Survey on Rawhides and Skins, CLRI, Chennai (2005).

Note: Field study was conducted adopting standard statistical analysis methods. The mortality reported is for young stock, not sex-wise. The above annexure provides state wise data on percent of calf deaths to the total deaths in a sample population selected for the study.

Buffalo accounts for about 25% of the total meat production in the country. Export of buffalo meat has increased significantly in the last few years (Table-3). It was 483478.3 metric tonne, valued at Rs.3549.78 crore in 2007-08, and has gone up to 495019.71 metric tonne valued at 5480.60 crore (54% increase)in 2009-10(APEDA,2011).In comparison to other products, buffalo meat and casings export has increased very high.

Table 3 : The export of meat and meat products during the last three years

Quantity in M.Ts
Value in Rs. Crores

Products	Year 2007-08 Qty.	Value	2008-09 Qty.	Value	2009-10 Qty.	Value
Buffalo meat	483478	3549.78	462749	4839.70	495019	5480.60
Sheep and goat meat	8908	134.10	37790	493.37	52868	747.20
Poultry products	1355246	441.08	1057016	422.05	1016783	372.11
Animal casings	619	6.84	1823	8.84	2020	31.52
Processed meat	1245	12.96	857	10.14	716	9.58
Swine meat	1710	24.63	817	9.17	1117	10.34
Total	1851206	4169.39	1561052	5783.27	1568523	6651.35

Source: DGCIS

The volume of global trade in leather stands at US$88 billion, with India contributing only US $2.4 billion thereof, despite having largest livestock population in world. For enlarging raw material base and improving leather availability in the country and boost buffalo veal export, there is great potential to salvage and rear male buffalo calves. Considering their economic value for meat, hide and other by-products, DADF, GOI has launched a scheme to assist farmers, NGOs, professionals and corporate bodies to rear male buffalo calves for meat production.

The potential states for implementation of the scheme, among others, are Andhra Pradesh, Bihar, Chhattisgarh, Jharkhand, Kerala, Madhya Pradesh, Maharashtra, Orissa, Rajasthan, Uttar Pradesh and West Bengal, keeping in view high buffalo population in these States.

Quality Concerns and Need for Modernization

For domestic consumptions, animals are slaughtered in municipal slaughterhouses, which have generally poor slaughter facilities. The quality of meat produced, in such slaughterhouses, is some times not good.

Legally slaughter of animals should be done only in licensed slaughterhouses. However, illegal slaughter is common. There are 5,520 registered slaughterhouses and more than 4,707 unregistered slaughterhouses operating in the country. Operating authorities are also responsible for giving licenses and therefore, there is laxity in adhering to operating standards.

To regulate the illegal slaughter and improve hygiene and sanitation, modernization of existing slaughterhouses is needed at a larger scale. Environmental and animal right's issues, through modernization of slaughter, could be addressed more effectively. This will not only help in providing safe and wholesome meat to the meat eaters but also in building the image of meat industry worldwide.

To provide safe and wholesome meat to the consumers, in smaller towns, cities and the rural areas and provide pollution free environment, Department of Animal Husbandry, Dairying and Fisheries is implementing Centrally Sponsored scheme on 'Establishment / modernization of rural slaughterhouses. The scheme aims to address those areas not specifically and fully covered by existing scheme of Ministry of Food Processing Industries (MFPI). Issue is of Public health importance with larger dimensions and the task is huge. Therefore, a multi-pronged approach is required to supplement the efforts of the States.

Scheme is initially implemented in three states i.e. AP,UP and Meghalaya, on pilot basis through NABARD.

Meat Food Safety, Quality control and Hygiene

In the interest of food safety and consumer protection, increasingly stringent hygiene measures are required at national and international trade levels. The key issues in this respect which needs to be addressed are meat food traceability, Good Hygienic Practices (GHP) and Hazard Analysis and Critical Control Point Schemes (HACCP).

Extensive knowledge of hazards, other than that of microorganisms, is indispensable in modern meat processing. Thus, along with meat processing hygiene including causes for meat product spoilage and food borne illnesses, stress to control the entry of harmful residues in product chain is equally important.

For the purpose of consumer protection and quality control of meat and products, simple test methods needs to be made available that can be carried out at the small enterprise level without sophisticated laboratory set-ups.

To remain competitive in the world market meat has to be produced adopting OIE and Codex guidelines and quality standards. While the mandate of the Codex is to develop international standards, guidelines and recommendations on food safety for international trade, OIE (World Organization for Animal Health) has the mandate to develop international standards, guidelines and recommendations on animal health including zoonoses.

For producing hygienic meat to be internationally acceptable for exports, Codex Alimentarius General Principles of Meat Hygiene needs to be followed.

The Department of Animal Husbandry Dairying and Fisheries and Ministry of Commerce and Industry through APEDA are regularly involved in various standards being formulated by the Codex Alimentarious Commission to ensure that India's interests are reflected in the decisions taken in the Codex Committee meetings.

With technical inputs from FAO, WHO and OIE, Codex established its first code that helps to ensure the safety of food for human consumption through adherence to good animal feeding practices at the farm level and good manufacturing practices during all phases of animal feeding.

Food Safety Regulations in India

There are following Food Safety Regulations in vogue in India:

(i) The Food Safety and Standard Act 2006 (Food safety and Standards Authority of India- FSSAI)

(ii) Milk and Milk Product Order, 1992.

(iii) Meat Food Product Order, 1973

(iv) Water (Prevention and Control of Pollution) Act 1974

(v) Air (Prevention and Control of Pollution) Act, 1981

(vi) Prevention of Food Adulteration Act, 1954

(vii) The Prevention of Cruelty to Animal Act, 1960

(viii) Export (Quality Control and Inspection) Act, 1963

(ix) Export (Quality Control and Inspection) Rules 1964

(x) Export of Raw Meat (Chilled/Frozen) Rules 1992

(xi) The Food Safety and Standards Authority of India (FSSAI) - Draft Safety Norms.

There is need for their harmonization so as to meet Codex standards.

Rules and Regulations for Export

The abattoirs and meat plants engaged in export production are required to be registered with APEDA, compulsory vide DGFT notification 12/(2004-

2005) dated 21st December, 2004. The plants are periodically inspected by a committee consisting of officials of various Government departments.

(a) Standards have been laid down for export of meat and meat products under Export (Quality Control and Inspection) Act, 1963. The export of Raw Meat (chilled and frozen) shall be allowed subject to the provision specified to the gazette notification on Raw Meat (chilled and frozen) under Export (Quality Control and Inspection) Act, 1963 in January, 1993. The notification lays down the Standards for abattoirs, meat processing plants and the products. Offal's too are subject to the same conditions of quality control and inspection.

(b) All consignments of Raw Meat (Chilled and Frozen) and export of canned meat products need to accompany with a Pre-shipment Inspection Certificate for which the Govt. has designated three agencies (i) All State Directorate of Animal Husbandry (ii) Export Inspection Agency (iii) Directorate of Marketing and Inspection, Government of India, to carry out the inspection in accordance with either the standards prevalent in the exporting country or standards prescribed under the Meat Food Products Order, 1973 under Export (Quality Control and Inspection) Act, 1963 or orders made there under.

(c) Export of meat and meat products will be allowed subject to the exporter furnishing a certificate to the customs at the time of export that the above items have been obtained/sourced from an abattoir/ meat processing plant registered with Agricultural and Processed Foods Products Export Development Authority (APEDA).

Export Policy

Export of Meat and Meat Products from India is, inter-alia, governed by the provisions of following Acts, Rules and Orders (Source: Indian Meat Industry: Red Meat Manual, APEDA) issued by Government of India:

(a) The Export (Quality Control And Inspection) Act, 1963;

(b) The Export of Raw Meat (Chilled/Frozen) (Quality Control And Inspection) Rules, 1992;

(c) Provision contained in Government of India Order issued vide S.O. 203, dated 15-01-1993;

(d) ITC (HS) Classification of Import and Export Items;

(e) Prevention of Cruelty Act, 1960 and Rules 2001;

(f) Various mandatory Indian Standards such as IS: 1982-1971: Code of Practice for Ante-mortem and Post-mortem Inspection of Meat Animals:

IS: 2537:1995: Meat and Meat Product-Beef and Buffalo Meat-Fresh, Chilled and Frozen-Technical Requirements; and Codex Alimentarius: Judgement Code for Slaughter Animals and Meat. There is need to have single window system for getting permission to set up the meat processing units.

The export of beef of cows, oxen and calf and offal's (includes heart, liver, tongue, kidneys and other organs) is prohibited and not permitted to be exported. Meat of buffalo (both male and female) and offal of buffalo except gonads and reproductive organs is free to export subject to the condition that exporter has to produce a certificate from the designated veterinary authority of the State, from which the meat or offals emanate, to the effect that the meat or offals are from buffaloes not used for breeding and milch purposes. The Quality control and inspection under (a) and (b) and (c) stipulated above under Rules & Regulations are required to be fulfilled. The meat and offal's of Indian sheep and goat is free for export subject to fulfilling the conditions (a) and (b) and (c) stipulated above.

Tallow, fat and/or oils of any animal origin excluding fish oil are prohibited for export.

Major bottlenecks in meat production and export

(i) Poor productivity of livestock

(ii) Livestock diseases

(iii) Hygiene and poor infrastructure

(iv) Food safety and traceability

(v) Least priority given by the states due to controversies involved with the subject.

Issues to be Addressed

- Country has made rapid strides in meat exports. On private sector we have modern integrated abattoirs where meat is produced adopting OIE guidelines and international quality standards for exports. State Government's need to take some bold decisions for modernization of municipal slaughterhouses as well others which caters to the need of domestic consumers. Environmental and animal rights issues through modernization of slaughter can be addressed more effectively. This will not only help in providing safe and wholesome meat to the meat eaters but also help in improving meat industry's image worldwide.
- The climate change and effect of biotic and abiotic stresses on livestock specially buffaloes production performances needs special attention for research.

- In most of the states only culled old and unproductive buffaloes are permitted to be slaughtered. It requires change in the state's bovine preservation policy so that such male calves when reared for meat purposes are allowed to be slaughtered.
- There is an urgent need for strengthening of quality testing and monitoring laboratories to carry out the testing and monitoring of meat and meat product samples for pesticide residues, toxic metals, veterinary drug residues and myco-toxins etc. More number of food and feed testing laboratories should be accredited with the laboratories of the developed countries to facilitate the export and build confidence among the meat exporters.
- To remain competitive in the world market, information about trade linked animal diseases, veterinary drug residues and other harmful residues in feed and products of animal origin, their maximum permissible limits set by Codex and consequences of their presence beyond permissible limits to human health, trade and industry needs to be disseminated to farmers, feed manufacturers, field veterinarians, animal product processors and the consumers by the States.
- The customs and regulatory mechanisms will require to be strengthened to check the flow of unwanted imported meat and meat products.
- The consumers needs to be educated through print and electronic media to remove their apprehensions about hygiene, sanitation and safety of meat and meat products and also importance of modernization of abattoirs in producing safe and wholesome meat and healthy environment.
- Processing of meat in to value added products, establishment of cold chains, modern storage facilities and packaging of products in durable and attractive packaging materials are the other important areas which will require greater attention by the industry in near future to meet the growing demand of quality ready-to-eat meat & meat products. Not more than 2% of the total meat produced is processed into value added meat products. Exports mainly comprise of chilled/frozen meats. The industry should seriously think of establishing backward linkages at primary livestock production level with the farmers and processing meat in to value added products to achieve real "pink" revolution.
- Industry should also think of playing a more active role in creation of more number of disease free zones, animal welfare issues, and the removal of deficiencies in the quality feed supply chain.

- There is no reputed manufacturer of meat processing equipments. Imported plants and machinery is subjected to import duty of 40-45 %.Waving off can reduce the cost of production.
- No taxes are imposed on fresh meat. For branded and packed meat products sales tax and excise duty is levied which needs to be exempted. The revenue Govt. gets from preparations of meat and marine products are not very high may be less than Rs 50.0 millions.
- There is need for harmonization of standards to meet the CODEX standards.

References

Agnihotri, M. K. and Rajkumar, (2008). Market trends in goat and sheep meat: national and international scenario. In: Small Ruminant Production in India. Karim, S.A., Tripathi, M.K. et al.(eds) Satish Serial Publishing House,Delhi.pp.423-434.

Agnihotri, M.K.,(2010).Meat Production, Export potential and SPS Measures. In: Climate Change and Stress management: Sheep and goat production. Karim, S.A., Joshi, Anil et al.(eds). Satish Serial Publishing House,Delhi.pp.643-650.

APEDA (2011). Agricultural and Processed Food Products Export Development Authority. Export Statistics 2011.Ministry of Commerce and Industry, Govt. of India, New Delhi.

Dastagiri, M.B. (2004). Demand and supply projections for livestock products in India. Policy Paper (21), National Centre for Agricultural Economics and policy Research (ICAR), New Delhi.pp.43.

FAO-STAT. (2007). www.fao.org.

□□□

10

Micronutrient as Immunomodulator in Poultry

R.P.S. BAGHEL AND ANKUR KHARE
Faculty of Veterinary Science and Animal Husbandry
Madhya Pradesh Pashu Chikitsa Vigyan Vishwavidyalaya, Jabalpur (M.P.)

Introduction

The role of nutrition in animal husbandry is not only for production or reproduction but also to minimize infectious diseases and their concomitant stresses. In context to Indian poultry industry, problem of immuno suppression has been felt very prominent due to various factors viz., managemental conditions, nutritional status, intensive production system, high density rearing and infectious diseases. Therefore, it is highly essential to find ways and means for enhancement of immune responses by nutritional manipulation. Further, as the use of antibiotics has been very limited, better use of supplementary immuno stimulatory nutrients has to be made in poultry feeding.

The bird's susceptibility to infectious challenges can be subdivided into two components, resistance and resilience. Resistance refers to the capacity of a variety of anatomical and physiological systems, including the immune system, to exclude pathogens. Resilience refers to the capacity of the bird to maintain productivity (e.g., growth, feed efficiency, egg production) during an infectious challenge. There are many situations in which diet that optimize resistance to infectious challenges are not optimal for resilience and maximal profitability (Klasing, 1997).

Nutrients which play important role in immunity include various amino acids, fatty acids, vitamins, minerals and other nutrients. Amino acids includes Glutamine, Arginine, Methionine, Isoleucine, Leucine and Valine whereas fatty acids includes á-linolenic acid and ã-linolenic acid while, vitamins includes â-carotene, Folic acid, Vitamin A, Vitamin B_{12}, Vitamin B_6, Vitamin C, Vitamin D, Vitamin E and minerals like Manganese, Iron, Selenium, Zinc and Copper. Some of the nutrients playing major role in immunity are described below:

Amino Acids and Immunity

Some of the amino acids which have very important role in the immune system are discussed below:

Arginine

Uricotelic species (i.e. birds) cannot synthesize arginine because they have an incomplete urea cycle. Identification of the arginine pathway that produces nitric oxide (Collier and Vallance, 1989) has led to research demonstrating that arginine is a potent immunomodulator. The nitric oxide has a potent role as tumriostatic (Hibbs *et al.*, 2003; Lepoivre *et al.*, 2005) and microbiostatic (Grager *et al.*, 1999; James *et al.*, 2000). It increases the production of macrophages (Sung *et al.*, 1991), improves the thymic weight and function, augments lymphocytes and macrophage functions and improves immunity against tumors and enhanced wound healing (Efron and Barbul, 1998; Evoy *et al.*, 1998). Effects of various ratio of arginine to lysine on body weight gain and mortality percentage is given in Table 1.

Table 1 : Impact of dietary arginine relative to dietary lysine on growth performance and mortality in 1-42 day old broiler chicks given a coccidia challenge at 28 day of age.

Arg:Lys	Weight gain (kg)	Mortality (%)
0.9 : 1	1.878	17.1[b]
1.1 : 1	1.964	17.9[b]
1.3 : 1	1.946	14.8[a]

Kidd *et al.* (2001) noted reduced mortality in mature broilers given a challenges of *Eimeria acervulina, Eimeria tenella* and *Eimeria maxima* when fed diets containing an Arg:Lys of 1.3:1 as compare to those birds receiving 0.9:1 or 1.1:1 Arg:Lys ratio in the diet.

Methionine

Methionine is the first limiting amino acid in practical chicken diet. The requirement of methionine according to NRC (1994) is 0.50%. It is important for proper functioning of the immune system and thymus cell proliferation (Lohakare *et al.*, 2005).

Liquid DL-Methionine hydroxy analogue free acid (MHA-FA) is a highly effective source of supplemental methionine (Richards *et al.*, 2005). MHA-FA is organic acid in nature so could lower the pH of the GIT and thus may suppress organic acid sensitive pathogenic bacteria, there by stimulating absorption of specific nutrients and enhances the immune response. Effect of various levels of methionine on antibody response is shown in Table 2.

Table 2 : Immune response of WL layer fed different levels of DLM and MHA-FA during summer 29°C-43°C.

Source	CBH*** response	SRBC titer (log2 value) (SRBC antigen) 32 weeks	40 weeks
DML*	1.91	7.5	8.04
MHA-FA**	1.98	7.54	8.08
Levels			
0.30	1.51[a]	6.88[a]	6.63[a]
0.36	2.15[b]	7.75[b]	8.75[b]
0.42	2.17[b]	7.93[b]	8.81[b]

DML* - DL-Methionine
MHA-FA** - Methionine hydroxy analogue free acids
CBH*** - Cutaneous basophil hypersensitivity test
SRBC - Sheep red blood cell antigen

Panda *et al.* (2007) compared MHA-FA to DLM as source of methionine and found both was equally effective in supporting immune competence. The immune response increased significantly, with increase in the concentration of methionine from 0.30 to 0.36% in diet indicating methionine requirement for immuno competence is higher.

Isoleucine

Isoleucine is categorized as a branched chain amino acid (BCAA). The BCAA consists of Valine, Isoleucine and leucine which are structurally related. Isoleucine is the most hydrophobic of the BCAA. It has been shown that a BCAA deficiency can significantly depress relative organ weights in chicken (Konashi *et al.*, 2000). Deficiency of BCAA caused the most severe decrease in thymus and bursa weights (Konashi *et al.*, 2000) compared with all other essential amino acids.

Glick *et al.* (1991, 1993) fed chicks at a diet deficient in all required amino acids and measured immune response of the chicks. Depressed delayed-type hypersensitivity responses and secondary IgG responses to Sheep Red Blood Cells (SRBC) were noted between adequately fed controls and deficient chicks. Different percent of Isoleucine and its effects on relative organ weight, is described in Table-3.

Table 3 : Impact of Isoleucine on relative lymphoid organ weight in 42 days old bird

Item	Bursa	Spleen (% of BW)	Thymus
Isoleucine (%)			
0.42	0.21	0.13	0.05
0.72	0.17	0.13	0.08+

Hale *et al.* (2004) fed broilers 0.42% isoleucine and observed reduced relative thymus weights (38% smaller in birds fed 0.72% Isoleucine). However, differences in relative bursa and spleen weights did not occur between Isoleucine treatments. Effect of Isoleucine on antibody response is described in Table-4.

Table 4 : Impact of isoleucine on cutaneous basophil hypersensitivity and primary antibody response to SRBC.

Item	Toe web swelling (mm)	Toe web swelling (%)	Titer
Isoleucine (%)			
0.42	0.17	15.3	8.43
0.50	0.23	18.9	6.93
0.58	0.33	27.7	9.93
0.66	0.32	24.8	8.33

Hale *et al.* (2004) also observed the impact of isoleucine on female broiler strain through cutaneous basophil hypersensitivity (CBH) test at day 38. The antibody titer increased as the isoleucine percent increased from 0.42-0.58 while, decreased on further increase in isoleucine percent.

Glutamine

Glutamine has long been recognized as an important metabolic fuel for the immune system (Ardawi *et al.*, 1985). Glutamine is primarily metabolized to generate energy for leukocytes, as well as reducing equivalents for synthesizing reactive oxygen intermediates (Newsholme, 2001). Glutamine can also be metabolized to arginine in murine macrophages and can spare arginine requirements for Nitric oxide (NO) synthesis (Murphy *et al.*, 1998). Since chicks lack the enzymes to synthesize arginine, glutamine cannot be metabolized to arginine, so this amino acid is likely to serves as an important energy substrate. In chicks, developing B and T cells express markers for glutamine utilization (Rudrappa *et al.*, 2007) suggests that this amino acid is used as an energy source to aid in the development of lymphocytes. Additionally, supplementing broiler diets with glutamine increased concentrations of serum IgA and IgG (Bartell *et al.*, 2007).

Polyunsaturated Acid (Pufa) and Immunity

Yang and Guo (2006) supplemented broiler birds with different sources of PUFA viz. fish oil, poultry oil and corn oil. The proportion of lymphocytes ($CD3^+$, $CD8^+$) of intestinal mucosa in corn oil group was higher on day 21 than that in fish oil group. The proportion of lymphocytes ($CD3^+$, $CD4^+$) of fish oil group was significantly higher on day 21, relative to poultry oil or corn oil group. The fish oil treatment enhanced the secretary immunoglobin A (sIgA) concentration in jejunum on d 42, compared with corn oil and poultry group. Fish oil and corn oil had similar effects on enhancing Interleukin-2 (IL-2) secretion of peripheral blood mononuclear cells (PBMC), and converse effects on IL-4 secretion. Compared with poultry oil group, chickens supplemented with fish oil or corn oil had greater concentration of intestinal mucosal membrane phospholipids on d 21 and d 42. In conclusion, Diet supplemented with corn oil or fish oil can affect cytokines secretion of PBMC in chickens, which works on systemic and mucosal immune response.

Vitamins and Immunity

Vitamins play an important role in immunity. Among various vitamins, vitamins which have important role in immunity are Vitamin A, Vitamin C and Vitamin E which are explained below.

Vitamin A

Vitamin A is also called infection resisting vitamin, because proper development of epithelium, Bursa of Fabricius and immunity is dependent on Vitamin A. Vitamin A in involved in the synthesis of muco-polysaccharides and mucus secretions in skin, deficiency of which causes atrophy of epithelial cells and keratinization which leads to the proliferation of infective layers of cells. Vitamin A maintains anatomical barriers of the body (non specific host responses). But once micro-organisms have penetrated this first line of defense Vitamin A plays a secondary role in systemic immune response (Davis and Sell, 1989).

It has a direct effect on immunoglobulin production by plasma cells (Friedman and Sklan, 1989). Some of the experiments showed the effect of vitamin A on fecal oocysts of *Eimeria acervulina* which is presented in Table 5.

Table 5 : Faecal oocyst (per kg BW) shed by birds infected with *Eimeria acervulina*

Diet	Total oocyst number (X 10^8)
Control	5.41±1.6
A-deficient	9.17±0.7

Control- 8000 I.U. Vit A/Kg of feed

Dalloul *et al.* (2002) inoculated birds with *Eimeria acervulina* on day 25, faecal samples collected on 6-9 days post inoculation. In Vitamin A deficient groups oocysts sheds were higher, indicating higher susceptibility of birds to parasite due to Vitamin A deficiency.

Friedman *et al.* (1990) divided the birds into two groups one as control i.e. normal vitamin A supplemented and another is vitamin A deficient. At 21 day age chicks were inoculated with 1x 10^9 CFU and 2x10^9 CFU *E. coli* and mortality was scored for 7 days. In this experiment, there was increased mortality in birds fed vitamin A deficient diet as compared to the control group (vitamin A- 0.85 mg/kg). Effect of Vitamin A on resistance of bird from *E. coli* is shown graphically (Figure 1).

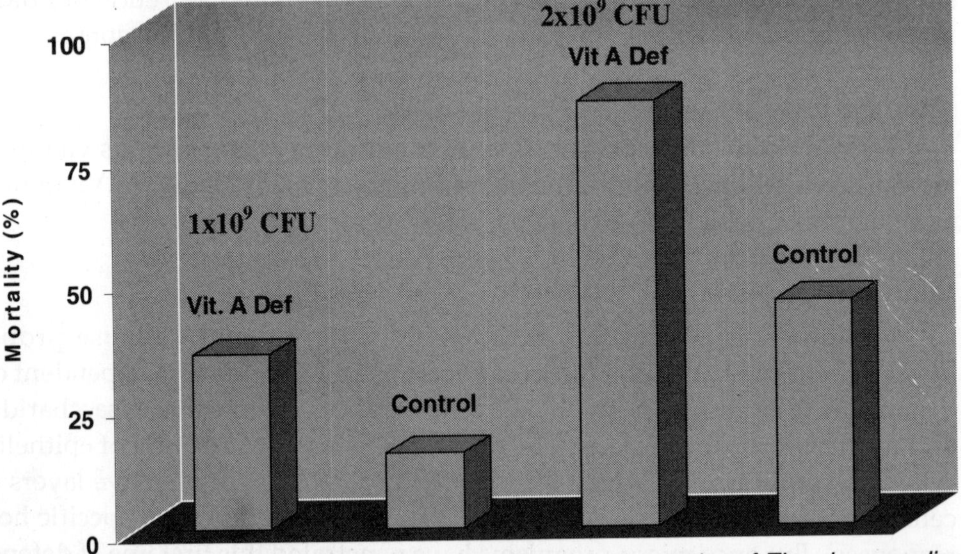

Fig. 1 : Mortality percentage in birds having two different concentration of *Eimeria acervulina* in Vitamin A deficient versus control.

Vitamin D

Vitamin D, whether from the diet or produced in the skin by irradiation of 7-dehydrocholestrol by ultra-violet light, is converted to its active hormonal form 1, 25-dehydroxycholcalciferol (1,25-$(OH)_2$ D_3 or calciterol) by two sequential hydroxylation reactions (Norman *et al.*, 1992). The first reaction occurs in the liver, forming 25-dehydroxycholecalciferol (25-$(OH)D_3$). Several studies have reported that the immune system of the chick, specifically monocyte and macrophage function, is negatively altered when diets are deficient in Vitamin D (Aslam *et al.*, 1998). It is also provided in the development of cell mediated immunity (CMI) in chicken through its role in the maturation and proper functioning of macrophages. Effect of Vitamin D on immune response of immune system and organ weight is explained in the Table-6 below.

Table 6 : Immune System response and weights of immune system organs

	Primary Antibody response			Secondary antibody response		
Antibody	Control	D def.	SEM	Control	D def.	SEM
Total	4.38	3.74	0.46	6.39	6.13	0.26
IgG	1.44	0.82	0.32	2.30	2.48	0.10
IgM	2.94	2.92	0.32	4.09	3.65	0.24

	Cutananeous basophil hypersensitivity response		
Time (h)	Control	D def	SEM
		Toe web swelling in mm	
20	0.84	0.52	0.069
24	0.78	0.49	0.054
28	0.77	0.42	0.050
		Organ weight at 24 day in gms	
Organs	Control	D def	SEM
Thymus	2.95	1.81	0.103
Bursa	2.60	1.88	0.153
Spleen	1.39	1.15	0.084

(NRC- 200 I.U./kg, control group- 800 I.U ./kg)

Aslam *et al.* (1998) observed that for the primary and secondary antibody responses, the total antibody titres, IgM and IgG were not different between the control and D deficient chicks. The response to Phytohemagglutinin-P (PHA-P) antigen by D deficient chicks was significantly depressed at each time period studied. The maximum cutaneous basophill hypersensitivity (CBH) response occurred at 20 hr after Phytohemagglutinin-P injection. At 20h, the average increase in interdigital thickness was 0.84 mm for the control group, compared to 0.52 mm for the deficient group. Thymus, spleen and bursa of fabricius weights were taken at 24 days of age. The vitamin D deficient chicks had significantly lower thymus weights than control group, whereas bursa and spleen weights were not different.

Vitamin E

Vitamin E is an immune booster. It is most likely that Vitamin E, like other nutritional factors, affects the development and maintenance of immunocompetence through multiple functions by acting directly on the immune cells or by indirectly altering metabolic and endocrine parameters, which in turn influence immune function (Gershwin *et al.*, 1985).

Although the mechanism of vitamin E is not fully understood, its bioactivity is mainly associated with its antioxidant activity. Vitamin E reduces free radical induced pathology during both normal metabolic states and inflammation. As a primary antioxidant of cell membranes, vitamin E is particularly important for the prevention of fatty acid peroxidation (Benedich, 1990). Fatty acids can act as immuno regulatory molecules that mediate cellular communication, membrane fluidity and second messenger elobration (Klasing, 1997; Watkins, 1991) and the effect of vitamin E on fatty acid stability may be immuno regulatory in itself. The standard vitamin E supplementation (16 mg Vitamin E/kg) was optimal for most aspects of macrophage functions. Effects of different concentration of vitamin E on the status of antioxidants and antibody response are described in Table 7.

Table 7 : Effects of supplemental Vit E on antioxidant status and immune response of heat stressed layers

	Supplementation of Vit E in diets (mg/kg)				
	5	25	125	250	500
Lipid peroxidase, nM/mg prot	1.92[c]	1.74[b]	1.66[a]	1.68[a]	1.66[a]
Catalase, K/g hb	222.7[a]	238.55[b]	252.8[c]	259.8[c]	252.6[c]
Glutathion peroxidase, unit/ml	219.5[a]	222.9[a]	246.9[ab]	236.9[b]	240.9[ab]
Antibody titer	4.9[a]	5.6[b]	6.3[c]	6.4[c]	6.3[c]

Panda *et al.* (2006) observed the effect of vitamin E on immune response and antioxidant status in heat stressed layer at different levels and find that the lipid peroxidase activity decreased while the activity of catalase and glutathione peroxidase increased by increasing the level of vitamin E from 5 to 125 mg/kg diet. No further improvement in the activity of antioxidant enzymes was observed by increasing concentration beyond 125 mg/kg diet.

Vitamin C

It is an anti stress vitamin. Corticosterone hormone which is released during stress is responsible for channeling of nutrients and body reserves away from economically important trait to vital physiological functions. Vitamin C functions metabolically to control the production of the corticosterone as a result restores some performance loss such as growth and immune response. This mechanism of effects is through inhibition of the 21-hydroxylase and 11-beta hydroxylase enzymes in the steroid biosynthetic pathway in the adrenal cortex. Vitamin C supplementation through the diet and water during periods of stress causes reduced synthesis of corticosterone (Brake, 1988). For the best result it should be given 24-48 hrs before stressful period. Effects of different levels of vitamin C supplementation on the proliferation of lymphocytes and on heterophill and lymphocytes ratio is described in Table 8 below.

Table 8 : Effect of supplemental vitamin C on lymphocyte proliferation assay and Heterophil:lymphocyte ratio during summer

	Control	Vitamin C (ppm)			
Time (hrs.)	0	10	50	100	200
24 h	2.45	2.48	2.39	2.45	2.50
48 h	2.08	1.91	2.16	2.13	2.13
72 h	2.18[ab]	1.90[c]	2.13[ab]	2.08[bc]	2.32[a]
H:L	0.425[a]	0.312[b]	0.370[ab]	0.394[a]	0.322[b]

Lohakare *et al.* (2005) studied the effect of supplemental vitamin C on lymphocytes proliferation and heterophill:lymphocytes (H:L) ratio and they observed that cell mediated immunity was increased at 200 ppm of vitamin C, and birds became resistant to infection. But no effect was noted at 24 and 48 hrs. Higher rates also lowered H:L ratio indicating reduction in heat stress as the experiment was carried out in summer.

Trace Minerals

The trace minerals that have been associated with an improvement in immunity are zinc, manganese, copper and selenium.

Selenium (Se)

Dietary Se interacts with vitamin E in antioxidant protection of cells because it is a component of glutathione peroxidase. In addition to antioxidant status, Se has been shown to impact diseases resistance. For example, broiler infected with *E. tenella* had improved resistance (i.e. reduced mortality and caecal lessions) when supplemented with selenium (Colnago *et al.*, 1994).

Effects of different levels of selenium with vitamin E on Haemagglutination inhibition (HI) titre and total immunoglobulin are shown in Table 9.

Table 9 : Effects of supplementing dietary vitamin E and selenium on HI titer and total immunoglobulin.

Vitamin E (mg/kg feed)	Selenium (mg/kg feed)		
	0	0.1	0.2
Log_2 HI titer			
0	4.00	4.00	4.00
100	4.75	5.75	6.75
200	5.50	6.25	7.50
Total Ig (g/dl)			
0	1.79[a]	1.81[a]	1.86[ab]
100	1.84[ab]	2.07[abc]	2.27[c]
200	1.87[ab]	1.98[abc]	2.20[bc]

Basal diet: Selenium-0.07 mg/kg diet, Vitamin E- 12.77 mg/kg of diet

Singh *et al.,* (2006) studied serum antibodies to NDV at 10 day post immunization and observed that vitamin E and Se were associated with an increase in HI titer. Maximum HI titre was obtained at 200 mg vitamin E and 0.2 mg Se. Se alone had no effect on HI titre. Maximum immunoglobulin was obtained with 100 mg vit. E and 0.2 mg Se. Recently, Khare and Baghel (2011) observed that the selenium @ 17.5 mg/Q of feed which was excess to the nutrient requirement (NRC, 1994), improved the performance as well as reduced the mortality percentage in the broiler birds from 0-6 weeks of age.

Zinc (Zn)

Zinc increases thrombocytes and peripheral T cell count, activity of natural killer cells and neutophills, macrophage and antibody production. The thymus synthesizes 9-amino acid peptide hormone, the thymulin, which is activated after having bound with zinc and this is required for T cell development. Enzymes like DNA and RNA polymerase are zinc containing enzymes which are necessary for T cell growth and multiplication. Supplementing zinc in the diet of broilers above 40 ppm (NRC, 1994) enhances antibody production (Stahl *et al.,* 1989). Bartlett and Smith (2003) performed an experiment to show the effect of three different levels of zinc on the antibody response against sheep red blood cell antigen and results are shown in Table 10.

Table 10 : Means of Anti SRBC antibody response of broiler fed different levels of zinc

Treatment	Primary Total Ab	IgM	IgG	Secondary Total Ab	IgM	IgG
Diet						
LZ (34 ppm)	3.76[c]	2.45[b]	1.31[b]	4.64[b]	1.44[b]	3.20[b]
AZ (68 ppm)	4.77[b]	2.92[b]	1.85[a]	6.50[a]	1.70[a]	4.80[a]
HZ (181 ppm)	5.80[a]	3.72[a]	2.08[a]	6.61[a]	1.86[a]	4.75[a]
Pooled SEM	0.16	0.17	0.13	0.24	0.12	0.21

Bartlett and Smith (2003) observed that average Zn (AZ) and high Zn (HZ) were similar with higher response for secondary challenge. Response of abdominal exudate cell and macrophage percent by three different levels of zinc is shown in Table 11.

Table 11 : Incidence of macrophage in abdominal exudate cell of broiler fed different levels of zinc under thermoneutral and heat stressed conditions.

Diet	Temperature	AEC (10^6)	Macrophages (%)
LZ	TN	5.38	95.22
	HS	5.91	92.40
AZ	TN	7.77	93.75
	HS	7.10	94.29
HZ	TN	8.09	95.86
	HS	9.64	94.93
Pooled SEM		1.10	0.53

HZ is 57% more than LZ

Abdominal exudate cell (AEC) was highest in HZ diet, which indicates Zn is important in maintaining integrity of the cells of the innate immune system. The number of AEC was not affected by Heat stress.

Shrivastava (2011) supplemented broiler birds with different concentration of zinc oxide in the diet and observed significant increase in WBC count in the group of broilers fed 80 ppm of zinc oxide in comparison to control (i.e. devoid of zinc supplementation). Weight of the spleen was also significantly higher in this group.

Copper (Cu)

Copper functions in the immune system through different ways like energy production, neutrophill production and activity, antioxidant enzyme production, development of antibodies and lymphocyte replication (Niederman *et al.*, 1994). The importance of copper for maintaining the functions of the immune system has been demonstrated in several studies. Copper containing ceruloplasmin serves as a protective antioxidant and is a necessary component of the acute phase response. The quantity of copper required to sustain this role is large relative to other function of copper (Butcher and Miles, 2002). Copper deficiency reduces the amount of ceruloplasmin which is released during an inflammatory stress (DeSilvestro and Marten, 1990). Percival (1998) described the effect of copper on the ceruloplasmin activity in adult broiler bird (Table 12).

Table 12 : Indicators of copper status in copper adequate and copper deficient birds

	Copper adequate	Copper def.	P value
Plasma copper (μmol/L)	12.0±4.2	1.22±0.71	<0.0001
Ceruloplasmin activity (μ/L)	17.08±4.52	0.16±0.31	<0.0001
Bone marrow Cu/Zn SOD	1533.4±384.1	934.7±271.5	0.022
Leukocyte Cu/Zn SOD	122.7±29.8	44.5±17.7	0.005

Cu/Zn superoxide dismutase (SOD) activity is expressed in μ/mg cell protein where 1 unit=50% inhibition of the oxidation rate of pyrogallol.

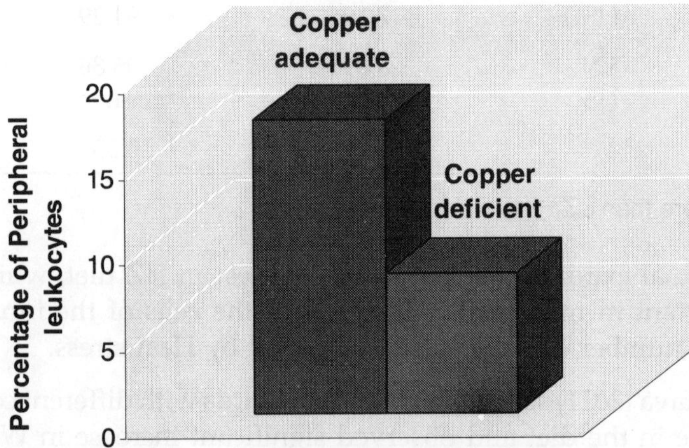

Fig. 2 : Percentage of peripheral leukocytes in relation to the copper adequate and copper deficient groups.

Manganese (Mn)

Manganese needs by the gastrointestinal tract, lungs and several other tissue in the birds are increased during an immune response. It serves as a cofactor of superoxide dismutase and ameliorates damage induced by the immune response itself. However, there is very little change in the circulating manganese levels in the plasma during stress (Klasing *et al.*, 1991). Virden *et al.* (2004) performed an experiment to describe the effect of different levels of manganese and zinc on different organ weights in 15 day old broiler breeder and is presented in Table 13.

Table 13 : Organ weight of 15 day old broiler breeder fed diets differing in Zn and Mn level sources.

Treatment	Bursa (%)	Thymus (%)	Spleen (%)
Control	0.13	0.12	0.11
Zn-Mn*	0.15	0.18	0.10
Zn-Mn**	0.12	0.16	0.10
Zn-Mn***	0.13	0.17	0.10
SEM	0.01	0.01	0.01

Bursa, thymus and spleen are expressed relative to BW
Control- Control diet containing 75mg/kg Zn and 83 mg/kg Mn.
* - Control plus 75mg/kg Zinc from Zinc sulfate and 80 mg/kg Manganese from Manganese Sulfate.
** - Control plus 75mg/kg Zinc from Zinc amino acid complex Availa Zinc and 80 mg/kg Manganese from Manganese Sulfate.
*** - Control plus 75mg/kg Zinc from Zinc amino acid complex Availa Zinc and 80 mg/kg Manganese from Manganese amino acid complex Availa Manganese.

Virden *et al.* (2004) observed that the weight of the spleen was constant in all the experimental diets while the weight of the bursa and thymus increase when the Zn-Mn diet is supplemented while it reduces afterwards.

Iron (Fe)

The role of iron in immunity can be appreciated by the sudden fall in iron concentration in the serum during the early phase of infection. Iron supplementation has been shown to increase the bactericidal activity of the macrophages in the liver and spleen of affected chicks. The survival rate increased in chicks inoculated with *Salmonella gallinarum* with additional supplementation of 100mg/kg iron in diets containing 200 mg/kg iron (Rao *et al.*, 2004).

Synergistic Effects of Micronutrients on Immunity

Vitamin E and Vitamin C

Nameghi *et al.* (2007) studied the effect of different levels of dietary vitamin E (0,50, 75 IU/ kg diets) and L-Ascorbic acid (0,500 and 1000 ppm in drinking water) in immune response of broilers birds. Immunity was assessed as antibody production to infectious bronchitis virus (IBV), New castle disease virus (NDV) and Sheep red blood cell antigen (SRBC). Chickens were inoculated (18 day) intramuscular with 0.5 ml of 5% SRBC. The injection of SRBC was repeated 12 day later. Lymphoid organ weights and antibody titer for primary and secondary response to SRBC were increased by 50 IU/kg Vit. E. Humoral immunologic response showed that antibody titer against NDV and IBV were highest in groups receiving 75 IU/kg diet Vit. E.

Adding 1000 ppm vitamin C in drinking water significantly increased antibody response to SRBC. Secondary response to SRBC, antibody titer to NDV and IBV were improved by supplemented 500 ppm Vit. C in drinking water. Optimum growth and humoral immune response may be achieved at supplemental level of Vitamin E of 50 IU/kg and Vitamin C at 50 ppm.

Vitamin C and Vitamin D

Lohakare *et al.* (2005) supplemented vitamin C at 0 or 200 mg/kg on the performance of commercial broilers fed vitamin D levels as per NRC recommendations (200 IU) or as per the levels followed in the commercial vitamin premixes (1,800 IU). Antibody titers to SRBC, cutaneous basophilic hypersensitivity response to phytohemagglutinin-P (Ph-P), and heterophil:lymphocyte (H:L) ratio did not show any difference within groups given supplemental Vit. C or Vit. D. It was concluded that the Vit. D levels as suggested by NRC (200 IU) promoted better performance of commercial broilers than 1,800 IU and that supplementing Vit. C at 200 mg/kg improved the performance under commercial growing conditions (Table 14).

Table 14 : Effects of vitamins C and D on antibody titres to SRBC and (H:L) Ratio

Parameter	0 mg/kg Vit C		200 mg/kg Vit. C	
	200 IU/kg Vit. D	1800 IU/kg Vit. D	200 IU/kg Vit. D	1800 IU/kg Vit. D
Anti-SRBC titers	236.67	93.33	128.33	330.0
H:L	0.313	0.280	0.297	0.310
TI*	0.168	0.274	0.199	0.169

*Thickness index: the thickness of the injected region at wattle was measured prior to injection and 24 h after injection using vernier calipers. The TI was calculated as (right wattle thickness due to phytohemagglutinin-P at 24 h post inoculation/corresponding right wattle thickness before inoculation)

There was no significant change on the H: L ratio and anti SRBC titres when vitamin D was supplied with or without vitamin C.

Vitamin E and Selenium

Vitamin E and Se play an important role in protecting against oxidative damage. Free radicals are scavenged by vitamin E as a first line of defense and then glutathione peroxidase of which Se is a part destroys any peroxides formed before they can damage the cell. Nutritional deficiencies of vitamin E or Se or both impair immune function as measured by humoral response to sheep red blood cells in young chicks. Se supplementation in its own was found less effective (Table 15).

Table 15 : Effect of supplementation of Vit E and / or Se on humoral immune response in commercial broilers.

Vitamin E (IU/ kg)	Selenium(mg/kg)		Ab titres (log_2) to				
	(I)	(O)	NDV		SRBC		
			28d	42d	5DPI	10DPI	15DPI
0	0	0	3.33^{b}	4.00^{d}	3.87^{c}	2.87^{b}	1.88^{c}
0	0.15	0	4.00^{ab}	4.33^{cd}	5.12^{b}	4.38^{a}	2.75^{b}
0	0	0.15	4.33^{ab}	4.67^{cd}	5.50^{ab}	4.25^{a}	2.88^{b}
150	0	0	4.33^{ab}	5.33^{abcd}	6.13^{ab}	4.63^{a}	3.00^{b}
300	0	0	4.00^{ab}	4.67^{cd}	5.75^{ab}	4.50^{a}	3.13^{ab}
150	0.15	0	4.67^{ab}	6.33^{ab}	6.38^{ab}	4.75^{a}	3.50^{ab}
300	0.15	0	4.00^{ab}	5.00^{bcd}	5.63^{ab}	4.75^{a}	3.25^{ab}
150	0	0.15	5.00^{a}	6.67^{a}	6.88^{a}	4.50^{a}	3.88^{a}
300	0	0.15	4.33^{ab}	5.66^{abc}	6.13^{ab}	4.63^{a}	3.38^{ab}

Shaik *et al.* (2005) supplemented two levels of Vit.E (150 and 300 IU/kg), two sources of Se (inorganic and organic each at 0.15 mg/kg) and their combinations. Cell mediated immune (CMI) response was significantly higher on Se diets, Vit.E at 150 IU/kg and the combination of Vit. E at 300 IU/kg with either of the sources of Se. Vit. E at 300 IU/kg lowered the H:L ratio while it increased the ratio when supplemented along with either of the sources of Se. The humoral immune response to SRBC was significantly higher on all experimental diets than reference. Vit. E or the sources of Se did not influence immune response to NDV. However, the combination of organic Se with either levels of Vit. E significantly increased immune response. It was concluded that Vit. E at 150 IU/kg and organic Se at 0.15 mg/kg may be supplemented to broiler diets for efficient immune response.

Arginine and Vitamin E

Abdukalykova and Feria (2006) supplemented 2 levels of arginine i.e. normal (NARG, 1.2% in the feed) and high (HARG, additional 0.3% ARG in the drinking water); and 3 levels of vitamin E (VE) (40, 80, and 400 IU / kg feed). Humoral immunity was measured as antibody responses to an I/P injection of sheep red blood cells (SRBC, 10% solution) at d 25 followed by agglutination assay. 4 d after SRBC injection the antibody titers were higher in HARG than in NARG birds, and in birds supplemented VE-80. Birds fed HARG showed a higher response than NARG birds, but after a second exposure, ARG levels did not have a significant effect. Birds fed VE-400 had a lower response to PHA than birds fed VE-40 and VE-80 birds at d 41. These results show that high levels of ARG accelerate antibody production whereas VE at 80 IU kg / feed maintains a proper immune function over time, suggesting that ARG and VE may have complimentary effects on the immune function and health of broiler chickens.

Zinc and Methionine

Moghaddam and Jahanian (2009) fed broiler chicks with different levels of organic zinc (zinc-methionine) supplementation to investigate partial or complete substitution of the organic zinc source for inorganic ones on the development of lymphoid organs and immunological responses. Dietary treatments consisted of two basal diets supplemented with 40 mg/kg added zinc as Zn sulfate or Zn oxide in which, Zn was replaced with zinc-methionine (ZnMet) complex at the levels of 25, 50, 75 or 100%. Among lymphoid organs, only thymus weight was affected by dietary treatments. The 10 days of age-assessed cutaneous hypersensitivity reaction was stronger in chicks fed ZnMet-containing diets. Dietary ZnMet supplementation caused an increase in proportion of lymphocytes and consequently a decrease in heterophil to lymphocyte (H:L) ratio. Diet fortification by zinc-methionine complex increased Newcastle antibody titer at 19 days of age. Also, a similar response was observed in antibody titers at 6 and 12 d after infectious bronchitis vaccine administration. At d 12 after vaccination, ZnMet-fortified diets improved antibody titer against IBDV. From the present findings, it can be concluded that dietary supplementation with organic zinc improves both cellular and humoral immune responses. It is necessary to replace 75% of supplemental inorganic zinc with organic ZnMet complex to achieve the optimum immunological responses in broiler.

Conclusion

Profitable poultry production needs better health status and livability of the birds. Problem of immuno suppression has been a problem in poultry with the increase in their production potential. Nutrients have been found to play important role in immunity. These include various amino acids (glutamine, arginine, methionine, isoleucine, leucine and valine), fatty acids (á-linolenic acid and γ-linolenic acid), vitamins (β-carotene, folic acid, vitamin A, vitamin B_{12}, vitamin B_6, vitamin C, vitamin D, vitamin E) and minerals (manganese, iron, selenium, zinc and copper) Table 16.

Table 16 : Influence of partial or complete substitution of zinc-methionine (ZnMet) for dietary inorganic zinc sources on antibody titers against Newcastle (log_2), Infectious bronchitis (IB) and Infectious bursal disease (IBD) viruses

Sources and levels of inorganic Zinc		Zn-Met	Newcastle	Infectious Bronchitis (IB)		Infectious bursal diseases (IBD)	
				6 dpi	12 dpi	6 dpi	12 dpi
Zinc	100	-	3.86	3.36	3.15	3.51	3.22
Sulfate	75	25	3.94	3.44	3.23	3.44	3.16
	50	50	4.21	3.33	3.31	3.55	3.23
	25	75	4.12	3.58	3.49	3.51	3.39
Zinc	100	-	4.05	3.41	3.11	3.41	3.21
oxide	75	25	4.01	3.39	3.16	3.45	3.18
	50	50	4.31	3.56	3.42	3.45	3.20
	25	75	4.45	3.79	3.60	3.52	3.43
	-	100	4.64	3.73	3.62	3.47	3.38

dpi: days post inoculation

Arginine through nitric oxide produced in the arginine pathway has potent role as tumriostatic and microbiostatic. While, methionine is needed for proper functioning of immune system and thymus cell proliferation. Similarly, isolucine is important for maintaining the thymus and bursa weights. Glutamine acts as an important metabolic fuel for the immune system and its supplementation increases the concentrations of serum IgA and IgG

Corn oil or fish oil can affect cytokines secretion of PBMC in chickens, which works on systemic and mucosal immune response. While, Vitamin A maintains anatomical barriers of the body and also A plays a secondary role in systemic immune response. Vitamin D has a direct effect on immunoglobulin production by plasma cells immune system of the chick, specifically monocyte and macrophage. Effect of vitamin E on fatty acid stability may be immuno regulatory in itself. While, vitamin C functions metabolically to control the production of the corticosterone as a result restores some performance loss such as growth and immune response.

Dietary Se interacts with vitamin E in antioxidant protection of cells because it is a component of glutathione peroxidase. Zinc increases thrombocytes and peripheral T cell count, activity of natural killer cells and neutophills, macrophage and antibody production. Copper functions in the immune system through different ways like energy production, neutrophill production and activity, antioxidant enzyme production, development of antibodies and lymphocyte replication It serves as a cofactor of superoxide dismutase and ameliorates damage induced by the immune response itself.

Thus, most of these nutrients play very important role as immunomodulator in poultry and their concentration in the diet should be on the higher side.

References

Abdukalykova, S. and C. Ruiz-Feria (2006). Arginine and vitamin E improve the cellular and humoral immune response of broiler chickens. *Int. J. Poult. Sci.*, 5(2): 121-127.

Ardawi, M.S. and E.A. Newsholme (1985). Metabolism in lymphocytes and its importance in the immune response. *Essays Biochem.*, 21:1-44.

Aslam, S.M., J.D. Garlich, and M.A. Qureshi (1998). Vitamin D deficiency alters the immune response of broiler chicks. *Poult. Sci.*, 77: 842-849.

Bartell, S.M. and A.B. Batal (2007). The effect of supplemental glutamine on growth performance, development of the gastrointestinal tract, and humoral immune response of broilers. *Poult. Sci.*, 86:1940-1947.

Barlett, J.R. and M.O. Smith (2003). Effects of different level of zinc on the performance and immunocompetence of broilers under heat stress. *Poult. Sci.*, 82:1580-1588.

Benedich, A. (1990). Antioxidant vitamins and their function in immune response. Advances in Experimental Medicine and Biology, Vol. 262. Plenum Press, New York., pp. 35–55.

Brake, J.T. (1988). Stress of birds, modern poultry management relationship defined. *Poultry Digest*, pp. 226-231.

Butcher., G. D and R. D. Miles (2002). Interrelationship of Nutrition and Immunity *http://edis.ifas.ufl.edu.*

Collier, J. and P. Vallance (1989). Second messenger role for NO widens to nervous and immune systems. *Trends Pharmacol.Sci.*, 10: 427–431.

Colnago, G.L., L.S. Jensen and P.L. Long (1984). Effect of selenium and vitamin E on the development of immunity to coccidiosis in chickens. *Poult. Sci.*, 63:1136.

Dalloul, R.A., H.S. Lillehoj, T.A. Shellem and J.A. Doerr (2002). Effect of Vitamin A deficiency on host intestinal immune response to *Eimeria acervulina* in Broiler chickens. *Poult. Sci.*, 81:1509-1515.

Davis, C. Y. and J. L. Sell (1989). Immunoglobulin concentrations in serum and tissues of vitamin A-deficient broiler chicks after Newcastle disease virus vaccination. *Poult. Sci.*, 68:136–144.

DeSilvestro, R. A. and J. T. Marten (1990). Effects of inflammation and copper intake on rat liver and erythrocyte Cu-Zn superoxide dismutase activity levels. *J. Nutr.*, 120:1223-1227.

Efron, D. T. and A. Barbul (1998). Modulation of inflammation and immunity by arginine supplements. *Curr. Opin. Clin. Nutr. Metab. Care*, 1: 531–538.

Evoy, D., M. D., Lieberman, T. J. Fahey and J. M. Daly (1998). Immunonutrition: The role of arginine. *Nutrition*, 14:611–617.

Friedman, A. and D. Sklan (1989). Impaired T lymphocyte immune response in vitamin A depleted rats and chicks. *Br. J. Nutr.*, 62:439–449.

Friedman, A., A. Meidovsky, G. Lettner and D. Sklan (1990). Decreased resistence and immune response to E.Coli infection in chicks with low and high intakes of Vit. A. *J. Nutr. & Immuno.*, 61:395-400.

Gershwin, M., R. Beach and L. Hurley (1985). The potent impact of nutritional factors on immune response. Nutrition and Immunity. Academic Press, New York, pp:1–7.

Grager, D.L., J.B. Hibbs, J.R. Perfect and D.T. Durack (1999). Metabolic fate of L-argenine in relation to microbiostatic capability of murine macrophage. *J. Clin. Invest.*, 85: 264-280.

Glick, B., E. J. Day and D. Thompson (1991). Calorie-protein deficiencies and the immune response of the chicken. I. Humoral immunity. *Poult. Sci.*, 60:2494–2500.

Glick, B., R. L. Taylor, D. E. Martin, M. Watabe, and E. J. Day (1993). Calorie protein deficiencies and the immune response of the chicken II. Cell mediated immunity. *Poult. Sci.*, 62:1889–1893.

Hale, L.L., G. T. Pharr, S. C. Burgess, A . Corzo and M. T. Kidd (2004). Isoleucine Needs of Thirty- to Forty-Day-Old Female Chickens: Immunity. *Poult. Sci.* 83:1979–1985.

Hibbs, J.B., R.R. Traintor and Z. Vavrin (2003). Macrophage cytotoxicity: role for L-argenine deaminase and imino nitrogen oxidation to nitrite. *J. immunol.*, 138:1979–1985.

James, S.L. and J. Glaven (2000). Macrophage toxicity against schistosoma masoni involves arginine dependent production of reactive nitrogen intermediates. *J. Immunol.*, 143:4208-4218.

Khare, A. and R.P.S. Baghel (2011). Effect of different levels of dietary selenium on growth performance and nutrient utilization of broiler birds. *Vety. World*, 4(4):173-175.

Kidd, M. T., S.K. Peeble, S. K. Whitmarsh, J. B. Yeatman and Jr. Wideman (2001). Growth and immuniy of broiler chicks as affected by dietary Arginine. *Poult. Sci.*, 80:1535-1542.

Klasing, D. C., B. J. Johnstone and B. N. Benson (1991). Implications of an immune response on growth and nutrient requirements of chicks. *In:* Recent Advances in Animal Nutrition (Haresign, W., Cole, D. J. A., ed), Butterworth Heinemann.

Klasing, K. C. (1997). Interaction between nutrition and infectious disease. *In*: Diseases of Poultry, B. W. Calnek, edn. Iowa State University Press, Ames, IA. Pp. 73–80.

Konashi, S., K. Takahashi and Y. Akiba (2000). Effects of dietary essential amino acid deficiencies on immunological variables in broiler chickens. *Br. J. Nut.*, 83:449–456.

Lepovire, M., H. Boubid and J.F. Petit (2005). Antiproliferative activity of gamma interferon combined with lipopolysaccharide on murine adenocarcinoma: dependence on an L-arginine metabolism with production of nitrite and citrulline. *Cancer Res.*, 49: 1970-1989.

Lohakare, J.D., M.H. Ryu, T.W. Hawn, J.K. Lee and B.J. Chae (2005). Effects of supplemental ascorbic acid on the performance and immunity of commercial broilers. *Poult. Sci.*, 82: 990-999.

Lohakare, J.D., M.H. Ryu, T.W. Hawn, J.K. Lee and B.J. Chae (2005). Effects of Vitamin C and Vitamin D Interaction on the Performance, Immunity, and Bone Characteristics of Commercial Broilers. *J. Appl. Poult. Res.*, 14:670–678.

Moghaddam, H.N. and R. Jahanian (2009). Immunological responses of broiler chicks can be modulated by dietary supplementation of Zinc-methionine in place of inorganic zinc sources. *Asian-Aust. J. Anim. Sci.*, 22(3): 396–403.

Murphy, C. and P. Newsholme (1998). Importance of glutamine metabolism in murine macrophages and human monocytes to L-arginine biosynthesis and rates of nitrite or urea production. *Clinical Science*. 95: 397-407.

Munir, K., M. A. Muneer, E. Masaoud, A. Tiwari, A. Mahmud, R. M. Chaudhry, and A. Rashid (2009). Dietary arginine stimulates humoral and cell-mediated immunity in chickens vaccinated and challenged against hydropericardium syndrome virus. *Poult. Sci.*, 88:1629–1638.

Nameghi, A.H.., H.N. Moghaddam, J.T. Afshari and H. Kermanshahi (2007). Effects of vitamin E and C supplementation on performance and immune response of broiler chicks. *J. Anim & Vety. Adv.*, 6(9): 1060-1069.

Newsholme, P. (2001). Why is L-glutamine metabolism important to cells of the immune system in health, postinjury, surgery or infection. *Journal of Nutrition*. 131:2515S-2522S.

Norman, A.W., J. Roth and L. Orci (1992). The vitamin D endocrine system: steroid metabolism, hormone receptor receptors, and biological response (calcium binding protein). *Endocr. Rev.*, 3(4): 331-366.

National Research Council (1994). Nutrient Requirements of Poultry. 9th edn. Washington, DC, National Academy research. Press. 27–31.

Niederman, J., K. Timberly and N. Jo (1994). Role of copper in cell mediated and humoral immunity. *Poult. Sci.*, 85:836-837.

Panda, A.K., M.V.L.N.Raju and S.V. Rama Rao (2006). Effect of vitamin E on laying bird under heat stress. *Asian-Aust. J. Anim Sci.*, 4:827-835.

Panda, A.K., S.V. Rama rao, M.V.L.N. Raju and S.K. Bhanja (2007). Relative performance and response in White Leghorn Layer fed liquid Dl-methionine Hydroxy Analogue and DL-methionine. *Asian Aust. J. Anim. Sci.*, 6:948-953.

Percival, S.S. (1998). Copper and immunity. *Am. J. Clin. Nutr.*, 67: 1064S-1068S.

Rao, S.V.R., M.V.L.N. Raju and D. Nagalakshmi (2004). Nutritional modulations to enhance immunity in chickens. *Poultry International*, 24-29.

Richards, J.D., C.A. Atwell, M. Vaqueez-Anon, and J.J. Dibner (2005). Comparative in vitro and in vivo absorption of 2-hydroxy-4 methylthio butanoic acid and methionine in the broiler chicken. *Poult. Sci.*, 54: 324-327.

Rudrappa, S.G. and B.D. Humphrey (2007). Energy metabolism in developing chicken lymphocytes is altered during the embryonic to posthatch transition. *J Nutr.*,137: 427-432.

Shaik, A., K.K. Reddy, R.V. Eswaraiah, A. Nageswara Rao and M.V.L.N. Raju (2005). Effect of supplementation of vitamin E and Selenium on the growth and immune response in broilers. *Indian J Poult Sci.*.,40(3):235-240.

Shrivastava, R. (2011). Effect of varying levels of zinc through different sources on the growth performance nutrient utilization and carcass traits of broilers. MVSc & A.H. Thesis M.P.P.C.V.V.

Singh, H., S Sodhi and R. Kaur (2006). Effects of dietary supplements of selenium, vitamin E or combinations of two on antibody responses of broilers. *Br. Poult. Sci.*, 47(6): 714-719.

Stahl, J. L., J. L. Greger and M. E. Cook (1989). Zinc, copper, and iron utilization by chicks fed various concentration of zinc. *Br. Poult. Sci.*, 30: 123–134.

Sung, Y., J. H. Hotchkiss, R. E. Austic and R. R. Dietert (1991). L-Arginine depenedent production of a reactive nitrogen intermediate by macrophages of a uricotelic species. *J. Leukocyte Biol.*, 50: 49–56.

Virden, W.S., J.B. Yeatman, S.J. Barber, T.L. Ward, and M.T. Kidd (2004). Immune system and cardiac functions of progeny chicks from dams fed diet differing in zinc and manganese level and source. *Poult. Sci.*, 83: 344-351.

Yang, X. and Y. Guo (2006). Modulation of intestinal mucosal immunity by dietary polyunsaturated fatty acids in chickens. *Food and Agricultural Immunology*, 17(2): 129-137.

Watkins, B. A. (1991). Importance of essential fatty acids and their derivatives in poultry. *J. Nutr.*, 121:1475–1485.

□□□

11

Breeding Policy and Action Plan for the Genetic Improvement of Cattle and Buffaloes of Chhattisgarh

MOHAN SINGH AND ANJALI SINGH
Department of Animal Genetics & Breeding, College of Veterinary Sci. & A.H., Anjora, Durg

Introduction

More than 90% of cattle and buffaloes of Chhattisgarh are of non-descript type. They have late maturity, shorter lactation length, poor milk production potential and longer calving interval, as compared to well known exotic dairy breeds and their crossbreds though they have an excellent capacity of heat tolerance, disease resistance and can thrive well under adverse conditions of feeding and management. The animals of Chhattisgarh state, particularly in rural areas, do not get adequate amount of feed and fodder. The nutritional requirements of the animals with respect to energy, protein, minerals and vitamins, are not fulfilled. Paddy straw forms the main source of staple fodder which is poor in carbohydrate and protein content. Moreover, due to high oxalate content it causes other health problems.

The main reasons for the poor productive and reproductive performance of the non-descript animals of Chhattisgarh are poor genetic potential coupled with inadequate feed and fodder availability, both, in quantity and quality, and also inadequate management and health care. According to a rough estimate, by improving the feeding conditions alone, the performance of the animals can be doubled but it can not go beyond the limit imposed by the genetic makeup of the animals. Moreover, the improvement thus effected, would be temporary in nature and, being non genetic, would not pass on to the progeny. Thus, to realize the sustainable enhancement in the productivity of animals, their very genetic constitution has to be changed by adopting proper breeding methods.

Objectives of Cattle and Buffalo domestication in Chhattisgarh

Before formulating any breeding policy it is imperative to understand the needs of the stakeholders and define the objectives. The animal husbandry in Chhattisgarh is a subsidiary occupation with agriculture being the main occupation of the farmers. To a large extent, it is in the hands of small and marginal farmers. The agriculture and animal husbandry complement each other in various ways. The objectives of cattle and buffalo rearing are different in rural and urban areas. In rural areas, the main purpose of cattle domestication is bullock production for various agricultural operations and transport. Milk is required only to meet the routine household needs. Commercial milk production is extremely rare in rural areas. Apart from that the dried cakes of cow dung form the main source of fuel. The surplus cow dung is used for preparation of organic manure. The rural farmers can not afford the high inputs required for sustaining the high production level of the exotic dairy breeds or their crosses. Therefore, in rural areas, the policy should be to produce dual purpose animals producing moderate amount of milk , say 6-8 liters per day, and at the same time generating powerful bullocks needed for various agricultural operations. In urban areas, on the other hand, the main purpose of the cattle and buffalo rearing is commercial milk production. Here, the farmers can afford high inputs required for maintaining high producing animals. Therefore, the breeding policies for the rural and urban areas should be framed to meet the objectives of the two areas.

Breeding policy for Cattle

A) For Rural Areas

As stated earlier, the objective of breeding policy in rural areas is to produce animals with moderate milk production potential (6-8 lit. per day) and bullocks required for various agricultural operations. The farmers can not afford to bear the high costs involved in the feeding, breeding, management and health care of crossbreds. Therefore, the most suitable breeding policy for the rural areas would be *Upgrading of local non-descript animals with Indian Dairy breeds.* Upgrading means mating the non-descript or graded females with bulls of a pure Indian dairy breed generation after generation. After 5-6 generations, the non descript females will almost be transformed into the improver breed. The upgrading has the following advantages over the crossbreeding.

Advantages of Grading up over exotic cross breeding

1. There is no restriction with regard to the level of inheritance of the improver breed. No problem, even if it goes up to 100%. On the other hand, there is linear increase in the performance of the graded animals with the increase in the level of the improver breed. In case of exotic crossbred, the level of exotic inheritance beyond 62.5% poses adaptability problem especially in rural areas.
2. The males as well as females, both are useful to the farmer. Males can be used as bullocks for cultivation whereas females will be better milk producer. The crossbred males, on the other hand, are not fit for agricultural purpose.
3. There is no adaptability problem with the graded animals. Feeding, management and health care do not necessitate special attention. It is almost the same as for the non descript animals. Graded animals with indigenous dairy breeds possess better immunity to diseases.
4. The performance of the graded animals is in no way inferior to the exotic crossbreds provided the bulls are of similar genetic merit.
5. The fat % in the milk of the graded cows will be higher than that in the milk of crossbred cows.

Choice of Breed for grading up

Any one of the below listed indigenous dairy breeds can be used for grading up-

1. Sahiwal
2. Red Sindhi
3. Gir
4. Tharparkar.

Ongole breed may also be used in Bastar region that forms border with Andhra Pradesh.

Though the choice of breed should be left on the farmers, however, it would be practically desirable not to use both, Sahiwal and Red Sindhi in the same region. Otherwise, problems may arise in distinguishing two kinds of graded animals. It is statistically desirable to replicate all the breeds in all the regions so that the comparative study could be made with regard to the growth, reproduction, production and adaptability of different genetic groups, viz- Sahiwal x local, Red Sindhi x local, Gir x local and Tharparkar x local. This will enable to determine the regionwise breed suitability and refining of the future breeding policy.

B. Cattle Breeding Policy For Urban Areas

In urban areas, cows and buffaloes are reared by the dairy owners for milk production on a commercial scale. For this, they need animals with high milk production potential. The dairy owners can afford the inputs in terms of feed and fodder, management and health care to sustain the high production level. To achieve this goal, the following breeding plan can be adopted

1. Hybridization with exotic dairy breeds to produce F_1 generation. For this either Jersey or Holstein Friesian breed can be used.
2. The F_1 generation should be bred with the bulls of Indian diary breeds to produce the II generation. For This, The breeds of choice are- Sahiwal, Gir, Tharparkar and Red Sindhi. Thus the II generation would be composed of 50% Indian dairy breed, 25% exotic breed and 25% local.

   The usual practice is to breed the F_1 with F_1 bulls (interse-breeding) to produce the F_2 generation. This results in sharp decline in milk production in F_2 because of 50% loss of heterosis and due to use of unselected F_1 bulls. But if the above scheme of breeding is followed, there is no decline in milk production. Rather, better reproductive efficiency and disease resistance is realized due to better adaptability. This experiment has been successfully conducted in Dhamtari District.
3. After F_2 generation a scheme of cris-crossing could be carried out between the exotic and the Indian dairy breeds. This scheme would have dual advantages- The milk production can be sustained to the F_1 level and secondly, the exotic level would never go beyond 67%. This will result in better adaptability and disease resistance thus cutting down the veterinary cost.

Breeding Policy for Buffaloes

A. *Urban Area:* In Urban areas mostly Murrah buffaloes are maintained by the dairy farms. They may be bred with Murrah bulls of high genetic merit.

Summery of the breeding policy

Species	Rural	Urban
Cattle	Grading up with Indian Dairy Breeds like Sahiwal, Gir, Tharparkar, Red Sindhi	Crossbreeding with HF, or Jersey followed by criss-crossing between Indian and exotic dairy breeds.
Buffalo	Hariana or Ongole. Grading up with Murrah or Jafarabadi breed.	Breeding of Murrah with Murrah and Jafarabadi with Jafarabadi.

B. *Rural Area*: The non- descript buffaloes of village area may be upgraded with Murrah or Jafarabadi breed. Both the improver breeds suggested are excellent and they may be used in different districts so that the two kinds of grades can be compared for their performance.

Action plan for implementation of the Breeding Policy

1. *Establishment of Bull mother Farms*: In order to cater to the need of the bulls required for the Central Semen Freezing Station for A.I. and for natural services it is imperative to establish the following bull mother farms.

S. No.	Breed	Location	Remark
1.	Sahiwal	Durg and Bilaspur	The existing farms may be strengthened.
2.	Gir	Dhamtari	To be established.
3.	Red Sindhi	Mahasmaund	To be established.
4.	Tharparkar	Ambikapur	To be established
6	Ongole	Jagadalpur	To be established.
8.	Jafarabadi	Rajnandgoan	To be established.

For the supply of Murrah and H.F. bulls the ABIS Dairy Farm at Rajnadgoan may be Collaborated. In every bull mother farm a minimum of 100 breedable cows should be maintained. This would ensure the supply of at least 20 breeding bulls per year and also 20 females as a replacement stock.

Some private breeders may be encouraged to establish the bull mother farms with an agreement to purchase their bulls provided they meet the fixed norms.

2. *Bull Rearing Farm*: A bull rearing farm may be established in order to maintain the young prospective bulls of different breeds by the state from one year of age to the breeding age. After attaining the breeding age the bulls may be transferred either to the Central Semen Freezing Station or for natural service. The bull rearing farm should have the capacity to maintain about 100 prospective bulls.

3. *Central Semen Freezing Station*: It has already been established at Anjora, Durg with all kinds of modern facilities for semen collection, evaluation, freezing and storage of semen. The centre is producing frozen semen of indigenous dairy breeds and buffaloes to meet the requirement of the entire state. It is in position to supply the semen to other agencies as well.

4. *Liquid Nitrogen Plant*: Some LN2 plants have already been established in the state but they are either non-functional or only partially functional. Efforts should be made to make them functional. The management of these plants may be privatized and the procurement of the LN2 from these plants may be guaranteed by the Govt.

5. *Transport Facility for LN2 and Frozen Semen From C.S.S. to A.I. Centers*: To ensure timely and efficient supply of LN2 and the frozen semen from the C.S.S. to different A.I. centers located throughout the state the transport facility should be created/strengthened. The failure in timely supply of LN2 and frozen semen may lead to the serious set back to the whole programme. For increasing the efficiency creation of regional/district level depots may be considered.

6. *Facility for storage of Frozen semen and LN2 in the A.I. Centers*: Every A.I. centre should be provided with the facility for storage of frozen semen as well as the LN2.

7. *Facility for door to door A. I. services*: The villages are generally located far awy from the A.I. centers/A.I. units and there is practical difficulty in bringing the animals to the A.I. centers. For this reason, the farmers generally become reluctant to A.I. and choose an easy option to go for natural service with the nearby available bull. Therefore, it is necessary to create the facilities for door to door A.I. services. Without this momentum to the breed improvement programme can not be gained. One A.I. center may be established for every 2000 breedable population of cows. A good network of information system between the farmres and the A.I. centers is the basic requirement for the success of the programme. For ensuring door to door A.I. service a model of public private partnership may be experimented.

8. *Plan for the follow-up and reporting*: A proper follow up is must for successful operation of the breeding programme particularly through A.I. An A.I. card should be issued to the farmer in respect of each inseminated animal mentioning the Date of A.I. Bull no. used, Breed of the Bull, ID. No. of the cow, Expected date of next heat incase of repeat, and date of P.D. in case of conception. The farmers should be categorically told to watch their cows on the expected date of repeat and inform the doctor/inseminator if the heat symptoms are noticed. In case, such an information is not received by the doctor, he should without fail, visit the farmer for P.D. on the scheduled date. The calvings should also be regularly recorded.

   A proper monthly reporting system should be followed by center in charge. The monthly progress report should consist of A.I. report, Semen utilization report, P.D. report, calving report and the report of expenditure incurred on P.O.L. and maintenance of vehicle. The modern information technology may be used for timely compilation of report by the Directorate from various districts.

9. *Administrative machinery for supervision and monitoring*: To supervise and monitor the entire breeding programme and to run the system smoothly and efficiently a suitable administrative set-up is needed. The whole Veterinary and Animal Husbandry Department should be bifurcated into two vertical divisions- The Animal Production Division and the Animal Health division.

   Apart from the proposed change in the administrative machinery there should be proper reward and punishment policy. The reward may be in the form of monitory incentive on the basis of per calf born or in the form of advance increment and promotion for the good workers. The punishment may be in the shape of cessation of further increment and promotion or some other punitive action for the non responders.

   The verification of the calves born should be made by some other independent and competent agency.

10. *Field performance recording and progeny testing*: A suitable system of field performance recording of animals should be developed and the progeny testing scheme should be started under the guidance of experts.

11. *Natural Service*: It is never possible to cover the entire population through A.I. alone. It is therefore necessary to identify the areas for the natural services and for the A.I. In the areas where N.S. is to be practiced, breeding bulls belonging to a particular breed should be distributed. Initially 2 bulls in each Gram Panchayat can be given to the volunteer Gosevak with a fixed monthly salary to him plus the fee for each service. The feed and the veterinary care may also be extended to popularize the scheme. In every three years the bulls may be rotated among the Gram Panchayats in order to avoid inbreeding.

12. *Formation of state level advisory committee on Animal Breeding*: An advisory committee may be constituted with an aim to monitor the work, identify the bottlenecks and suggest the remedial measures. The committee may be chaired by the Director, Veterinary services. The other members may be Professor, Animal Breeding & Genetics, M.D., Dugdh Sangh, Joint Director, Animal Production and Joint Director, Farms. One Dy. Director, incharge of animal breeding , may be the member secretary. This committee should meet at least once in 3 months.

□□□

utilization report, P.D. report, calving report and the report of expenditure incurred on P.O.L. and maintenance of vehicle. The modern information technology may be used for timely compilation of data by the Directorate from various districts.

Administrative machinery for supervision and monitoring: To supervise and monitor the entire breeding programme and to run the system smoothly and efficiently a suitable administrative set-up is needed. The Veterinary and Animal Husbandry Department should be bifurcated into two vertical divisions. The Animal Production Division and the Animal Health division.

Apart from the proposed change in the administrative machinery there should be proper reward and punishment policy. The rewards may be in the form of monthly incentive on the basis of per calf born or in the form of advance increment and promotion for the good workers. The punishment may be in the shape of cessation of further increment and promotion or some other punitive action for the non-performers.

The evaluation of the entire programme should be made by some other independent and competent authority.

10. *Field performance recording and progeny testing:* A suitable system of field performance recording of animals should be developed and the progeny testing scheme should be started under the guidance of experts.

11. *Natural service:* It is never possible to cover the entire population through A.I. alone. It is therefore necessary to identify the areas for the natural services and for the A.I. In the areas where A.I. is not in practice, breeding bulls belonging to a particular breed should be distributed. Initially 2 bulls in each Gram Panchayat can be given to the volunteer Gosevak with a fixed monthly salary to him plus the fee for each service. The feed and the veterinary care may also be extended to popularize the scheme. In every three years the bulls may be rotated among the Gram Panchayats in order to avoid inbreeding.

12. *Formation of state level advisory committee on Animal Breeding:* An advisory committee may be constituted with an aim to monitor the work, identify the bottlenecks and suggest the remedial measures. The committee may be chaired by the Director, Veterinary services. The other members may be Professor, Animal Breeding & Genetics, M.D., [illegible], Joint Director, Animal Production and Joint Director, Farms. The Dy. Director, incharge of animal breeding, may be the member secretary. This committee should meet at least once in 3 months.

12

Business Ventures for Youth in Livestock Sector

RUPASI TIWARI
Senior Scientist and I/C, ATIC, Indian Veterinary Research Institute
Izatnagar, Bareilly, UP-243122

Introduction

India possesses one of the largest livestock populations in the world, which is more than 535million with the top position in cattle (199 million), buffalo (105 million), goat (140 million) and sheep (71 million),pigs (11 million) and poultry (505 million) (DAHD, 2007). Further, the country has 16.49 percent of the world's cattle population and 56.78 percent of the world's buffalo population. Out of the total livestock in the country, around 38.2 percent are cattle, 20.2 percent are buffaloes, 12.7 percent are sheep, 25.6 percent are goats and only 2.8 percent are pigs. All other animals are less than 0.50 percent of the total livestock population. India has a large genetic diversity of livestock containing 30 breeds of cattle, 10 breeds of buffaloes, 42 breeds of sheep, 20 breeds of goats and 7 breeds of camels. Further, the country has 13 percent of the world's cattle population and 57 percent of the world's buffalo population and is on top in terms of the buffalo population and at 2nd position in terms of the total cattle population in the world. Of the total buffalo and cattle breeds of the world, approximately 75% and 20% respectively are available in Asia and 15 and 5% in India. The country possesses 5.78 percent of world sheep and 14.76 percent of goat population, ranking second in goat and third in sheep population. India accounts for nearly 3.00 percent of the world poultry population and stands at 5th position in the world. The poultry which was considered as a backyard venture in the early 60's has now been transformed into strong agro-based. farming activity. With an annual production of about 112million tones of milk and 59.8 billion eggs India ranks 1st and 5th in the world, respectively, and is one of the top ten broiler producers in the world. Dairy enterprise is considered a "treasure" of the Indian economy, particularly for rural systems. It provides nutrition, draft animal power, organic manure, supplementary employment, cash income, and a 'cushion' for 'drought proofing' in India. The sector involves millions of resource-poor farmers, for whom animal ownership ensures critical livelihood, sustainable farming, and economic stability. According to National Sample Survey Organization's data, the livestock sector provides employment to 22 million people including 18.5 million workers in dairying and another 3.5 million in poultry and meat industry.

Economic Contribution

About 24.72 per cent of the agricultural GDP in this country is contributed by livestock sector and contribution of national GDP is about 4.36 percent. In the arid areas, the contribution of livestock to Agriculture GDP is as high as 70 per cent while in Semi-arid areas the contribution is over 40 per cent. India has been making steady progress in livestock sector with annual growth at the rate of more than 3.5%. The gross value of output from livestock comes to around Rs. 2, 40,601 Crore (2007-08) which is about 26.9 % of the total value of agricultural output (8, 94,420 Crore). With a total annual milk production of around 112.5 million MT and meat production of 4 million tonnes and wool production of 43.2 million kgs, it has a huge impact on Indian economy. The total earning from milk alone comes to Rs. 1, 62,136 Crore which is more than that of paddy (95,038 Crore), wheat (71,579 Crore) and sugarcane (33,691 Crore) (DAHD Annual Report, 2007-08). Further the earning from meat group is around 34,310 Crore. Export earning from livestock, poultry and other related products is Rs. 8,656 Crore, which reveals the growing importance of the livestock sector in the country's economy and food security.

Contribution to Food Security

The per capita availability of the livestock produce has also remarkably increased during the last decades. The per capita availability of the milk rose from 112 gm/head / day in 1970-71 to 258 gm /head / day now. Further the per capita availability of eggs has also risen from 5.32 eggs/head /year in 1961 to 30 eggs in 1994 to 42 eggs/head /year now. Still there is a big gap that remains to be fulfilled to achieve the food security in terms of animal protein requirement. Although per capita consumption of animal products has increased but still we are not able to provide minimum amount of animal protein recommended by WHO i.e. 25 gm/person/day. At present it is available only 10gm/person/day. In fact per day per person requirement is 60 gm out of which at least 25 gm should be from animal origin.

Employment Scenario Worldwide

Employment and income generation are the buzz words in all the developmental sectors. With the increasing population there seems to be extreme scarcity of employment in the government sectors and further the government is also burdened thus trying to cut off the already existing posts in various departments to meet the financial burden. In such a scenario the youth employment has become the major cause of concern. Unemployment rates have been growing annually at more than 15% all over the world. According to a United Nation 2000 report on youth unemployment, the problem is worse in Asia which accounts for 54 percent of world's unemployed youth population and major portion of this population is in India. By 2001, there were 212 million young people in India, but only 23.6 percent could be absorbed in the labour force. Simultaneously there's been a marked decrease in the number of jobs on offer from the organized sector (less than 10 percent). The gravity of the situation can be judged from the fact that India's labour force totals to approximately 40 crore, which is 10 times of the number registered in the exchanges. *(http://www.financialexpress.com)*

The Human Development Index ranking, based on 2007 data, finds India at a shocking 134th place out of 182 countries.. The Human Poverty Index (HPI) places India at 88th among 135 countries (a steep decline from 62nd place among 155 countries in the last HDR). The HDR 2009 tells, that 41.6% of India's population earns below $ 1.25 a day, and 75.6% earns below $ 2 a day *(http://www.cpiml. Org)*

According to ILO youth unemployment has increased by over 10 million in the last two years, the worst surge since the agency began compiling global statistics in 1991. The global unemployment rate was 6.6 percent in 2008, but that the true scope of the problem was much worse because over 600 million workers and their families were surviving on less than $1.25 a day. Another 200 million were hovering just above the international poverty line. *(http://sify.com)*

Employment in Agriculture in India

Agriculture is the predominant occupation in India, accounting for about 52% of employment. Agricultural and allied sectors accounted for about 60% of the total workforce in 2003 same as in 1993-94. While agriculture has faced stagnation in growth, services have seen a steady growth. Of the total workforce, 8% is in the organised sector, two-thirds of which are in the public sector. The NSSO survey estimated that in 1999-2000, 106 million, nearly 10% of the population were unemployed and the overall unemployment rate was 7.3%, with rural areas doing marginally better (7.2%) than urban areas (7.7%). India's labor force is growing by 2.5% annually, but employment only at 2.3% a year. Official unemployment exceeds 9%. Almost 30% of workers are casual workers who work only when they are able to get jobs and remain unpaid for the rest of the time. Only 10% of the workforce is in regular employment. Unemployment in India is characterized by chronic underemployment or disguised unemployment. Government schemes that target eradication of both poverty and unemployment (which in recent decades has sent millions of poor and unskilled people into urban areas in search of livelihoods) attempt to solve the problem, by providing financial assistance for setting up businesses, skill honing, setting up public sector enterprises, reservations in governments, etc. (http://en.wikipedia.org).

Future scenario of unemployment

Unemployment may reach 29% by 2020 in India. Over 40% of our workforce is the working poor (make enough money to live but not enough to pull out of poverty) 50% of the workforce is marginally self-employed; 70% of workers generate only 18% of GDP. *(http://www.teamlease.com)*

Open unemployment is not a true indicator of the gravity of the unemployment problem in an economy such as India, characterised as it is by large-scale underemployment and poor employment quality in the unorganised sector, which accounts for over 90 per cent of the total employment. The organised sector contributes only about 9 per cent to the total employment. (http://www.indiaonestop. Com)

Enhancing employment and ensuring livelihood security

In the present era of shrinking land holding and increasing unemployment of youth in rural areas, agri-business and micro enterprise promotion has evolved as an answer to the employment crisis facing the world. As a result, the emphasis on job creation has shifted to the informal sector. Generation of self-employment opportunities, especially for the rural youths, is a must for ensuring true development of the rural masses. Livestock Sector offers a very attractive opportunity for such business ventures.

Employment in livestock sector

In India, livestock sector remains one of the mainstays of agriculture which is a source of livelihood for over 68 per cent of the population. Table 1 provides a view of the employment in livestock vis-à-vis other sectors.

Table 1 : Sectoral distribution of rural workers in India (%)

Sector description	Total persons 1983	Total persons 1993-94	Total persons 1999-2000	Male 1983	Male 1993-94	Male 1999-2000	Female 1983	Female 1993-94	Female 1999-2000
Crop production	70.5	70	68.1	70.2	68.4	66	71	73	72
Livestock production	8.5	5.3	4.9	4.8	2.4	2.2	14.8	10.4	9.8
Plantation	1.7	1.8	1.4	1.8	1.9	1.3	1.6	1.6	1.6
Forestry and logging	0.3	0.3	0.3	0.4	0.3	0.2	0.2	0.3	0.4
Fishing	0.4	0.5	0.3	0.5	0.6	0.4	0.2	0.2	0.1
Agricultural services	0.1	0.6	1.2	0.09	0.5	1.1	0.1	0.7	1.3
Non-farm sector	18.5	21.6	23.8	22.2	25.9	28.9	12.2	13.9	14.7
Total	100	100	100	100	100	100	100	100	100

Source: Results on Employment and Unemployment Situation in India (various issues), NSSO, Ministry of Statistics and Program Implementation, Govt. of India.

Though the share of agricultural sector in gross domestic product is declining the share of livestock sector to the Agricultural. GDP is continuously rising. The role of livestock sector in employment generation needs no emphasis. Rural women play a very important role in animal production and participate actively in areas like animal feeding, milking, breeding, cleaning and providing health care to the animals. As an adjunct to agricultural, livestock production contributes substantially to poverty alleviation and creates employment opportunities, particularly in rural areas. This sector has great potential for bringing about socio-economic transformation in rural India. According to the recent estimates about 22.45 million people work in the livestock sector out of which 16.84 million are female. Further animal husbandry sector employs 11.44 million people in principal status and 11.01 million in subsidiary status. About 5.50% of the total working population of the country is engaged in animal husbandry sector.

Apart from being an important contributor to national income, the sector has been considered as one with high potential for alleviating rural poverty and unemployment in rural areas. Over 70% of rural house holds own livestock. A large majority (65%) of livestock owners comprises of small marginal farmers and landless agricultural workers. The overall distribution of livestock is much more equitable than that of land. The bottom 60% of rural households owns 65% of all livestock leading to more equitable distribution of gains from livestock production.

Challenges facing livestock sector

One of the major challenges facing our livestock industry is the launching of the WTO due to which we have to be more cautious about the quality of the livestock produce if we have to compete in the international market. The major SPS concerns for India include the quality and safety of Dairy and Meat products. It is imperative that the principle of Hazard analysis critical control point (HACCP) systems, Code of practices on good animal feed, good hygienic practices (GHP) and good manufacturing practices (GMP) and cold chain system are followed. India should also put in place Prevention of Infectious and contagious diseases in Animals Act and take effective measures to eradicate "A" category diseases as notified by OIE. For the hygienic practices for milk production, Codex standards are required not only for the livestock products for export conform to stipulated safety and suitability standards but also that the raw milk used in the manufacture of the products is produced using GHP and GMPs. Extensive extension programs should be implemented to ensure this. Better physical infrastructure for reference laboratories for monitoring and surveillance of the contaminants and their levels and strengthening of information systems for risk analysis are needed.

In this era of WTO, there is a tremendous scope of promoting the backyard livestock keeping in India into commercial micro enterprises through entrepreneurship development programmes and entrepreneur favourable government policies. Apart from rearing of livestock, the livestock based industry has vast scope of generating additional income and employment through its various allied enterprises such as the commercial livestock rearing units, livestock input industry, livestock product processing units and organic livestock production units which can be harnessed for increasing employment and income in the rural areas.

Eleventh Plan Proposals

The Planning Commission had indicated an outlay of Rs 8174.00 crore for the DAHD&F Department for the Eleventh Plan. The approach identified for the livestock sector in the 11th Plan is to achieve an overall growth between 6 to 7 percent per annum for the sector as a whole, with milk group achieving a growth of 5% per annum and meat and poultry achieving a growth of 10% per annum. The benefit of higher growth should be equitable, benefiting mainly the small and marginal farmers and landless labourers who maintain bulk of the livestock in the country. *(http://business.gov.in)*

Commercializing the Livestock Enterprises

Livestock rearing is the major subsidiary occupation in most part of our country. But keeping in view its potentiality for generating employment and providing food security to the country it needs to be taken up as a main occupation. For starting any livestock enterprise commercially on scientific lines the rural youth can avail loan from banks. For obtaining bank loan the farmers / entrepreneurs can apply to the nearest branch of commercial, cooperative or regional rural banks in the prescribed application form, which is available in the branches of the financing banks. There are various livestock enterprises, which can be practiced on commercial scale and can be started with small investment.

Development of Commercial Dairy Farms

In starting dairy farm it is essential to decide which animal is to be taken for this purpose. Normally Cow/Buffalo is the choice for dairy enterprise. Both the animals are milch animal but they differ in many aspects in production. The cow can yield high amount of milk and can be very economical at high production level. They breed regularly, giving one calf at every 13-14 month intervals. Buffalo breed is also suitable for a commercial dairy farm. There is a greater demand for buffalo milk in the country because of its higher fat contents and its suitability for making ghee and other milk products. Other plus point in buffalo is that they can utilize crop residues with better efficiency than cows, and are more resistant to diseases. However, buffalo largely mature late and have longer calving intervals (16-18months). These animals also need additional cooling facilities eg. Wallowing tank or showers/ foggers with fan. Thus in a commercial farm, a combination of cow and buffalo could work better than growing cow or buffalo alone. Cross bred cow and buffalo should be kept in separate row under one shed.

The minimum economic size of commercial dairy farm under Indian condition should contain a minimum 20 (10 cows & 10 buffalo) especially for a suburban area. The economic viability of the unit will depend on the production performance of dairy animals and the rates of various items including feed, fodder and milk. As far as economics of small dairy unit concern, Walli et al. (2005) suggested that a livestock owner may get near about Rs. 10000 as net income /animal/year.

Economic of small dairy unit (Rathore & Sharma, 2007)

Capital investment (Rs.)

1.	Cost of animal (10cow+10buffalo)	:	4,50,000
2.	Building construction cost	:	6,53,175
3.	Cost of equipments	:	3,20,000
	Total capital investment	:	14, 23,175

Non-recurring/ fixed expenditure (Rs.)

1.	Interest on capital investment @ 10 percent / annum	:	1,42,317
2.	Depreciation on livestock @ 12.5 percent / annum	:	56, 250
3.	Depreciation on building @ 3.0 percent /annum	:	19,595
4.	Depreciation on equipment @ 10.0% per annum	:	32, 000
5.	Insurance @ Rs. 800/cow or buffalo /year	:	16,000
	Total (Rs.)	:	2, 66,162

Recurring expenditure (Rs.)

1.	Cost of farm grown green fodder	:	62,415
2.	Cost of purchased dry fodder	:	24, 966
3.	Cost of concentrate mixture	:	2,33, 016
4.	Labour charges	:	60,000
5.	Animal health care and reproduction charges @ Rs.400/- per animal/year	:	9,000
6.	Miscellaneous expenses including repair, electric bill, phone bill, purchase of chain, rope, etc.Rs.700/- per animal/year	:	15,750
	Total expenditure (Rs.)	:	4, 05, 147
	Grand total	:	6, 71,309

Income from sale

7.	Sale of cow milk (12.5x7x365x15)	:	4,79,063
8.	Sale of buffalo milk (10x6x365x18)	:	3,94,200
9.	Sale of manure @ Rs 500/- per animal/ year	:	11,400
10.	Sale of 4 buffalo male calves at 10 month of age @Rs.500/- per animal	:	2,000
	Total sale proceed (Rs.)	:	8, 86,663
	Net income / year	:	2, 15,354
	Net income /month	:	17946
	Net income/animal/year	:	9529 say 10000/-

Development of Commercial Sheep Farms

Keeping in view the ever-increasing population of our country there is tremendous pressure on our natural resources such as land and water. Especially in the light of the marginalization of agricultural land holding sheep rearing is a better option as compared to other livestock, more so, in the semi arid and the arid zones of our country. The sheep produce wool and meat. In spite of the fact that the country is endowed with 11.5 percent of the world livestock population it contributes little over 2.26 percent (5.74 million tones) to the world total meat production of 245 million tones. Considering 70 percent of human population non-vegetarian, the annual per capita availability of meat is roughly 8 Kg. as against the recommended intake of 11 Kg. Of the total meat production more than 70 percent comes from cattle (old bullocks), buffalo and pigs and for that preference is limited to socio religious factors. Therefore burden lies on goat and sheep meat, and in the recent years the domestic market price for mutton has increased from Rs. 50 per Kg. to Rs. 100 –120 per Kg. Moreover expected huge increase in demand for meat in developing countries (by 100 percent) especially in East and South East Asia in next 20 years presents an excellent opportunity for enhancing export of live goat / sheep and their meat from India. Therefore there is immense potential for entrepreneurship development through commercial sheep rearing in our country.

Development of Commercial Goat Farms

Goat is a multidimensional animal and plays a significant role in the economy and nutrition of landless, small and marginal farmers in the country. Goat rearing is an important subsidiary occupation especially practiced by the small marginal and landless farmers since it requires small amount of investment. The small and landless youth can start a small scale goat farm of 10 goats with a small initial investment of Rs. 30000 -35000 only and this unit will yield him a net income of Rupees 15,000 - 20000/ year. For starting a large-scale goat farm of 100 goats 1000 sq. meter of land will be required in addition to an initial investment of Rs. 3 to 3.5 lakhs and this enterprise can yield him a net income of Rupees 1.5 lakh / year i.e., Rs. 12,500/ month. The rural youth can get practical training on commercial goat rearing from either at IVRI Izatnagar or Central Goat Research Institute, Makhdoom, Mathura. In fact, Goat rearing under intensive and semi intensive system for commercial production is economically viable and gaining momentum in the country.

Prospects of meat export of goat and other animals

There is great potential to increase the quantum of meat export from India even at present level of production. Even under more competitive WTO regime India has got several advantages in meat export like proximity to importing countries, leanness of meat, good upcoming modern infrastructure, lower cost of production, safer meat from toxic residue point of view and CJ disease. Total quality management systems has assumed a greater significance under the changed world meat trade scenario. This would assure the finished products to be of high laid quality and standards. The typical choice of 'hot' meat purchased by the Indian meat eaters shall play a decisive role in protecting Indian meat industry through frozen meat imports.

- Goat meat produced and exported from India is lean in character and good for fat and energy conscious people. Contrary to this, the lambs produced in Australia and New Zealand, which are the major competitor, contains high carcass fat. This is the reason that in future, demand for sheep/goat meat from India shall continue to increase. The basic reason for the lean character of meat produced from goat is mainly the extensive system of rearing the animals unlike New Zealand and Australia where the animals are primarily reared adopting the intensive system of management.
- Since our animals' graze/browse in the pastures/range-lands hence the meat produced is relatively safer from any feed additive residue point of view and is nearer to organic system of meat production. Because of the closer proximity to the Gulf countries, the meat from India reaches to the destinations in a relatively fresh condition at a cheaper cost. This could be another advantage.
- Processing of meat is crucial for its value addition and for enhancing the profitability of exports. Processed meat constitutes merely 0.25 percent of the total value of meat exported from India. Establishment and up-gradation of meat processing facilities therefore need to be encouraged and supported.
- Presence of large number of ethnic Indians through out the world provides a niche for the export of meat and meat products especially from goat and sheep. India can enjoy the benefit its richness in spices and condiments, which adds to flavour and taste to ethnic consumers.
- Expected huge global increase in demand for meat especially from East and Southeast Asia would be an excellent opportunity for enhancing export of meat from India.
- Vast genetic variability in Indian livestock consisting numbers of breeds of buffalo, cattle, goat and sheep provides an opportunity for productivity enhancement through breed improvement programme for sustainable meat production.

However an important consideration would be to meet the sanitary and phyto-sanitary standards strictly. It is mandatory under the provisions of WTO for meat exporters to adopt 'Hazard Analysis Critical Control Point' (HACCP) and certified as ISO 9002. Until recently only few Indian Companies had adopted HACCP. More number of modern slaughterhouses including municipal slaughterhouses adopting Good Manufacturing Practices (GMP) need to be established.

Establishing Commercial Poultry Farms

Today India is the 5th largest egg producer and one of the top ten broiler producers in the world. This has been achieved due to the commercialization of the poultry sector. But, in spite of the considerable growth in the egg production (2.5 million to 30000 million during 1950 to 2000 and broiler production, the per capita availability of poultry products is considerably low; 42 eggs and 500 gm. meat / annum as against the requirement of 180 eggs and 10 kg. meat per annum, which shows that there is great potentiality for the development of poultry sector in the country thereby presenting higher opportunities of entrepreneurship development in rural areas.

For development of entrepreneurship in poultry sector following points to be kept in mind

i. The agro-climatic conditions must be suitable for rearing birds in the area.

ii. It should be ascertained that the applicant has knowledge/experience in raising poultry.

iii. Selected site should be away from main roads and free from water logging conditions.

iv. The poultry shed should be adequate to accommodate the number of birds to be raised. The poultry house should be according to standard requirements and should give protection to birds from sun, rain, wind and predators.

v. Suitable arrangements should be made for purchase of high quality one day old chicks or layers from reputed sellers at reasonable prices.

vi. Sufficient clean water should be available for birds. It should also be ascertained that the poultry feed is available from close proximity at reasonable price.

vi. Proper Veterinary services must be available near the farm for treating the birds. Birds should be vaccinated against poultry diseases.

vii. Firm arrangements must be made for marketing of eggs/broilers/culled birds.

vii. Arrangements should be made for insurance of birds and the insurance policy should be made in favour of the bank. Layers @ Rs. 4.23% birds, Broilers @ Rs. 0.71/ birds, building and Equipments @ 0.40% of cost.

viii. Proper records of all purchases and sales should be maintained.

Rural youth can earn attractive profits if they start the enterprise commercially. Further the two enterprises layer and broiler farming can be started on small scale with low investment also. A broiler farm of 1000 birds can be started with a covered land size of 1000 sq. ft. and an initial investment of Rupees 50,000 as fixed cost for shed and other equipment. Around Rupees 50,000 will be required for the variable expenditure on chicks, feed and other miscellaneous expenses. The broiler birds are ready within 42 days with an average body weight of 1.5 to 1.8 kg. and can yield a minimum profit of Rs. 10,000 per batch of 1000 birds (@ Rs. 40 / Kg market price and 1.5 Kg live weight of bird) which amounts to around Rs. 70,000 per year (if the entrepreneur puts 7 batches of 1000 birds in a year) i.e., a net profit of Rupees 5800 per month. The profit from a batch of 1000 bird can increase to Rs. 20,000 with the increase in live weight of birds to 1.8 kg./ bird. Further profits can be earned if the market prices are higher.

Development of Piggery Farm

In India pig rearing is mainly carried out by the socially and economically backward class of our society. The pig can play a very important role in increasing meat production and thereby to meet the protein hunger. They excel all other farm animals in respect of edible flesh The pig rearing gives high returns with a low investment, so the popular name "mortgage lifter" is often give to them. The major advantages of pig rearing over the other livestock enterprises are its short generation interval, big litter size (6-7 in case of indigenous breed, 8-12 in case of exotic breed, 5-9 in case of cross bred pigs), can be fed on cheap feed and food by products, High food conversion efficiency, quicker increase in body weight, 1 kg body weight at birth become 80-100 kg only in 7-10 months of age. Before starting a piggery, a suitable site is required to be selected. As feed cost accounts for about 70 percent of the total expenditure, the pig farm should either be established near to metropolitan city, where left food from hotel/mess/hostel is available or near a village where cheap by product from agriculture are plenty. A good land with out ditches at higher level should be arranged near road side. Water and electric supply must be arranged. The animals should preferably be purchased with following characteristics.

1. Pure bred Large White, Middle White and Landrace (white)
2. Physically strong and healthy with good condition
3. Normal body temperature (101° F)
4. Female of exotic and crossbred must have 7 & 6 pairs of teats and belong to dams with good litter size.
5. Male should have good libido and semen quality.
6. Female of regular oestrus cyclicity.

Daily routine jobs in piggery is to perform like cleaning of all pigsties, feeding and water trough, farm premises along with disposal of dung/urine, checking the herd for spotting out the sick animals, spotty of sows/gilts in heat, if in heat then necessary breeding is to be planned and carried out, isolation of near parturition sows/gilts into furrowing pens or suitable place so that she is not disturbed by other animal. Whereas periodical jobs are also necessary like weighing of stock, which help the farmers to know the gain per unit for given inputs. Cutting of needle teeth which will prevent infection of wound from fighting or causing injuries to the teat of mother, piglets should be castrated when they are 2-3 weeks of age, weaning of piglets at 8 week of age, deworming periodically, culling & disposal of piglets as and when needed and vaccination against infectious diseases.

Economic of small piggery unit (2 male+10 female)

A. Total input (Rs.)

1. Cost of construction of two sheds : 50,000
2. Cost of 12 pigs. : 28,000
   (Large White Yorkshire or Landress 60 kg) @ Rs. 40/kg live wt
3. Feed cost ;
   - Feeding of adult animal average concentrate 2 kg/day @ 4.0/kg for one year : 35,040
   - Cost of creep feed for piglet of first farrowing : 2,000
   - Cost of grower feed 70 gms (for 5 months @ 1.5 kg /day/Rs. 4.00 /kg.) : 63,000
   - Creep feed for 2nd farrowing : 2,000
4. Other expenses;
   - Labour charges annually : 30,000
   - Vet. Med. Including vaccine : 5,000

Total expenditure : 2, 15, 040

Interest @ 6%/annum : 12, 542

B. Total out put

1.	Sale of 12 adult pigs of appx. 100 kg bwt.	:	48,000
2.	Sale of 70 growers of 1st farrowing of about 60 kg bwt	:	1, 68,000
3.	Sale of 70 weaners @ Rs. 100/- each	:	70,000
4.	Cost of manure	:	5,000
	Total receipt	:	2, 91,000
	Net income	:	63, 418 say 63500/-

The profit will be increased in 2nd year onwards as number of breed able sows will be more giving birth to piglets.

Buffalo Calves Rearing for Meat Purpose

Buffalo calves rearing for meat purpose is a very attractive entrepreneurship for rural youth as those buffalo calves can be reared partially on grazing and partially on the left out feed of the lactating animals. Later on fattening diet can be given to get proper body weight and good quality of meat. For meat purpose buffalo calves may be purchased from urban and peri urban dairy on throw away prices at the age of 2-6 month. These calves should be castrated at 3-6 month of age for good growth of meat. For rearing of 10 buffalo calves an economic estimation is given below.

The cost of 10 buffalo calves @ Rs 300/- each will be (Rs 3000/-). Rearing cost of these 10 buffalo calves for 24 months to gain 250-300 kg body weight including feed, fodder and medication etc., will be Rs, 39,000 (excluding fixed cost of shed & land). The total returns after 24 months will be Rs 1, 00,000 @ Rs 40/ kg rate of buffalo meat. Thus net profit will be 61,000 & per calf Rs 6,100 per month.

Commercial Dry Cattle/ Buffalo Rearing Units

Those animals which are in their productive age but dry are mostly sold off or given to the villagers on contract by the commercial dairy farmers especially in the peri urban and urban areas as these farmers rear only the milch animals to have a stable amount of milk production all round the year. The rural youth can use this as an opportunity and can set up dry buffalo / cattle rearing farms and can purchase / take on contract dry animals and at parturition can sell them at higher prices. The practice of giving dry animals on contract to villagers presently exists among the commercial dairy farmers in the urban area but this can be used as an opportunity by the rural youth and they can take up this enterprise in an organized manner commercially and can start such type of farms in the rural areas.

Commercial Cattle / Buffalo Calf Rearing Units

It has been found that in the commercial dairy farms the management of calves is very poor leading to a high calf mortality rate. This is leading to a heavy loss to the farmers as well as to the nation in form of loss of good quality germplasm. Therefore such units can be established by the rural / urban youth and they can purchase cow / buffalo calves from these farmers and rear them till parturition and then can sell them at attractive prices to the same dairy owners. Further, the male buffalo calves can be fattened / reared especially for meat purpose.

Integrated Livestock Farming

In this type of farming two or three livestock species are reared together and each species supplements the other. In fact it can be said that this type of farming is symbiotic in nature. Various types of livestock integration are practiced in our country such as Pig- Fish integration, Poultry- fish integration, Pig-poultry-fish integration, Pig-poultry-fish- duck integration and Dairy-fish Duck- integration.

In these types of livestock rearing the waste products of one species are utilized by the other therein enhancing the productivity of both the species in terms of waste utilization and lower expenditure on feed. For example; In the case of pig - fish integration the excreta of the pig is used for manuring the pond which give rise to various planktons and phytoplankton's which are eaten by the fish thereby reducing the expenditure on manuring of pond. Further, the dead fish can be utilized for making the ration of pigs. Also it has been found that an individual can get a fish production of 6000 Kg. per hectare through the integration of livestock with fish by spending only on the purchase of fish seeds. Further such type of integration help in the use of barren and unproductive lands and water bodies, thereby effectively utilizing the natural resources.

Livestock Input Industry for Entrepreneurship Generation

Various forms of inputs are required for the livestock enterprises such as feed and fodder, medicines, breeding services etc. and practicing these enterprises commercially can generate good amount of income and employment for rural youth. Various livestock input enterprises, which can be taken up by youth in rural areas, are:

Commercial Feed and Fodder Production

Feed and fodder account for the major cost of livestock products and are the major components of the livestock industry. Keeping in view the growing shortage of feed and fodder in our country, promoting these enterprises on commercial scale can solve both the problem i.e., removing unemployment and developing adequate feed resources for our livestock. This industry has various avenues, which can be harnessed by the rural youth for entrepreneurship development.

1. Establishment of Area Specific Mineral Mixture Unit

It is well established fact that area specific mineral mixture is more profitable to our livestock community for increase in milk production and body weight in young animals. It will be a very good venture to establish unit for product of area specific mineral mixture and by this unit one can earn a lot of profit by sale of this product. The technology can be purchased from IVRI & Commercial production can be started.

2. Commercial Dry Fodder Enrichment Unit (Preparing Urea Treated Straw)

Further, dry fodder enrichment units can be set up, wherein the nutritional quality of the crop residues can be enhanced thereby raising the market value of the poor quality roughages The Urea enriched dry fodder can be prepared on commercial level and can be sold to the dairy farmers at the time of shortage of green fodder which can fetch attractive prices.

3. Commercial Hay / Silage Preparation

The basic principal of hay making is to reduce the moisture concentration in the green forages sufficiently as to permit their storage without spoilage or further nutrient loss. The moisture content in hay must be less than 15% at storage time. Crop with thin stem and many leaves are better suited for hay making as they dry faster than those having pithy stems and small leaves. Crop harvesting at flowering of pre-flowering stage is good since it contains maximum nutrients. The harvested forage should be spread in the field and raked a few times for quick drying. The dried forage should be collected and baled when the moisture concentration becomes lower that 15%. Bailing the hay helps in storage and requires less space

The term silage refers to any wet and/ or green fodder, preserved by organic acids, chiefly lactic acid, that is produces naturally by bacterial fermentation of sugars in the plants under anerobic conditions. Silage making is commonly recommended in most parts of India, but it has lot been established for the number of reasons e.g. lack of surplus fodder during rainy season; unreliable rainfall pattern, making farmers reluctant to ensile a forage surplus during the rainy season, since the actual feed shortage during the dry season will than also vary considerably and its being labour intensive.

During the flush season when fodder prices are low, these can be preserved in form of hay and silage. And during the lean period (especially summer) when there is heavy shortage of green fodder, the hay and silage can be sold to the dairy farmers at attractive prices, which can fetch additional returns to the commercial fodder growers.

4. Growing Fodder Crops Commercially Round The Year

Another option is to grow high yielding fodder crops commercially round the year and supply it to the urban and peri -urban areas, wherein there is heavy demand for green fodder as most of the commercial dairy farms are situated in these areas and can fetch the rural entrepreneurs good price for their fodder.

Estimated Economics of Green Fodder Production in Peri-urban Area

Since berseem is being commonly used in cities as a green fodder source, the economics of berseem production in periurban area is presented. If we assume price seed @ Rs. 50/kg and rate of green berseem @ Rs. 50/q., than total income and benefit cost ratio from berseem production from one hectare of land in periurban areas will be as mentioned below.

Characters	Price (Rs.)
Input	
• Cost of seed (25kg/ha)	1250
• Fertilizer (N,P,K)	1400
• Irrigation (water)	800
• Transport of fodder	1000
• Labour wages	
1. Irrigation (@Rs. 100/labour)- (for 10 irrigation)	1000
2. Field making, sowing, bund making	1500
3. Cuttings (4 cuts)	8000
4. Seed harvesting, threshing and transport	2500
5. Seed clearing and packaging	1550
Cost of cultivation	**19,000**
Output	
Income from green fodder (yield from four cuts- 600q/ha	30,000
Income from seed sale(seed production 50q/ha)@ Rs. 50 / Kg	25,000
Total income	**55,000**
Benefit Cost ratio	**1.89**

Mishra, S. (2006)

5. Establishment of Cattle/ Poultry Feed Unit

A rural youth can start the cattle / poultry feed unit with a small initial investment of Rs. 2,00,000 including fixed and variable cost, wherein he can get a bank loan of Rs. 1,67,500 and rest he has to invest himself. This unit will earn him a yearly profit of Rs. 1,16,600 i.e., Rs. 9717 / month.

Commercial Breeding Units

For commercial livestock rearing one of the essential components is the availability of good quality breed of livestock viz., cattle, buffalo, goat, pig or poultry. Keeping in view the importance of the breeding services, such activity can be taken up commercially and various types of commercial enterprises can be started in rural areas such as:

1. Livestock breeding farms

Another important input for the commercial livestock rearing is the availability of high yielding breeds of animals like cows Sahiwal, Red sindhi, Tharparker, Gir etc and of buffalo like buffalo like Murrah, Nili, Ravi etc.. It has been found that the dairy farmers have to go to other places especially other states viz., Haryana, Punjab and Gujrat to get good quality cow & buffaloes. Further, most of them who are not able to afford bringing animals from distant places just purchase the animals from the local market. For smaller livestock species such as goat, sheep and pigs the farmers do not bother to make many efforts for procuring a good breed of animal.

This gap between demand and availability of good breed of livestock poses excellent opportunity in front of rural youth, to establish livestock breeding farms in their areas and sell the young ones at good prices. Different types of livestock breeding farms can be established viz.,

1. Cattle/ Buffalo breeding farms
2. Sheep / goat breeding farms
3. Pig breeding farms

But the major requirement is of getting appropriate scientific training in running a livestock-breeding farm. Opening up of poultry hatchery is also a proposition that can be taken up by educated rural youth.

2. Providing private doorstep artificial insemination (A.I) services

The rural youth can be employed effectively for providing doorstep A.I services by providing them a short para vet training on A.I. from the state government, Krishi Vigyan Kendras or other NGO's after which they can purchase the necessary equipments viz., the moped, A.I. Kit, Liquid Nitrogen (LN) container etc., and provide doorstep services to the livestock owners thereby upgrading the non descript stock on one hand and generating additional income on the other. The rural youth can start the mobile A.I. unit with an initial investment of Rs. 45,500 for which they can get loan from banks. In fact this activity is very successful in china.

3. Establishing commercial livestock service centers

Commercial livestock service centers can be established by the unemployed rural youth in the villages wherein they can provide both the natural services as well as the Artificial insemination services for the livestock. Such type of activity is being practiced in rural areas but the farmer do not maintain good breed of cow / buffalo bull and charge Rs. 50 / to 100/- service. Whereas in urban areas with good quality bulls the charges are Rs. 100 / to 200/- service and this type of enterprise can yield good return to the rural youth also. (Rupasi & Sharma, 2007).

Commercial Livestock First Aid Clinics

Timely health care is an important input required for any commercial livestock enterprise. In urban areas there are a number of private doctors and clinics available for livestock , but such facilities are not available in the rural areas. Further, the government health care machinery is not so efficient as to provide adequate health coverage to all the livestock population. Therefore, two types of livestock first aid clinics can be established in the rural areas

- Allopathic treatment Clinics
- Indigenous treatment Clinics or Alternate System of treatment
- Combined system of treatment

The rural youth can be provided six month or one year training in first aid treatment of the livestock, through state government, NGO's, K.V.K's, Dairy cooperatives, which will have dual benefits. On one hand it will generate employment for rural youth and on the other hand it will help in boosting the commercial livestock enterprise in rural areas through timely health care measures. Also in rural areas a number of indigenous treatment are practiced for livestock . The rural youth can learn the effective and time-tested indigenous treatment from their elders and can practice them in their areas to earn a living.

Organic Livestock Production Units

In the past decade there has been an increasing awareness about the use of organic products especially in developed countries. The demand for organic products has created new export opportunities for the developing world. The organic products are sold at impressive premiums often at prices 20 percent higher than the identical traditional products. Therefore, there exists tremendous opportunities of entrepreneurship development through organic livestock production in our country. The major characteristic of the organic food is that it is produced in a naturally defined ecosystem without the use of any artificial means. But production of organic food especially in developed countries is a tough task as there is a heavy use of chemicals such as fertilizer, pesticide and herbicides. India has an edge over the developed countries in this aspect as still in most parts of our country the agricultural production is chemical free and the farmers are very close to being organic. The only difference is that they are not aware about the standards and procedures so as to get their products certified as organic products. Therefore the major requirement is of making our farmers aware about the national standards for organic production developed by apeda, ministry of commerce, goi, so as to help them fetch higher price for their produce. Such an effort will in turn generate additional employment and income in the livestock sector.

Livestock Product Post Harvest Processing Units

In India the revenue from livestock sector is mostly generated by the raw livestock produce i.e., milk, meat and eggs. Hardly a small percent is being processed and value added. Post harvest processing helps in enhancing the shelf life of livestock products, which are a highly perishable commodity and also helps in reducing contamination thereby enhancing the palatability and market value of the livestock products. The annual production of meat and poultry products in India is estimated to be almost 4 million tones per annum, whereas about 1 percent of meat produced is converted into value added products. There is a tremendous opportunity in the livestock sector for employment generation through livestock product processing and value addition. The rural youth can establish various type of livestock product processing and value addition units to earn a livelihood Viz., Milk chilling, storage and packaging units, Meat freezing and packaging units,Milk pasteurization units, Commercial milk product (Ghee, paneer, Khoa etc.) production, Commercial meat products value addition unit for preparing nuggets, soup powder, papad, sausage, pickle, crackles, patties, samosa etc. from mutton, chicken, fish pork and eggs and processing unit for important organs of dead animals or slaughter house by products.

Processing Units for Important Organs of Dead Animals

In India many million animals die every year and there is no proper processing place or unit in rural area where remaining body parts of dead animals (skin, hides, hair bristles, horn, hoof, intestine, bones etc), can be processed and can be converted in to value added products. Processing techniques are easy and rural youth can get the training from IVRI or any veterinary college. Collection of various glands from slaughter animals are also very beneficial to prepare various kinds of hormones, enzymes, medicines. The processed organ or parts of dead animals are in great demand not in our country but abroad also. Although these practices are already in vogue in villages and slaughter houses but in crude form not scientifically.

Organic Waste Management and Entrepreneurship Generation

Animal waste management is most essential from economic and empowerment angle and this involves production, collection, storage, process and utilization. Addressing each stage by adequate technological help is expected to reduce the impact on global warming and to improve the profitability of dairy farming. A better balanced feed not only improves the production but also reduce harmful effects through livestock waste. Improving manure collection process and improved manure storage help to improve soil fertility and to prevent water contamination. Composting is a aerobic process that allows the return of nutrients to the soil for future use. Drying of solid manure is another option to reduce the volume. Improved utilization of manure like feed production for fish in aquaculture, energy (methane gas) or algal growth as fertilizer will also help to improve profitability. Manure application increases soil organic matter improves soil structure, fertility and stability, reduces soil vulnerability to erosion and improves water holding capability. Dung is essential for vermiculture and organic agriculture. Animal wastage like dead skin is utilized in leather industries. Blood and bones could be used efficiently in bone meal, blood meal, etc. Efficient usage of animal wastage using appropriate technological interventions will earn revenue to farmers and reduce ill effects on environment. There is enormous scope for entrepreneurship development in the area of animal waste management.

Loan from Banks

Various Banks are providing loan for livestock based enterprises, here one model i.e., financing for Dairy unit has been given. However, time to time, and bank to bank financing terms and conditions may vary.

Employment opportunities for the professional in the Livestock sector

The professionals engaged in the livestock sector have immense scope of employment and income generation in various sub sectors of the livestock sector. These mainly include Health care in the Dairy farms and Stud farms, expert opinion on AI and related matters, Hygienic milk management, Drug inspection and consultancy for GMP, private and the govt. dairy farms, feed manufacturers, development of veterinary hospitals, disease diagnosis, organic livestock production, pharmaceuticals, livestock breeding farms, fodder growers, fodder enrichment and conservation, development of slaughter house, Livestock product processing units, NGO dealing with livestock development programmes, bank and insurance companies for livestock related matters, animal welfare issues, Zoos and at Airports and sea ports for animal quarantine.

Conclusion

Livestock sector is the backbone of Indian agriculture and it is having potential to increase percent annual growth rate and G.D.P., for making livestock sector potential enterprise. Government of India should also provide subsidy to animal sector as well as frame such policies which develop the interest of farmers in livestock sector. Support of technocrat is highly needed to train the rural masses so that they can apply the latest technical knowledge for developing proper enterprise in this sector.

References

Birthal, P.S. & Rao, P. (2002). Technology options for sustainable livestock production in India. Proceedings of the workshop on Documentation, Adoption & Impact of livestock technologies in India., 18-19 Jan . 2001, ICRISAT, Patancheru, Hyderabad, pp: 12-19.

Chabbra, A.K., Tiwari, C & Tripathi, H. (2002). Shukar Palan- Labhdayak vyavsay. Joint Directorate of Extension Education, IVRI, Izatnagar. Pp: 11-12.

DAHD Annual Report, (2007-08). Available online @ dahd.nic.in/Annual%20 Report%20-2007-08%20 (English).pdf

DAHD, (2007). State wise livestock population (2007). Aavailable online@ www.dahd.nic.in

Desai, Anuradha (2004). Poultry problems and prospects. The Hindu survey of Indian Agriculture. Pp: 104-105.

Haleem, M.A. (2003). Prospects and constraints of Indian meat industry for export. In proceedings of the 4th Asian Buffalo Congress held at New Delhi during Feb. 25-28, 2003.

Jabir Ali (2007). Livestock sector development and implications for rural poverty alleviation in India. Livestock Research for Rural Development, 19 (2) 2007. http://www.cipav.org.co/lrrd/lrrd19/2/cont1902.htm

Jaryal, G.S. & Bedi, T. (2004). Pashu aahar/ Murgi dana nirman kee Ikai. *Udyamita*. 13(4): 67-69.

Jaryal, G.S. (2004). Dairy farm kee ikai kee yozana. *Udyamita*. 12(9): 36-38.

Kumar, S. Deoghare, P.R. (2004). Bakari palan ke vyavsayik pahlu. *Udyamita*. 12(9): 59-60.

Mishra, S., Sharma, S., Vasudevan Padma, Pandey, S. and Meena, B.S. (2006). Fodder supply micromodels for periurban farming systems. In Sharma, J.P., Singh, C.B., Chaudhari, M. and Singh R. eds. Microenterprise promotion in agriculture. Ambica Book Agency, Shastri Nagar, PB No. 1, Jaipur, pp: 59-68.

Rathore, M.S. and Sharma, M.C (2007). Development of livestock enterprises. In Sharma, M.C., Tiwari, R. Singh, B.P. and Rathore, M.S. eds. Microentrepreneurship promotion in livestock sector. 134-141.

Sharma, N. and Kumar, S. (2004). Yawning productivity gap. The Hindu survey of Indian Agriculture. Pp: 115-118.

Singh, Lalji (2008). Role of banks in rural development. In Sharma,M.C., Tiwari, R. Singh, B.P. and Rathore, M.S. eds. Microentrepreneurship promotion in livestock sector.:191-207

Singh, R. Saxena, V.K. and Sharma, D. (2002). Technological developments in the poultry subsector. In Birthal & Rao(Eds) Technology options for sustainable livestock production in India. Proceedings of the workshop on Documentation, Adoption & Impact of livestock technologies in India., 18-19 Jan . 2001, ICRISAT, Hyderabad

Singh, S.P. and Tiwari, N. (2003). New horizons in livestock development, Diversified Agriculture Support Project, pp- 1.

Tiwari, Rupasi, Singh, B.P. & Mandape, M.K. (2004). An Indepth analysis of commercial dairy farming in urban areas. Project report. IVRI. Izatnagar.

□□□

13

Role of Dietary Antioxidants on Performance and Self Life of Meat with Special Reference to Broiler

M. V. DHUMAL, M. G. NIKAM AND K. K. KHOSE
Department of Poultry Science, College of Veterinary and Animal Science, MAFSU, Parbhani - 431 402 (MS)

Introduction

As part of adaptation from marine life, terrestrial plants began producing non marine antioxidants such as ascorbic acid (Vitamin C), polyphenols and tocopherols. Further development of angiosperm plants between 50 and 200 million years ago, particularly during the Jurassic period, produced many antioxidant pigments evolved during the late Jurassic period as chemical defenses against reactive oxygen species produced during photosynthesis. The term antioxidant originally was used to refer specifically to a chemical that prevented the consumption of oxygen. In the late 19th and early 20th centuries, extensive study was devoted to the uses of antioxidants in important industrial processes, such as the prevention of metal corrosion, the vulcanization of rubber, and the polymerization of fuels in the fouling of internal combustion engines.

The possible mechanisms of action of antioxidants were first explored when it was recognized that a substance with antioxidative activity is likely to be one that is itself readily oxidized. Vitamin E prevents the process of lipid peroxidation led to the identification of antioxidants as reducing agents that prevent oxidative reactions, often by scavenging reactive oxygen species before they can damage cells.

An oxidation occurs in feeds and feedstuffs, resulting in rancidity of fats, destruction of vitamins A, D, E, and pigmenters (carotenoids) and amino acids with resultant lowered biological energy values for the diet. If this destruction is allowed to proceed unchecked in a feed, or even in a single ingredient, a lowered feed consumption may result in disastrous nutrient deficiencies. Researchers in a number of fields have been studying the various problems resulting from uncontrolled oxidation and have been developing ways of bringing these oxidation processes under control. It is noted that oxidative rancidity or lipid peroxidation, as contrasted with hydrolytic rancidity, results in a serious decrease in the energy value of a fat or oil. Antioxidants are specific organic compounds that are active in the prevention of very rapid harmful chemical chain reactions with oxygen or nitric oxide, i.e. oxidation reactions. In the body of birds, oxidation reactions generally involve highly reactive molecules called free radicals. Free radicals reside primarily in the mitochondria of cells. When free radicals are released from the mitochondria in numbers sufficient to overwhelm the protective biochemical systems of the body, they become a threat to some cellular structures such as lipids, proteins, carbohydrates, and nucleic acids in cell membranes. Compromised cellular structure alters cellular function, and may lead to the initiation of the disease process.

Mode of action of Antioxidants

An antioxidant is a molecule capable of slowing or preventing the oxidation of other molecules. Oxidation is a chemical reaction that transfers electron from a substance to an oxidizing agent. Oxidation reactions can produce free radicals which start chain reaction that damage cells. Antioxidants terminate these chain reactions by removing free radical intermediates, and inhibit other oxidation reactions by being oxidized themselves. As a result, antioxidants are often reducing agents, as illustrated in stages of oxidation.

Oxidised fat in diet increased the exposure to free radicals, including stress in the intestine and increasing antioxidant requirement to prevent damage to tissues. Chicken diet include fat, and undergone high temperature treatment, resulting peroxidases can contribute substantially to oxidative stress (Surai, 2002).

The three stages of Oxidation

1) Initiation phase

RH ----------→ $R^o + H^o$

Fat molecule Free radical

2) Propagation phase

$R^o + O_2$ ---------→ ROO^o (peroxide)

ROO^o + RH --------→ ROOH + R^o

3) Termination phase

$ROO^o + ROO^o$ ------→ stable end products

(aldehydes, ketones, short chain fatty acids)

Oxidation Process involving Oxygen & lipids

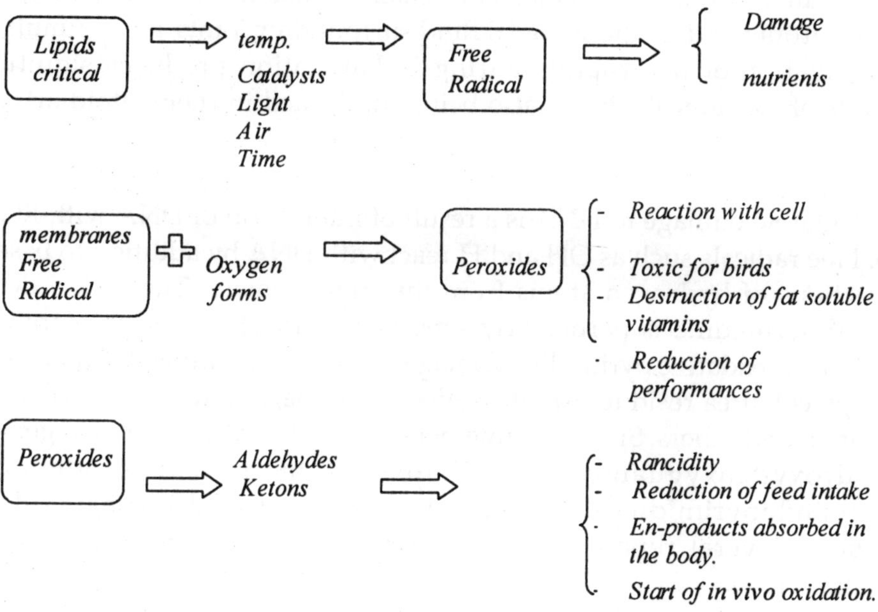

Effects of oxidation process on lipid, carbohydrate, DNA and protein

Lights and Lipid Peroxidation

Membrane lipids present in subcellular organelles are highly susceptible to free radical damage. Lipids when reacted with free radicals can undergo the highly damaging chain reaction of lipid peroxidation (LP) leading to both direct and indirect effects. During LP a large number of toxic byproducts are also formed that can have effects at a site away from the area of generation, behaving as 'second messengers". The damage caused by LP is highly detrimental to the functioning of the cell (Devasagayam et al 2003).

Lipid peroxidation is a free radical medicated process. Initiation of a peroxidative sequence is due to the attack by any species, which can abstract a hydrogen atom from a methylene group (CH2), leaving behind an unpaired electron on the carbon atom (+CH). The resultant carbon radical is subsidized by molecular rearrangement to produce a conjugated Diane, which then can react with an oxygen molecule to give a lipid petoxyl radical (LOO). These radicals can further abstract hydrogen atoms from other lipid molecules to form lipid hydroperoxides (LOOH) and at the same time propagate LOP farther. The peroxidation reaction can be terminated by a member of reactions.

Carbohydrates

Free radicals such as OH react with carbohydrates by randomly abstracting a hydrogen atom from one of the carbon atoms, producing a carbon centered radical. This leads to chain breaks in important molecules like hyaluronic acid. In the synovial fluid surrounding joints, an accumulation and activation of neutrophils during inflammation produces significant amounts of oxyradicals that is also being implicated in rheumatoid arthritis.

DNA

Oxidative damage to DNA is a result of interaction of DNA with ROS or RNS. Free radicals such as OH and H react with DNA by addition to bases or abstractions of hydrogen atoms from the sugar moiety. The C4-C5 double bond of pyrimidine is particularly sensitive to attack by OH, generating a spectrum of oxidative pyrimidine damage products, including thymine glycol, uracil glycol, urea residue, 5-hydroxydeoxyuridine, 5-hydroxydeoxycytidine, hydantion and others. Similarly, interaction of OH with purines will generate 8 hydroxydeoxyguanosine (8-OHdG), 8-hydroxydeoxyadenosine, formamindopyrimidines and other less characterized purine oxidative products. Several repair pathways repair DNA damage (halliwell and Aruoma, 1993).

Proteins

Oxidation of proteins by ROS / RNS can generate a range of stable as well as reactive products such as protein hydroperoxides that can generate additional radicals particularly upon interaction with transition metal ions. Although most oxidized proteins that are functionally inactive are rapidly removed, some can gradually accumulate with time and thereby contribute to the damage associated with ageing as well as various diseases.

Suitability of antioxidants in poultry feed

(a) It must be effective in preserving animal and vegetable fats, vitamins, and other feed qualities subject to oxidative destruction;

(b) It must be non-toxic to man and to the birds

(c) It should be effective at very low concentrations

(d) It must be low enough in cost to be economically practical

(e) It should have stability against temperature

Commonly used antioxidants in poultry diet and their molecular structure

(a) Ethoxyquin (generic term: 1,2-dihydro-6-ethoxy-2,2,4- trimethylquinoline)

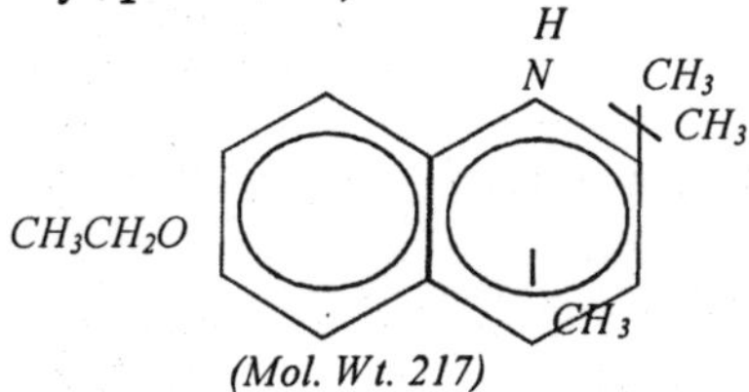

(b) BHA (butylated hydroxyanisole);

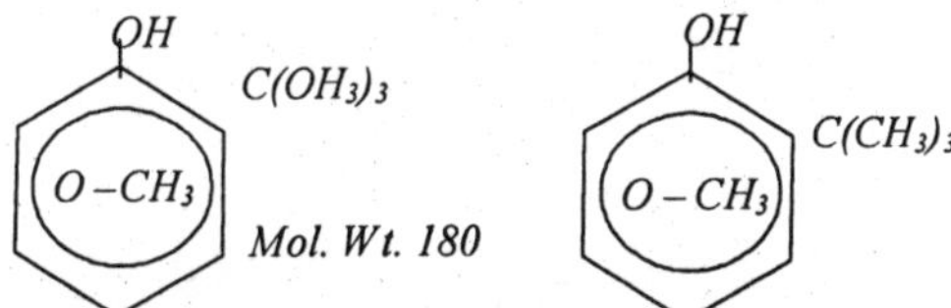

(c) BHT (butylated hydroxytoluene)

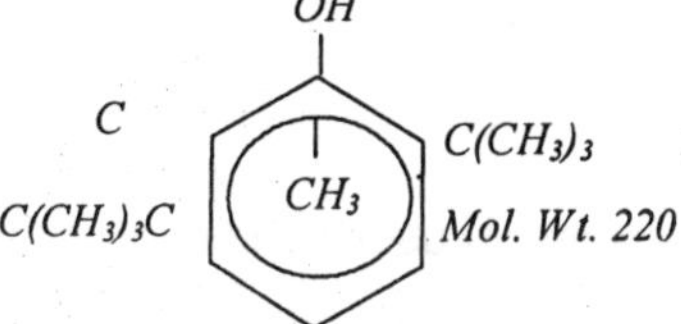

(d) vitamin E (structure of tecopherols)

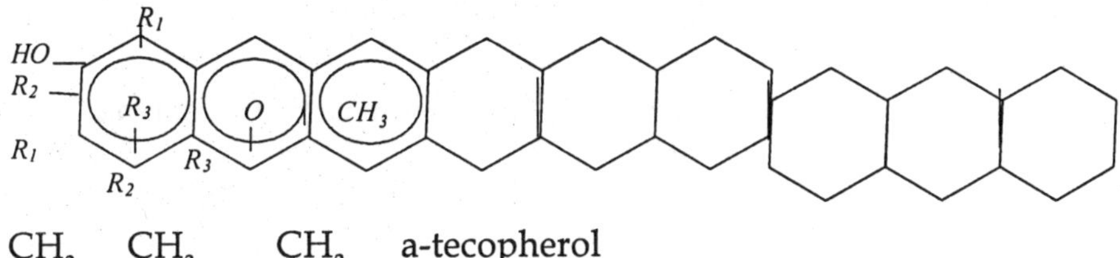

CH_3	CH_3	CH_3	a-tecopherol
CH_3	H	CH_3	b-tecopherol
H	CH_3	CH_3	c-tecopherol
H	H	CH_3	d-tecopherol

(e) vitamin C (structure of ascorbic acid)

CH_2OH
H – C – OH
O
= O
H
HO
OH

(f) Propyl gallate

O
$C – O – CH_2 – CH_2 – CH_3$
OH
OH
OH

Mol. Wt. 212

(g) TBHQ - (Tertiary-butylhydroquinone)

OH
$C(CH_3)_3$
OH

Mol. Wt. 166

(h) Selenium

Table 1 : Properties, applications and regulations of commonly used synthetic anti oxidants a) BHA

S No	Category	Particulars
1	Name	Butylated hydroxyanisole (BHA)
2	Formula	$(CH_3)_3CC_6H_3OCH_3OH$
3	Function	Antioxidant preservative by terminating free radicals
4	Alternative	BHT,PG,TBHQ
5	Synergists	BHT, PG, methionine,lecithin,citric acid,phosphoric acid, thiodipropionic acid
6	Food safety	Not subjected to great criticism, suspected for tumor formation in animals
7	legislation	USA : 0.02%-0.01 of weight of fat UK AND EROPPE,CANADA, JAPAN, AUSTRALIA/PACIFIC RIM JAPAN – Approved

b) BHT

S No	Category	Particulars
1	Name	Butylated hydroxytoluene (BHT)
2	formula	$\{(CH_3)_3C\}_2C_6H_2CH_3OH$
3	function	Antioxidant preservative by terminating free radicals,Antimicrobial Activity
4	Alternative	BHA,PG,TBHQ
5	synergists	BHA,
6	Food safety	Not subjected to great criticism, over safety
7	legislation	USA : 0.02%- of weight of fat UK and Eroppe, Canada, Japan, Australia / Pacific Rim Japan – Approved

c) TBHQ

S No	Category	Particulars
1	Name	Tert-Butylhydroxyquinonetoluene (TBHQ)
2	formula	$(CH_3)_3CC_6H_3(OH)_2$
3	function	Antioxidant preservative by terminating free radicals,
4	Alternative	BHA,BHT
5	synergists	BHA, Citric acid
6	Food safety	Mutagenicity in vivo,
7	legislation	USA : 0.02%- of weight of fat but not allowed to use in combination with PG.

d) Propyl gallate (PG)

S No	Category	Particulars
1	Name	Propyl gallate (PG)
2	formula	$(OH)_3C_6H_2COOCH_2CH_2CH_3$
3	function	Prevents oxidation rancidity development in lipid by terminating free radicals,
4	Alternative	BHA,BHT, TBHQ,octyl gallate,dodecyl gallate
5	synergists	BHA, BHT
6	Food safety	Not subjected to great criticism, over safety
7	legislation	USA : 0.02%- of weight of fat but not allowed to use in combination with TBHQ

Source : Fereidoon and Ying Zhong, 2005

Levels of antioxidants in food

Table 2 : ADIs of some antioxidants permitted in foods.

Antioxidant	ADI (mg/kg bw)
Propyl gallate	0 - 2.5
BHA	0 – 0.5
BHT	0 - 0.125
TBHQ	0.02
Tocopherols	0.15 – 2.0
Ethoxyquin	0.0.06
Vitamin C	Not limited

BW = body weight (*Source :* Fereidoon Shahidi and Ying Zhong, 2005)

Efficacy of antioxidants illustrated by graphical presentation

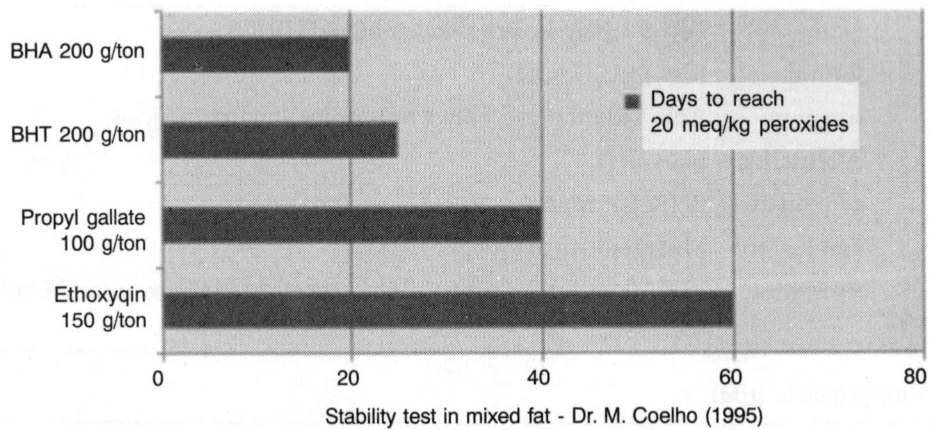

Functional Effects of Antioxidants in Broilers

Nutrient deficiency prevention

Dietary deficiencies of vitamins A and E seem to be ameliorated in certain circumstances and ethoxyquin promotes higher levels of vitamin A storage in the liver. Repletion/deletion experiments show that in both monogastric and ruminant animals, a diet containing an anti-oxidant protects fat soluble vitamins throughout ingestion and metabolism. The important benefit of antioxidants most probably lies in their conservation of essential nutrients and their improved utilization by the birdsl. It has been shown in diets designed for chicken and turkey breeders that ethoxyquin has a vitamin E sparing effect thereby improving the performance of birds.

Table 3 : Regulatory approval status of Major antioxidants in different countries.

Country	Antioxidants BHA	NHT	Gallates	TBHQ
Afghanistan	+	+	-	-
Argentina	+	+	1	+
Australia	+	+	+	+
Bahrain	+	+	+	+
Belgium	+	+	-	-
Brazil	+	+	+	+
China	+	+	+	-
Colombia	+	+	+	+
Denmark	+	+	+	-
Finland	+	+	+	-
France	+	+	+	-
Germany	+	+	+	-
Greece	-	-	+	-
Hongkong	+	+	-	-
India	+	-	+	+
Indonesia	+	+	-	-
Iran	+	+	+	+
Italy	+	+	+	-
Japan	+	-	-	-
South Coria	+	+	+	+
Malaysia	+	+	+	+
Mexico	+	+	+	+
Netherlands	+	-	-	-
New Zealand	+	+	+	+
Nigeria	+	+	-	-
Pakistan	+	+	-	-
Peru	+	+	-	-
Philippines	+	+	+	+
Saudi Arabia	+	+	+	+
South Africa	+	+	+	+
Sweedam	+	+	+	-
Switzerland	+	+	+	-
Taiwan	+	+	+	+
Thailand	+	+	+	+
Turkey	-	-	+	+
United Kingdom	+	+	+	-
Zimbabwe	+	-	-	-

Source : Fereidoon Shahidi and Ying Zhong, 2005

Body weight gain / growth rate

Waldroup et. *al.*, (1961) carried out an experiment to determine the effects of ethoxyquin on broiler performance and concluded dietary supplementation of ethoxyquin produced significantly higher weight gain after four weeks, Cabel et *al.* (1988) revealed supplementation of 62.5 and 125-ppm ethoxyquin in broilers resulted in significantly heavier birds at 49 days of age. Beneficial effects of ethoxyquin supplementation were evident at higher peroxide levels. The study showed that at least 4 meq peroxide/kg feed was required to significantly affect bird performance, and that the addition of ethoxyquin could alleviate the deleterious effects of dietary peroxide. Lin et *al.* (1989) carried out an experiment in broilers fed on diets containing oxidised sunflower oil, sunflower oil and sunflower oil supplemented with alpha-tocopherol, butylated hydroxyl anisole (BHA) or butylated hydroxyl toluene (BHT). Oxidised oil caused a significant reduction in broiler body weights, however alpha-tocopherol and BHA/BHT supplementation improved growth performance. Lauridsen and Jensen (1995) carried out two feeding experiments with broilers by addition of BHT and Ethoxyquin and compared with feed prepared by different technology procedures and concluded a significant interaction between antioxidants and feed technology was revealed as per growth performance of broilers, similarly they also revealed that activity of ethoxyquin seemed to be better to the activity of BHT with respect to growth performance of broilers. Sui-ying et *al.* (1997) reported Ethoxyquin exhibited greater weight gains during starter and grower period. Wang et *al.* (1997) reported that there is a slight increase (6-7%) in the body weight after 3 weeks of treatment, but not after 7 weeks. Mitsuaki et *al.* (1999) conducted an experiment using seven-day old chicks were allocated to six treatments and fed dietary ethoxyquin up to 125 mg, and 350 mg/ kg for 2 weeks. Dietary ethoxyquin up to 125-mg/ kg improved body weight gain from 88 to 98 g and gain per feed from 0.44 to 0.46 although the differences were not significant. However, levels of ethoxyquin in the diet higher than 350-mg/ kg significantly reduced the body weight gain, Sahin and Kucuk (2002) revealed that increased supplemental vitamin E linearly increased live weight gain ($P< 0.01$).

Yuming et *al.* (2003) supplementation of vitamin E tended to improve growth of broilers during 0-3 weeks of age, but the performance from 0 to 6 weeks of age were not influenced. Bolukbasi et *al.* (2006) reported highest weight gain after a 42-day feeding period in male broilers by dietary vitamin E. Lad.(2010) Reported significant ($P<0.01$) influence of various antioxidants on body weight of broilers and concluded that the detrimental effect of xidation process can be prevented through addition of antioxidant compounds.

In contrast, Bartov and Frigg (1992), Jakobsen et *al.* (1995), Soren et *al.* (1999), Coetzee and Hoffman (2001), Bolu et *al.* (2006), Goni et *al.* (2007), Habib et *al.* (2008)and Dhumal et *al.* (2009) reported non significant effect of dietary antioxidants in broilers. Similarly, Patil (2011) reported non significant effect of supplementation of selenium and BHT on body weight of broilers except first week.

Feed consumption

The most of report from literature indicate non significant influence of antioxidants on feed consumption of broilers. Bartov and Weisman (1991) revealed Vitamin E and Ethoxiquine did not affect feed efficiency. Jakobsen et *al.* (1995) reported non significant differences between the antioxidants supplemented groups with respect to feed consumption, Soren et *al.* (1999) revealed non significant differences among the eight antioxidants experimental groups with respect to feed intake in broilers. Also, Mitsuaki et *al.* (1999) reported dietary ethoxyquin up to 125 mg/ kg, feed consumption differences were not significant, Bolu et *al.* (2006) revealed broilers were fed diets containing anti microbial, terramycin, and anti-oxidant, butylated hydroxy toluene (BHT) and natural vitamin premix (NVP) and commercial alternative. Feed intake was similar for all the treatments. Leonel et *al.* (2007) concluded non significant differences (P>0.05) among treatments with respect to the feed intake when diet supplemented with vitamin E from 1 to 15, 1 to 30, 1 to 45, 14 to 45 and 30 to 45 days of age in broilers, Habib et *al.* (2008) inferred that feed intake not significantly affected by experimental diets. Niu et *al.* (2009) showed that feed intake was not significantly influenced by dietary vitamin E (P>0.05) in broilers.

Dhumal et *al.* (2009) revealed that by supplementation of Ethoxyquin and Vitamin E at the dose rate of 0.2 gm/100kg of feed and 50mg/kg live body weight, respectively, the cumulative feed consumption was non-significant among the treatment groups. Lad (2010) reported the non significant differences for weekly feed consumption in various antioxidant treatment group and concluded that the antioxidants used in present study had not imparted any adverse effect on palatability, taste and flavor of feed. Patil (2011) reported no significant effect of supplementation of selenium and BHT on feed consumption of broilers except first week. Wangang (2011)concluded that addition of antioxidants did not show significant effects on feed consumption in broilers.

The literature citated significant influence of antioxidants on feed consumption/feed efficiency: Lauridsen and Jensen (1995) concluded a significant interaction between antioxidants and feed technology, increased in the feed consumption during the time interval, 7-15 days of age. Sui-ying *et al.* (1997) revealed that birds fed on NF/E or NF exhibited greater feed efficiency in the starter period. Yuming *et al.* (2003) reported that supplementation of vitamin E tended to improve feed utilization of birds during 0-3 weeks of age, but the performance from 0 to 6 weeks of age was not influenced, Lohakare (2004) showed that feed intake was significantly higher in antioxidant supplemented groups as compared to control. Bolukbasi *et al.* (2006) reported the best feed efficiency in birds that were fed the E200 diet. Based on the results of this study, they advised to supplement broiler feed with 200 mg/kg of thyme oil as an antioxidant. Cimrin *et al.* (2008) reported that antioxidants NC diet adversely affected (P<0.05) feed intake in broilers.

Feed conversion ratio (FCR)

From economic point of view, narrow the FCR more is the profit because minimum quantity of feed is converted to more amount of meat. The studies carried out by various workers on feed conversion ratio have observed significant influence on FCR of broilers. Kennedy *et al.* (1992) reported increased net income by a significantly improved feed conversion ratio in broilers with use of antioxidants (P < 0.05). Lauridsen and Jensen (1995) observed significant interaction between antioxidants and feed technology for feed conversion at 15 and 29 days of age. Gonzalo (2002) revealed that Vitamin E-supplemented diets resulted in better growth performance, lower rates of feed conversion, content. Vitamin C-supplemented diets resulted in lower feed consumption and lower rates of feed conversion. Yuming et *al.* (2003) observed supplementation of vitamin E tended to improve feed utilization of birds during 0-3 weeks of age, but the performance from 0 to 6 weeks of age were not influenced. Bolukbasi *et al.* (2006) inferred the best feed efficiency and feed conversion rate in birds that were fed the E200 diet. Based on the results of this study, advised to supplement broiler feed with 200 mg/kg of thyme oil as an antioxidant. Lad (2010) reported significant to highly significant (P<0.05 to 0.01) influence of various antioxidant on FCR of broiler during Ist and IInd week, respectively however non significant influence was observed in IV, V and VI week.

In contrast, Niu *et al.* (2009), Cabel *et al.* (1988), Bartov and Frigg (1992), *Jakobsen et al. (1995)*, Coetzee and Hoffman (2001), Hayat *et al.* (2002), Leonel *et al.* (2007), Dhumal *et al.* (2009) reported non significant influence of different antioxidants on FCR of broilers. Patil (2011) reported non significant effect of supplementation of selenium and BHT on FCR of broilers.

Prevention of Rancid Oxidation of Fats in Feed and Improving Shelf life of Meat of Broilers

Antioxidants stabilize critical oxidation-susceptible nutrients that are naturally present in a poultry feed composed of several feedstuffs so that losses are minimal from mixing and storing. The literature citated in this regard is discussed in the foregoing para.

Lin *et al.* (1989) evaluated oxidative stability of meat samples from broilers stored at 4 degrees C and -20 degrees C. dietary alpha-tocopherol and BHA/BHT supplementation increased alpha-tocopherol and BHA/BHT concentrations in meat and significantly ($P< 0.05$) improved the oxidative stability of meat during refrigerated and frozen storage. Bartov and Weisman (1991). Observed vitamin E significantly and consistently decreased TBA values and restricted their increase, particularly in the drumstick meat. Bartov and Frigg (1992) found that the stability of meat of birds fed the various combinations of vitamin E was significantly ($P<0.05$) higher. Ann De Winne and Patrick Dirinck (1996) shown that vitamin E supplementation had a beneficial effect on oxidative stability of the meat as measured by TBA. Sui-ying *et al.* (1997) concluded that ethoxyquin-supplemented diet fed to birds exhibited higher duodenal and ileal GSH, indicating the enhancement of antioxidant mechanism of intestinal cell against detrimental effect of oxidative stress.

Juan *et al.* (1999) suggested that the antioxidant effect of β-carotene requires the presence of vitamin E in tissues. Taniguchi *et al.* (1999) concluded that CTC induces oxidative stress, hypercholesterolemia and growth inhibition, and these effects of CTC are minimized by vitamin E. Coetzee and Hoffman (2001) concluded TBARS values increased with increasing storage time, but decreased with increasing vitamin E levels. Herranz *et al.* (2002) evaluated three feed antioxidants on the oxidative stability of chicken meat under different storage conditions. Two concentrations of ethoxyquin were assessed, as well as the potential synergistic effect in combination with vitamin E. There was a significant decrease in MDA in uncooked breast meat, from the addition of any antioxidant in the feed., it can be stated that 150 mg/kg of ethoxyquin (T2) in feed was more effective than 75 mg/kg (T3), addition of 50 mg/kg of vitamin E to 75 mg/kg of ethoxyquin (T4) was more effective than 150 mg of ethoxyquin alone, Yuming *et al.* (2003) revealed a significant inverse relationship between TBARS value in the thigh meat and the dietary vitamin E level ($R^2 = 0.93$, $P < 0.01$). Supplementation of vitamin E significantly improved the meat quality stability substantially against oxidative deterioration.

Carreras and Guerrero (2004) investigated the effect of dietary -tocopheryl acetate and -carotene supplementation on lipid oxidation of breast meat from broilers fed lard as the fat source. The results show the effectiveness of dietary -tocopheryl acetate supplementation in protecting broiler meat against lipid oxidation. Lohakare (2004) conducted a trial to compare the effects of vitamin E (VE) when supplemented in either feed or water on the performance and meat quality of broilers. The TBARS values measured after 5 and 10 days of storage, showed significantly lower levels in antioxidant supplemented diets. They inferred that supplementation of VE was beneficial.

Waheed et *al.* (2004) concluded that oxidation of oil in ration increased significantly ($P<0.05$) with increasing period. Higher storage temperature also significantly affected the oxidation of fat. Supplementation of ration with high levels of antioxidant significantly ($P<0.05$) improved the stability of corn oil in ration. Fellenberg and Speisky (2005) concluded that supplementation of antioxidant provides quality and safety of meat for human consumption, and in turn the prevention and/or delay of several oxidation processes would allow its management for an optimal quality and self life conservation. Njobeh *et al.* (2006) revealed synthetic antioxidants have demonstrated efficacy in reducing the rate of oxidative rancidity in broiler diets.

Goni *et al.* (2007) concluded that Grape pomace and vitamin E diets reduced the lipid oxidation of meat during refrigerated storage and increased liver alpha-tocopherol concentration, Danka *et al.* (2007) showed that the rosemary powder was effective in delaying lipid oxidation compared to the control diet at all time points, but less effective than α-tocopherol. Leonel *et al.* (2007) observed the TBARS values at 3 day of storage significantly different ($P<0.01$) of treatments with vitamin E supplementation for leg muscles.

Kanatte *et al.* (2008) reported TBA values and carbonyl content for irradiated samples of ground chicken meat higher than for non irradiated samples. Addition of antioxidants tocopherol (natural) or BHT (synthetic) resulted in retardation of oxidative rancidity ($p<0.05$). Meat treated with antioxidants prior to irradiation had lower TBA values as compared to untreated irradiated counterparts. Free fatty acid (FFA) values decreased after irradiation. Addition of antioxidants prior to irradiation showed a synergistic effect in decreasing FFA content. TLC of muscle lipids indicated a reduction in the triacylglcerols content with concomitant increases in FFA of all samples during storage. All irradiated meats were acceptable for consumption up to 4 wk of storage. Reddy *et al.* (2009) concluded that dietary supplementation of ocimum and it's combination with selenium (0.3ppm) can combat oxidative stress in broilers.

Lad (2010) showed significant (P,0.01) differences among treatment groups for TBA values on 3rd, 7$^{th\ day}$ of refrigeration storage and the superior TBA values were recorded for BHT antioxidant. Wangang (2011)concluded that addition of antioxidants significantly arrested protein oxidation in blood, and breast meat quality parameters.

Effect of Antioxidants on Mortality Pattern of Broilers

Sui-ying *et al.* (1997), Bolu *et al.* (2006), Leonel *et al.* (2007), reported similar mortality pattern for all the treatments groups. However, lowest mortality (2.67%) in Vit. E supplemented group, followed by ethoxyquin group (5.33%) and control (8.00%) as reported by Dhumal *et al.* (2009), Lad (2010) reported lower mortality in broiler, supplemented with antioxidants compared to control group.

Conclusion

1. The various antioxidants like Ethoxiquin, BHA, BHT, TBHQ, Vitamin E, Vitamin C and selenium have proved efficacy in reducing the rate of oxidative rancidity in broiler diets.
2. The various antioxidants are functioning as an inhibitor to oxidation reactions through various mechanisms and prevent the deterioration in performance of broiler.
3. Use of dietary antioxidants is also beneficial for prevention of oxidative changes during meat storage and thereby improves self life of meat, which is important from trading point of view.
4. Dietary antioxidants are important as they enrich meat for human health.
5. Future research is expected on various combinations (synergistic effects) of antioxidants and their level of incorporation.

Hence coordinated research involving high levels of antioxidant properties in food/ meat (functional food) can make significant difference to broiler industry in coming decades. No Indian belly should remain without designer meat -should be the motto of poultry nutritionist.

References

Ann De Winne and Patrick Dirinck, (1996). Studies on Vitamin E and Meat Quality. 2. Effect of Feeding High Vitamin E Levels on Chicken Meat Quality. *J. Agric. Food Chem.*, 44 (7): 1691-1696.

Bartov and Weisman (1991). Effects of high concentrations of dietary vitamin e and ethoxyquin on the performance of laying hens. *British Poultry Science*, 32: 525-534.

Bartov and Frigg (1992). Effect of high concentrations of dietary vitamin e during various age periods on performance, plasma vitamin e and meat stability of broiler chicks at 7 weeks of age. *British Poultry Science*, 33: 393-402.

Bolu, Bologun and Akilu. (2006). Effects of improved natural vitamin premix on the histology and specific enzyme activities of broilers Department of Animal Production, University of Ilorin, Ilorin (Nigeria).

Bolukbasi S.C, Erhan M.K and zkan A. A. (2006). Effect of dietary thyme oil and vitamin E on growth, lipid oxidation, meat fatty acid composition and serum lipoproteins of broi Volume: 36.

Cabel, M.C., P.W. Waldroup, W.D. Shermer and D.F. Calabotta (1988). Effects of ethoxyquin feed preservative and peroxide level on broiler performance. *Poultry Sci.* 67: 7125-1730.

Carreras and Guerrero (2004). Vitamin E levels, thiobarbituric acid test and sensory evaluation of breast muscles from broilers fed -tocopheryl acetate- and -carotene-supplemented diets. *Journal of the Science of Food and Agriculture*, 84(4): 313-317.

Cimrin Tulay, Demire and Murat (2008). Effect of Dietary Phytase and Some Antioxidants on the Fattening Performance of Broilers. Animal Science Department, Agricultural Faculty, Yüzüncü Yil University, 65080, Van-Turkey.

Coetzee and Hoffman (2001) Effect of dietary vitamin E on the performance of broilers and quality of broiler meat during refrigerated and frozen storage. *South African Journal of Animal Science* 2001: 31(3).

Danka Pernakova, Dionyzmate, Hanna rosanska, and Gabriel Kovac (2007). Effects of dietary rosemary extract and alpha tocopherol on the performance of chickens, meat quality, and lipid oxidation in meat storage under chilling conditions. *Bull Vet Inst Pulawy* 51: 585-589.

Devasagayam TPA, Tilak J.C., Boloor K.K., Sane. K.S., Ghaskadb. S.S and Lele. R.D, (2003). Free radicals and antioxidants in human health :Current status and future prospects.JAPI-52:794-804.www.Japi.org.

Dhumal M.V., Siddiqui, M.F. Nikam M.G., Avari P.E., Surjuse P.D. and Lad R.G. (2009). Studies on performance of broilers supplemented with different antioxidants. *Ipsacon* pp. 191: abstract 131.

Fellenberg, M.A. and Speisky H. (2005). Antioxidants: their effects on broiler oxidative stress and its meat oxidative stability mafellen@puc.cl

Goni I, Brenes A, Centeno C, Viveros A, Saura-Calixto F, Rebole A, Arija and Estevez R (2007). Effect of dietary grape pomace and vitamin E on growth performance, nutrient digestibility, and susceptibility to meat lipid oxidation in chickens. *Poult Sci.* 2007 Mar; 86(3): 508-16.

Gonzalo (2002). Effects of dietary supplementation with vitamin C or vitamin E on cardiac lipid per oxidation and growth performance in broilers at risk of developing ascites syndrome. *American Journal of Veterinary Research*, Vol. 63(5), doi: 10.2460/ajvr.2002.63.673.

Habib Aghdam Shahriar, Kambiz Nazer Adl, Yahya Ebrahim Nezhad, Ramin Salamat Doust Nobar and Alireza Ahmadzadeh (2008). Effect of Dietary Fat Type and Different Levels of Vitamin E on Broiler Breeder Performance and Vitamin E Levels of Egg http://scialert.net/abstract/? doi=ajava.2008.147.154

Herranz, Pla, Calafat and Vila (2002). Oxidative stability of chicken meat with natural and synthetic feed antioxidants IRTA, Animal Nutrition, c/Licorices 42, 43800 Val's, Spain.

Jakobsen, Engberg and Andersen (1995). Supplementation of broiler diets with all-rac-alpha- or a mixture of natural source RRR-alpha-, gamma-, delta-tocopheryl acetate. 1. Effect on vitamin E status of broilers in vivo and at slaughter. *Poult Sci.* 74(12): 1984-94.

Juan, Anna, perez and Enric (1999). Effect of â-Carotene and Vitamin E on Oxidative Stability in Leg Meat of Broilers Fed Different Supplemental Fats. *J. Agric. Food Chem.*, 47(2): 448–454.

Kantte S. R. Pushpa Paul, S.F. D'Souza, Paul, Thomas (2008). Lipid peroxidation in Chicken meat during chilled storage as affected by Antioxidants combined with low dose gamme irradiation. *Journal of Food.* 63 (2) : 198-200.

Kennedy, Rice and Bruce (1992). Economic effects of increased vitamin E supplementation of broiler diets on commercial broiler production. *British Poultry Science*, 33(5): 1015-1023.

Lad, R.G. (2010). Comparative studies on performance of broilers supplemented with various antioxidants through feed. Thesis submitted to Maharashtra Animal and Fishery Science University, Nagpur, for award of M V Sc degree.

Lauridsen and Jensen (1995). Effects of synthetic antioxidants in feed of different technological treatments on the performance of broilers. Royal veterinary agricultural univ., dep. animal sci. animal health, 1870 Frederiksberg, Danemark

Leonel FR, Oba A, Pelicano ERL, Zeola NMBL, Boiago MM, Scatolini AM, LimaTMA, Souza PA and Souza HBA (2007) Performance, Carcass Yield, and Qualitative Characteristics of Breast and Leg Muscles of Broilers Fed Diets Supplemented with Vitamin E at Different Ages. Brazilian Journal of Poultry Science. 9(2): 91-97.

Lin, Asghar, Gray and Booren (1989). Effects of oxidised dietary oil and antioxidant supplementation on broiler growth and meat stability. *Br Poult Sci.* 30(4): 855-64.

Lohakare (2004). Effects of Feeding Methods (Feed vs. Water) of Vitamin E on Growth Performance and Meat Quality of Broilers. *Asian-Australasian Journal of Animal Sciences.* 17 (No.9).

Mitsuaki Ohshima, Dolores V. Layug, Hiro-omi Yokota and Henry T. Ostrowski-Meissner (1999). Effect of graded levels of ethoxyquin in alfalfa leaf extracts on carotenoid and cholesterol concentrations in chicks. *Animal Feed Science and Technology.* 62(2-4): 141-150.

Niu ZY, Liu FZ, Yan QL, Li WC. (2009). Effects of different levels of vitamin E on growth performance and immune responses of broilers under heat stress. *Poult Sci.* 88(10): 2101-7.

Njobeh, P.B., P.A. Iji and I.V. Nsahlai. (2006) Influence of composition andstorage conditions on the concentrations of free fatty acids and peroxides in broiler diets. *Intl. J. Poultry Sci.* 5(3): 279-283.

Patil, S.R. (2011). Studies on performance of broilers supplemented with antioxidant and different forms of selenium through feed. Thesis submitted to Maharashtra Animal and Fishery Science University, Nagpur, for awards of M V Sc degree.

Reddy L.S.S. Vara Prasad, A. Thangavel, V. Leela and K.V.S. Narayana Raju(2009) Antioxidant enzyme status in broilers: Role of dietary supplementation Tulsi Ocimum sanctum and selenium. *Tamilnadu J. Veterinary & Animal Sciences* 5(6) : 251-256.

Sahin and Kucuk (2002). Optimal dietary concentration of vitamin E for alleviating the effect of heat stress on performance, thyroid status, ACTH and some serum metabolite and mineral concentrations in broilers Vet. Med. - Czech, 47 (4): 110–116.

Soren, K. Jensen, Ricarda M. Engberg and Mette S. Hedemann (1999) All-rac--Tocopherol Acetate Is a Better Vitamin E Source than all-rac – Tocopherol Succinate for Broilers. The American Society for Nutritional Sciences. *Journal of Nutrition*. 129:1355-1360.

Sui-ying wang, Walter Bottje, Philip Maynard, Julia Dibner, and William Shermer (1997). Effect of Santoquin and Oxidized Fat on Liver and Intestinal Glutathione in Broilers. *Poultry Science* 76:961–967

Surai, P.F. (2002). Natural Antioxidants in Avian Nutrition and Reproduction. Nottingham University Press, Nottingham.

Surai P.F. (2000). Natural antioxidant in poultry nutrition: New developments. 16th Eropean symposium on poultry nutrition. 669-676.

Taniguchi.N, Ohtsuka.A,Hayashi K (1999). Effect of dietary Corticosterone and Vitamin E on growth and oxidative stress in broiler chickens. *Ani. Sci. Journal*. 70: 195-200.

Waheed, A., T. Ahmad, A Yousaf and I. J. Zaefr (2004). Effect of various levels of fat and antioxidant on the quality of broiler rations stored at high temperature for different periods. *Pakisthan Vet. J*.24 (2):70-75.

Waldroup, P.W., C.R. Douglas, J.T. McCall and R.H. Harms. (1961). The effects of Santoquin on the performance of broilers. *Poultry Sci*. 39:1313-1317.

Wang, S.Y., Bottje, W., Maynard, P., Dibner, J. and Shermer, W. (1997). Effect of Santoquin ® and Oxidized Fat on Liver and Intestinal Glutathione in Broilers. *Poultry Science* 76: 961-967.

Wangang Zhang,Shan Xiao,Eun Joo Lee and Dong (2011). The book is published in Iowa State University Animal Industry report.

Yuming, Quing, Jianmin and Zirong. (2003). Effects of source and level of magnesium and Vitamin E on prevention of hepatic peroxidation and oxidative deterioration of broiler meat Animal feed science and technology ISSN 0377.

□□□

14

Prospects of Integrated Helminth Parasite Management in Dairy Animals in India using Medicated Urea Molasses Block Technology

P.K. SANYAL
Professor & Head
Department of Veterinary Parasitology, College of Veterinary Science & Animal Husbandry, Indira Gandhi Krishi Vishwavidyalaya, Anjora, Durg-491 001, Chhattisgarh

ABSTRACT

Gastrointestinal helminth parasites continue to be major constraints to efficient production of milk in cattle and buffaloes throughout the world including India. This probem is exacerbated in production systems, where nutritional inputs are sub-optimal and helminth parasites are not adequately controlled. To optimise the production potential in these areas, there is an urgent need to gather epidemiological information on helminth parasitism so that appropriate control measures can be put in place. In situations where urea molasses blocks are considered benefical as nutrient supplementation in dairy animals, blocks containing anthelmintic can then be introduced for short periods during times when parasite challenge is high or during periods of lowered host immunity caused by immaturity or physiological stresses such as reproduction and lactation. For these reasons, it is likely that medicated blocks would form an integral part of strategic parasite control programmes in India where urea molasses block technology has been shown to offer substantial nutritional benefits.

Introduction

The continuing growth of the human population makes it necessary to search for new ways to increase food production. Approaches aiming to reduce losses caused by pests and diseases may be one of such. Current estimates put global losses caused by pests at US$ 300 billion annually (Thamsborg *et al.*, 1999), which equals around 30-40% of potential global food, fibre, and feed production with substantially higher proportion in developing countries. Ecologically sustainable development has become a major international concept of importance, which aims to meets the needs of the present without compromising the ability of future generations to meet their own needs. The most important effect is the realisation of the urgency and magnitude of the world's problem and of the environmental and consumer concerns. The demand for milk, meat and fibre in the developing world is growing consistently not only because of increasing human population but also due to rise of per capita income. The need is not only to feed more people but also to address the challenges of undernourishment. Ruminants play a crucial role in the conversion of low quality plant material and crop residues to high quality human food as well as by returning valuable plant nutrients to the soil and thus, appear sustainable.

Attempts to increase productivity of ruminants generally encounter two principal constraints, nutrition and health. Depending on the environment and production system, undernutrition interacts with infectious diseases, parasitic diseases in particular, to limit animal performance. Nutrition of ruminant animals in India is constrained by the low quality available forages that influences animal productivity unless supplements are offered. In such a scenario, urea molasses blocks can provide a low cost means of providing deficient nutrients and would optimise productivity from the available feed resources. Of the health constraints, bacterial and viral diseases can be successfully controlled through conventional vaccination and quarantine measures. However, for parasitic diseases, chemotherapy is the only option available. As a parasitologist it is worthwhile for us to better define our potential contribution within a broad understanding of the global problem. As sustainable development is a compromise between reducing environmental degradation and positive economic growth, sustainable parasite control should aim towards less intensive, lower input, lesser risk of parasite induced losses with greater opportunities for integration of all available control resources (Sanyal, 2001). Parasitic helminthoses are regarded as major impediments to profitable ruminant production. The haematophagous abomasal parasite *Haemonchus* spp. and *Fasciola gigantica* are the dominant species in both small and large ruminants in India and the degree of infection is more in grazing livestock than tethered animals. Rainfall governs the severity of infection which favour development and survival of preparasitic (Sanyal, 1996a). Veterinarians and animal health workers tend to recognise the seasonality of the problem and accordingly treat the animals with anthelmintics. In many instances, lengthy periods of high rainfall require regular and frequent treatment.

The primary focus of this paper is to describe the potential for using urea molasses blocks (UMB) for the delivery of anthelmintic medication to control gastrointestinal parasites, nematode and liver flukes in particular, in cattle and buffaloes so as to achieve both chemotherapeutic and nutritional control of these great menaces. However, before application it is desirable to discuss on parasite epidemiology in different agroclimatic zones of India and the impact of parasitoses on milk production of cattle and buffaloes.

Parasite Epidmiology

Studies on parasite epidemiology in seven Veterinary Colleges, each representing a geographic zone, during 1994-1996 reveal greater infection intensity in the host and higher larval burden on pasture following the advent of monsoon rains. However, the month and duration of peak infection varied from zone to zone. Haematophagous abomasal nematode, *Haemonchus contortus*, and *Fasciola gigantica* are the predominant parasites encountered in all geographical and agroclimatic zones. The principal recommendation of an international workshop, where these epidemiological findings were discussed, is to use medicated blocks at the onset of monsoon rains for strategic and sustainable parasite control in dairy animals (Sanyal and Singh, 1995a).

Impact of Gastrointestinal Parasites on Milk Production

Production losses due to helminths at subclinical levels of infection can appear as lower growth rates and lower yield of milk. Studies indicated that per-parturient anthelmintic treatments could result in 11% increase in milk yield of crossbred cattle (Sanyal *et al.*, 1992) and 13% in dairy buffaloes in India (Sanyal *et al.*, 1993).

Anti-nematode Medicated Urea Molasses Blocks (MUMB)

Anthelmintic pharmacokinetics studies undertaken in dairy cattle and buffaloes provided the dose of the selected anthelmintic to be targeted in UMBs, so that the animals could receive the desired dose of the drug on a daily basis. Fenbendazole (FBZ) was found most suitable for incorporation in UMBs as the drug was stable in blocks, do not require milk withholding period and has a safety index of 67 in cattle and 1000 in small ruminants. Moreover as the drug is not patented, it can be bulk procured from the open market.

A series of studies on FBZ pharmacokinetics on single and continuous intraruminal dosing, confirm that effective concentration of oxfendazole (OFZ), the anthelmintically active principal metabolite of FBZ in plasma could be achieved by daily intraruminal administration of FBZ at 0.5 mg kg^{-1} body weight (Sanyal, 1993a, Sanyal, 1994; Sanyal and Singh, 1992). The effective level was reached between day 4-6 of drug administration and a plateau was maintained thereafter. The OFZ disposition profile reveals typical zero order absorption-elimination from day 4-6. In other words, by daily low level dosing the parasites would be exposed to the toxic concentration of the drug for much longer periods without additional use of the drug. Successful incorporation of FBZ in UMBs at 0.5 gm kg^{-1} block materials is demonstrated by solid phase extraction and reverse phase high performance liquid chromatography (HPLC). The medicated blocks offered to the animals reveal sustained levels of the parent drug and its metabolites in the plasma, resulting in selection of drug doses to be incorporated in UMBs that would ensure the desired plasma concentrations of the anthelmintic in cattle and buffalo (Sanyal and Singh, 1993a; Sanyal, 1993b).

Trials conducted in calves experimentally infected with *Haemonchus placei* for evaluating the efficacy of FBZ incorporated MUMBs demonstrate that the medicated blocks could effectively remove established adult parasites and also prevent establishment of infection by killing incoming larvae (Sanyal and Singh, 1993b). The anthelmintic delivery device could thus be highly effective for the treatment as well as prevention of gastrointestinal nematodosis in cattle and buffaloes.

Farm and large-scale field trials conducted on replacement heifers and lactating crossbred cattle and buffaloes in Gujarat reveal improvement in animal productivity. Farm-bred heifers of 20-33 months of age and weighing 165-240 kg, licking MUMB for 4 months, exhibit consistent zero egg counts with a weight gain of 60 gm per day (Sanyal and Singh, 1995b). On-farm lactating buffaloes offered MUMB, produce more milk with a net gain of 1.0 litre milk per buffalo per day (Sanyal and Singh, 1995c). Sustained parasite control could also be achieved in farm-bred lactating crossbred cattle with an average increase of 0.57 litre milk per animal per day (Sanyal *et al.*, 1995).

Field trials involving buffaloes and cattle in Surat and Ahmedabad cooperative milk unions of Gujarat indicate that the animals with access to MUMB could withstand parasite challenge even a month after MUMB withdrawal. The farmers report improvement in body coat texture and overall health of animals. A field trial conducted by Surat District Cooperative Milk Producers' Union Ltd., Surat involving 2000 dairy cattle and buffaloes indicate an average intake of block of 210.0 gm per day. An increase in fodder consumption by the animals following MUMB offer resulting in improved health and hair coat and an average increase of 0.5 litre milk per animal per day, are some of the farmer's observations.

Anti-fluke MUMB

For developing a flukicide incorporated MUMB using the principle of prolonged low-level administration, triclabendazole (TCBZ; Fasinex, Ciba-Geigy, Switzerland) is the drug of choice as this is the only drug available in India, which is effective against early immature liver flukes. Pharmacokinetic studies on TCBZ in dairy animals reveal very poor anthelmintic uptake in buffaloes compared to cattle (Sanyal, 1995). Critical efficacy of TCBZ against experimental bovine and bubaline fasciolosis reveal high efficacy of the drug against both immature and mature fasciolosis in cattle at the recommended dose rates of 12.0 mg kg^{-1} body weight (Sanyal, 1996b), while buffaloes require 24.0 mg kg^{-1} body weight or above to control immature and mature fasciolosis (Sanyal and Gupta, 1996a). Daily low-level administration of TCBZ against experimental bovine and bubaline fasciolosis indicate that daily dosing for 10 days is required to eliminate mature liver flukes in cattle and buffalo at the rate of 0.5 and 1.5 mg kg^{-1} body weight, respectively (Sanyal and Gupta, 1996b). Thus, different drug dose rates are targeted in TCBZ MUMBs for cattle and buffaloes, to ensure delivery of a minimum daily dose of 0.5 and 1.5 mg kg^{-1} body weight, respectively and prove their efficacy against experimental bovine and bubaline fasciolosis (Sanyal and Gupta, 1998).

Conclusion

Control of parasitic disease in India, at least in the foreseeable future, will depend primarily on the use of chemotherapeutic agents. At the advent of escalating problem of anthelmintic resistance, food residues and environmental concerns, MUMBs in combination with UMBs could become effective tools for anthelmintic and nutrional management. This is particularly important as sustained low level administration of benzimidazole anthelmintics has also been found efficacious against larvae of benzimidazole-resistant strains of nematode parasites (Barger *et al.*, 1993). Prolonged low level administration of anthelmintics through UMBs would have the following benefits :

1. The involvement of labour and spillage of medicines that occurs during conventional oral drenching could be avoided.
2. The low but prolonged administration of the drug would not only increase its efficacy against existing worms but also prevent reinfection.
3. The urea, molasses and minerals incorporated in the blocks, would greatly improve nutritional status of the animals, which makes them more tolerant to parasites and in turn increase productivity of the animals.
4. The emergence of anthelmintic resistant parasites would likely to be delayed and the larvae of already resistant parasite strains would likely

to be killed, thereby extending the effective life of existing anthelmintic drugs.

5. Strategic application of MUMBs would help in reduction of worm egg output in the faeces of the animals resulting in reduced level of pasture contamination and finally reduced level of parasitic challenge to young calves which are highly susceptible to worm infections.

Thus, MUMB could effectively be used as a tool for integrated parasite management for sustainable development of dairy animals.

Acknowledgement

The research was the result of two collaborative projects between the National Dairy Development Board (NDDB), India and CSIRO Division of Animal Production, Australia under the aegis of Australian Centre for International Agricultural Research, Australia (ACIAR Project Nos. 8523 and 9132).

References

Barger, I.A., Steel, J.W. and Rodden, B.R. (1993). Effect of a continuous release albendazole capsule on parasitism and production of grazing merino ewes and lambs. *Australian Veterinary Journal*, 70: 41-48.

Sanyal, P.K. (1993a). Plasma levels of fenbendazole metabolites in buffalo and cattle after long-term intraruminal administration. *Veterinary Quarterly*, 15: 157-159.

Sanyal, P.K. (1993b). The uptake of fenbendazole by cattle and buffalo following long-term low-level administration in urea-molasses blocks : further studies on block formulations. *Veterinary Research Communication*, 17: 325-331.

Sanyal, P.K. (1994). The pharmacokinetic behaviour of fenbendazole in buffalo and cattle. *Journal of Veterinary Pharmacology and Therapeutics*, 17: 1-4.

Sanyal, P.K. (1995). Kinetic disposition of triclabendazole in buffalo compared to cattle. Journal of Veterinary Pharmacology and Therapeutics, 18: 370-374.

Sanyal, P.K. (1996a). Gastrointestinal parasites and small ruminant production in India. Australian Centre for International Agricultural Research Proceedings No. 74 on Sustainable Parasite Control in Small Ruminants. ACIAR, Canberra, Australia, pp. 109-112.

Sanyal, P.K. (1996b). Kinetic disposition and critical efficacy of triclabendazole against experimental bovine and bubaline fasciolosis. *Journal of Veterinary Parasitology*, 10: 147-152.

Sanyal, P.K. (2001). Integrated management of parasitic gastroenteritis in ruminants. In : Perspectives on Helminthology (Eds. N. Chowdhury and I. Tada), Oxford & IBH Publishing Co. Ltd., New Delhi, pp. 439-460.

Sanyal, P.K. and Gupta, S.C. (1996a). Efficacy and pharmacokinetics of triclabendazole in buffalo with induced fasciolosis. *Veterinary Parasitology*, 63: 75-82.

Sanyal, P.K. and Gupta, S.C. (1996b). The efficacy and pharmacokinetics of long-term low-level intraruminal administration of triclabendazole in buffalo with induced fasciolosis. *Veterinary Research Communications*, 20: 461-468.

Sanyal, P.K. and Gupta, S.C. (1998). Pharmacokinetics and efficacy of long-term low-level administration of triclabendazole in urea molasses blocks against induced bovine and bubaline fasciolosis. *Veterinary Parasitology*, 76: 57-64.

Sanyal, P.K. and Singh, D.K. (1992). Plasma oxfendazole profile in buffalo and cattle : a marker of pharmacokinetics of fenbendazole. *Buffalo Journal*, 8: 157-161.

Sanyal, P.K. and Singh, D.K. (1993a). The uptake by cattle and buffalo following long term low level administration in urea molasses block. *Veterinary Research Communications*, 17: 137-142.

Sanyal, P.K. and Singh, D.K. (1993b). Prophylactic and therapeutic efficacy of long term low level administration of fenbendazole through urea molasses block against experimental haemonchosis in calves. *Journal of Veterinary Parasitology*, 7: 71-80.

Sanyal, P.K. and Singh, D.K. (1995a). Proceedings of the workshop on control strategy against gastrointestinal parasites in dairy animals using medicated urea molasses blocks, Anand, National Dairy Development Board, 47 p.

Sanyal, P.K. and Singh, D.K. (1995b). Effect of fenbendazole in urea molasses block on nematode infection and growth of heifers of cross-bred cattle. *Journal of Veterinary Parasitology*, 9: 79-85.

Sanyal, P.K. and Singh, D.K. (1995c). Administration of fenbendazole in urea molasses block to dairy buffaloes of India. *Tropical Animal Health and Production*, 27: 186-190.

Sanyal, P.K., Singh, D.K. and Knox, M.R. (1992). The effect of peri-parturient anthelmintic treatment on the productivity of dairy cattle in subtropical Western India. *Veterinary Research Communications*. 16: 445-450.

Sanyal, P. K., Singh, D. K. and Knox, M. R. (1993). Effect of peri-parturient anthelmintic treatment on milk yield of dairy buffaloes in subtropical Western India. *Buffalo Journal*. 9: 265-270.

Sanyal, P.K., Srivastava, S.M., Panchal, A.G. and Singh, D.K. (1995). Effect of feeding fenbendazole incorporated urea molasses block on nematode infection and milk yield of dairy cattle. *Journal of Veterinary Parasitology*, 9: 11-16.

Thamsborg, S.M., Roepstorff, A. and Larsen, M. (1999). Integrated and biological control of parasites in organic and conventional production systems. *Veterinary Parasitology*. 84 : 169-186.

□□□

15

Strategic Feed Supplements for Health and Production of Livestock

USHA R.MEHRA
Ex- Director cum Head, Center of Advanced Studies in Animal Nutrition, IVRI
Izatnagar, 243 122 (U.P.)

The problem of feeding urea to animals has been overcome in India by the introduction of feed supplementation blocks in the form of urea-molasses mineral block (UMMB) licks developed at Indian Veterinary Research Institute, Izatnagar, (1990) by cold process technology. National Dairy development board (NDDB), Anand, India developed hot process technology (Kunju, 1986 a,b) The slow ingestion of urea provided through such licks ensures its efficient, non toxic utilization However the formulation , packing and feeding of UMMB licks require critical attention to ensure their regular and proper use by farmers.

The preparation of UMMB is cost-effective and can easily be adopted by the skilled farmers, at their own door, The methodology is based on confirmatory evaluation of improved performance (growth, digestibility, N and mineral balances etc) in different species of ruminants i.e. cattle and buffalo and different categories i.e. growing and adult animals (Mehra *et al* 2007). The supplementation of UMMB licks appeared to be a simple way of improving the efficiency of utilization of fibrous feeds, which constitute the bulk of the diets of ruminants in most of the developing countries.

These blocks can improve the growth performance, nutrient intake and nitrogen utilization in growing buffalo calves. (Tiwari *et al* 1990).

The Composition of the block is given as under in table 1.

Table 1

Ingredient	Percent
Wheat bran	40
Molasses	38
Urea	10
Cement Portland	10
Mineral Mixture	1
Common Salt	1
Vitamin A & D_3	@10g /quintal

The blocks prepared by cold process technology is given in Fig 1.

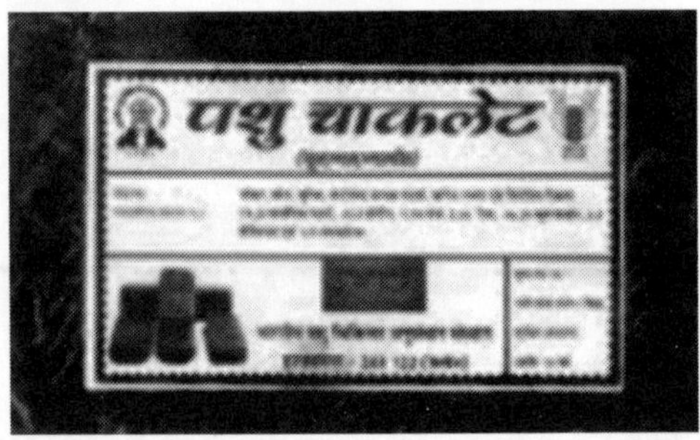

Assessment for valuation of UMMB in respect of growth and metabolic activities

An experiment was conducted on male growing male buffalo calves of 9-13 months of age. These calves were randomly divided into five groups of four animals in each, following completely randomized block design. The initial average body weights of the animals are given in Table 2. The animals were individually offered wheat straw *ad libitum* and wheat bran and oil extracted rice bran at the rate of 500g each day. Animals of groups 3, 4 and 5 were given UMMB lick *ad libitum*. In addition, animals in groups 3, 4 and 5 were given supplements of fish meal @ of 50, 100 and 150g, respectively. A growth trial was conducted for a period of 131 days.

Effect of UMMB feeding on Body weight gain

The initial body weight of animals as well as gain in body weight (g day^{-1}) are presented in Table 3. The lowest gain in body weight was recorded in group I (90±16.00g day^{-1}) where animal were offered wheat straw *ad libitum* and wheat bran and deoiled rice bran at the rate of 500g each day^{-1}. There was appreciable improvement in gain in group 2 (166±20.52 g day^{-1}) owing to supplementation of *ad libitum* UMMB in the basal diet. The maximum growth was attained by the animals of group 4 where in addition to UMMB lick 100g fish meal was incorporated in the diet. There are several reports of incorporating by pass protein in the diet of ruminants resulting in significantly increased daily gain in body weight. It appears from the data that daily gain in body weight depends on the plane of nutrition of the animal. The total digestible nutrients were 1.52, 2.17, 2.27, 2.48 and 2.57 kg day^{-1} in group 1, 2, 3, 4 and 5 respectively against a recommended intake of 2.53kg day^{-1} (Kearl, 1982). Similarly the actual intake of digestible crude protein in the five groups was 53, 237, 255, 318 and 359g day^{-1}, (Kearl, 1982). The animals in groups 4 and 5 received sufficient nutrients (energy and protein) for growth of body tissues. The nitrogen, calcium and phosphorus retention in the animals were maximum in group 4 where UMMB and fish meal (100g day^{-1})were supplemented in the basal diet.

Table 2 : Intake of feed ingredients and UMMB by buffalo calves under various groups (Mean ±S.E.)

Groups	Initial Body weight (kg)	Wheat straw intake (DM kg/day)*	Concentrate intake (g/day)**	Fish meal intake (g/day)	UMMB intake (g/day)	Total Dry matter intake (kg/day)
I	202.75±23.75	2.86±0.18	1000	-	-	3.78±0.18
II	218.00±18.02	3.12±0.11	1000	-	746.13±79.01	7.70±0.16
III	223.25±8.84	3.36±0.25	1000	50	823.48±83.46	4.82±0.07
IV	227.75±11.55	3.38±0.12	1000	100	854.53±102.64	5.28±0.08
V	225.25±9.81	3.28±0.14	1000	150	851.09±29.45	5.19±0.17

The results revealed that supplementation of UMMB alone to the control group increased the daily gain in the body weight of about 80g/day. However the incorporation of a catalytic amount of fish meal (100g day^{-1}) further increased it 1.5 fold. This was probably owing to the fact that fish meal, being a high quality protein supplement, might have supplied some indispensable amino acids for the growth of rumen microbes. In addition, fish meal might have increased the availability of amino acids at the sight of absorption, which might have supplied the desirable numbers and proportions of amino acids for the synthesis of body proteins and resulted in the better growth of the animals.

Table 3 : Intake of feed ingredients and UMMB and daily body weight gain by buffalo calves under various groups

Groups	Initial Body weight (kg)	Wheat straw dry Matter intake (kg day^{-1})[1]	Concentrate intake (g day^{-1})	Fish meal intake (g day^{-1})[2]	UMMB intake (g day^{-1}) (g day^{-1})	Live weight gain
1	202.8±23.8	2.86±0.18	1000	-	-	90±16.00
2	218.0±18.0	3.12±0.11	1000	-	7.46±79.01	166±20.52
3	223.3±8.8	3.36±0.12	1000	50	8.23±83.46	179±24.63
4	227.8±11.6	3.38±0.12	1000	100	855±102.64	288±16.60
5	225.3±9.8	3.28±0.14	1000	150	8.51±29.45	275±38.29

Urea entry, degradation and excretion rate

On a low N diet, the ruminants conserve nitrogen by utilizing indogenous urea, which may be of sufficient magnitude to sustain rumen function, Urea recycling in the rumen is under physiological control and is of considerable significance in the nitrogen economy of the ruminants. In this study, experiment was conducted to assess the extent of nitrogen utilization form urea. Urea molasses mineral block (UMMB) in the rumen of buffalo calves fed on poor quality crop residues. Twelve male growing buffalo calves were randomly divided into 3 groups of 4 animals each. All the animals were offered wheat straw *ad libitum* and wheat bran and deoiled rice bran at the rate of 500g each daily (gr. Diet). Animals of gr. II and gr. III were supplemented with fish meal (100 g/d). A metabolism trial of 7 days duration was conducted after a feeding period of 131 days. Urine samples were analysed for nitrogen. Urea entry and degradation rate were measured on three animals form each group, using C14 urea.14 urea (100 to 120 uci) in saline was injected into each animal intravenously through jugular vein catheter and total amount of urine excreted in 24hr was also measured. Urea was estimated in plasma and in urine after treating it with washed permutit. Specific radioactivity of urea in the plasma was calculated. The samples were counted for radioactivity on Packard Tricarb Liquid Scintillation Spectrometer Model 3320 using Brays' scintillation fluid.

Results revealed significantly (P<0.01) more entry and degradation rate of urea in group 1 as compared to group II and III. However, the urea excretion rate was maximum in group III and minimum in group III and minimum in control group in table 4.

Table 4: Urea entry and degradation rates in buffalo calves supplemented with UMMB

Groups	Plasma urea concentration (mg/100ml)**	Specific radioactivity at zero time (SR 0 dpm/mg urea)	Pool size of Urea (g)	Half life (t1/2) (Minutes)	Urea entry rate (mg/minute)*	Urea excretion rate (mg/minutes)**	Urea degradation rates (mg/minute)**	Per cent urea entering body pool which is degraded **
I	9.65±0.69^{a}	13557±979.74	16.53±1.13	236.00±0.58	49.41±3.31^{a}	13.68±1.09	35.73±2.22^{a}	72.36±0.36
II	14.39±0.61^{b}	15036.67±500.15	17.76±0.59	317.00± 4.93	38.89±1.10^{b}	23.83±0.83	15.06±0.72^{b}	38.72±1.36
III	16.97±0.9^{b}	16112±535.52	16.57±0.55	309.33±15.64	37.32±1.68^{b}	24.86±0.57	12.46±1.13^{b}	33.25±1.52

The supplementation of blocks in the diet of adult ruminants fed on crop residues can form a maintenance diet. The device used for the preparation of blocks is simple, cost effective, light weight and can easily be transported to villages as well as draught/flood affected areas. The methodology will certainly help in uplifting the socio-economic status of our farmers.

Feed Blocks as Catalytic Supplements for Animals on Tannin-rich Diets

Woody vegetation is often the main diet of ruminant animals raised in arid, semi-arid and mountainous zones. The low nutritive value of these diets-due to low levels of energy and nitrogen or the presence of tannins results in reduced animal performance. In many situations, farmers use considerable quantities of concentrate feeds as supplements for their animals. The replacement of these expensive supplements with alternative feed sources would decrease the cost of feed. Feed blocks seem to be an interesting alternative.

However, very little is known about the effect of feed blocks on the nutritive value of tannin rich diets and consequent livestock production. Ben Salem, Nefzaoui and Ben Salem (2000) concluded that supplementing with olive-cake-based blocks for goats grazing shrubland dominated by tannin-rich shrub species (*Olea europea, Pistacia lentiscus, etc.*) did not affect their feeding behavior, but increased their daily gain by 60 percent compared with those not receiving supplements. The growth rate was further increased when a mixture of small amounts of spineless cactus pads (100g dry matter) and fresh foliage of Atriplex nummularia (100g dry matter) was offered to goats. Gartner and Niven (1978) showed beneficial effects with several minerals (phosphorus, sulphur, etc.) given to sheep on Acacia aneura, a tannin-rich shrub species. Increased intake, digestion, daily gain and wool growth suggest that blocks may be used successfully as a carrier for these minerals. The enormous advantage in this case is the possibility of providing a supplement to animals on tanniniferous shrub species whilst they are still in the rangeland.

Table 5 : Effect of feed block supply on behavioural activities and growth of goats on shrublands.

Parameter	No. Supplement	Treatment Feed blocks(1)	Cactus + atriplex	Standard Error (Significance)
Browsing time (2)	41.9	38.0	43.7	2.76(NS)
Grazing time(2)	45.7	48.7	44.5	2.72(NS)
Walking time(2)	6.7	7.3	6.3	0.68(NS)
Resting time(2)	5.8	5.9	5.4	0.78(NS)
Daily gain (g)	25	41	60	5.02(*)

Source: Ben Salem, Nefzaoul and Ben Salem, 2000

Feed blocks as a cost-effective carrier of PEG to de-activate browse tannins

Using hard feed blocks could be a way to ensure continuous and slow release of PEG to the animal. Ben Salem et al. (2000) confirmed the enormous advantage of PEG- containing feed blocks for sheep on a tannin-rich browse foliage, namely fresh leaves of Acacia cyanophylla. These authors include graded levels of PEG 4000 (0, 6, 12, 18 and 24 percent) in olive cake based feed blocks (see Formulas 1 and 2 in Table 6). Linear increases were recorded in acacia intake, and in organic matter, crude protein and fibre in vivo digestibilities of the diet. An improvement was evident in the nitrogen value of the diet, as reflected by an improved nitrogen balance and increased microbial nitrogen supply.

Table 6 : Formulas of feed blocks given to sheep or goats fed tanniniferous shrubs and trees.

Item	Formula								
	1	2	3	4	5	6	7	8	9
Ingredients (as percentage of DM)									
Olive cake	38.0	31.2	40.1	38.0	35.6	36.7	33.1	13.8	10.2
Wheat bran	28.0	23.0	25.1	23.7	22.2	24.3	21.8	36.5	30.3
Wheat feeds	11.0	9.0	12.3	11.6	10.9	-	-	-	-
Molasses	-	-	-	-	-	-	-	9.5	9.3
Opuntia fruit	-	-	-	-	-	9.0	8.0	-	-
Urea	5	4.1	7.3	-	6.4	7.3	6.6	11.4	11.2
Cement	-	-	-	-	-	-	-	11.6	11.2
Quick lime	12.0	9.9	9.2	8.7	8.1	15.4	13.9	-	-
Salt	5.0	4.1	7.3	-	6.4	7.3	6.6	5.8	3.6
Di-calcium Phosphate	-	-	-	-	-	-	-	5.7	5.5
Mineral vitamin Supplement	1.0	0.8	1.3	1.0	1.0	-	-	5.7	5.5
PEG 4000	-	18.0	-	12.5	11.7	-	10.0	-	11.2

Sources for formulas: 1 and 2-Ben Salem *et al.*, 2000b. 3,4 and 5-Ben salem *et al.*, 2002; 6 and 7-Ben salem *et al.*, 2003; 8 and 9-Moujahed *et al.*, 2000

Medicated feed supplements for health and production

Deaths due to parasitism can occasionally reach catastrophic proportions and represents only the tip of the iceberg of production losses. There is

25-40% reduction in weight gains in infected animals and their productivity is considerably reduced (Suttle 1994). The present day concept of worm control programme is 'to live with worms' and worm burden is not allowed to rise to that level which hampers productivity. Administration of benzimidazole anthelminthics in medicated urea molasses block (MUMB) reduces the labour involved in treating individual animals, spreads the dose ever days and obviates the possibility of ruminal by- pass (Blagurn etal,1987). Tannin has biological effects that may aid in the control of gastrointestinal nematodes. The condensed tannin (CT) binds proteins and other molecules tightly at near neutral pH ,such as occurs in the rumen, with dissociation in the acidic pH of the abomasum, freeing them for digestion. Plant CT may have direct or indirect effects on gastro-intestinal nematodes. Direct effects might be mediated through CT- nematode interactions, thereby affecting physiological functioning of gastro- intestinal nematodes (Min and Hart 2003). Saponin have practical use as anthelmintics in the traditional medicine of certain countries In fact, a large number of saponin exhibit an anthelminthic activity, but many find no practical application due to parallel irritation of mucous membranes. Therefore research and development programmes must be undertaken to improve the health and production through these medicated feed supplements.

Medicated Urea Molasses Block

Collaborative research projects were initiated in 1990 by National dairy development board and commonwealth Scientific and Industrial Research Organization (CSIRO) under the auspices of the Australian Centre for International Agricultural Research (ACIAR). The projects aimed to develop a self medication device for prolonged low level administration of anthelmintics, using UMMBS,as the carrier. Anthelmintic pharmacokinetics studies undertaken in dairy cattle and buffaloes provided the dosage needed for the anthelmintic selected for use in UMMBS so that the animals could receive the desired dose of the drug on a daily basis. Following successful formulation and demonstration of effective nematode parasite control in dairy animals, nationwide data on parasite epidemiology were generated for formulating regionbased strategic nematode parasite control programmes using medicated UMMBS (MUMMBS).Outside the oborative umbrella, technology for the production of UMMBs incorporating flukicide was also developed to control liver flukes in dairy animals.

Anti nematode MUMMB

Fenbendazole (FBZ) bas been found most suitable for incorporation in UMMBS as the drug is stable in blocks, does not require a milk with holding period and has a safety index of 67 in cattle and 1000 in small ruminants.

Moreover, as the drug is not patent protected it can be procured in bulk from the open market . A series of studies on FBZ pharmacokinetics on single and continuous intraruminal dosing, confirm that effective concentration of oxfendazole (OFZ) the anthelmintically active principal metabolite of FBZ in plasma could be achieved by daily intraruminal administration of FBZ at 0.5mg/kg body weight (Sanyal 1994). The effective level was reached between days 4 and 6 of drug administration and a plateau was maintained thereafter. The OFZ disposition profile reveals typical zero order absorption elimination from day 4-6. In other words, by daily low level dosing the parasites would be exposed to the toxic concentration of the drug for much longer periods without additional use of the drug. Successful incorporation of FBZ in UMMBS at 0.5g/kg block material has been demonstrated by solid phase extraction and reverse phase high performance liquid chromatography (HPLC). The medicated blocks offered to the animals give sustained levels of the parent drug and its metabolites in the plasma resulting in selection of drug doses to be incorporated in UMMBS that would ensure the desired plasma concentrations of the anthelminthic in cattle and buffalo. 52 urea molasses blocks for dairy animals Indian experiences Trials conducted in calves experimentally infected with Haemon clius placei for evaluating the efficacy of MUMMBS incorporating FBZ demonstrated that the medicated blocks could effectively remove established adult parasites and also prevent establishment of infection by killing incoming larvae.

Anti fluke MUMMB

For developing MUMMBs incorporating fluckicide exploiting the principle of prolonged low level administration triclabendazole (TCBZ, Fasinex TM, Ciba Geigy, Switzerland) is the drug of choice as this is the only drug available in India effective against early immature liver flukes. Pharmacokinetic studies on TCBZ in dairy animals revealed very poor Urea Molasses Multi Nutrient blocks 53 anthelmintic uptake in buffaloes compared with cattle . Critical efficacy of TCBZ against experimental bovine and bubaline fasciolosis reveal high efficacy of the drug against both immature and mature fasciolosis in cattle at the recommended dose rats of 12.0 mg /kg body weight , while buffaloes require 24.0mg/kg body weight or more to control immature and mature fasciolosis (Sanyal and Gupta, 1996). Daily low level administration of TCBZ against experimental bovine and bubaline fasciolosis showed that daily dosing for 10days is required to eliminate mature liver flukes in cattle and buffalo when ingested at a rate of 0.5 and 1.5mg/kh body weight respectively Thus, different drug dose rates are required for TCBZ MUMMBS for cattle and for buffaloes to ensure that delivery of the appropriate minimum daily dose for efficacy against experimental bovine and bubaline fasciolosis.

Multifaceted Role of Plant Secondary Compound on Parasitized Hosts

Plant seeardary metabolites (PSM) are organic compounds that do not seem to have a role in primary plant metabolism i.e. growth, reproduction or development of plants, but involved in plant defence mechanism against herbivory.

Tannins

Alternative nondrug parasite control strategies have recently been suggested based on forages that contain condensed tannins (CT) (Niezen etal., 1995). CT may have direct effects on internal parasites themselves or may indirectly control the parasites by increasing the resistance and resilience of animals to gastrointestinal parasite (GIP) infections through improved protein nutrition. Possible direct effects could be mediated through CT- nematode interactions, which reduced nematode viability. The CT complex with nutrient availability for larval growth or decrease GIP metabolism directly through inhibition of oxidative phosporylation , causing larval death. Direct effects of CT on GIP accounts for reduced faecal egg count (FEC) and nematode burdens in lambs that grazed sulla compared to Lucerne (Niezen *et al,* 1995). Goats grazing an Sericea Lespedeza ,a tannin rich legume, showed a 60% reduction in FEC and daily egg output compared to those grazing on low tannin forages. CT may destroy the parasite sheath making parasites more susceptible to host defenses (Hoste *et al,* 2006). PSM also effect the host gut environment in which parasites resides, by affecting the pH of rumen (Osoro *et al,* 2007).

Dietary CT may benefit parasitized ruminants by improving the protein nutrition which in turn may enhance animal's immune response to the parasite infection. The potential of CT as a promising alternative in the control of GIP was reported in the studies of Cenci *et al* (2007). The consumption of tannins has been associated with reduction of feed intake, dry matter digestibility and the impairment of rumen metabolism when included at more than 4-5% of dry matter.

Saponins

Saponins are naturally occurring surface active glycosides. It consists of a sugar moiety usually containing glucose, galactose, glucteronic acid, xylose or rhamnoase glycosidically linked to a hydrophobic aglycone (sapogenin) which may be triterpenoid or steroid in nature, Saponin occurs in many plant species either as triterperoid or steroid in nature saponins.

Some saponin preparations have practical use as anthelmintics in the traditional medicine of certain countries. In fact a large number of saponin exhibit and anthelmintic activity but many find no practical application due to parallel irritation of mucous membranes. The evaluation of Filix type vermicidal activity of Albizzia anthelmintica and one of its saponin, musennin has confirmed the use of bark of this tree as a nematocidet in Ethiopia Musennin is a linear tetra sacharide of echinocystic acid. Both a saponin preparation and alpha hedlrin from the leaves of Hedera helix (Araliaceae) killed the liver flukes the liver flukes F. hepatica and Dicrocoelium spp. at a concentration of around 0.005mg/ml in vitro. The saponin preparation also eliminated the trematodes of Dicrocoelium spp from sheep. Ghosh etal(1996) reported the effect of saponin Acacia side A and B from Acacia auriculiformis on rat cestode.Saponins acaciaside A and B have been to damage parasite membrane by forming peroxide link.

Dietary saponins have significant effect on all phases of metabolism from the ingestion of feed to the excretion of waste in ruminants and other domestic animals . The extract of the plant, Y. schidigera, a saponin rich plant has been found to improve growth feed efficiency and health in ruminants Saponin containing S. Saponaria fruit had no effect on total tract digestibility of organic matter (OM), N or neutral detergent fibre (NDF) (Abreu etal, 2004). Similarly saponins reduce protein digestibility probably by the formation of sparingly digestible saponin protein complexes (Potter etal 1993) . Besides these negative effects, a positive effect of saponins on digestibility was reported with a silage based diet supplemented with sara saponin (Goetsch and Oweno, 1985) and high concentrate diet supplemented with alfalfa saponins.

Deoiled mahua cake as a functional feed

Significant inflammatory activity of Mahua cake (M. Longifolia) saponins was observed in chronic inflammation (Gaikwad etal. 2009) Deoiled mahua cake (DOMSC) in the ration of buffaloes (5 and 10% level in concentrate mixture) counteracted the development Fasciola gigantica infection in buffaloes as indicated by reduction in EPG count and improvement in growth and nutrient utilization DMSC fed animals (Singh etal 2008). The Hb and PCV values of the F. gigantica infected buffaloes were improved due to 10% DMSC supplementation. Lower antibody titre in the supplemented groups indicated that the infection was less severe in DMSC fed animals. It is evident that feeding of DMSC containing condensed tannins and saponins has clearly helped to combat the adverse effect of fasciolosis resulted from the ingestion of 800 metacercaria of F. gigantica (Singh *et al* 2008).

Future of UMMB technology in India

The fast increasing human population pressure is reducing the land available for fodder production. However, the increased cereal production leaves abundant agro-industrial by - products, simultaneously reducing potential environmental pollution. Apart from the importance of UMMB in reproduction, there is a great potential role to play in meeting the nutritional needs of animals in drought-prone western states and in flood affected eastern states of India. The use of medicated blocks for control of endoparasites should be exploited in small ruminants. It is already started exploring the use of UMMB in solving the major problem of "delayed puberty" in buffaloes in India. The use of UMMB as carrier to deliver many herbal digestive stimulants, herbal galactagouges, herbal ecbolics, ionophores and anthelmintics is under consideration.

References

Ben Salem, H., Nefzaoui, A., Ben Salem, L.& Tisserand, J.L. (2000). Deactivation of condensed tannins in Acacia cyanophylla Lindl. Foliage by polyethylene glycol in feed blocks. Effects on feed intake, diet digestibility, nitrogen balance,microbial synthesis and growth by sheep. *Livestock Production Secience*, 64: 51-60

Ben Salem, H., Atti, N., Priolo, A.&Nefzaoui A. (2002). Polyethylene glycol in concentrate or feed blocks to deactivate condensed tannins in Acacia cyanophylla Lindl. Foliage. 1-Effects on feed intake, digestion and growth by Barbarine lambs. *Animal Science*, 75:127-135

Ben Salem, H., Ben Salem, I., Nefzaoui, Nefzaoui, N.&Ben Said, M.S. (2003). Effect of PEG and olive cake feed blocks supply on intake, digestion and health of goats given kermes oak (Quercus coccifera L.) foliage. *Animal feed Science and Technology*. (in press).

Berger, I.A. Steel, J.W. and Rodden, B.R. (1993). Effect of a continuous release albendazole capsule on parasitism and production of grazing merino ewes and lambs. Aust. Vet. J. 70: 41-48.

Blagburu, B.L., Hanraham, L.A. Hendrix, C.M. and Lindsay D.S. (1987). Efficacy of Fenbendazole medicated feed blocks against gastrointestinal nematode infection in calves. *American Journal of Veterinary Research* 48:1017-19.

Cenci, F.B, Louvandini, H., McManus, C.M, Duel Porto, A., Costa, D.M, Argujo, S.C., Minho, A.P. and Abdalla, A.L. (2007). Effects of condensed tannin from Acacia mearnsii on sheep infected naturally with gastrointestinal helminths. *Vet. Parasitol*, 144:132-137

Gaikwad, R.D., Ahmed, M.D, Khalid, M.D., and Swamy, P. (2009). Antiinflammatory activity of Madhuca langifolic seed saponin mixture. *Pharmacent. Biol*, 47: 592-597.

Ghosh, N.K, Sinha Babu, S.P., Sahul, N.C and ITO, A (1996). Cestocidal activity of Acacia Auriculifarmis. *J. Helminthol*, 70:171-172

Hoste, H., Jackson, S., Athanasiaden, S.M. Thamsborg, S.O. and Hoskin (2006). The effects of tannin rich plants on parasitic nematodes in ruminants. *Trends Parasitol*. 22: 253-261.

Kearl, L.C. (1982). Nutrient Requirements of Ruminants in Developing Countries. International Feed stuffs. Institute Utah, Agricultural experimental Utah State University, logan, Utah.

Kunju , P.J.G. (1986b). Urea molasses block lick: A future animal feed supplement. *Asian Livestock,* 11:154-157.

Kunju, P.J.G. (1986a) . Urea molasses block lick: a feed supplement for ruminants. PP. 261-274 in : M.N.M Ibrahein & J.B. Schiere (eds). Rice straw and related feeds in ruminant rations. Proceedings of an International Workshop kandy Sri Lnka, 24-28March 1986.

Mehra, Usha R., Dass, R.S. and Pathak N.N., (2007). "Cold process Technology for the preparation of Urea Molasses Mineral Block" IVRI, Patent No. 210528.

Min, B.R., and Hart, S.P. (2003). Tannins for suppression of internal parasites. *Journal of Animal Science* 81(E.Suppl 2):E 102-E109.

Moujahed N, Kayouli C, Thewis A, Beckers Y and Rezgui S. (2000). Effects of multinutrient blocks and polyethylene glycol 4000 supplies on intake and digestion by sheep fed Acacia cyanophylla Lindl. foliage-based diets. *Animal Feed Science and Technology* 88: 219-238.

Niezen, J.H., Waghorn, T.S., Charleston, W.A and Waghern G.C. (1995). Growth and gastrointestinal parasitism in lamb grazing one of seven herbages and dosed with larval for six weeks. *J.Agric. Sci.,* 125:281-289.

Osoro,K., Mateos-Sanz, A, Frutos, P, Garcia, U. Ortega-Mora, L.M, Ferreira, L.M.M., Celaya, R. and Ferre, I. (2007). Anthelmintic and nutritional effects of heather supplementation on Cashmere goats grazing perennial ryegrass white clover pastures. *J. Anim. Sci.* 85: 861-870.

Potter, S.M, Jimenez-Flores, R, Pollack, J, Lone, T.A and Berber-Jimenez, M.D. (1993). Protein saponin interaction and its. Influence on blood lipids. *J Agric . Food chem.,* 41:1287-1291G.

Sainyal, P.K. (1994). The pharmacokinetic behavior of fenbendazale in buffalo and cattle. *Journal of veterinary pharmacology and Therapeutics.* 17:1-4.

Sanyal, P.K. and Gupta, S.C. (1996). Efficacy and pharmacokinetics of triclabendazole in buffalo with induced fasciolosis. *Veterinary Parasitology,* 63:75-82.

Singh, P., Mehra, U.R, Verma, A.K. and Gupta, S.C. (2008). impact of nutritional status of fesciolosis A.P. Cess fund Project report submitted to ICAR, New Delhi, India.

Suttle, N.F. (1994). Seasonal infection and nutritional status. *Proceedings of Nutritional Society.* 53:545-55.

Tiwari, S.P., Singh, U.B and Mehra, U.R. (1990). Urea molasses mineral block as a feed supplement : effect on growth and nutrient utilization in buffalo calves. *Anim. feed Sci. and Technol.,* 29: 333-338.

□□□

16

Designing Poultry Meat and Eggs through Dietary Approaches

A.B. MANDAL AND PRAVIN K TYAGI
Central Avian Research Institute, Izatnagar-243 122

Introduction

Poultry production has gained momentum during the last four decades. Consequently it has taken a shape of industry. Presently the industry has emerged as the most dynamic and fast growing segment in animal husbandry sector in India with an annual growth rate of 6% in 1980s, 11% in 1990s, 19% in 1997-2002, about 6% from 2002-2008 in broiler chickens and 5-7% in egg production. The productivity of meat-type chickens and eggs have also dramatically improved due to the concomitant progress in rearing methods, nutrition, genetics, disease prevention, medication and bio-security that resulted in the reduction of slaughter age and pre-harvest losses. Poultry industry, being most organized one has the potential to solve the malnutrition and unemployment problems and augment rural economy in a state where in agricultural production has reached nearly to a plateau. The present society is very much concerned on clean and safe environment besides animal welfare and production of safe products akin to customers demand. The poultry products like meat and eggs have already gained a healthy image. These products are also being designed to perform a particular function or set of functions effectively and reliably, to suit the purposes and the attitudes of the consumers. With the self-sufficiency and adequate levels of quantitative food production, increasing capacity of purchasing power of consumers with more earnings, change in life style, and public demand for food of specific quality and purpose, the quality and designing aspects have got emphasis in many developed and underdeveloped countries. In the integrated production system, designer products may play an important role in providing additional profit to the producers, if quality commands premium price in a given market. Though, India is still deficient in quantitative supply to meet the demand of the poultry products, but designing aspects can also be exploited for improving long-term market prospects. Moreover, in the competitive market, who respond successfully remains always gainer. Improving consumers' health and nutritional status by designing nutritional profile of poultry meat and eggs through dietary approaches is relatively simple concept. Nutrition of birds influences meat qualities in terms of nutritive value, acceptability, human health and processing. Similarly, eggs can be designed through dietary approaches either through feed intrinsic factors, supplementation of specific nutrients or certain herbs or specific drugs. Designing eggs is important as the per capita egg consumption in world is decreasing due to presence of high cholesterol and problems associated with Salmonella in eggs. Moreover, eggs can be enriched with certain specific nutrients or agents that have functional and therapeutic properties.

Dietary Approaches for Designer Meat

The major changes in meat that can be brought through nutritional manipulation are increase in protein with concomitant decrease in fat and cholesterol, enrichment of meat with specific fatty acids, fat-soluble vitamins and probably certain minerals. The chemical composition of white and red meat is different. The white meat contains 74.41% moisture, 23.40% protein, 0.80% fat, 1.14% ash, 0.005% calcium and 0.273% phosphorus, while red meat contained 75.26% moisture, 19.11% protein, 4.12% fat, 1.04% ash, 0.005% calcium and 0.186% phosphorus. Breast meat was 21.94% of live body weight and breast meat gain to mass of cut carcass was 29.70%, while leg and thigh meat to live weight was lower at 15.57%, while the leg and thigh meat to cut carcass weight was 21.09% (Alibegovic *et al.*, 2003). Manipulating energy to protein ratio and amino acid concentration in diets can increase the breast yield, and relative concentration of protein and moisture in breast and thigh muscles. Cr supplementation (0.2 mg Cr per kg food dry matter) improved protein accretion and lowered fat deposition in meat (Amatya *et al.*, 2004). Supplementation of Cu (35 to 126 mg/kg feed) increased oleic acid content and reduced meat cholesterol (Skrivanova *et al.*, 2004). The higher oleic acid content in breast meat and skin of Peking ducks was reflected on feeding high oleic corn (Lu *et al.*, 2004). Probiotics together (*Lactobacillus acidophilus, L. casei, Bifidobacterium bifidum, Aspergillus oryzae, Streptococcus faecium* and *Toluropsis*) @ 100mg/kg diet improved moisture, protein, ash and decreased fat content in leg and breast meat of chickens (Khaksefidi and Rahimi, 2005). Reduction of serum cholesterol levels has also been reported in broilers fed lactobacillus culture (Jin *et al.* 1998).

There are growing public concern over consumption of poultry meat having more cholesterol and saturated fatty acids. Coronary heart disease and arterioscelorosis are strongly related to the dietary intake of cholesterol and saturated fatty acids. Chicken meat is relatively low in fat and cholesterol, and thus considered healthier than other animal protein sources. Numerous including dietary factors have been demonstrated to alter fat deposition and cholesterol contents in meat. Dietary supplementation of methionine; lysine, glycine, tryptophan and amino acid mixtures can reduce body fat deposition (Takahashi *et al.,* 1994). Dietary fiber also reduces fat concentration and facilitates lean meat production. Dietary supplementation of garlic, copper and omega-3 fatty acids has been used successfully to reduce cholesterol content in poultry meat. Dehydrated alfalfa is a good source of hypocholesterolaemic compounds such as saponins. It was possible to produce chicken lean breast meat with reduced cholesterol content by feeding free choice alfalfa (Ponte *et al.,* 2004).

The omega-3 group of polyunsaturated fatty acids (PUFA) has received attention from health professionals and nutritionists in recent past due to their beneficial effect on human health. Higher intake of PUFA decreases the risk of heart diseases and strokes, and also exerts immunological and neurological effects and has positive effects in the prevention of heart beat irregularities, cancers, aging and even depression, and improving blood lipid profile and blood coagulation. The (decosahexaenoic acid) DHA is a major component of brain tissues and retina. Its intake is positively correlated in learning process and deficiency is related to impaired retinal function (Mellor, 2005). Broiler chicken is an excellent alternative source of PUFA. Many studies are also being directed towards the manipulation of the fatty acid composition of broiler chicks further to augment human health. Cod liver oil positively affected performance, but even at 1% supplementation rate, an off-flavour was detected. The diet supplemented with linseed oil had a negative effect both on performance and carcass quality. No significant difference was found between poultry fat and olive oil supplementation. Pumpkin seed oil resulted in significantly higher abdominal fat deposition, but improved organoleptic parameters the best. Feeding olive oil significantly increased the oleic acid; pumpkin seed oil the linoleic acid, linseed oil the linolenic acid and cod liver oil the EPA, DHA and docosapentaenoic acid (DPA) concentration in the tissues (Bartos *et al.,* 2004).

The main sources of PUFA are fish oil, linseed, millets and sea algae. The sea algae are the best sources to enrich meat with omega-3 fatty acid. Moreover, the PUFA of algae origin are more stable and in more active form than that in plant oils. Certain cereals like corn, barley and oats are also rich in linolenic acid. The combination of animal (fish) and vegetable (rapeseed, linseed) oils viz. is also effective. Enrichment in n-3 fatty acids results in higher rate of oxidation that could be controlled by the antioxidants such as alpha-tocopherol or vitamin E as discussed later. Dietary supplementation of linolenic acid showed an increase in its content in dark meat, but had little effect on white meat. Supplementation broiler diets with EPA enhanced the levels of the fatty acid in white meat, but only to a limited extent in the dark meat. White meat rather is a far richer source of phospholipids, in which EPA and DHA are more concentrated (Mellor, 2005). Fish oil in diet at the rate of 1.5% as source of n-3 fatty acids (Basmacoglu *et al.*, 2004) was beneficial. Chicks fed with omega-3 PUFA rich cod liver or linseed oil supplemented diets showed significantly higher total n-3 fatty acid content in all tissues as compared to other oils. The best source of long chain n-3 PUFA was the cod liver oil, but the linseed oil, due to its high linolenic acid content, also resulted in significantly higher EPA, DPA and DHA deposition in the tissues, compared to the other treatments. The best omega-6/omega-3 ratio from a human health aspect was detected by the linseed oil and cod liver oil supplementation (Bartos *et al.*, 2004). The effect of feeding fish oil, linseed oil, sunflower oil and soybean oil and different oil levels on fatty acid composition, long chain omega-3 polyunsaturated fatty acids, n-6/n-3 ratio and oxidation stability as malondialdehyde (MDA) levels of Cobb broiler chicken muscles was studied (Kahraman *et al.*, 2004). It was shown that dietary fat source influenced lipid composition of thigh meat more than dietary fat level. According to the fat source added to the diet, significant differences of thigh meat fatty acid levels were observed. Thigh meat from broiler groups fed with 8% oil showed a different fatty acid profile to the other oil levels (2 and 4%). Broilers fed with fish oil had statistically higher EPA and DHA levels in thigh meat than broilers fed with soybean oil. The thigh meat of the soybean oil fed group also showed a high-level of n-6 group fatty acids, while the fish oil group's thigh meat showed a high level of n-3 fatty acids. The n-6/n-3 ratio was lowest for fish oil and the PUFA level changed depending on the type of oil and dietary level. The MDA level in the thigh meat was more affected by the dietary fatty acid source than by the level of fat. MDA level in thigh meat was increased with increasing percentage of the dietary oil. However, using fish oil and vegetable oil rich in long chain unsaturated fatty acids in broiler diets may result in an increased fatty acid oxidation in muscle tissues (Kahraman *et al.*, 2004). Similarly, the oleic acid content in feed containing the high oil, high oleic corn was reflected to the composition of breast meat and skin of Peking ducks (Lu *et al.*, 2004). Conjugated linoleic acids (CLA) are the natural components of animal foods derived from linoleic acid, also have been proved as beneficial. Numerous health beneficial effects have been attributed to CLA in experimental animal models over the past two decades that include ameliorating carcinogenesis, atheroscelerosis, onset of diabetes and body fat mass or obesity. CLA is also a potent regulator of body fat accumulation and retention (Chin *et al.,* 1994).

Intestinal colonization of Salmonella, Campylobacter and Coliforms in the chickens is the source of carcass contamination during slaughter. Salmonella and Campylobacter cause gastro-enteritis in human beings. Nutritional manipulation that affects colonization of these bacteria may reduce their contamination in carcass. Administration of *Bacillus subtilis* C -3102 to chickens reduced the number and incidence of Salmonella and Campylobacter in the intestinal tract of broilers (Maruta *et al.,* 1996). Carcass of broilers fed with probiotic had significantly lower Salmonella, Campylobacter and aerobic count than birds fed control diet (Frittis *et al.,* 2000). The chicken carcasses fed diets with prebiotics had low Campylobacter and coliforms (Khaksefidi and Rahimi, 2005). The prebiotics and probiotics in diet and fasting hour also influenced micobiological meat quality (Mandal, *et al.,* 2005; Elanovan, *et al.,* 2005).

Poultry meat is highly susceptible to oxidative rancidity or lipid oxidation during frozen storage. Lipid oxidation is a complex process that accounts for the appearance of rancidity during fresh meat storage and causes the development of warmed-over flavours when cooked meat is stored or reheated. Moreover, the oxidative stability of cholesterol is also less. It is easily converted to oxidative products in presence of light and molecular oxygen, which are potent carcinogen and atherogen. Similarly the unsaturated fatty acids are also susceptible to oxidative rancidity. The process is believed to begin at the cellular membrane level and particularly affects the polyunsaturated fatty acids and cholesterol resulting in loss of membrane integrity and generation of compounds affecting the flovour, colour, and texture of the meat, nutritive value of meat and the acceptability of the product by the consumer. The oxidation of unsaturated lipids leads to formation of hydroperoxides as the primary products which are then broken down to produce volatile and nonvolatile compounds. Volatile compounds are related to acceptability or rejection of food products, while the nonvolatile compounds mainly affect the safety of the consumers as oxidative stress is involved in the pathology of cancer, arteriosclerosis, malaria, and rheumatoid arthritis and plays a role in neurodegenerative diseases and aging process. The cells have protective agents that guard against damage induced by oxygen reactive species. The enzymes glutathione peroxidase, catalase, superoxide dismutase constitute an antioxidant cellular enzyme system.

Naturally occurring antioxidant - vitamin E or alfa-tocopherol had been reported to be effective in improving self-life of poultry meat and meat products through delaying lipid oxidation. Thigh meat is more susceptible to lipid oxidation than breast meat (about 22% of live body weight or 30% of carcass mass). The oxidative stability of poultry meat is related to tissue concentration of tocopherol. As the level of vitamin E in diet increases there is concomitant increase in its concentration in tissues and having following order of deposition in descending order: egg yolk, liver, adipose tissue and muscle. Higher levels of vitamin E in poultry not only improve the oxidative stability but also prevent excessive drip loss as it is believed that ?-tocopherol, by maintaining the integrity of cellular membranes, reduces leakage of sacroplasmic components from muscle cells thereby reduces drip. The sensory quality of meat assessed from scoring of aroma, flavour, taste, etc. is reported to be improved by adding vitamin E in diets of broilers. Even vitamin E decreased the production of fishy flavour because of fishmeal oil supplementation in diet and warmed over flavour in refrigerated cooked meat and raw frozen meat. The stability of the meat has been correlated with the tissue concentration of a-tocopherol. For poultry, levels of 7mg/kg a-tocopherol in muscle are recommended to prolong the keeping quality of meat. The supplemented tissues were more stable in cold store. Feeding of vitamin supplemented diets (10 to 20ppm) showed significantly lower levels of thiobarbituric acid reactive substances (TBARS) in the meat measured after 5 and 10 days of storage (Lohakare *et al.*, 2005).

The role of dietary selenium (Se) in influencing the quality of poultry meat and meat products appears to have not been studied to a great extent so far. Nevertheless, based on the knowledge of Se deficiency conditions in poultry, which causes exudative diathesis, muscular dystrophy and other deficiency syndromes, it is possible to assume that Se may have a significant role on the quality of poultry meat and meat products. The dietary selenium may have a significant role on the quality of poultry meat and meat products (Tyagi et. al. 2005). The thiobarbituric acid reactive substances reduced in the breast meat of broilers in diets containing vitamin A (12 000 IU/kg diet) and E (100 IU/kg diet) and methionine 20% higher than the requirements (Lohakare, *et al.*, 2005).

Feeding of alpha -tocopheryl acetate (20 mg, 400 mg or 1000 mg /kg feed) from day-old white Peking ducklings (Russell *et al.*, 2004) revealed significantly (P<0.05) increased concentrations of vitamin E in breast, thigh, liver and heart tissues in a dose-dependent manner. Supplementation also enhanced oxidative stability of duck muscle. However, breast muscle was more susceptible to lipid oxidation than thigh for all groups, even though breast muscle contained higher alpha -tocopherol levels than thigh muscle (Russell *et al.*, 2004).

Combinations of oregano and rosemary essential oils (150mg/kg each) had a greater effect than those fed individually or alpha-tocopheryl acetate (200 mg/kg) on inhibiting lipid oxidation, and protecting alpha alpha-tocopheryl acetate concentration in refrigerated meat enriched with n-PUFAs stored for 15 days. (Basmacoglu *et al.*, 2004). This combination of essential oils also proved as effective as alpha -TA in retaining the sensory qualities of breast meat after 15 days storage, and was more effective than when these essential oils were fed individually or at 300 mg/kg. There is a possible synergistic effect between oregano and rosemary essential oil in preventing lipid oxidation in stored meat enriched with n-3 PUFAs.

The production of lipid peroxides in the carcasses of broiler chickens during storage could be delayed by astaxanthin. Therefore, astaxanthin (chemical 45 mg/kg feed or biological from the red yeast Xanthophyllomyces dendrorhous 22.5 mg/kg feed) could be used as an antioxidant as well as a colourant for broiler chickens (An *et al.*, 2004). Xanthophyll (natural or synthetic) sources to chicks could improve colour intensity of and inhibit lipid oxidation in leg meat (Kim *et al.*, 2004). The antibacterial agent, lasalacid sodium salt (LS) added to the diet affected not only their growth performance but also their meat yield and stress response. Withdrawal of LS increased the plasma 2-thiobarbituric acid reactant value, an indicator of lipid peroxidation (Matsushita *et al.*, 2004).

Dietary Approaches for Designer Eggs

The eggs have been described as "Nature's original functional food" (Hasler, 2000) packed with thirteen important vitamins and minerals. The quality of egg protein is also considered better than many animal protein sources. Eggs are also the cheapest sources of quality nutritional package. One large egg contributes about 70-80 kcal of energy, 7 g of protein, total fat 4.5 g, saturated fat 1.5 g, polyunsaturated fat 0.5g, monounsaturated fat 2.0 g, cholesterol 200-250 mg, sodium 65 mg, potassium 60 mg, total carbohydrate 1 g, choline (300 mg) and significant quantity of vitamin B12, folate, selenium, riboflavin, vitamin D, phosphorus, vitamin E and vitamin A. The nutritive composition can be altered through dietary approaches. Consumers can now find eggs with less cholesterol and saturated fat than conventional one with additional vitamin E and omega-3 fatty acids as bonus.

Egg yolk is the excellent, highly bio-available source of the carotenoids, lutein and zeaxanthin (Handelman *et al.*, 1999). Recent research demonstrated the link between these dietary compounds and the macular pigment of the retina of the eye (Landrum and Bone, 2001). Lutein and zeaxanthin are the primary carotenoids found in the macular region. Sufficient quantities of these nutrients in the diet are thought to reduce the risk of age-related macular degeneration, a leading cause of old-age blindness. Besides reducing the risk of macular degeneration, lutein has a protective effect for early atherosclerosis. Increased amounts of dietary lutein from green leafy vegetables and egg yolks could help in protecting against atherosclerosis by slowing the progression of atherosclerotic lesions in humans and animals (Dwyer et al, 2001). Early arteriosclerosis was inversely related to levels of plasma lutein which were affected by dietary intake indicating an inverse relationship between dietary lutein and arteriosclerosis development.

To cater the growing demands of health conscious consumers, the eggs are being designed but yet a small percentage of eggs are sold as designer eggs. The possibilities for designing eggs are limitless. The eggs may be designed for enhanced nutritionally, value addition and added processing. Free range eggs are produced by hens that are not kept in cages. Hens have daily access to outdoors, depending on the climate. The nutrient content of free-range eggs is identical to conventional eggs provided not kept in different feeding regimen. Organic eggs are produced by hens kept under the norms of organic farming. The eggs produced from hen fed completely vegetarian diet are generally termed as vegetarian eggs suitable for lacto-ovo-vegetarians.

Eggs marketed with low cholesterol or modified fat, contains less cholesterol, less saturated fat, more omega-3 fatty acids and vitamin E in comparison to conventional generic shell eggs. The cholesterol and saturated fat contents can be reduced to an extent of about 30% through dietary manipulations. Linolenic acid is the major acid in egg yolk. The egg yolk is a good vehicle for DHA, arachidonic acid and EPA. The hens fed diets or feedstuffs (linseed oil, fish oil, etc.) containing high in omega-3 fatty acids produce eggs with high omega-3 fatty acid content in the yolks. The hens fed flax seed oil through diet resulted in increase in omega-3-fatty acids amounting 7-12% of egg yolk and the different fatty acids in order were LNA- linolenic acid>DHA>DPA>EPA (Sim and Guang-Hai, 1995). The possibility of conversion of LNA to EPA, DPA and DHA through desaturation and elongation has also been suggested (Garg *et al.* 1988). A series of studies (Sim et al. 1992, Jiang and Sim, 1992, Sim, 1993) indicated that the chicken egg can be enriched with omega-3 fatty acids to an extent of 500-600 mg per egg leading to significant elevated polyunsaturated FA : saturated fatty acids (from 0.6-1.02), and lowering the omega 6:omega-3 FA ratio from 10:1 to 1:1. The studies also claimed that about 600 mg of total omega-3 fatty acids balanced with DHA< DPA and EPA equivalent to approximately 100 g of serving fish.

The hens fed guggul alone or herbs in combination (Arjuna, guggul, cinnemon and Amla) in diets reduced egg yolk cholesterol by 16-20% and 14-18% from 6th or 8th weeks onward (Sharma, *et al.* 2009). Some of the recent work initiated at CARI, Izatnagar on the production of low cholesterol eggs by the supplementation of layer diets with the combination of either pharmacological drugs or minerals indicated that layer diet with Atorvastatin 0.03% + Niacin 375 ppm + ethylene diamine tetra acetic acid-EDTA 0.5% reduced egg yolk cholesterol content up to 35% (Tyagi *et al*, 2009). In an another study, a dietary level of 300mg Cu/kg together with 3200 µg chromium-Cr/kg in the diet of laying hens was found adequate for the production of low cholesterol eggs (Tyagi et al, 2009). Similarly, enrichment of diet of with iodine or vitamin E increases their concentration in eggs. Probiotic (*Saccharomyces cerevisiae, Enterococcus faecium and Lactobacillus acidophilus* @ 4 g/kg diet) inclusion significantly reduced yolk cholesterol and total lipids (Osman, 2003).

Lutein is a xanthophyll carotenoid present in dark green leaves, leaf meal, leafy vegetables, corn gluten meal and egg yolk. These are widely distributed in tissues and are the principal carotenoids in the eye lens and macular region of the retina (Ribaya-Mercado and Blumberg, 2004). It has potential for the prevention of numerous diseases in human. An inverse relationship was reported based on epidemiological studies between xanthophyll intake or its status in the body and cataract as well as age-related macular degeneration. Moreover, these xanthophylls may help in reducing the risk of certain types of cancer (particularly those of the breast and lung) and prevention of heart disease and stroke (Ribaya-Mercado and Blumberg, 2004). There is also role of lutein and zeaxanthin in disease prevention. Dietary lutein stimulated the antibody response to infectious bronchitis virus vaccination in laying hens (Bédécarrats and Leeson, 2006). The lutein content in eggs is directly correlated with the lutein concentration in hens diet. Adding lutein to the layers' diet resulted in a significant improvement in yolk color score within 7 d of supplementation and lutein was transferred into the yolk increasing from a basal level of 0.3 mg to 1.5 mg/60 g of egg (Leeson and Caston, 2004). Corn gluten meal and alfalfa also increased the lutein content up to a level of 2.2 mg/60 g of egg with dietary lutein of 500 ppm. However, adding flax to these diets depressed yolk lutein content (Leeson and Caston, 2004, Bédécarrats and Leeson, 2006).

Feeding human volunteers designer egg enriched in vitamin E (26 times), carotenoids/lutein(16 times), selenium (over 7 times) and DHA (6 times) one daily for . eight week resulted in significant increase in alpha-tocopherol (vitamin E), lutein and DHA in the plasma (Surai *et al.*, 2000). In another study (Farrell, 1998), feeding of enriched eggs with omega-3 fatty acids to human volunteers for twenty-two weeks (consumed seven eggs/week for first 20 weeks and approximately 10 eggs/ week for last 2 weeks) resulted in significant increase in levels of EPA, DHA, total omega-3 fatty acids and HDL in blood without increase in total blood cholesterol and triacylglycerol levels.

Similarly, volunteers consuming four egg yolk per day, and possibly two egg yolks per d for five weeks benefited macular health in older adults with low macular pigment optical density (MPOD) (Vishwanathan et al. 2009). Additionally, serum high-density lipoprotein (HDL) cholesterol increased without an increase in low-density lipoprotein (LDL) cholesterol in the study population, most of whom were taking cholesterol-lowering statins. Serum lutein increased by only 16 percent and 24 percent compared with increases of 36 percent and 82 percent in serum zeaxanthin (n=52) after consumption of two and four egg yolks, respectively. Serum HDL cholesterol increased by 5 percent after consumption of two and four egg yolks. Serum LDL cholesterol did not change with either egg yolk treatment.

Conclusion

Designer meat and eggs provide options for consumers who want those products with different nutritional benefits than generic eggs. With the advent of more knowledge on interaction of different dietary intrinsic (nutrients) and extrinsic factors (herbs/drugs) on the quality of eggs and meat in terms of nutritive value, acceptability, human health aspects, processing, etc. indicate that the dietary approaches will be a safe and user-friendly tool for designing eggs and meat. The major changes that can be brought in meat and egg through nutritional manipulation are increase of protein with concomitant decrease in fat, enrichment of meat with fatty acids, fat-soluble vitamins and probably certain minerals. Numerous nutritional and non-nutritional factors have been demonstrated to alter fat deposition and cholesterol contents in meat and egg. Such designing will help to remove phobia for high cholesterol and fat and thus will certainly help in increasing consumption of poultry products. Moreover, the heart patients will have scope for enjoying delicious poultry meat and eggs. However, designer poultry products should be produced economically, salable profitably, and safe for human consumption. Designing must take into consideration the particular production facilities, available materials, know-how, and economic resources of the producers. Moreover, the welfare aspects and production potentiality of birds and environmental issues must also be taken care of in the process of designer eggs and meat.

References

Alibegovic Z. F., Gagic, A., Piplica, S., Aklovica, F., Residbegovic, E., Kavazovic, A. and Crnkic, C. (2003). *Veterinaria Sarajevo*. 52: 137-146.

Amatya, J. L., Haldar, S. and Ghosh, T. K. (2004). *Anim. Sci.* 79: 241-253.

Bartos, A., Pal, L., Banyai, A., Horvath, P., Wagner, L. and Dublecz, K. (2004). *Allattenyesztes es Takarmanyozas*. 53:63-78.

Basmacoglu, H., Tokusoglu, O. and Ergul, M. (2004). *South African J. Anim. Sci.* 34:197-210.

Bédécarrats, G. Y. and Leeson S. (2006). *J. Appl. Poult. Res.* 2006. 15:183-189.

Chin, S.F., Storkson, J.M., Albright, J.A., Cook, M.E. and Pariza, M.W. (1994). *J. Nutr.* 124:2344-2349.

Dwyer, J.H.; Navab, M.; Dwyer, K.M.; Hassan, K.; Sun, P.; Shircore, A.; Hama-Levy, S.; Hough, G.; Wang, X.; Drake, T.; Bairey Merz, C.N.; Fogelman, A.M. (2001). The Los Angeles Atherosclerosis Study. *Circulation*. 103: 2922-2927.

Elangovan, A.V., Mandal, A.B., Yadav, A. S. and A.K. Ashrivastav. (2006). *CARI News Letter*. 11 (1): 6.

Elangovan, A.V., Yadav, A. S. Mandal, A.B. Tyagi, Praveen K., Tyagi Pramod K.and Saroj Toppo (2005). *Indian J. Anim. Nutr.* 22:129-131.

Farrell, D. J. (1998). *American Journal of Clinical Nutrition*. 68: 538-44.

Frittis, C. A., Kersey, J.H., Motl, M. A., Kroger, E.C., Yan, F., Si, J., Jiang, Q., Compos, M.M., Waldroup, A.L. and Waldroup, P.W. (2000). *J. Appl. Poult. Sci.* 9:149-155.

Garg, M.L., Sebokova, E., Wierzbicki, E., Thompson, A.B.R. and Clandinin, M.T. (1988). *Lipids*, 23:847-852.

Handelman, G.J.; Nightingale, Z.D.; Lichtenstein, A.H.; Schaefer, E.J.; Blumberg, J.B. (1999). *American Journal of Clinical Nutrition*. 70: 247-251.

Hasler, C.M. (2000). *Journal of the American College of Nutrition*. 19: 499S-506S.

Jiang, Z., and Sim, J.S. (1992). *Lipids* 27: 279-284.

Jin, L.Z.; Ho, Y.W.; Abdullah, N.; Jalaludin, S. (1998). *Poult.Sci.* 77: 1259–1265.

Kahraman, R; Ozpinar, H; Abas, I; Kutay, H.C., Eseceli, H. and Grashorn, M A. (2004). Archiv fur Geflugelkunde. 68: 77-86.

Khaksefidi, A. and Rahimi, Sh. 2005. Asian-Austr. J. Anim. Sci. 18: 1153-1156.

Landrum, J.T., Bone, R.A. (2001). *Archives of Biochemistry and Biophysics*. 385: 28-40.

Lee, J.L., Kim, Y.D., Kim, D. Y., Choi, Y.I., Ahn, J.N., Chae, H.S. and Choi, J.H. (2002). *Proc. J. Anim. Sci. Technol.* p34.

Leeson, S. and Caston, L. (2004). *Poultry Science*, 83(10): 1709-1712.

Liao YuYing, and Qin, ShiShan (2003). *China Poultry* 25: 12-13.

Lohakare, J.D., Choi, J.Y., Kim, J. K., Yong, J.S., Shim,Y.H., Hahn, T.W. and Chae, B.J. (2005). *Asian Aust. J. Anim. Sci.* 18: 516-523.

Lohakare, J.D., Hahn, T.W; Shim, Y.H; Choi, J Y, Chae, B. J. (2004). *Asian Australasian Journal of Animal Sciences*. 17(9): 1260-1265.

Lu Lin, Ji Cheng; Luo XuGang; Liu Bin; Yu ShunXiang. (2004). 37(12): 1917-1924.

Mandal, A. B., Yadav, A. S., Elangovan, A.V., Tyagi, Praveen K., Tyagi Pramod K. and Saroj Toppo (2005). *Indian J. Poult. Sci.* 40: 285-87.

Matsushita, K; Takahashi, K; Akiba, Y. (2004). *Japanese Poultry Science*. 2004; 41(2): 57-67.

Mellor, S. (2005). *World Poultry*. 21(7):12-13.

Osman, M. (2003). *Egyptian Poult. Sci. J.* 23: 283-297.

Ponte, P.I.P., Mendes, I., Quaresma, M., Aguiar, M. N. M., Lemos, J.P.C., Ferreira, L.M.A., Soares, M.A.C., Alfaia, C.M., Prates, J.A.M., and Fontes, C.M.G.A. (2004). *Poultry Science* 83: 810-814.

Ribaya-Mercado, J.D. and Blumberg, J. B. (2004). *J. Am. Coll. Nutr.* 23:567S-587S.

Rohini Vishwanathan, Elizabeth F Goodrow-Kotyla, Billy R Wooten, Thomas A Wilson, and Robert J Nicolosi, (2009). *Am. J. Clin. Nutr.* 90: 1972-79.

Russell, E.A; Lynch, P.B; O' Sullivan, K; Kerry, J.P. (2004). *International Journal of Food Science and Technology*. 39(3): 331-340.

Sharma, R.K., Elangovan, A.V., Mandal, A.B., Tyagi, Praveen K.,.and Shrivastav, A.K. (2009). *Indian J. Poult. Sci.* 44 (press).

Sim, J.S. (1993). Proc. 54th Minnesota Nutr. Conf. & National Renders Technical Seminar, Bloomington, Minnesota, pp 275-286.

Sim, J.S. and Guang-Hai, Qi (1995d). In: Flaxseed in Human Nutrition, Thompson, L.U. and Cunnane, S. (Eds), AOCS, pp 315-333.

Sim, J.S., Cherian G. and Jiang, Z. (1992). *Int.J. Applied & Basic Nutritional Sci (Nutrition)* 8: 221-222.

Skrivanova, V., Skrivan, M., Tumova, E., and Sevcikova, S. (2004). *Czech J. Anim. Sci.* 49: 71-79.

Surai, P.F.; MacPherson, A.; Speake, B.K.; Sparks, N.H.C. (2000). *European Journal of Clinical Nutrition*. 54: 298-305.

Takahashi, K., Konashi, S., Akiba, Y. And Horiguchi, M. (1994). *Anim. Sci. Technol.* 65: 244-250.

Tyagi *et al.* (2009). Personal communication.

Tyagi, Praveen K., Tyagi Pramod K., Singh, R.P. Elangovan, A.V. and Mandal, A.B. (2005). *Anim. Nutr. Feed Technol.* 5:53-60.

❑❑❑

17

Methane Mitigation in Respose to Climatic Change

S.P.TIWARI*, KIRAN KUMARI, M.K.GENDLEY, DILIP CHOUDHARY AND SMITA

Professor & Head*, Department of Animal Nutrition, College of Veterinary Science & AH, Anjora, Durg-491001 (C.G.)

Introduction

Climate change is a reality with a warming of the earth as result. Current trends in the most relevant climate indicators are inline with what can be expected from climate models, e.g., the global heat content of oceans has increased significantly in the last decades, the global average sea level is rising, the global average surface temperature has an increasing long-term trend. If nothing is done to reduce the emissions of greenhouse gases the global average surface temperature is estimated by the Inter governmental Panel on Climate Change (IPCC) to increase between about 2 and 7 degrees Celsius above the pre-industrial level by year 2100 and with continuing warming thereafter (IPCC, 2007; Solomon *et al*, 2009). Temperature scenarios at the higher range of the interval would both imply a global average temperature level and a rate of change in the temperature not witnessed for millions of years (Jansen *et al*, 2007). Even for less severe, and more likely temperature scenarios, serious negative impacts on ecosystems and society are expected to occur. Even though there may be some positive economic impact for small changes in the climate, these will mainly occur in developed countries, while developing countries, which in general are more dependent on agricultural activities, already have a warmer climate and have less resource for adapting to changes in it, are expected to suffer already from small changes in the climate. The overall picture concerning the negative impacts of climate change is more serious today than it was about a decade ago.

A significant portion of forage is used by the cattle industry as a source of feed for cows, bulls and growing/young stock. Microbial breakdown of forage and other feedstuffs in the rumen, also known as enteric fermentation, results in the production of methane. Greenhouse gases trap heat in the Earth's atmosphere affecting climate change. Some greenhouse gases such as carbon dioxide and water vapour occur naturally and are emitted to the atmosphere through natural processes and human activities. Other greenhouse gases are emitted mostly through human activities. The principal greenhouse gases caused by human activities are:

Carbon Dioxide (CO_2) : Carbon dioxide enters the atmosphere through the burning of fossil fuels (oil, natural gas, and coal), solid waste, trees and wood products, and also as a result of chemical reactions. Carbon dioxide is also removed from the atmosphere (or "sequestered") when it is absorbed by plants as part of the biological carbon cycle.

Methane (CH_4) : Methane is emitted during the production and transportation of fossil fuels such as coal, natural gas, and oil. Methane emissions also result from raising livestock and agricultural practices, the decay of organic waste in solid waste landfills, and small amounts during the combustion of fossil fuels in transportation.

Nitrous Oxide (N_2O) : Nitrous oxide is emitted during agricultural and industrial activities, as well as small amounts during combustion of fossil fuels and solid waste.

Fluorinated Gases : Hydrofluorocarbons, perfluorocarbons, and sulfur hexafluoride are synthetic, greenhouse gases that are emitted from a variety of industrial processes. Fluorinated gases are sometimes used as substitutes for ozone-depleting substances (i.e., CFCs, HCFCs, and halons). These gases are typically emitted in smaller quantities, but are potent greenhouse gases based on their global warming potentials.

Indian Perspective

Majority of livestock in India are fed on agro-industrial by products and poor quality crop residues which is one of the reasons not only for low productivity but also contributing towards higher methane production.On a global scale, agriculture and in particular enteric fermentation in ruminants (predominantly cattle and small ruminants) produces between 21 and 25 per cent of the total anthropogenic emission of methane. In India, out of the total 27 per cent Green House Gas (GHG) emission from agriculture sector, 50 per cent is estimated to be the contribution from its 485 million livestock which amounts to about 10.4 million tons, the major contribution coming from cattle and buffalo (92%) and rest from small ruminants (7%). Climate change is expected not only to impact livestock at the species level but also decide sustainability of a breed or a species to a particular climatic condition. This has emerged as a major challenge to researchers not only to provide mechanisms for adaptation to the immediate change in climate but also to vision and forecast technologies for its mitigation.

Generation of a database on methane production under different production systems adopting a common protocol would be useful in drawing mitigation strategies. Enhancing the bio-availability of nutrients from crop residues through treatment or strategic supplementation would stimulate microbial protein synthesis and reduce methanogenesis. Use of alternate hydrogen sinks (electron acceptors) like inclusion of unsaturated edible oils in the ration would help in reducing methane production. A technology that holds some promise in the long-term of diverting electrons from methanogens is the production of acetic acid by acetogens. Increasing the population of acetogens through exogenous inoculation could be useful for competing against methanogens. The other strategies could be exploring molecular techniques to assess the effect of methane inhibitors, use of feed additives and secondary plant metabolites, ration balancing and strategic supplementation of feeds through total mixed rations and feed blocks to reduce methanogenesis are some of the technologies that have been discussed. Replacing low producing animals with high producers could be a viable approach to enhance livestock productivity without much increase in methane production, where livestock number is the major contributing factor as in India.

The Intergovernmental Panel on Climate Change (IPCC) predicts more floods, intense storms, heat waves and droughts due to global warming. Its study forecasts a rise of 1.4 to 5.8 degrees Celsius in the global mean surface temperature over the next 100 years, with developing countries most vulnerable. Other studies are even more apocalyptic. A report commissioned by the World Wildlife Fund predicts "dangerous" warming of the earth's surface in as little as 20 years, with the Arctic warming so much that its polar ice could melt in the summer by the year 2100, pushing polar bears close to extinction. The Arctic Climate Impact Assessment predicts that caribou, musk ox and reindeer would find their habitats severely reduced. Northern aboriginal peoples around the world would find their way of life changed forever, the study said.

Considerable evidence of climate change associated with emissions of greenhouse gases (GHG), mainly carbon dioxide (CO2), methane (CH4) and nitrous oxide (N2O), in the atmosphere has resulted in international efforts to reduce GHG emissions. Methane is the second major GHG after CO2 and it is 20 times more potent than CO2 contributing about 15-20 per cent of the total greenhouse gases. The annual global methane production from livestock is about 80 Tg from enteric fermentation and India's contribution is about 10.4 Tg per year, which corresponds to 13 % of the global influx of methane. Methane production by Indian cattle, buffalo, sheep and goat was 76.7, 97.0, 11.6 and 10.1 g/head/d, respectively. The notable fact is that by 2012 India shall be bound by the restrictions of the Kyoto protocol that makes us mandatory to restrict our methane emission to a specified level and this might be much lower than the present level of methane emission.

India houses 16.10, 56.50 and 16.50 percent respectively of world's cattle, buffalo and goat population occupying first position in milk, 3rd in egg and 5th in broiler production in spite of the production system being predominantly based on agro-by-products and crop residues. Medium to large herds of cattle and buffalo, however exist in the periphery of large towns and cities mainly for supply of milk (peri-urban system). Small ruminants and pigs are reared under extensive and semi-intensive systems of production. Resource-poor small and marginal farmers and landless labourers' are the main custodian of the livestock owning 71% of cattle, 63% of buffaloes, 66% of small ruminants, 70% of pigs and 74% of poultry. Intensification of production system has occurred only in poultry and on a limited scale in dairy industry. Intensive pig farming has been initiated at a low scale. The vast number of livestock numbers associated with production systems based on crop residues and agricultural wastes is a cause of major concern as this is going to add to the total pool of green house gases.

Methane (CH4) is a colorless, odorless gas generated as a by-product of microbial fermentation of feed in the gastrointestinal tract of ruminant animals. Methane producing bacteria, commonly referred to as methanogens, use the hydrogen and carbon dioxide produced as end products of microbial digestion to generate energy for growth, with CH4 as an end product. Energy losses associated with enteric CH4 emissions range from 2 to 11.3 % of gross energy intake. Numerous mitigation strategies have been suggested in the literature, including: manipulation of rumen microfloral populations, diet manipulation to provide alternate hydrogen acceptors, diet manipulation to shift the fermentation pathway, management for improved productivity, and genetic selection for low methane emitting animals. There are opportunities to reduce enteric methane emissions in commercial production systems. Many of these mitigation strategies will influence carbon sequestration opportunities and nitrous oxide emissions associated with manure handling and storage, and will require evaluation and validation at a systems level.

Principles and Background of Enteric CH_4 Production

Methane originates from anaerobic microbial fermentation processes in the gastrointestinal tract of ruminant animals. This fermentation occurs particularly in the reticulorumen, rumen in short. In an adult cow, the rumen occupies a volume of over 100 litres of which usually 85 to 90% is fluid. The high moisture content and a temperature that is kept rather constant at around 37° C makes this an eminently suited environment for microbes to survive and grow, provided the microbes are regularly supplied with a suitable substrate. Substrates needed by the microbes are provided through the ingestion of feed by the host animal. The feed ingested by a ruminant is attacked by the microbes and degraded in a wide range of end products. The anaerobic condition in the rumen and hindgut limit the oxidation of organic substrate into carbon dioxide (CO2) and water (H2O), but an internal rearrangement of the carbon (C), hydrogen (H) and oxygen (O) present in the feed, between microbial biomass and the end products, keeps the system going. During this process reducing equivalents (H2) are generated. To prevent the accumulation of H2, which by itself is poisonous to the microbes, a H2 sink is needed. Various H2 sinks are present in the rumen of which the conversion of H2 and CO2 into CH4 is by far the most important. An accumulation of CH4 is prevented by eructation and respiration, and the CH4 is emitted to the environment. Other important end products of fermentation are microbial mass and volatile fatty acids (VFA).

The rumen resembles a microbial population cultured in a buffered semi-continuous chemostat with a semicontinuous inflow of substrates from ingested feed as well as inflow of drinking water, and continuous outflow and mixing of contents. There is also a continuous inflow of urea in saliva and by absorption from blood to the rumen. Buffering is maintained by the continuous inflow of saliva and due the process of VFA absorption. Simultaneously, an outflow of unfermented substrates, of synthesized microbial matter and of rumen fluid and solutes occurs. The majority of the VFA (about two thirds) leave the rumen through absorption by the rumen wall to the blood. Mixing of rumen contents takes place by frequent rumen contractions.

The main part, usually some 60 to 65%, of the dry matter entering the rumen is carbohydrates, 15 to 20% is protein, 10 to 15% minerals and less than 10% lipids. Several types of carbohydrates (sugars, starch, pectins, hemi-cellulose and cellulose) are degraded by the micro-organisms in the rumen. Also degradation of proteins occurs and a significant proportion of their amino acids is either incorporated in microbial protein or degraded further in VFA and ammonia (NH_3). Lipids and free long-chain fatty acids are hardly fermented, but, to some extent, long chain fatty acids may be incorporated in microbial matter (Harfoot & Hazlewood, 1997). Within the rumen several classes of micro-organisms degrade substrates, synthesize microbial matter, and ferment substrate to VFA, CO_2, H_2 and NH_3. The purpose of the degradation is to generate energy for maintenance and energy and precursors for synthetic processes.

Mostly, a pragmatic and rather global distinction is made between sugar and starch utilizing bacteria, cell wall utilizing bacteria and protozoa, of which the latter predate on bacteria. These microbial classes not only distinguish themselves in the type of substrate they use, but also in the fractional rate of their rumen outflow, together with their preferred types of substrate. Protozoa are capable to retain themselves within the rumen and flow out with a much lower fractional rate than bacteria.

Methanogens co-exist with the substrate degrading micro-organisms and produce CH_4 from CO_2 and H_2. By far the major part of the H2 formed in the rumen is converted into CH4 (Mills *et al.*, 2001). Besides methanogenesis, H2 and CO_2 can be converted to acetate by acetogens, which are also present in the rumen environment (Johnson & Johnson, 1995; Demeyer & Fievez, 2000; Moss *et al.*, 2000). Based on thermodynamics, Kohn & Boston (2000) argued that under normal fermentation conditions in the rumen, methanogenesis is feasible (reduction potential below -0.3 Volt), but for acetogenesis to occur more reducing conditions are required. This means that acetogenesis does not play an important role in the rumen hydrogen balance and the quantities of CH_4 produced.

Contribution of hindgut fermentation

In addition to that in the rumen, also fermentation in the hindgut contributes to enteric CH_4 production. This contribution appears generally to be less than 10% and slightly lower than the contribution of the hindgut to the digestion of organic matter (Kebreab *et al.*, 2006b). The opposite would be expected because hindgut fermentation yields relatively less propionate and, as will be explained in section 1.3, hence more H2 is formed than in the rumen. Apparently, the stoichiometry of VFA production differs between rumen and hindgut. A possible explanation is a higher contribution of acetogenesis to remove the H2, because in comparison to the rumen conditions, fermentation conditions in the hindgut may be more favourable for acetogenesis than for methanogenesis (De Graeve & Demeyer, 1988). With acetogenesis, acetate rather than CH4 is formed from CO_2 and H_2 (Kohn & Boston, 2000; Offner & Sauvant, 2006). Hence, removal of H_2 by acetogenesis reduces CH_4 yield.

VFA yield, hydrogen balance and CH_4 yield

Together with the production of VFA, and depending on the type of VFA, H_2 is either generated or utilized With acetate and butyrate production, H_2 is produced, whereas with propionate and valerate production, H_2 is utilized. Acetate is the main VFA resulting from rumen fermentation of fibre, starch, sugars and protein (Bannink *et al.*, 2006a), and therefore a net excess of H_2 is produced in the rumen. Although some other sinks of H_2 can be identified (microbial synthesis with NH_3 as the N source and the biohydrogenation of unsaturated fatty acids), the type of VFA produced is the major determinant of the amount of H2 produced. The specific addition of other.

H2 sinks to the diet may further affect the size of the H2 excess, and hence CH4 yield. Reversely, the addition of compounds such as ionophores, which affect the viability of specific classes of micro-organisms (Chen *et al.*, 1977), may force a shift in the rumen fermentation patterns towards more propionate and a lower H2 excess (Kohn & Boston, 2000; Offner & Sauvant, 2006). It is generally assumed that the excess H2 is almost completely converted into CH4 by methanogens. As a result, the partial gas pressure of H2 remains low under normal fermentation conditions (Moate *et al.*, 1997).

Factors influencing CH_4 yield

Factors that can be identified as influencing CH_4 yield include dietary characteristics as well as the fermentation conditions in the rumen. Important dietary characteristics are daily feed intake and the resulting rumen fill (1), the proportion of concentrates in dietary dry matter (2), and the composition and the rate and extent of degradation of individual feed fractions (the types of carbohydrate and protein) in dietary dry matter (3). Among important fermentation conditions are acidity (pH) of rumen fluid (1), the presence of unsaturated long chain fatty acids (2),the composition of the microbial population within the rumen (3), the dynamics of the passage of particles, fluid and the microbial population (4), the inflow of saliva (5) and the absorption capacity of the rumen wall. The combined effect of both types of factors is represented in conditions that characterize the ruminant, such as production level (1), stage of lactation (or other physiological conditions like pregnancy) (2), and management related interventions (3) such as grazing regime, feeding regime (diet supplementation, concentrate feeding, use of by-products like beet pulp, and protein sources), housing and milking. Methane yield can thus be related to many and different categories of factors. However, these factors are often interrelated and so are their effects on CH_4 yield in the rumen. This complicates the use of such factors to predict the course of fermentation in the rumen, the extent of organic matter digestion and the productive response of the ruminant. Due to these interrelationships, the contribution of a single feed component or type of carbohydrate to CH4 yield is not necessarily constant but may vary with a change of the dietary characteristics and the fermentation conditions in the rumen (Mills et al., 2001; Bannink et al., 2005a). Changing the level of feed intake, the dietary characteristics or the fermentation conditions in the rumen affect the extent of substrate degradation by micro-organisms and the efficiency of microbial synthesis. As a consequence, amounts of microbial matter as well as undegraded feed substrate flowing out of the rumen to the small intestine change. For example, a higher fractional outflow rate of feed substrate and their associated microbes leads to less degraded substrate but, because of its reduced rumen residence time, it may be accompanied with an increased efficiency of microbial synthesis (Dijkstra et al., 1998 & 2005). Because of the multiple factors that may have changed simultaneously and have affected rumen fermentation and hence CH4 yield, the effect of nutritional measures on VFA and CH4 production may be difficult to predict and interpret. The observed effect of a nutritional intervention on CH4 yield is therefore strongly confounded with the concomitant changes brought about in these factors. Some of the principal factors affecting rumen function and CH4 production will be discussed below.

Feed Intake

Changes in dry matter intake not only affect the amount of substrate available for microbial degradation, but it also changes fermentation conditions and the size of the microbial population. For example, the fate of ingested starch changes with changes in the amount of dry matter ingested, as increased intake levels will lead to a proportionally higher amount of starch digested in the small intestine rather then fermented in the rumen. Aspects which need to be considered are the storage of starch by micro-organisms with increasing concentrations in the rumen, or an altered passage rate which alters the time available for microbial degradation.

Microbial degradation of substrates in the rumen depends primarily on intrinsic characteristics that determine the susceptibility of the substrate to be attacked, degraded and utilized by micro-organisms. These characteristics differ between types of substrate and between types of feedstuffs that are used as dietary components Obviously, intrinsic characteristics are important determinants of substrate degradation and utilization by microorganisms,VFA production and the concomitant CH_4 yield. Passage rate of substrate together with their intrinsic degradation characteristics determines the fraction of a substrate that becomes degraded in the rumen or escapes to the small intestine. In present day dairy nutrition, feedstuffs are often selected to increase the quantity of starch and protein escaping rumen fermentation, hence contributing to the nutrient supply of the cow without generating VFA and CH4. Hence, a higher passage rate ue to a higher feed intake level as well as a less degradable substrate may both increase the escape of substrate and lead to a decrease in CH_4 yield.

Type of substrate fermented and type of diet

Different types of fermented carbohydrate give different profiles of VFA production and hence CH4 yield. With higher levels of milk production, basal rations of dairy cows are supplemented with concentrates. Independent of the effect of fluid acidity, an analysis of VFA profiles showed about 25 and 15% lower CH4 yields for fermented sugars and starch, respectively, on concentrate-rich diets compared to forage-rich diets (Bannink & Dijkstra,2005).

Fermentation rate and fluid acidity

The acidity of rumen fluid (pH) influences rumen fermentation in two ways. Firstly, pH values lower than 6.2 appear to reduce the activity of fibrolytic micro-organisms degrading cell walls (Argyle & Baldwin, 1988; Dijkstra *et al.*, 1992). Therefore, pH determines cell wall degradability and its contribution to microbial growth, and VFA and CH4 yields. Secondly, pH determines the profile of VFA produced (separate from the type of substrate and the type of diet as was discussed in section 1.5.3). An increased rate of substrate fermentation, as a result of an increased feed intake or due to large concentrate meals, leads to increased rates of VFA production, to higher VFA concentrations and a more acidic rumen fluid. As a result, also the profile of VFA shifts towards a propionate oriented fermentation (Dijkstra et al., 1994). This will cause a lower H2 excess and lower CH4 yield. In an analysis of in vivo data on rumen fermentation, a decrease of the pH of the rumen fluid from 6.5 to 5.5 was estimated to lead to about 15% less CH4 produced from both fermented sugars and starch (Bannink et al., 2005a & 2005b). Not only VFA concentrations determine rumen fluid pH (Baldwin, 1995; Mills et al., 2001), but also the bufferingcapacity of saliva flowing into the rumen (Pitt et al., 1996; Imamidoost & Cant, 2006; Bannink & Dijkstra, 2006).Buffering of rumen contents is enhanced by the inclusion in the diet of ingredients that stimulate rumination (such as straw), by feeding mixed rations, by frequent feeding (particularly of concentrates), and by preparing the rumen wall for strong increases in concentrate intake during the first weeks of lactation. If buffering processes are stimulated at the same time, an increased feed intake rate does not necessarily lead to a strong acidification of rumen fluid.

Methane is the second most important anthropogenic greenhouse gas only preceded by carbon dioxide. Methane has a relatively short atmospheric short-life time and therefore it has other economic characteristics than carbon dioxide. For example, if the ultimate aim of international climate policy is to stabilise the global average surface temperature to 2 K above the pre-industrial level at lowest possible cost, the current relative value of reducing methane as compared to carbon dioxide should be lower than its Global Warming Potential (GWP) value used in the Kyoto Protocol. However, this result is changed to the opposite if one adopts a cost-benefit approach.

Methane is also an important precursor to tropospheric ozone. Tropospheric ozone has in turn serious consequences on human health, agricultural production and ecosystems. Taking into account this in social cost/shadow price estimates of methane can increase the value considerably, in the order of 100 %. Consequently, the benefit cost ratios of methane mitigation are strongly dependent on which approach is adopted when valuing methane's economic impacts and if the tropospheric ozone co-benefit of methane mitigation is considered or not. Many sources of methane are non-point emission sources. This makes it harder to regulate and control methane emissions than most carbon dioxide emissions. The most important single sector emitting methane is livestock production.

Methane Mitigation Strategies

Mitigation of rumen CH4 emission is essential and can be effectively achieved by strategies that improve the efficiency of animal production. The dietary/nutritional strategy that improve productivity with no potential negative effects on livestock health and production and are cost effective has a better chance of being adopted. The approach for mitigation also depends on the production systems and agronomic practices in the region.

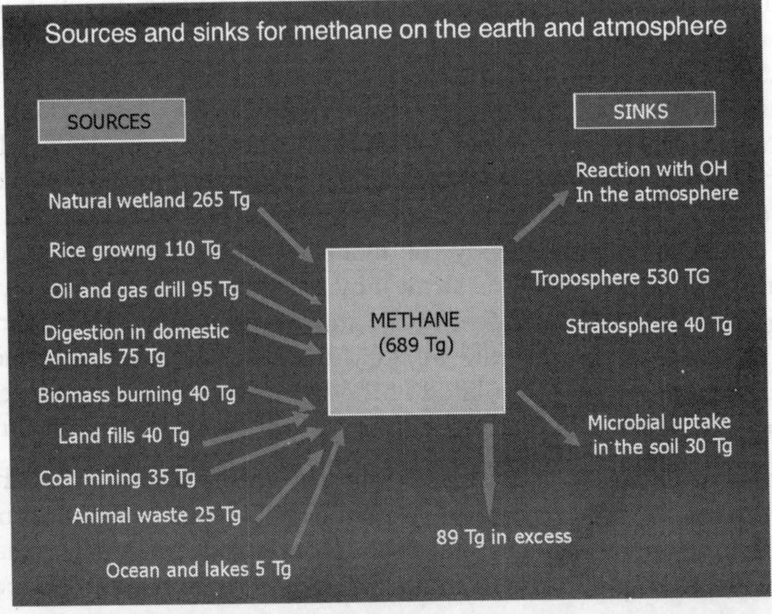

Enteric Fermentation

Enteric methane emission is produced as a result of microbial fermentation of feed components. Primary digestive microorganisms (bacteria, protozoa and fungi) hydrolyze proteins, starch and plant cell wall polymers into amino acids and sugars. These simple products are then fermented to volatile fatty acids (VFA), hydrogen (H2) and carbon dioxide (CO2). Acetate, propionate and butyrate, which are the major VFA, are then absorbed and utilized by the host animal. The major producers of H2 are the organisms which produce acetic acid in the fermentation pathway. Acetate and butyrate production results in CH4 production, while propionate formation serves as a competitive pathway for H2 use in the rumen. Under feeding situations where poor quality roughages form the major constituent of animal diet the production of acetate is more contributing to higher methane production. Particularly low producing animals on straw based diets produce higher quantities of methane per unit dry matter intake.

Within livestock production about two thirds of methane emissions stem from enteric fermentation of ruminant animals, mainly cattle with the rest from animal waste. Methane production in the rumen occurs as a consequence of the presence of a group of microorganisms called methanogens that reside in the reticulo-rumen and large intestine of ruminant livestock. These organisms play an important role in converting organic matter to methane. As described in a detailed review by McAllister *et al.* (1996).Proteins, starch and plant cell-wall polymers consumed by the animal are hydrolyzed to amino acids and simple sugars by the bacteria, protozoa and fungi which reside in the rumen. Primary and secondary digestive microorganisms further ferment the amino acids and sugars into volatile fatty acids, hydrogen, carbon dioxide and other end products. Methanogens then reduce carbon dioxide to methane, preventing the accumulation of hydrogen. Excessive quantities of hydrogen ions or protons, when allowed to accumulate in the rumen environment, result in a decline in pH, and subsequent inhibition of many organisms that are essential for fibre digestion.

Approximately, 87% of enteric methane originates in the reticulo-rumen while the remainder is produced in the hindgut. A significant portion of the latter, approximately 89%, is absorbed and expired through the lungs, with the remainder being excreted through the anus (Murray et al, 1976,Torrent et al.,1994). Losses in gross energy intake associated with methane production range from 2-3% of gross energy intake (GEI) when animals are fed high grain diets and 11.3% of GEI when consuming low quality forage (Ominski *et al.* 2004). An understanding of the microbial processes responsible for the production of enteric methane production, coupled with the identification of management strategies leading to reduced methane emissions and improved animal performance will help facilitate the efforts of the Government to achieve a 6% reduction in greenhouse gas emissions by 2008-2012, as outlined in the Kyoto Protocol.

Several mechanisms influence the availability of hydrogen in the rumen and subsequent production of enteric methane emissions by cattle. Processes that yield propionate act as net proton-using reactions while those that yield acetate result in a net increase in protons. That is, the proportion of volatile fatty acids, specifically acetate: propionate, produced as a consequence of microbial fermentation in the rumen has a significant influence on methane production. This ratio may, for example, be influenced by the type of carbohydrate consumed by the animal. Cereal-based diets that are high in starch favour propionate production and consequently tend to produce less methane per unit of feed consumed than forage-based diets (McAllister, 1996).In addition to the type of carbohydrate in the diet, other dietary factors influence the acetate:propionate profile in the rumen, including residence time in the rumen. Okine *et al.* (1989) have demonstrated a 29% reduction in methane production when weights were added to the rumen to stimulate contraction of the rumen wall in order to decrease residence time of the feed in the digestive tract Digestibility of dietary energy may also influence enteric methane production. When intake was restricted to 2% of body weight, an increase in methane production, expressed as a percent of GEI, was no longer evident. As changes in diet digestibility and residence time in the rumen are associated with intake, it is not unexpected that level of intake also influences enteric methane emissions. Johnson and Johnson (1995) concluded that feeding highly available carbohydrates at limited intakes, results in high fractional methane losses while feeding highly available carbohydrates at high intakes leads to low fractional methane losses. Further, (Blaxter,1967) has described an increase in total production of methane with increases in intake, from maintenance to twice maintenance. However, when expressed as amount of energy lost per unit of feed, a reduction is realized. Another mechanism by which methane production may be reduced during the rumen fermentation process is through the provision of alternative hydrogen acceptors or sinks. Compounds such as unsaturated fatty acids provide alternative hydrogen acceptors, consuming hydrogen in limited quantities, during biohydration (Boadi, 2004). Dicarboxylic acids (such as fumaric and malic acids), which are intermediates in the propionic acid pathway, may also serve as alternative electron sinks for H2,. Bayaru *et al.* (2001) observed a 23% reduction in methane production, and increased propionic acid formation with no effect on DM digestibility when fumaric acid was added to whole crop sorghum silage fed to Holstein steers.

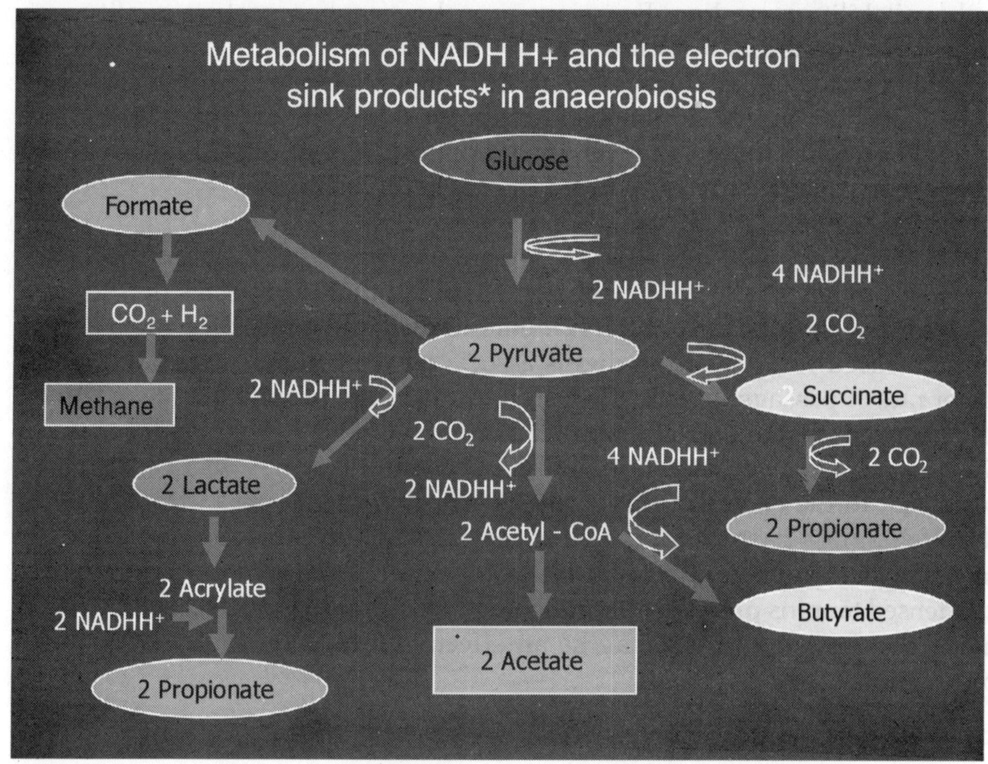

Management Strategies Leading to a Reduction in Enteric Methane Emissions

These management strategies may be categorized as follows: forage utilization, feed additives, and improved production efficiencies. Each will be addressed in the subsequent section.

Forage utilization

Quality

Steers grazing during the early period of the grazing season had 44% and 29% less energy lost as methane than steers grazing during the mid and late grazing periods respectively. Further, steers experienced a 54% reduction in enteric emissions upon entry vs. exit of a paddock. Efficiency of forage fermentation was linked to biomass availability and quality of pasture. The impact of pasture forage quality and availability on enteric methane emissions from cattle in grass-based production systems has been studied by Ominski *et al.* (2004). Enteric methane emissions measured early and late in the grazing season were influenced by pasture type and season of grazing. Further, it appeared that emissions were influenced by pasture dry matter availability and quality, in that emissions were highest (11% of GEI) when pasture quality and availability were low. Emissions were lower when pasture quality was high and availability was low (6.9% Unfortunately, neither pasture ever attained a status of high forage quality and high pasture availability. It can be concluded that enteric emissions are highest when the animal is presented with poor quality forage and has limited opportunity to select higher quality forage as a consequence of reduced dry matter availability.

Species

McCaughey *et al.* (1999) have demonstrated that the species present in a pasture may significantly influence enteric methane emissions. Inclusion of legume-based forages in the diet is associated with higher digestibility and faster rate of passage resulting in a shift toward high propionate in the rumen and reduced methane production. The improved feed utilization observed in the cow as a consequence of the reduced enteric emission proved to be beneficial to the calves in this study as calf growth rate was 11% higher on the alfalfa-grass pasture compared to the grass only pasture. Species selection may play an important role in reducing enteric methane emissions, also condensed tannins present in several forage species are associated with reduced methanogenesis and thus may be an effective technique to lower methane production.

Pasture management

Boadi *et al.* (2002) examined the use of supplemental grain as a means of reducing enteric methane emissions in an alfalfa-grass pasture environment. The benefits of grain supplementation in terms of mitigation potential on good quality pasture are limited, as pasture quality had a greater impact on methane production than did grain supplementation.

Forage preservation and processing

A decrease in methane production as a consequence of ensiling has been reported.

Feed additives

Ionophores are frequently utilized in beef cattle production systems to improve animal performance, as well as to reduce the incidence of bloat and prevent outbreaks of coccidiosis. Improvements in feed efficiency of 5-6% have been attributed to a shift in the fermentation pathway from acetate to propionate (Goodrich, 1984). Ionophore supplementation may reduce methane emissions by 20-25%.The use of ionophores to reduce enteric methane emissions on pasture has been examined by McCaughey *et al* 1997. Neither voluntary intake nor methane production was affected by the presence of monensin. Research conducted by Müller-Özkan (2002) has demonstrated that the addition of calcium ions in vitro had a tendency to reduce activity of methane-producing bacteria, as evidenced by a decrease in methane production. The addition of fat supplementation in high-energy finishing diets has been examined in several commercial production systems. Mathison (1997) demonstrated that daily enteric methane emissions could be reduced by 33% when canola oil was added to an 85% concentrate feedlot diet. Further, a demonstrated a 30% reduction in daily enteric methane emissions when comparing a typical feedlot diet (88.5% concentrate) with a ration of equal energy density containing a 44:42:14 ratio of concentrate, silage and whole sunflower seed. These studies demonstrate that fat supplementation may effectively reduce enteric emissions for finishing cattle. The mitigation potential of supplemental fat in low quality forage diets has not been addressed. Although this strategy of reducing enteric methane emissions may not seem viable from an economic perspective at the present time, future trading of carbon offsets may prove otherwise. In addition to economic viability, other factors that require exploration include practical application techniques in forage based production systems and appropriate levels of supplementation to ensure that fibre degradation is not compromised.

Reductive acetogenesis

In the gut of termites and rodents, acetogens convert excess H2 to acetic acid, which is then utilized by the host. However, in the rumen the number of acetogens is few and cannot compete effectively with methanogens for H2 ions, because they have a lower affinity for H2 than methanogens. Increasing the populations of acetogens through exogenous inoculations into the rumen could be useful for competing against methanogens. However, previous attempts at inducing acetic acid by inoculation with acetogens were not successful.

PROPOSED MECHANISM OF ACTION OF GOS ON REDUCTION IN CH_4 EMISSION

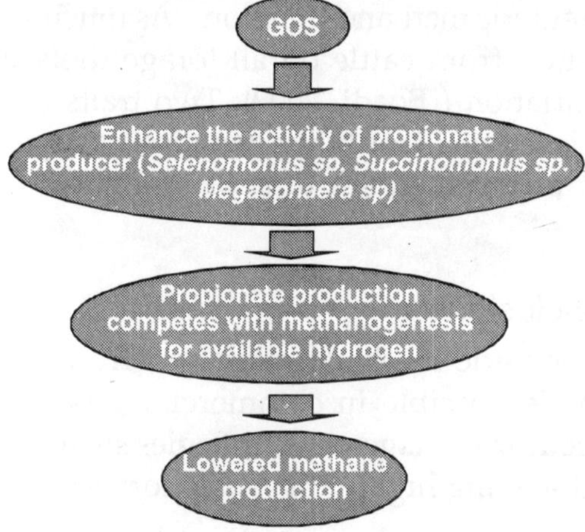

Improved Production Efficiencies

Methane losses (% GEI) in commercial situations do not deviate considerably from 6%. The best strategy for mitigation is to decrease methane loss per unit of product. Using this approach, strategies to decrease methane emissions in the cattle industry should include effective management of feed resources other than forage, such as water quality, mineral supplementation and ration balancing. The impact of water quality on cattle performance has been demonstrated in a series of trials conducted by Willms *et al*. (2002). Calves from cows having access to water from a natural water source delivered to a trough (clean water) gained 9% more than calves from cows that had direct access to a pond. Yearling heifers having access to clean water gained 23% and 20% more weight than their counterparts drinking directly from a pond, or from a pond pumped to a trough, respectively. Thus, adopting management strategies that serve to improve water quality and subsequent animal performance should serve to reduce methane emissions per unit of product. Adequate mineral supplementation is another avenue by which the cattle industry may realize a net reduction in enteric methane emissions. Minerals, which serve numerous functions in the body - structural, physiological, catalytic and regulatory - are necessary if optimal growth, health and productivity of the animal are to be achieved It is anticipated that lack of mineral supplementation or inadequate intake of supplemental mineral on the pastures would result in less than optimal performance and thus increased emissions per unit of product. Other than effective management of feeding programs, there are several other management strategies that would serve to improve animal productivity. These include animal selection for improved production, management for improved reproduction, and use of growth promoting agents.

Genetic selection of animals that consume less feed or produce less methane per unit of feed is another management strategy that may be employed to reduce enteric methane emissions. As much as 27% of the variation in methane production from cattle on all-forage diets was associated with animal-to-animal variation (Boadi, 2002). Two traits that are actively being investigated as a means of identifying genetically superior animals are net feed efficiency and mean retention time of digesta in the rumen(Hegarty, 2002).

Summary and Conclusions

A reduction in enteric methane emissions from cattle in forage-based production systems is possible in commercial production systems. These strategies include feeding management strategies such as inclusion of legumes in forage mixes and feeding highly digestible forages. Adoption of strategies that serve to improve production efficiency including feed analyses and ration balancing, pregnancy testing and provision of good quality water, will not only serve to reduce enteric methane emissions but will also prove to be economically beneficial. The mitigation potential of several commercially accepted practices, including the use of ionophores, probiotics, and silage-based feeding systems requires further evaluation, as does the use of novel production practices such as the inclusion of fat in forage based diets. In addition, long-term research support is required to examine the potential for selection of low-methane emitting animals in forage-based production environments.

References

Argyle, J.L. & R.L. Baldwin, (1988). Modeling of rumen water kinetics and effects of rumen pH changes. *J.Dairy Sci.* 71: 1178-1188.

Baldwin, R.L., (1995). Modeling Ruminant Digestion and Metabolism. Chapman & Hall Ltd, London, UK.

Bannink, A. & S. Tamminga, (2005). Rumen Function. Pages 263-288 In: Quantitative Aspects of Ruminant Digestion and Metabolism, 2nd Edition. Eds. Dijkstra, J., J.M. Forbes & J. France. CAB International,Wallingford, UK.

Bannink, A., Dijkstra, J., Mills, J. A. N., Kebreab, E. & J. France, (2005a). Nutritional strategies to reduce enteric methane formation in dairy cows. In: Emissions from European Agriculture, pp. 367-376

Bannink, A. & J. Dijkstra, (2006). Voorspelling van de zuurgraad van pensvloeistof. ASG report 12. ASG,Lelystad

Bannink, A., Kogut, J., Dijkstra, J., Kebreab, E., France, J., Tamminga, S. & A.M. Van Vuuren, (2006a). Estimation of the stoichiometry of volatile fatty acid production in the rumen of lactating cows. *J. Theoret.Biol.*, 238: 36-51.

Boadi, D., Wittenberg, K.M., and McCaughey, W.P. (2002). Effects of grain supplementation on methane production of grazing steers using the sulphur hexafluoride (SF6) tracer gas technique,*Can. J. Anim. Sci.*, 2: 151.

Boadi, D., Benchaar, C., Chiquette, J., and Massé, D. (2004). Mitigation strategies to reduce entericmethane emissions from dairy cows: Update review, *Can. J. Anim. Sci.*, 84: 319.

Bayaru, E., Kanda, S., Kamada, T., Itabashi, H., Andoh, S., Nishida, T., Ishida, M., Itoh, T.,Nagara, K., and Isobe, Y. (2001). Effect of fumaric acid on methane production, rumen fermentation and digestibility of cattle fed roughage alone, *Animal Science J.*, 72: 139.

Blaxter, K.L., *The Energy Metabolism of Ruminants,* Hutchinson and Co. Ltd., London,UK, (1967). 332 p.

Chen, M. & M.J. Wolin, (1979). Effect of monensin & lasacoid-sodium on the growth of methanogenic &rumen saccharolytic bacteria. *Appl. Environ. Microbiol.* 38: 72-77.

Czerkawski, J.W. (1972). Fate of metabolic hydrogen in the rumen, *Proc. Nutr. Soc.*, 31: 141.

De Graeve, K. & D.I. Demeyer, (1988). Rumen and hindgut fermentation: differences for possible explanation? Med. Fac. Landbouww. Rijksuniv. Gent

Demeyer, D. & V. Fievez. (2000). Ruminants et environment: la méthanogenèse. *Ann. Zootech* 49: 95-112.

Dijkstra, J., Neal, HD.St.C., Beever, D.E., & J. France, (1992). Simulation of nutrient digestion, absorption and outflow in the rumen: model description. *J. Nutr.* 122: 2239-2256.

Dijkstra, J. (1994). Production and absorption of volatile fatty acids in the rumen. *Livest. Prod. Sci.*, 39: 61-69.

Dijkstra, J., France, J. & D.R. Davies (1998). Different mathematical approaches to estimating microbial protein supply in ruminants. *J. Dairy Sci.* 81: 3370-3384.

Dijkstra, J., Kebreab, E., Bannink, A., France, J. & S. Lopez, (2005). Application of the gas production technique in feed evaluation systems for ruminants. *Anim. Fd. Sci.Technol.*, 123-124, 561-578.

Goodrich, R.D., Garrett, J.E., Gast, D.R., Kirick, M.A., Larson, D.A., and Meiske, J.C. (1984). Influence of monensin of the performance of cattle, *J. Anim. Sci.*, 58: 1484.

Harfoot, C.G. & G.P. Hazlewood, (1997). Lipid metabolism in the rumen. Pages 382-426 In: The Rumen Microbial Ecosystem, Second Edition, Eds: P.N. Hobson & C.S. Stewart. Blackie Academic & Professional, London.

Hagarty, R.S. (2002). Strategies for mitigating methane emissions from livestock – Australian options and opportunities, in *Greenhouse gases and animal agriculture*, Takahashi, J. and Young, B.A., Eds., Elsevier Science.

Imamidoost, R. & J.P. Cant, (2005). Non-steady-state modeling of effects of timing and level of concentrate supplementation on ruminal pH and forage intake in high-producing grazing ewes. *J. Anim. Sci.* 83: 1102-1115.

IPCC, 2007: *Summary for Policymakers. In: Climate Change 2007: The Physical Science Basis. Contribution of Working Group I to the Fourth Assessment Report of the Intergovernmental Panel on Climate Change* [Solomon, S., D. Qin, M. Manning, Z. Chen, M. Marquis, K.B. Averyt, M.Tignor and H.L. Miller (eds.)]. Cambridge University Press, Cambridge, United Kingdom and New York, NY, USA.

Jansen, E., J. Overpeck, K.R. Briffa, J.C. Duplessy, F. Joos, V. Masson-Delmotte, D. Olago, B. Otto-Bliesner, W.R. Peltier, S. Rahmstorf, R. Ramesh, D. Raynaud, D. Rind, O. Solomina, R. Villalba and D. Zhang, (2007). Palaeoclimate, *Climate Change 2007: The Physical Science Basis. Contribution of Working Group I to the Fourth Assessment Report of the Intergovernmental Panel on Climate Change* [Solomon, S., D. Qin, M. Manning, Z. Chen, M. Marquis, K.B. Averyt, M. Tignor and H.L. Miller (eds.)]. Cambridge University Press, Cambridge, United Kingdom and New York, NY, USA.

Johnson, K.A, & D.E. Johnson, (1995). Methane emissions from cattle. *J. Anim. Sci.* 73: 2483-2492.

Kebreab, E., France, J., McBride, B.W., Bannink, A., Mills J.A.N. & J. Dijkstra, (2006a). Evaluation of models to predict methane emissions from enteric fermentation in North American Cattle. In: Modelling NutrientUtilization in Farm Animals, Eds, E. Kebreab, J. Dijkstra, J. France, A. Bannink & W.J.J. Gerrits,. CAB International, Wallingford, UK.

Kohn, R.A. & R.C. Boston, (2000). The role of thermodynamics in controlling rumen metabolism. Pages 11-24 In Modelling Nutrient Utilization in Farm Animals. Eds. J.P. McNamara, J. France & D.E. Beever. CAB International, Wallingford, UK.

Kuczynski, U. Dämmgen, J. Webb and A. Myczko, editors]. Wageningen Academic Publishers, Wageningen,the Netherlands.

Mathison, G. (1997 abstr). Effect of canola oil on methane production in steers, *Can. J. Anim. Sci.*, 77: 545.

McAllister, T.A., Okine, E.K., Mathison, G.W., and Cheng, K.J. (1996). Dietary, environmental and microbiological aspects of methane production in ruminants, *Can. J. Anim. Sci.*, 76: 231.

McCaughey, W.P., Wittenberg, K.M., and Corrigan, D. (1997). Methane production by steers on pasture, *Can. J. Anim. Sci.*, 77: 519.

McCaughey, W.P., Wittenberg, K., and Corrigan, D. (1999). Impact of pasture type on methane production by lactating beef cows, *Can. J. Anim. Sci.*, 79: 221.

Mills, J.A.N., Dijkstra, J., Bannink, A., Cammell, S.B., Kebreab, E. & J. France, (2001). A mechanistic model of whole-tract digestion and methanogenesis in the lactating dairy cow: Model development, evaluation, and application. *J. Anim. Sci.* 79: 1584-1597.

Moate, P.J., Chalupoa, W., Jenkins, T.C. & R.C. Boston, (2004). A model to describe ruminal metabolism and intestinal absorption of long chain fatty acids. *Anim. Feed Sci. Technol.*, 112: 79-105.

Moss, A.R., Jouany, J.P. & J. Newbold, (2000). Methane production by ruminants: its contribution to global warming. *Ann. Zootech.*, 49: 231-253.

Müller-Özkan, E. (2002). Investigation of the effects of anion rich diets on the carbohydrate metabolism in the bovine rumen (in vitro), Ph.D. thesis, School of Veterinary Medicine, Hannover.

Murray, R.M., Bryant, A.M., and Leng, R.A. (1976). Rates of production of methane in the rumen and large intestine of sheep, *Brit. J. Nutr.*, 36: 1.

Offner, A. & D. Sauvant, (2006). Thermodynamic modelling of ruminal fermentations. *Anim. Res.* 55: 1-23.

Okine, E.K., Mathison, G.W., and Hardin, R.T. (1989). Effects of changes in frequency of reticular contractions on fluid and particulate passage rates in cattle, *Can. J. Anim. Sci.*, 67: 3388.

Ominski, K.H., Wittenberg, K.M., and Boadi, D., Examination of economically and environmentally sustainable management practices in forage-based beef production systems, presented at the CCFIA Final Workshop, Winnipeg, January 2004.

Pitt, R.E., Van Kessel, J.S., Fox, D.G., Pell, A.N., Barry, M.C. & P.J. Van Soest, (1996). Prediction of ruminal volatile fatty acids and pH within the net carbohydrate and protein system. J. Anim. Sci., 74: 226-244.

Solomon S., Plattner G.K., Knutti R., Friedlingstein P. (2009). Irreversible climate change due to carbon dioxide emissions, *Proceedings of National Academy of Sciences*, 106(6): 1704-1709.

Torrent, J. and Johnson, D.E. (1994). Methane production in the large intestine of sheep, in *Energy Metabolism of Farm Animals,* Aquilera, J.F., Ed., EAAP Publication No. 76: CSIC Publishing Service, Spain.

Willms, W.D., Kenzie, O.R., McAllister, T.A., Colwell, D., Veira, D., Wilmshurst, J.F.,Entz, T., and Olson, M.E. (2002). Effects of water quality on cattle performance, *J. Range Manage.*, 55: 452.

□□□

18

Nutrition in Relation to Yak Production

K. K. BARUAH[1] AND N.N.PATHAK[2]
[1]National Research Centre on Yak (ICAR), Dirang-780 101, West Kameng District Arunachal Pradesh, India [2] Izatnagar

Introduction

Livestock rearing is an age old activity in hilly regions of India. Among the livestock, the yak (*Poephagus grunniens* or *Bos grunniens*) is one of the most remarkable domestic animals adapted to living in high altitude mountain terrains in harsh conditions. The yak is inherently associated with the culture, religion and social life of the pastoral nomads of highlands for their food and livelihood security. The yak production system followed by highlanders is different from other livestock. Yaks are usually reared under free-range system by the highlanders. It is a multipurpose animal adapted for living at high altitudes between 3,000 to 4,500 m above msl. It can even thrive at an altitude of 6,000 m above msl.

Yak belongs to the order Artiodactyla, family Bovidae, sub-family Bovine, genus *Bos* and species *grunniens*. It is domesticated from the wild yak (*Bos mutus*) which is still found in the remote Quinghai-Tibet plateau and neighbouring regions. This animal inhabits in very high-altitude elevations of Himalayas viz., Tibetan plateau and entire Indian Territory in Ladakh, Western China, Pakistan, Northern Afghanistan, Bhutan, Mongolia, Nepal and Soviet Union. In India, yaks are highly valued by Himalayan people because of its contribution to human economy as milk, meat, wool, leather, dung for fuel and manure, and as pack animal. Of the 14.2 million domesticated yaks in the world about 13.3 million are found in China. Whereas, in India 83,080 yaks are found in the hilly tracts of Arunachal Pradesh (14,000), Sikkim (5,000), Jammu and Kashmir (62,000), Himachal Pradesh (2,000), Uttrakhand (50) and Sandakufu area of West Bengal (30).

In Arunachal Pradesh, *'Monpa'*, a mongoloid Buddhist tribe is the only tribe rearing yaks. Yaks in Ladakh region of Jammu and Kashmir are reared by the Buddhist tribe as well as Muslim nomads. In Sikkim, *Aho*, *Bho* and *Bhutia* tribes (mostly Buddhist) are rearing yaks. In Himachal Pradesh, they are reared by Buddhist tribes in Lahual-Spiti and Kinnuar districts, and Hindu tribes in Chamba district (Ramesha and Bhattacharya 2008). In Arunachal, the yak lives predominantly on the hills of West Kameng and Tawang districts at the altitudes of 2,000 to 4,000 m above from msl. The yak herders locally called *'Brokpas'* predominantly occupies these areas. The yaks in Sikkim were originated from Bhutan and Tibet, which are presently found in Lachung, Lachen, Thangu and Muguthang valleys in North, Nathula, Kupup, Gnathang, Thegu in East and Yuksom-Dzongri in West Sikkim. The yak herders in Sikkim are called *'Dokpas'*. *Brokpas* and *Dokpas* migrate with their livestock from one hill to another and live in a transhumance.

Yak is a unique genetic resource with an ability to survive in severe cold at low temperature even at -40°C. They have a thick coat of hair with outer coarse hair and inner dense fine hair, better lung capacity and ability to climb on hilly terrains. They have good adaptation to the hypoxic condition of the high altitude as haemoglobin content is higher as compared to cattle. Red blood cells (RBC's) are larger in yaks (4.83µm) than local cattle (4.38µm) and RBC number is also higher, thus increasing its blood capacity to retain more oxygen (Zhang *et al.*, 1994). A low pulmonary vasocontraction (Anand *et al.*, 1988) and high oxygen affinity of hāemoglobin (Weber et al., 1988) favour yak survival at high altitude. Cup-shaped hooves in yaks help them to walk on steep hills and also on the slippery snow covered grounds for carrying load. The surface area of yak is relatively less per unit of body weight which is quite useful adaptive characteristics for living at high altitude hills.

Yak Types

Indian yaks are categorized into five types (i) Common (ii) Bisonian (iii) Bareback (iv) Hairy forehead and, (v) White yaks. Based on the geographical area of inhabitation of India yaks, they are classified into Ladakh yaks, Arunachal yaks, Himachal yaks and Sikkim yaks (Pathak, 1994).

Utility of Yaks

The milk production of yaks ranged from 129-282 kg in a lactation ranging from 120 days to 300 days. The age of puberty among the India yaks ranged between 38-42 months under the field conditions. The age at first service is around 3-4 years in all the states and gestation period is about 258 days in yaks (Ramesha *et al.*, 2008). The major source of income for the yak farmers comes from yak milk. Yak milk is one of the richest sources of fat with a range of 5.8-7.9% (Jain and Yadav, 1985). The principle milk products which are prepared from yak milk are Butter, Ghee, Churpi (Cheese), Khoa, Churkum, Sour milk and Whey. Yak cheese contain 24.8% higher (P<0.01) level of total long-chain saturated fatty acids (c17:0- c26:0) and 3.2 times higher (P<0.01) content of total n-3 PUFA than cow cheddar cheese. Yak cheese had 2.8 times higher total trans-18:1 content. Yak meat is fine textured and scarlet in colour. It is very palatable (Jialin *et al.*, 1998). It is devoid of marbling. The meat yield is between 70-190kg. The yak meat is nutritionally superior since it contains 24.7% protein, 16-20% fat and 1.33% total ash (Sarbagisher *et al.*, 1989). Its delicious flavour comes from the unique distribution of fatty acid percentage. Yak meat is very lean and low in saturated fat. Yaks when compared to mules are efficient in carrying the load during winter season but are slow when compared to mules. Yaks weighing 250 to 350kg are suitable for carrying the loads at high altitudes and can carry about 60kg upto a distance of 4.5 to 7.5 km (Ramesha *et al.*, 2008).

Feeding and Nutrition

The yaks receive their nutritional supply through grazing on alpine pastures and other herbages of high altitudes. In India, yak farmers practices two-pasture utilization strategy. During hot and humid season when lush growing pastures are available they migrate to the high altitudes (8,500-14,000ft. above msl) or even to the 16,000 ft. above msl. The summer pasture extends for about 190 days (May to October) and the winter pasture for about 138-150 days (November to April). The rest period is spent on transit from winter pasture to summer pastures. The traditional way of maintaining the animals is to allow them to put on weight as much as possible in summer and utilize the fat as an energy reserve for survival in winter months, when there is scarcity of feed. An experiment conducted at Sela in Tawang district of Arunachal Pradesh revealed that there were fourteen plant species in this grassland. However, two most dominant species were *Brachypodium spp.* and *Aletris peciflora* contributing about half of the total plant population. No legume species was found. Average plant height was 2cm and average plant density (No. of plants/m^2) was 11294 ± 2195.2 and the total herbage production was 50.07 ± 3.98 q/ha. The average DM, CP, EE, CF, NFE, NDF, ADF and ADL silica and total ash contents of the mixed herbage were 12.83, 11.9, 1.65,

22.89, 45.96, 21.37, 23.82, 8.71, 7.84 and 17.60 %, respectively (Basu *et al.*, 2005). The voluntary DM intake was 2% of body weight and digestibility of DM was 41.05 ± 2.42% (average). All animals gained an average body weight 95.29± 33.05 g/day indicating that grazing alone could maintain yaks with little gain in body weight during summer from May to September (Basu *et al.*, 2005). However, higher DM digestibility and body weight gain was reported on feeding feed blocks prepared with locally available tree fodder and maize stover (Baruah *et al.*, 2010) Due to non-availability of feed resources during winter months (November to March) a substantial loss (25-30%) in body weight of yaks occurs. The performance of yaks in terms of production and reproduction are also affected. Recent experiment conducted at Mandala (10000 ft.) above msl of West Kameng district of Arunachal Pradesh revealed that yak could grow at optimum rate even during winter if they were fed adequately. Two types of CFB viz CFB 1 (50% maize stover, 47% concentrate and 3% molasses) and CFB 2 (25% maize stover, 25% Salix leaves, 47% concentrate and 3% molasses) alongwith area specific mineral mixture were fed to growing yak calves average body weight 153 kg could grow at the rate of 347-422 g/d (Annon, 2011).

Rate of passage

The rate of passage of ingesta through the gastro-intestinal tract of yak is much slower in comparison to cattle. Average retention time of feeds in the gastro-intestinal tract of yak is about 78 hours. It is similar to 79 hours in the bison but 9-13 hours more than in cattle on the some feeding regimen. Longer retention time of feeds in the gastro-intestinal tract of the yaks is a very important factor in the utilization of nutrients of the feeds. This provides more opportunity for the action of the digestive microbial enzymes of the gut and longer time for the absorption of the digestive nutrients. This is also advantageous for the more efficient utilization of dietary nitrogen available as non-protein nitrogen through recycling (Schaffer *et al.*, 1978). Under natural feeding on pastures it may be possible that the feed retention time is further increased due to less availability and fibrous nature of the herbages.

Water requirement

Quantitative estimate is not available for the water requirement of yaks for drinking. However, yaks like to drink running water and satisfy their thirst by eating snow in the winter.

DM requirement

Dry matter intake in yak varies due to different factors viz. age and body weight, sex, the nature of the feed, climatic conditions and to certain aspects of management. Yak generally consume less dry matter than cattle and buffaloes, probably because of their smaller rumen capacity. There is a linear correlation between the DMI of yak and their body weight. (Liu *et al.*, 1997) evolved an equation to estimate the DMI kg/day in growing yak.

DMI kg/day=0.0165 w + 0.0486 (r= 0.959) Where w is body wt. in kilograms.

Han *et al.*, (1990) studied on feed intake of two to three year old castrated yak in stall fed condition and observed that the dry matter intake (DMI) of roughage decreased with the increasing level of concentrates in the diets. They also observed that feed intake in yak increased at lower temperature both in stall fed and grazing on natural pasture. It is interesting to note that yak can graze normally when temperature is as low as -30^{0} to -40^{0}C or even lower. But at higher temperature they grazes less and as a result feed intake falls.

Dry matter intake varies from 1.63-2.42 kg/d when different complete feed blocks were fed to growing yak calves (AICRP, 2010).

Protein and energy requirement

Saikia *et al* (2007) reported 450 g daily gain and FCE 9.70 on feeding 100% of Kearl requirement of growing cattle. In an another experiment conducted for 150 days on feeding 2 levels of protein and energy 100% and 75% of NRC (1989) it was observe that average daily gain in body weight was highest ($P< 0.01$) in high protein high energy (504g/d), followed by high protein low energy (456 g/d), low protein high energy (408 g/d) and low protein low energy (356 g/d) respectively. From the experiment it is assumed that growing yaks require 80.5 g DM, 10.7 g DCP and 50.6 g TDN per kg metabolic body weight to support growth rate of 431g ADG (Annon, 2011).

Mineral requirement

No information is available about the mineral requirement of yak but there is a possibility of mineral deficiency due to non-availability of feed during winter months and also leaching during summer in draining water of melted snow.

Carotenes utilization

The conversion of carotenes into vitamin A activity is less efficient is yaks as in cattle. It is evident from the high yellow pigmentation of butter fat in the yak milk.

Salt feeding

Yaks have great craving for salt. This habit has been used to attract the animal and they return from the pasture for obtain their salt on the fixed day and time. Salt is fed at weekly or fortnightly intervals.

Conclusion

Since adequate information's are not yet available on the different aspects of nutrition, it may be advantageous to provide some supplements of proteinous feeds and complex mineral mixture to take care of deficiency, if any.

References

Anand, I., Health, D., Williams, D., Dean, M., Perrari, R., Bergel, D. and Harris, P. (1988). The pulmonary circulation of some domestic animals at high altitude. *International J. Biotechnology*, 32: 56-64.

Annon (2011 Yak News), 8: 1.

Baruah, K.K., Chakravarty, P., Paul, V., Sarma, H. Ahmed, F.A. and Das, K.C. (2010). Effect of feeding complete feed block based on unconventional feeds on growth performance and a nutrient utilization of yak calves. *Indian Vet. J.* (In press).

Basu, A., Chatterjee, A, Baruah, K.K. and Bhattacharya M. (2005). Voluntary feed intake and live weight gain in yaks (Poephagus grunniens L.) grazed on high altitude grassland. *Indian J. Anim. Sci.* 75 (1): 81-83.

Han X, Xie, A. and Hu, L. (1990). Feed intake of growing yak. *Journal of Qinghai Animal Husbandry and Veterinary Medicine*, 20(6): 5-6, 39.

Jain, Y.C. and Yadav, R.S. (1985). Yield and composition of milk of Himachali yak, yak hybrid and hill cow. *Indian J. Anim. Sci.* 55: 223-224.

Jialin, B., Minggiang, W., Zhonglin, L. and Chesworth, J.M. (1988). Meat production from crossbred and domestic yaks in china. *Anim. Sci.* 66: 465-469.

Liu Shujie *et al.* (1997). Study on the forage intake at different phonological periods in grazing yak. *Journal of Qinghai Animal Husbandry and Veterinary Medicine*, 27(2): 4-8.

Pathak, N.N. (1994). An introduction to yak husbandry, Pub. No.26, IVRI, Izatnagar.

Ramesha, K.P., Kataktalware, M.A., Das, S., Pourouchottamane, R., Bandopadhyay, S., Sarvanan, B.C., Krishnan, G., Sarkar, M., Battacharya, M. (2008). Performance and body measurements of yaks and their hybrids under field condition. *Indian J. Anim. Sci.* 78 (9): 1032-33.

Ramesha, K.P. and Bhattacharya, M. (2008). Domestication, distribution and genetic characterization. In Yak-Moving treasure of the Himalayas edited by K.P. Ramesha. NRC on Yak publication, Dirang, India.

Saikia, P.K.; Saikia, B.N.; Ghosh, M.K.; Baruah, K.K.; Chakravarty, P. and Bhattacharya, M. (2007). Effect of different levels of dietary protein on growth and nutrient of yaks (Poephagus grunniens L.). *Proc. VI Biennial Conf. of Animal Nutrition Assoc.* Jammu, 15-17 Sept., 2006.

Sarbagisher, B.S., Rabochev, V.K., Terebaev, A.I. (1999). Yak in : Animal Genetic resources of the USSR, FAO, Animal Production and Health Paper No. 65, Rome, pp 357-364.

Schaffer, A.L.; Young, B.A. and Chimwano, A.M. (1978). Ration digestion and retention time in digesta in domestic cattle (Bos Taurus). American Bison bison) and Tibetan yak Bos grunniens). *Canad. J. Zool.* 56:2355.

Weber, R.E., Lalthantlnanga, R., Braunitzer, G. (1988). Functional characterization of fetal and adult hemoglobin : an oxygen binding cascade and its molecular basis. Archives of Biochem. *Biophys.* 263: 199-203.

Zhang, R.C., Wu, J.P., Han, J.L., and Yang, P. (1994). Anatomical physiology of yak adapting to low oxygen content on the high plateau. Proceedings of the 1st international Congress on Yak held on August 1-6, 1994, Lanzhou, P.R. China, pp. 236-240.

❑❑❑

19

Climatic Stress and Mitigation Strategies in Dairy Animals

U.K. MISHRA
Director of Instruction and Dean, College of Dairy Technology IGKV, Raipur

Introduction

Stress is a common term that is often associated with negative situations and settings. Climate change poses formidable challenge to the milk production potential of elite cows and buffaloes in India (Singh, *et al.*, 2009). The rise in temperature together with increased precipitation and humidity aggravate the heat stress in dairy animals, adversely affecting their milk production and reproductive performance. The effect of extreme hot dry or hot humid weather is quite large and devastating for the low-income rural farmers due to substantial loss of milk production. Besides this, climate also has a negative impact on feed and fodder shortages in summer. India has become the largest milk producers in the word but livestock sector requires intensive and innovative tools to ameliorate climate stress to further boost the milk production of lactating animals by 10-20%.

Thermoneutral zone : The range of environmental temperatures over which the heat produced by a 'warm-blooded' animal remains fairly constant. Hence, it is the range in which the animal is 'comfortable', having neither to generate extra heat to keep warm nor expend metabolic energy on cooling mechanisms, such as panting. Animals adapted to cold environments tend to have broader thermoneutral zones than ones living in hot environments.

Temperature Humidity Index

To evaluate the combined effect of temperature and humidity is to use the temperature -humidity index (THI). It is considered that at THI higher than 72, the animals would begin to suffer stress (Hahn, 1985, 1993). It is also very important to determine the number of hours of stress along the day and the number of days. As environmental temperature and the relative humidity increase, the loss of heat of the cow from skin diminishes and its corporal temperature increases (temperature of > 25°C and humidity to > 50%). To evaluate the environmental impact on the comfort, the THI (Temperature-Humidity Index) is used i.e. the relationship between the temperature and humidity. This relationship causes a condition that affects directly the animal and their production. To improve their comfort, the animals move towards the wind, looking for a fresh or humid place or natural or artificial shades (Hahn *et al.* 1993). These mechanisms are necessary to maintain the normal operations of the body. The most productive, mature and heaviest animals are more susceptible to heat stress.

The upper critical temperature range for high producing exotic dairy cows and calves has been reported between 25 and 26°C (Berman *et al.*, 2005; Webster, 1994). When animal can no longer dissipate enough metabolic heat to maintain homeothermy, vasodilation, sweating, and panting mechanisms are invoked to dissipate body heat (Curtis, 1983). At this time, feed intake during heat stress is also voluntarily reduced (Armstrong, 1994; West, 2003) resulting in less heat generated by digestion and absorption of nutrients. Additionally due to the U-shaped relationship of the nutrient energy requirement for maintenance and temperature in lactating cows, there is an increase in the energy requirement of maintenance with the temperature rising above (and below) 18 to 20°C (National Research Council,1981). Thus, as the temperature rises the energy requirement needs for maintenance increases, whereas feed intake is suppressed. Death can occur when the body temperature is 3°C higher than normal, but it depends on the duration of heat stress, acclimation, body weight, and production level among other factors (Curtis, 1983). Strategic planning of shelter management and feeding practices can mitigate heat stress to a great extent.

Effect on Milk Production and Composition

Hot weather reduces milk production in cows with high genetic merit for milk production. With the extensive crossbreeding, the average milk production per cow has doubled, the metabolic heat output per animal has increased substantially rendering animals more susceptible to heat stress (Collier *et al* 2006).

Numerous studies have examined the physiology, production, genetics, and management tools of heat stress, under both climatic laboratory and on-farm conditions. (Armstrong *et al*, 1999; West, 2003; Berman, 2005). Lactating cows suffering from heat stress seek and remain in shade, reduce feed intake, drink more water, and shows an immediate drop in daily milk yield (Fig. 1).

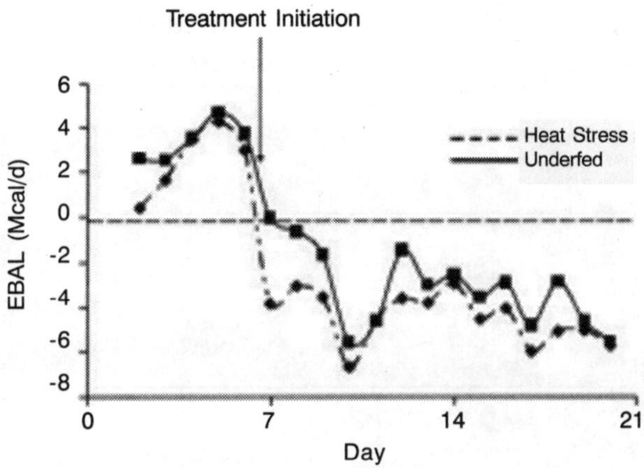

Fig. 1 : Effects of heat stress and pair-feeding thermal-neutral conditions on calculated net energy balance in lactating Holstein cows. (Adapted from Wheelock *et al.*, 2006.)

The milk production of the crossbred cows declines faster than the indigenous Sahiwal and Tharparkar cows (Singh *et al.*, 2003). During the hot dry season the drop in milk yield can be checked effectively, if crossbred cows are offered *ad. lib.* green fodder and water. Elite cows and buffaloes cannot withstand rigors of high ambient temperature and a significant reduction in milk yield occurs (20-30 %) due to decline in metabolic hormones, feed intake and increase of respiration, pulse rate and body temperature (Aggarwal and Singh, 2005). Somatic cell counts and incidence of mastitis rise due to unhygienic condition during hot humid climate. It is not known how much of the reduction in milk yield is due to hot conditions alone and how much improved management, nutrition and health could overcome reduced production. The reduction in milk yield in dairy cattle in hot environments is not the result of a simple process and is an interaction of metabolic, hormones and adaptive changes; however understanding of the exact causes and effects is not complete.

Innovative Methods to Mitigate Heat Stress

Shelter Management

Shelter for the animal is one the most important prerequisite for the expression of their full genetic potential. Shelter management under normal condition has no meaning for the small landless farmers as later have no priority of animal shelter due to lack of resources. One of the best and cheapest ways of mitigating the heat stress is to keep the animals under trees or in mud houses, which is a very old and traditional practice in many parts of our country. But this practice is feasible only to a limited number of cows and buffaloes and that too for medium and low milk producing animals. The provision of tress in a loose housing system provides effective cooling against heat stress by lowering the ambient temperature (4 to 6°C), (Fig. 2).

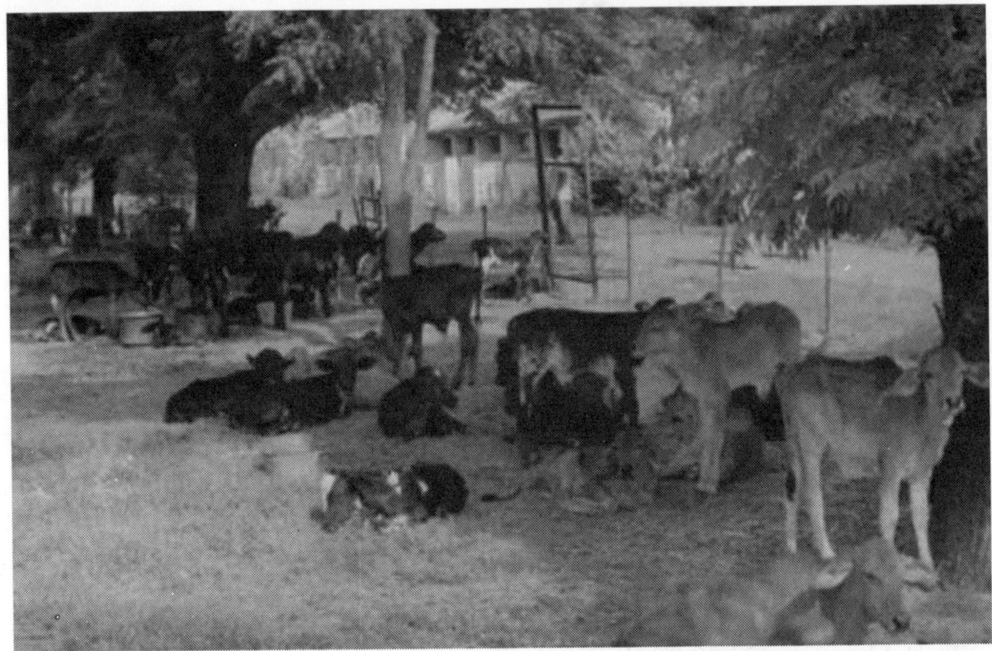

Fig. 2 : Use of tree shaddow to Mitigate summer stress

In West Bengal farmers use many types of shelters which are made up of bamboos and paddy straws/thatch roof. Such houses are quite cheap, economical and comfortable to animals during hot dry and hot humid seasons (Singh *et al.*, 2007). The use of paddy straw bedding (6 inches) over the asbestos roof during hot humid season has been found to reduce the heat stress and improves milk yield of cows (Singh *et al.*, 2008). Use of sand bedding and fan during hot dry and hot humid climate is also effective and economic way of minimizing the heat stress (Singh *et al.*, 2003).

Photo : Use of sand bedding and mist to alleviate stress of hot humid climate.

Photo: Bamboo and thatch roof shelter in hot humid climate of West Bengal.

Use of Mister/ Water showers

Successful cooling strategies for lactating dairy animals are based on maximizing available routes of heat exchange, convection, conduction, radiation, and evaporation. Provision of fans, wetting the animal's body surface, high pressure mist to cool the air in the animal shed, and facilities designed to minimize the transfer of solar radiation (use of sprinklers, thatch material over the roof of the shed) are used for heat abatement (Aggarwal and Singh, 2006). Due to more awareness and ever increasing population density in urban areas, the progressive/commercial farmers now keep elite cows in group of 50 or more. In such farms, summer induced dramatic decline in milk yield, associated with low feed intake during summer could be checked effectively by use of mister or shower system. The efficacy of the mister system is further improved by use of fan. These systems have been shown to decrease losses in milk yield, decrease mortality in post-parturient cows, improve reproductive parameters (services/conception, conception rate, days open), and improve appetite (Shultz and Morrison, 1987). Cooling pre-parturient dairy cows with shades, fans, and sprinklers compared with sprinklers alone improved total 60-d milk production by 84.3 kg/cow, and increased profitability per cow (Urdaz et al, 2006; Ludri and Singh, 1987,1989). There is a dearth of scientific information on the specific effects of rainfall (Fox and Tylutki, 1998). Excessive moisture in the ground or bedding of dairy cattle has various effects on their behavior and physiology. Rainy or wet conditions have been shown to drastically reduce the time dairy cattle spend lying down (Tucker *et al.*, 2007). Besides, there is a much greater level of energy expenditure when walking in muddy and wet conditions (Dijkman and Lawrence, 1997), along with a reduction in feed intake (Fox and Tylutki, 1998). The lack of cleanliness associated with wet environments affects health conditions in dairy cattle including an increase in uterine and intra-mammary environmental pathogens (Schreiner and Ruegg, 2003) that predispose dairy cattle to endometritis (Lewis, 1997; Heuwieser *et al.*, 2000) and mastitis, respectively, the latter leading to milk contamination (Anderson and Walker, 1998). Lameness is one of the most costly diseases on dairy farms (Kossaibati and Esslemont, 1997), and wet conditions contribute to softer hooves and an increase in lameness (Boderas *et al.*, 2004; Amstel *et al.*, 2004). Though cost of mist system installation is met within 3 months and farmers get quite a reasonable profit through its use, but important constrains is the availability of water under rural condition. Some measure needs to be taken to recycle the same water in mist cooling system. The other important considerations lie with the disease incidence like mastitis. The wetness/ dampness of floor renders the microenvironment favorable for the growth of the bacteria and thus hygiene has to be maintained to minimize the risk of udder health. Short term studies in crossbred cows indicated no adverse effect of mist+fan use on udder health (Aggarwal and Singh,

2006).The floor of the house therefore should have better slope for effective drainage and drying. The progressive farmers now are using fan and mister system to mitigate the heat stress. However, use of fan is effective only in hot humid climate for better evaporative cooling in comparison to hot dry condition (Aggarwal and Singh, 2005, 2006, 2008).

Economical aspects of mist system

Table : Cost of establishment of infrastructure for six animals (Mister/showersystem)

Name of item	Unit/No.	Cost (Rs.)
1. GI Pipe	20 ft.	320.00
2. Mist fogger/shower	3	195.00
3. GI T	3	45.00
4. Socket	2	18.00
5. GI albow	2	24.00
6. GI union (1/2²)	1	35.00
7. Gate valve (1/2²)	1	125.00
8. Pump (0.25 hp)	1	2000.00
9. Miscellaneous		100.00
10. Fan (48²)	2	1800.00
	Total	**4662.00**

Feeding Management

Energy is one of the most important limitation in milk synthesis and secretion. Hot and hot humid conditions interfere in heat dissipation, increase heat loads on animals resulting in less feed intake and low milk yields. Heat stress reduces both feed intake and milk yield. The decline in nutrient intake has been identified as a major cause of reduced milk synthesis (Fuquay, 1981); however, the exact contribution of declining feed intake to the overall reduced milk yield remains unknown. At high ambient temperature feed intake decrease, increased gut fill, decreased rate of passage of ingesta, increased water intake occurs. The heat stressed animals behavior also change and cows prefer to have intake in nights when temperature decline. Night feeding during cooler time increase feed intake of cows. Heat-stressed cows had an average rectal temperature of ~ 105°F during the afternoons of the treatment implementation. Heat-stressed cows had an immediate reduction (5 kg/d) in dry matter intake (DMI) with the decrease reaching nadir at ~ d 4 and remaining stable. Reduction in DMI can only account for ~ 40-50% of the decrease in milk production when cows are heat-stressed and that ~ 50-60% can be explained by other heat-stressed induced changes.

During summer, feeding of concentrate mixture, straw and water mixture improves the milk yield, and meets the water requirements ((Singh *et al.*, 2007). High feed intake by elite cows results in raised metabolic heat increment which requires effective thermoregulatory mechanisms to maintain body temperature in a thermoneutral zone and in physiological homeostasis. Cows can succumb to hyperthermia if they fail to maintain thermoneutrality. Accurate measurement of time when cows enter heat stress is complicated because the responses to heat stress affect not only the energy balance, but also water, sodium, potassium and chlorine metabolism. Water, sodium, potassium and chlorine are important constituents of sweat, and sweating is a major, if not the most important, thermoregulatory mechanism used to dissipate excess body heat. Due to high metabolic heat increment, and especially in the warmer months, high-producing dairy cows may enter heat stress much earlier than their lower-producing counterparts and than currently thought or extra heat has been accommodated by physiological adaptations. Should this be the case, then strategies to reduce heat stress must be developed to enable the elite cows to express their full genetic potential.

Hormone release

Climate has a major effect on endocrine system due to alteration in metabolism. The release of hormones is controlled by the hypothalamus which is affected by high ambient temperature through input signals of cold and warm receptors. During cold stress, the basal metabolic rate increases, feed intake increases and the thyroxine release is more. Thus cold stress stimulate thermo-sensitive cells in the anterior hypothalamus and affect secretion of glucocoroticoids. Growth hormone concentration increase in rats, but in cows no seasonal variation occurs in GH level. Plasma prolactin levels decline due to less photoperiod and reduced water intake. It is considered that PRL is involved in water/ osmoregulation. Epinephrine and nor-epinephrine secretion increase due to change in deep body temperature that influences both neural and hormonal thermoregulatory mechanism (non-shivering thermogenesis). The mode of action of these effects is probably via the eyes to the pineal gland which, in turn, influences the secretion of hormones. During summer secretion of prolactin is consistently elevated by long days due to increased photoperiod, and their role in water and electrolyte metabolism. The increased water intake increase prolactin secretion. Growth hormone and insulin are unaffected by day length, whereas there is conflicting evidence for effects of day length on thyroxine and corticosteroids. Thyroid hormone, glucocorticoids, epinephrine and nor-epinephrine hormone decline at high ambient temperatures. Aldosterone concentration increase which conserves the sodium at the expense of potassium, but aldosterone decrease in cattle due to more postassium secretion in sweat. The cortisol level increase initially in response to high ambient temperature but decline subsequently in long term exposure.

Milk temperature, somatic cell count and milk prolactin concentration increase with increasing environmental temperatures. Milk growth hormone concentration also increase with lactation level and declined significantly during summer heat. Milk temperature and PRL level may serve as indicators of the impact of the climatic environment on lactating cattle.

Blood Glucose

Mammary gland requires glucose to synthesize milk lactose. Lactose is the primary osmo-regulator and determinant of milk yield. However, at high ambient temperature, body (primarily skeletal muscle) utilizes glucose at an increased rate to generate less metabolic heat. As a consequence mammary gland may not receive adequate amounts of glucose; thus mammary lactose production and subsequent milk yield are reduced. This may be the primary mechanism which accounts for the additional reductions in milk yield that cannot be explained by decreased feed intake. Heat-stressed cows require special attention with regards to heat abatement and other dietary considerations (i.e. concentrate: forage ratio and HCO3-, etc.). Cows also have an extra requirement for dietary or rumen-derived glucose precursors. During heat stress, propionate is primarily converted into glucose by the liver. Highly fermentable starches, such as grains, increase rumen propionate production. Although propionate is the primary glucose precursor, feeding additional grains can be risky, as heat-stressed cows are already susceptible to rumen acidosis.

Nutritional amelioration

The average body weight of dairy cows has increased over time as cows have been selected to produce more milk. Larger cows have larger gastrointestinal tracts that allow them to consume and digest more feed. This in turn provides more substrates for milk synthesis. The lactating cow uses ME for milk production at an average efficiency (q) of 65% (Moe et al 1970). Heat increment during milk synthesis is also dependent on the quality and quantity of feed that the animal consumes. On roughage diets rumen fermentation yields a large molar excess of acetate compared with propionate and if the latter is insufficient to provide enough $NADPH_2$ then acetate may need to be converted, by some form of futile cycle, to heat in order to prevent a metabolic excess (MacRae and Lobley 1982). On a concentrate diet the molar proportion of propionate increases while that of acetate decreases and so supply of $NADPH_2$ is not rate limiting. Thus increased milk production is related to elevated HI. Total milk production and HI have increased over time, although the rate of increase of HI has been slower than of milk production.

The biological mechanism by which heat stress impacts production and reproduction is partly explained by reduced feed intake, but also includes altered endocrine status, reduction in rumination and nutrient absorption, and increased maintenance requirements (Collier et al 2005; Aggarwal and Signh,2009) resulting in a net decrease in nutrient / energy availability for production. Reductions in energy intake during heat stress result in a majority of lactating cows entering into negative energy balance. Such cows largely depend on nonesterified fatty acids (NEFA) for energy. Despite having much greater energy content, oxidizing fatty acids generates more metabolic heat (about 2 kcal / g or 13% on an energetic basis) compared to glucose. Hence precursors for gluconeogenesis such as amino acids, propionate is in greater need.

During periods of heat stress protein excesses aggravate the situation because protein itself is calorigenic, and nitrogen excretion requires energy. Hence diet needs to be balanced for amino acids to prevent the feeding of excess crude protein. Recent advances in animal nutrition, including the feeding of ruminally-protected fats and protected proteins are among other endeavours to reduce metabolic heat production and supply the correct profile of nutrients to high producing cows in early lactation. Supplemental fat, as rumen-inert fat, is used as an effective source of energy with low heat increment on straw-based diets in tropical environment. An adequate supply of nutrients must also include well-balanced mixture of dietary minerals, especially of Na, K, Cl and SO^{2-}_{4}. These play a pivotal role in the thermal physiology of the cow and are influenced by the heat stress (Singh *et al.*, 2008).

Rumen protected protein and fat produced from oilseeds provide a practical feeding strategy to regulate nutrient and energy partitioning and augment essential / bioactive fatty acids (linoleic and alpha-linolenic acids) and conjugated linoleic acid content of meat and milk (Gulati et al 2005). Feeding of 1 kg of formaldehyde-treated oilseed protein meal supplement increased milk yield by 10% compared with untreated protein meal supplements in cows and buffaloes of India, which were fed on straw based diets (Garg et al 2002; 2003). Improving productivity in dairy animals exposed to adverse environmental conditions may be achieved by improving the environment around the animals and improving their nutritional management. Feeding of non-hormonal substances like choline chloride and milkofeed also prevents decline in milk yield of cows during summer (Singh *et al.*, 2006).

Stress Response Pathways

Stress on animal and human being occurs is response to a stressor in different ways. Any stressor result in release of Nor epinephrine hormone in body to counter or control the challenge, and therefore the "fight" hormone predominantly released is epinephrine. If strength/ intensity of stress arousal increases and a possible loss of control is felt by the individual, then epinephrine, another "flight/anxiety" hormone is released. When stress is prolonged and seen as hopeless, the individual becomes more distressed and defeated. This activates the hypothalamus in the brain resulting in the final release of cortisol, a steroid hormone from the adrenal cortex (of the kidney). It is a steroid (compound based from a steroid nucleus) hormone that is produced in the cortex of the adrenal glands located on top of each kidney. Fasting, food intake, exercising, awakening, and psychosocial, climatic stressors cause the body to release cortisol. Animal and human studies have demonstrated that cortisol injections are associated with increased appetite, cravings for sugar, and weight gain. Cortisol indirectly influences appetite by regulating CRH (corticotrophin releasing hormone), leptin, and neuropeptide Y (NPY) released during stress. Fight or "flight" stress responses cause the heart to beat faster and harder as well as release more free fatty acids (disassembled triglycerides) into the blood, and suppression of the immune system.

Cold Stress

Lactating animals are more prone to heat stress than the cold stress. The following factors affect an animal's ability to withstand the cold climatic conditions.

- *Acclimation*: Cattle do adjust or acclimate to colder weather by growing a longer, thicker coat. This provides additional insulation against cold weather. The coat must be clean and dry to provide maximum protection to the cow. Dirt or moisture on the coat reduces its insulation value dramatically.
- *Fat Layer*: Cattle in good condition with a thick fat layer are better able to withstand the cold than thin cattle. The fat layer acts as another insulating layer between the animal's core and the environment.
- *Metabolic Rate*: Cows will also increase their metabolic rate to increase heat production and help maintain body temperature. This increases the need for dietary energy, so appetite is usually increased and cows eat more (www.omafra.gov.on.ca)

Hypothermia occurs when the body temperature drops well below normal. In general terms, with cattle, mild hypothermia occurs with a body temperature of 30°C–32°C, (86°F–89°F), moderate hypothermia at 22°F–29°C, (71°F–85°F) and severe hypothermia below 20°C (68°F). As rectal temperature drops below 28°C (82°F), cows are not able to return to normal temperature without assistance through warming and the administration of warm fluids. As hypothermia progresses, metabolic and physiological processes slow down, and blood is diverted from the extremities to protect the vital organs. Teats, ears and testes are prone to frostbite. In extremes, respiration and heart rate drop, animals lose consciousness and die.

In most situations, a more insidious and costly problem occurs. Cows are subjected to an environmental temperature below the lower critical temperature, but without obvious signs of hypothermia. This increases the maintenance energy requirement of these animals as they adjust to the conditions and divert more energy to maintaining body temperature.

Key management factors to limit the effects of cold stress

- Monitor the weather conditions, ambient minimum and maximum temperature, increase feeding quantity and frequency in response to cold weather. Late pregnant cows require additional grain feeding when the effective temperature falls below the lower critical level.
- Protect animals from cold wind as later markedly reduces the effective temperature and increase cold stress on animals.
- Bed cows well. Lactating animals may be provided with paddy straw dry bedding (6 inches) which provide warmness against ground floor and increase ability of cattle to withstand cold stress.
- Keep cows clean and dry. Cows should be dry and clean so that effect of cold weather is reduced. Wet coats greatly reduce insulating properties and make cows more susceptible to cold stress. Mud-caked coats also reduce the insulating properties of the hair.
- Provide additional feed. Feed more hay (wheat/ paddy straw) and grain which help in heat production and sufficient energy is provided to animals to withstand the cold stress.
- Provide water. Make sure cows have ample water available at all times. Limiting water will limit feed intake and make it more difficult for cows to meet their energy requirements. Excessively cold water seriously limit water intake.

We can't control the weather but we can do everything reasonably possible to reduce the effects of cold on cows. This will help reduce costs and improve production efficiency.

References

Aggarwal, A. and Mahendra Singh (2005). Physiological response, milk production and composition in crossbred cows with and without mister system during hot humid season. *Egyptian Journal of Dairy Sciences.*, 32 (1): 175-186.

Aggarwal. A. and Mahendra Singh (2005). Impact of micro-climatic modification on *milk production,* composition and physiological responses in Murrah buffaloes during winter. Indian *Journal of Dairy Sciences,* 58 (4) : 269-274.

Aggarwal, A. and Mahendra Singh (2006). Impact of microclimatic modification on production of dairy animals during summer. *Indian Dairyman,* 58 (3): 49-59.

Aggarwal, A. and Mahendra Singh (2007). Economics of using mist and fan system during summer and houses during winter for alleviating environmental stress in dairy animals. *Ind. J. Agric. Economics,* 62: 272-279.

Aggarwal,A., Mahendra Singh and R.C. Chopra (2008). Minerals in milk and plasma of cows during early lactation provided with mister and fan cooling during hot-dry season. *Indian J. Dairy Sci.,* 61 (1): 88-89.

Aggrwal. A. and Mahendra Singh (2008). Changes in skin and rectal temperature in lactating buffaloes provided with showers and wallowing during hot-dry season, *Tropical Animal Health and Production,* 40 (3) : 223-228.

Aggarwal, A. and Mahendra Singh (2009). Effect of in-house shelter during winter on plasma hormones in cows and buffaloes. *Indian Journal of Dairy Science,* 62 (1): 35-38.

Aggarwal, A. and Mahendra Singh (2009). Effect of in-house shelter during winter on plasma hormones in cows and buffaloes. *Indian Journal of Dairy Science,* 62 (1): 35-38.

Armstrong, D.V. (1994). Symposium - Nutrition and Heat-Stress. Heat-Stress interaction with shade and cooling. J. *Dairy Sci.* 77:2044–2050.

Berman, A. (2005). Estimates of heat stress relief needs for Holstein dairy cows. *J. Anim. Sci.* 83:1377–1384.

Berman, A., Y. Folman, M. Kaim, M. Mamen, Z. Herz, D. Wolfenson, A. Arieli, and Y. Graber. (1985). Upper critical-temperatures and forced ventilation effects for high-yielding dairy-cows in a subtropical climate. *J. Dairy Sci.* 68:1488–1495.

Borderas, T.F., B. Pawluczuk, A.M. de Passille, and J. Rushen, (2004). Claw hardness of dairy cows: Relationship to water content and claw lesions. *J. Dairy Sci.* 87: 2085-2093.

Brumby P E, Storry J E, Bines J K and Fulford R L (1978). Utilization of energy for maintenance and production in dairy cows given protected tallow during early lactation. *Journal of Agriculture Science.* 91: 151-159.

Collier R J, Dahl G E and VanBaale M J (2006). Major advances associated with environmental effects on dairy cattle. *Journal of Dairy Science.* 89: 1244-1253.

Curtis, S.E. (1983). Environmental Management in Animal Agriculture. Iowa State University Press, Ames.

Dijkman, J. T., and P. R. Lawrence, (1997). The energy expenditure of cattle and buffaloes walking and working in different soil conditions. *J. Agric. Sci.* 128:95–103.

Fox, D. G., and T. P. Tylutki, (1998). Accounting for the effects of environment on the nutrient requirements of dairy cattle. *J. Dairy Sci.* 81:3085–3095.

Garg M R, Sherasia P L, Bhandari B M, Gulati S K and Scott T W (2002). Effect of feeding rumen protected nutrients on milk production in crossbred cows. *Indian Journal of Animal Nutrition*. 19: 191-198.

Garg M R, Sherasia P L, Bhandari B M, Gulati S K and Scott T W (2003). Effect of feeding rumen protected protein on milk production in lactating buffaloes. *Animal Nutrition and Feed Technology* 3: 151-157.

Henry, J.P. Biological basis of the stress response. (1993). NIPS 8: 69-73.

Heuwieser, W., B. A. Tenhagen, M. Tischer, J. Luhr, and H. Blum, (2000). Effect of three programmes for the treatment of endometritis on the reproductive performance of a dairy herd. *Vet. Rec.* 146:338–341.

Jenkins T C and Palmquist D L (1984). Effect of fatty acids or calcium soaps on total nutrient digestibility of dairy rations. *Journal of Dairy Science*. 67: 978-986.

Kadzere C T, Murphy M R, Silanikove N and Maltz E (2002). Heat stress in lactating dairy cows: a review. *Livestock Production Science* 77: 59-91.

Kossaibati, M. A., and R. J. Esslemont, (1997). The costs of production diseases in dairy herds in England. *Vet.J.* 154: 41–51.

Lewis, G. S. (1997). Uterine health and disorders. *J. Dairy Sci.* 80: 984–994.

McEwen, B.S. The brain as a target of endocrine hormones. In Neuroendocrinology. Krieger and Hughs, Eds.: 33-42. Sinauer Association, Inc., Massachusetts, 1980.

MacRae J C and Lobley G E (1982). Some factors which influence thermal energy losses during the metabolism of ruminants. *Livestock Production Science* 9: 447-456.

Ludri, R.S. and Mahendra Singh (1987). Feed and water intakes and milk production by crossbred cows during summer. *Indian Journal of Animal Sciences*. 57: 1310-1313.

Ludri, R.S. and Mahendra Singh (1989). Efficiency of milk production in crossbred cows during summer and winter seasons. *International Journal of Animal Sciences*. 4: 52-55.

Singh, Mahendra, A.K. Tyagi, R.K. Mehla and Charan Singh (2003). Milk production performance of cows under two sets of management during summer. *Indian Journal of Animal Sciences*, 73 (6) :117.

Singh,Mahendra, D.K. Sharma, S. Dutta and A. Ghosh, (2008). Effect of modified management on milk production, composition and physiological responses in crossbred cows in Eastern region, *Indian J. Dairy Science*, 61(4): 295-297.

Singh, Mahendra and Dang, A.K. (2006). Milko Feed to augment lactation in dairy cows. *Livestock International*, 7: 11-14.

Singh, Mahendra, R.A. Dey and D.K. Sharma, (2007). Sustainability of Buffalo Dairy Production System in Peri-Urban Areas of North-East Region: Constraints and Scope of Development, *Indian Dairyman* 60:40-44.

National Research Council, (1981). Dairy Cattle. Effect of Environment on Nutrient requirements of Domestic Animals. National Academy Press,Washington, DC, Pages 75–84.

Schreiner, D. A., and P. L. Ruegg, (2003). Relationship between udder and leg hygiene scores and subclinical mastitis. *J. Dairy Sci.* 86:3460–3465.

Shultz, T.A., and S.R. Morrison, (1987). Manger misting improves dairy cows appetite. *Calif. Agric.* 41:12–13.

Tucker, C. B., A. R. Rogers, G. A. Verkerk, P. E. Kendall, J. R. Webster, and L. R. Matthews. (2007). Effects of shelter and body condition on the behaviour and physiology of dairy cattle in winter. *Appl.Anim.Behav.Sci.* 105: 1-13.

Twisk, J. and W. de Vente, (2002). Attrition in longitudinal studies: How to deal with missing data. *Clin. Epidemiology*, 55:329-337.

Twisk, J. W. R. (2003). Applied Longitudinal Data Analysis for Epidemiology: A Practical Guide. Cambridge University Press, Cambridge, UK.

Urdaz, J. H., M. W. Overton, D. A. Moore, and J. E. P. Santos, (2006). Technical note: Effects of adding shade and fans to a feed bunk sprinkler system for preparturient cows on health and performance. *J. Dairy Sci.* 89:2000–2006.

□□□

20

Implications of Nutritional Regimen on Urolithiasis Pathophysiology in Ruminants and its Dietary Management

R.K. SHARMA, ANKUR RASTOGI, A.K. PATHAK AND PRATIKSHA RAGHUWANSHI*
Division of Animal Nutrition, FVSc & AH, SKUAST-J, R S Pura, Jammu-181 102
* Division of Veterinary Biochemistry, FVSc & AH, SKUAST-J, R S Pura, Jammu

Introduction

Ruminant urolithiasis is considered primarily a nutritional disease. Uroliths are routinely formed and excreted in many animals without causing any obvious discomfort or disorder. However, obstructive urolithiasis is considered to be the most economically significant urinary tract disease of farm ruminants. It is a common and frustrating problem for owners and Veterinarians in terms of limited treatment options and frequent recurrence, especially in small ruminants. It has been attributed to be the fifth most prevalent cause of death in feedlots (Singh *et al.*, 1981).

Formation of calculi (stones or crystals) within the urinary tract of ruminants is primarily a metabolic process and is attributed to multitude of interrelated features stemming from nutritional regimen of the affected herd.

Types of uroliths and their pathophysiology

Urinary calculi, or uroliths, are solid crystalline formations in the urine which are composed of organic matrix and organic and inorganic crystalloids

(Osborne *et al.*, 1985). The composition of urinary stones varies with geographic location and dietary regimen, but the most common uroliths are magnesium ammonium phosphate (struvite), calcium phosphate (apatite) and calcium carbonate (VanMetre and Divers, 2002). Silicate stones are also seen occasionally.

Urinary calculi formation is not consistent or predictable and usually results from a combination of physiologic, nutritional and management factors (Udall and Chow, 1965). It is mainly attributed to excessive or imbalanced intake of minerals (McIntosh, 1978; Larson, 1996; Radostits *et al.*, 2000) but numerous additional factors like heavy concentrate-low roughage diets, limited water intake, deprivation of water or dehydration, urine alkalinity, mineralized artesian water, alkaline water supplies, excess of sodium bicarbonate in the diet, vitamin imbalances e.g. hypo vitaminosis A and hyper vitaminosis D and high-protein rations have been incriminated as contributing causes for the development of calculi with resultant obstructive urolithiasis (Drolet and Dee, 1999; Radostits *et al.*, 2000).

Phosphatic Calculi

Urolithiasis is commonly seen in animals fed high grain rations, with the most common stone compositions in this setting being struvite (magnesium ammonium phosphate) and apatite (calcium hydrogen phosphate dihydrate). These hard masses are normally formed because of an environment of high-concentrate feed, low-roughage, and feed with low calcium-to-phosphorus ratio, high magnesium diets and alkaline urine. Payne (1989) reported that the feedstuffs which contain phosphorus and magnesium in excess, but relatively low levels of calcium and potassium, predisposes to occurrence of the disease.

A diet mainly made up of cereal grains, is high in phosphorus and results in urine with large amounts of phosphorus in it. High phosphorus diets overwhelm the salivary excretion mechanism and result in high urinary excretion of phosphorus (Bushman *et al.*, 1965). Moreover, as calcium opposes phosphorus absorption in the gut, phosphate absorption, and therefore the urinary phosphate load, are increased if the dietary calcium: phosphorus ratio is skewed towards phosphorus (less than 1.5:1 calcium: phosphorus) (Emerick and Embry, 1963; VanMetre and Divers, 2002; Kimberling, 1988; Floyd, 1999; Pugh, 2002; Hay, 1990).

Consumption of high dietary magnesium even with normal (2:1) calcium: phosphorus ratio has been shown to increase the incidence of struvite and apatite formation (Kallfelz *et al.*, 1987; Poole, 1989; Hay, 1990; Pugh, 2002). However, the contribution of magnesium to calculogenesis is not easily predictable (Cuddeford, 1987) and it has been suggested that it may be aided by high amount of phosphorus (Poole, 1989). Again, both these conditions are fulfilled by concentrate rations as magnesium is more available and absorbed more efficiently from concentrate rations than from roughage diets (Hay, 1990).

Feeding of pelleted ration is also a predisposing factor for development of struvite calculi. Dietary phosphorus is secreted in saliva of ruminant animals, thereby making faecal excretion as primary excretory route for phosphorus. In theory, ruminants fed pelleted rations produce smaller volumes of saliva, which reduces phosphorus excretion through faeces and increases urinary phosphorus excretion. Similar condition may occur with animals kept on low roughage regimen as it also results in less rumination and therefore less amount of salivation (VanMetre and Divers, 2002; Hay, 1990). Further, Radostits *et al.* (2000) suggested that this regimen of heavy concentrate-low roughage or pelleted rations also results in increased production of mucoprotein, which may act as a cementing agent favoring the formation of calculi.

Wang *et al.* (1997) reported prismatic crystals, with granules associated with feeding of high level of cottonseed meal diet to water buffalo calves. These crystals were rich in potassium and similar to struvite in crystal structure. These were identified as potassium magnesium phosphate ($KMgPO_4.6H_2O$).

Calcium-carbonate calculi

Calcium calculi in ruminants occur as calcium carbonate calculi and not calcium oxalate calculi. In man and dogs, inherent defects in calcium homeostasis and glycine metabolism have been reported to contribute to calcium oxalate urolithiasis. However, in ruminants, calcium oxalate uroliths are rare.

Most of the published information on calcium - based uroliths in ruminants comes from Australia, where the disease is seen most commonly in sheep grazing lush, rapidly-growing clover pastures. These forages are rich in calcium, low in phosphorus, and have high oxalate content. With adaptation to oxalate-containing diets, rumen bacteria start efficiently metabolizing oxalate to bicarbonate and this increases the availability of dietary calcium. These factors combine to increase urinary calcium excretion and alkalinize urine, thereby promoting calcium carbonate calculogenesis.

Calcium-based urolithiasis has also been reported in small ruminants fed on legume hay. Legume hays contain far more calcium than a mature male sheep or goat needs for maintenance. As a result, urine calcium excretion can increase to the point of precipitation of calcium-based crystals.

Silicate Calculi

Silicate calculogenesis occurs when animals are fed plants grown in sandy areas or water containing high levels of silica. Feeds with high calcium-to-phosphorus ratios and supplemented with sodium bicarbonate may also result in silicate Calculi. This can be the scenario with cereal hays. Deficiency of either copper or zinc along with high intake of silica may also contribute to silica urolithiasis (Stewart *et al.*, 1993).

Silica urolithiasis is primarily a problem of sheep and cattle that graze grasses high in silcates. The silica content of these grasses tends to increase as the grasses mature, and can continue to increase even after growth ends. In some areas, 4-8% of total plant dry matter may be silicon compounds. Non-polymerized silicic acid in the rumen is absorbed into the bloodstream and excreted unchanged in the urine. During the periods of water deprivation as in summer and during traditional livestock migration in hilly areas such as Jammu and Kashmir; the kidneys of range ruminants perform avid water and sodium reabsorption, creating highly concentrated urine. Concentrated silicic acid may polymerize, bind to urinary mucoproteins, and become insoluble under such conditions (Bailey, 1981).

Miscellaneous etiological factors related to nutrition

Irrespective of the type of calculi, some factors are common to uroliths formation. These are urinary pH, water quality and availability and continuity of epithelial lining of urinary ducts.

Urolithiasis is seen most often during winter in animals on full feed, or on pasture during severe weather conditions with limited water intake, especially when the water has a high mineral content. It has been suggested that the mineral composition of water, in concert with dietary mineral imbalances, probably contributes more to initiating urolith formation than does the lack of water itself (Swingle and Marsh, 1953).

Another significant factor in availability of urolith components and their binding ability is urine pH (Floyd, 1999). Alkaline pH promotes the precipitation of minerals in the urine, thereby aiding calculogenesis. Struvite, apatite and calcium carbonate uroliths are known to precipitate in alkaline urine (Jacobs *et al.*, 2001; Sheldon and Smith, 1982; Osborne and Kruger, 1984). Although, animals under both acid or alkaline urine conditions formed uroliths, but crystal growth rate is increased in alkaline conditions (Udall, 1962).

Urine of cattle or sheep is normally alkaline, and the extent that a given feed contributes to urine alkalinity cannot be surmised from the initial acidity or alkalinity of the ration ingredients. The acids associated with plants or plant fermentation products (silage etc.) are metabolized in the body and do not reach the urine. Most forage contributes toward alkaline urine, cereal grains have little influence on urine pH and feeds having a high content of natural protein (soybean meal, lucerne etc.) contribute some degree of acidity to urine pH. Animals with diets rich in cations (e.g. legumes and grass hays) or animals with urinary infections are both prone to have alkaline urine. In sheep fed high levels of dietary phosphorus, the addition of the urinary acidifier ammonium chloride was found to prevent the increased incidence of calculi formation (Bushman *et al.*, 1967). Thus it was concluded that pH was of greater importance than dietary phosphorus level in the development of urinary calculi.

Vitamin A deficiency also predisposes animals to calculi formation. This occurs as the damaged epithelium interferes with the normal secretion and elimination of urine and the sloughed keratinised cell may form foci for the formation of stones (Packett and Coburn, 1965). Vitamin A deficiency, however, is considered to be a minor factor in urolith formation in ruminants (Eveleth *et al*, 1948; Lindley *et al.*, 1953; Swingle and Marsh, 1956).

Urolith formation occurs as a two-step process beginning with the formation of an organic matrix followed by deposition of minerals on that matrix (Floyd, 1999). Deficiencies in several macromolecules (Organic acids, magnesium, inorganic pyrophosphate, urea, mucopolysaccharides, glycosaminoglycans etc.) that inhibit crystallization of matrix in urine have also been suggested as a contributory factor to calculogenesis (Griffin, 1998; Atmani and Khan, 1999).

Prevention and control

A definitive diagnosis of urolithiasis in a single animal suggests that all males in the population are at risk for the disease. The treatment of obstructive urolithiasis is primarily surgical but in large flock it may not be feasible and moreover, surgical management of urolithiasis has been plagued by a high rate of postoperative recurrence of urethral obstruction and therefore postoperative dietary changes to control the disease needs to be stressed upon.

For preventive measures the chemical composition of uroliths together with environmental and dietary factors should be considered. Due to the important role of metabolic by-products and minerals in the pathophysiology of urolithiasis, diet serves as a large contributor to urolithiasis and is therefore the primary focus of disease prevention. Risk factors addressed in preventative strategies include high dietary phosphorus and magnesium, low dietary calcium, low fiber content of rations, low urine output and an alkaline urine pH.

Maintaining Calcium: phosphorus ratio

Maintaining the calcium to phosphorus ratio (2:1) by the addition of calcium containing mineral supplements and reducing the dependence on oilseed cakes/meals and cereal grains like maize and oat (with abnormally low calcium-to-phosphorus ratio: 1:4 to 1:6) in ration can help in maintaining the calcium: phosphorus ratio in intensively fed animals. Increasing the level of calcium in the diet markedly decreased the incidence of urolithiasis, probably due to competition with phosphorus for intestinal absorption and matrix binding (Hoar *et al.*, 1970). The ratio of Ca:P should never be allowed to go below 1:1.

Intensive concentrate feeding, such as in many finishing programs, frequently leads to urolith formation and urethral obstruction. Thus, any feeding program incorporating concentrate feeding must include appropriate calcium supplementation. However, calcium over-supplementation should be avoided as increased calcium excretion in the urine may contribute to calcium-containing uroliths (Pugh, 2002).

Magnesium level

In the case of struvite stones, an increase in magnesium excretion into the urine is contributory to crystallization. It is recommended that magnesium make up less than 0.6% of the total ration of ruminants (Pugh, 2002). A level of or very near to 0.2-0.3% (DM basis) has been recommended to significantly limit phosphatic urolithiasis. For this purpose, inclusion of cereal grains and their by-products in ration needs to be restricted as they result in increased magnesium and peptides in the urine (Matthews, 1999; Kimberling, 1988). It is recommended that neither magnesium nor phosphorus should be added to concentrate diets.

Increasing salivation

Urine phosphorus excretion is greater in animals fed pelleted rations as compared to meal-type rations (Crookshank *et al.*, 1965) due to less amount of salivation. Reducing pelleted diet and increasing roughage component are important from this standpoint (Hay, 1990) as it increases rumination, thus increasing faecal output of phosphorus and decreasing urinary output of phosphorus.

Common salt supplementation

Due to an ability to alter acid-base balance and body water balance, salts have been widely used and recommended for the prevention of urolithiasis. Anionic salts containing primarily chlorides have been popular and used extensively for the prevention of urolithiasis, as they induce acidic urine and an increase in water intake and diuresis. Chloride ions compete with magnesium and phosphate for binding sites on the matrix and decrease the incidence of urolith formation (Udall and Chow, 1963). They may therefore prevent nucleation, but have also shown characteristics of inhibition of crystal growth (Chow *et al.*, 1968).

Chlorides with various cation attachments, namely NaCl, KCl, $CaCl_2$ and NH_4Cl, have traditionally been used to prevent calculi formation (Udall and Chow, 1965; Bushman *et al.*, 1968; Gohar and Shokry, 1981; Bushman *et al.*, 1967; Stewart *et al.*, 1991; Udall, 1959; Crookshank, 1966).

Sodium chloride (NaCl) has been shown to increase urine volume at levels as low as 0.5% and 1.5% (Bushman *et al.*, 1967). With the increase in urine volume with NaCl, there was also a decrease in urine hexosamine and protein (Udall, 1959). However, NaCl has been associated with decreased average daily gain and decreased ration palatability at levels as low as 4%. Therefore, it is recommended that common salt supplementation to diets is an effective strategy that can be used when urolithiasis is a herd problem, but its introduction should be slow to allow adaptation and its level should be limited to 1-4% of diet (Pugh, 2002).

All time *ad libitum* water availability is very important, when adding salt to the diet. However, salt should not be added to the water source, since lambs and kids will find it unpalatable and drink less water.

Provision of multiple salt sources and multiple waterers, when possible, are the most common means of control for silica calculi in animals on range.

Increasing urine output

Increasing water intake and urine volume is an important preventive measure for urolithiasis. Provision of adequate palatable water at desirable temperatures according to the ambient environment is highly recommended. Adding sugar-free flavoring to the water may encourage increased intake. The water containers should be regularly and vigorously cleaned to maintain water palatability. Allowing access to pasture or browse may increase dietary water intake. Additionally, a reduction in urine output has been noted when sheep were changed from an lucerne hay diet to a concentrate pellet (Swingle and Cornelius, 1962), demonstrating a reduction in water intake for grain feeding over roughage feeding.

Provision of a balanced ration in one or two feedings per day induces significant changes in body fluid homeostasis in ruminants. Meal feeding induces a surge in the production of ruminal volatile fatty acids, which exert an osmotic "pull" on the extracellular fluid (ECF). Water from the ECF is drawn into the rumen. Antidiuretic hormone is released in response to loss of free water from the ECF. A marked, albeit transient increase in urine concentration results, which promotes calculogenesis. These marked changes in urine concentration can be limited by frequent or ad libitum feeding. (VanMetre and Divers, 2002).

Acidifying the urine

Dietary supplements that acidify the urine and/or reduce urinary tract infection may be useful in stone prevention. Ammonium chloride (NH_4Cl) has been administered to ruminants (Bushman *et al.*, 1967; Crookshank, 1970; Stewart *et al.*, 1991; Mellau *et al.*, 2002), with varied success at reducing urine pH and the rate of urolithiasis. NH_4Cl may be preferred over other salts for growing animals as the ammonium may be used for metabolic processes, leaving chloride available to exert its urinary actions (Udall and Chow, 1969). Historically, NH_4Cl has been recommended and used in rations as a source of anion at a rate of 0.5%of the ration (VanMetre and Divers, 2002; Kimberling, 1988; Floyd, 1999; Pugh, 2002; Kimberling and Arnold, 1983; Hay, 1990; Matthews, 1999) for at-risk ruminants. However, NH_4Cl at a rate of 1.0% of the ration has been shown to reduce average daily gain (Bushman *et al.*, 1967).

Acidification of the urine should be maintained for > 1 week due to the probable presence of multiple calculi in the bladder, while antibiotics may be used to control bacterial uterine infection, thus reducing urinary alkalinity. However, this salt is unpalatable and needs masking of flavour, which should not be performed by molasses as it is a rich source of potassium.

Increasing crystallization inhibitors

Urolith formation occurs as a two-step process beginning with the formation of an organic matrix followed by deposition of minerals on that matrix (Floyd, 1999). It is important to understand and prevent both the formation of matrix as well as the mineral components.

The presence of crystallization inhibitors are important to consider, as urine is normally a supersaturated solution. Crystalloids are consistently maintained in solution in urine at higher concentrations than they could be held in water. Organic acids, magnesium, inorganic pyrophosphate, urea, mucopolysaccharides, glycosaminoglycans, an RNA-like substance, and many unidentified substances are suspected to inhibit crystallization. These protective substances allow super-saturation without precipitation. The addition of calcium citrate to a calculogenic diet reduced urine volume, but also reduced urine protein excretion, mucoprotein and tyrosine (Packett and Coburn, 1965). These crystallization inhibitors have been identified as having a role in inhibition of calcium oxalate and calcium phosphate crystallization, but have not been definitively identified for struvite and silica uroliths.

Conclusion

Nutritional regimen appears to be the single most important etiological factor for urolithiasis. For feedlot animals, balancing of ration in terms of calcium: phosphorus ratio; concentrate: roughage ratio; legume: non-legume roughage ratio; magnesium, potassium and other dietary cations content needs to be carefully controlled to reduce the risk of uroliths formation. Provision of common salt supplementation, all time availability of clean drinking water and increasing feeding frequency can be practiced both for intensively fed and animals kept on grazing. Ammonium chloride supplementation can be an effective way of controlling the incidences of urolithiasis in an animal population at risk. Further, supplements should not be haphazardly added to otherwise balanced rations.

References

Atmani, F. and Khan, S.R. (1999). Role of inter-alpha-inhibitor and its related proteins in urolithiasis. Purification of an inter-alpha-inhibitor related protein from the bovine kidney. *Urol. Res.*, 27: 57-61.

Bailey, C.B. (1981). Silica metabolism and silica urolithiasis in ruminants: A review. *Can. J. Anim. Sci.*, 61: 219-235.

Bushman, D.H., Emerick, R.J. and Embry, L.B. (1965). Experimentally induced ovine phosphatic urolithiasis: relationships involving dietary calcium, phosphorus, and magnesium, *J. Nutr.*, 87: 499-504.

Bushman, D.H., Embry, L.B. and Emerick, R.J. (1967). Efficacy of various chlorides and calcium carbonate in the prevention of urinary calculi. *J. Anim. Sci.*, 26(5): 1199-1204.

Bushman, D.H., Emerick, R.J. and Embry, L.B. (1968). Effect of various chlorides and calcium carbonate on calcium, phosphorus, sodium, potassium and chloride balance and their relationship to urinary calculi in lambs. *J. Anim. Sci.*, 27(2): 490-496.

Chow, F.H.C., Hamar, D.W. and Udall, R.H. (1968). Studies on urolithiasis: XI. Interaction of urine polyelectrolytes and inorganic ions. *Invest. Urol.*, 5(6): 557-567.

Crookshank, H.R., Packett, L.V. Jr. and Kunkel, H.O. (1965). Ovine urinary calculi and pelleted rations. *J. Anim. Sci.*, 24: 638-642.

Crookshank, H.R. (1966). Effect of sodium or potassium on ovine urinary calculi. *J. Anim. Sci.*, 25(4): 1005-1009.

Crookshank, H.R. (1970). Effect of ammonium salts on the production of ovine urinary calculi. *J. Anim. Sci.*, 30(6): 1002-1004.

Cuddeford, D. (1987). Role of magnesium in the aetiology of ovine urolithiasis in fattening store lambs and intensively fattened lambs. *Vet. Rec.*, 121: 194-197.

Drolet, R. and Dee, S. (1999). Diseases of the urinary system. In: Diseases of Swine, VIII Ed. (*Eds.* Straw, B.E., Allaire, S., Mengeling, W.L. and Taylor, D.J.), Iowa State University Press, Ames, IA. pp. 959–976.

Emerick, R.J., Embry, L.B. (1963). Calcium and phosphorus levels related to the development of phosphate urinary calculi in sheep. *J. Animal. Sci.*, 22: 510.

Eveleth, D.F., Bolin, F.M., Goldsby, A.I. and Ford, K.D. (1948). Urinary calculi of lambs. *N. Dakota Agr. Expt. Sta. Bimonthly Bull.*, 10: 149-157.

Floyd, J.G. Jr. (1999). Urolithiasis in food animals. In: *Current Veterinary Therapy 4: Food Animal Practice.* (Howard, J.L., Smith, R.A., Eds.), Philadelphia: Saunders. pp. 621-624.

Gohar, H.M. and Shokry, M. (1981). Efficacy of sodium chloride in prevention of sheep urolithiasis. *Bull. Anim. Hlth Prod. Afr.*, 29: 321-324.

Griffin, D. (1998). Feedlot diseases. *Vet. Clin. North Am. Food Anim. Pract.*, 14: 199-231.

Hay, L. (1990). Prevention and treatment of urolithiasis in sheep. *Vet. Record Suppl.: In Practice*, 12: 87-91.

Hoar, D.W., Emerick, R.J. and Embry, L.B. (1970). Influence of calcium source, phosphorus level and acid-base-forming effects of the diet on feedlot performance and urinary calculi formation in lambs. *J. Anim. Sci.*, 31(1): 118-125.

Jacobs, D., Heimbach, D. and Hesse, A. (2001). Chemolysis of struvite stones by acidification of artificial urine. *Scand. J. Urol. Nephrol.*, 35: 345-349.

Kallfelz, F.A., Ahmed, A.S. and Wallace, R.J. (1987). Dietary magnesium and urolithiasis in growing calves. *Cornell Vet.*, 77: 33-45.

Kimberling, C.V. and Arnold, K.S. (1983). Diseases of the urinary system of sheep and goats. *Vet. Clin. N. Am. Large Anim. Pract.*, 5(3): 637-655.

Kimberling, C.V. (1988). Diseases of the urinary system: Calculosis. In: *Jensen and Swift's Diseases of Sheep.* III ed. Philadelphia: Lea and Febiger. pp. 205-208.

Larson, B.L. (1996). Identifying, treating, and preventing bovine urolithiasis. *Vet. Med.*, 91: 366-377.

Lindley, C.E., Fayson, E.D., Ham, W.E. and Schneider, B.H. (1953). Urinary calculi in sheep. *J. Animal Science*, 12: 704-714.

Matthews, J. (1999). Urolithiasis. In: *Diseases of the goat.* II ed. Malden, MA: Blackwell Science Ltd. pp. 234-238.

McIntosh, G.H. (1978). Urolithiasis in animals. *Aust. Vet. J.*, 54: 267-271.

Mellau, L.S.B., Jorgensen, R.J. and Kambarage, D.M. (2002). The influence of short-term anion salt exposure on urine pH and on resistance to experimentally induced hypocalcemia in cows. *J. Vet. Med.*, 49: 225-229.

Osborne, C.A. and Kruger, J.M. (1984). Initiation and growth of uroliths. *Vet. Clin. N. Am. Sm. Anim. Pract.*, 14(3): 439-454.

Osborne, C.A., Polzin, D.J. and Abdullahi, S.U. (1985). Struvite urolithiasis in animals and man: Formation, detection and dissolution. *Adv. Vet. Sci. Comp. Med.* 29:1-45.

Packett, L.V. and Coburn, S.P. (1965). Urine proteins in nutritionally induced ovine urolithiasis. *Am. J. Vet. Res.*, 26(10): 112-119.

Payne, J.M. (1989). Metabolic and Nutritional Diseases of Cattle. Blackwell, Oxford, pp. 41-44.

Poole, D.B.R. (1989). Observations on the role of magnesium and phosphorus in the aetiology of urolithiasis in male sheep. *Irish Vet. J.*, 43: 60-63.

Pugh, D.G. (2002). Lower urinary tract problems. In: *Sheep and goat medicine.* I ed. (*Ed.* Pugh, D.G.) Philadelphia: Saunders. pp. 267-276.

Radostits, O.M., Blood, D.C., Gay, C.C. and Hinchcliff, K.W. (2000). Veterinary Medicine: a textbook of the diseases of cattle, sheep, pigs, goats and horses. Baillière Tindall, London. pp. 493-498.

Sheldon, C.A. and Smith, A.D. (1982). Chemolysis of calculi. *Urol. Clin. N. Am.*, 9: 121-130.

Singh, S., Gera, K.L. and Nigam, J.M. (1981). Hematological and biochemical studying obstructive urolithiasis in bovine. *Ind. J. Vet. Surgery*, 2: 72-79.

Stewart, S.R., Emerick, R.J. and Pritchard, R.H. (1991). Effects of dietary ammonium chloride and variations in calcium to phosphorus ratio on silica urolithiasis in sheep. *J. Anim. Sci.*, 69: 2225-2229.

Stewart, S.R., Emerick, R.J. and Kayongo-Male, H. (1993). Silicon-zinc interactions and potential roles for dietary zinc and copper in minimizing silica urolithiasis in rats. *J. Anim. Sci.*, 71: 946-954.

Swingle, K.F. and Cornelius, C.E. (1962). Ruminant urolithiasis V. Excretion of certain urinary biocolloid fractions by sheep on alfalfa and grain rations. *Am. J. Vet. Res.*, 23: 9726.

Swingle, K.F. and Marsh, H. (1953). The relation of limited water consumption to the development of urinary calculi in steers. *Am. J. Vet. Res.*, 14: 16-18.

Swingle, K.F. and Marsh, H. (1956). Vitamin A deficiency and urolithiasis in range cattle. *Am. J. Vet. Res.*, 17: 415-424.

Udall, R.H. and Chow, F.H.C. (1963). Ion-competition and the formation of phosphatic uroliths. *Ann. New York Acad. Sci.*, 104: 612-620.

Udall, R.H. and Chow, F.H.C. (1965). Studies in urolithiasis. VII. The effects of sodium, potassium, or chloride ions in the control of urinary calculi. *Cornell Vet.*, 55(4): 538-544.

Udall, R.H. and Chow, F.H.C. (1969). The etiology and control of urolithiasis. *Adv. Vet. Sci. Comp. Med.*, 13: 29-57.

Udall, R.H. (1959). Studies on urolithiasis. The control by force feeding sodium chloride. *Am. J. Vet. Res.*, 20: 423.

Udall, R.H. (1962). Studies on urolithiasis V. The effects of urinary hydrogen excretion of proteins and the incidence of calculosis. *Am. J. Vet. Res.*, 23: 1241-1245.

VanMetre, D.C. and Divers, T.J. (2002). Diseases of the Renal System: Urolithiasis. In: *Large animal internal medicine.* III ed. (Ed. Smith, B.P.) St. Louis: Mosby. pp. 853-861.

Wang, X., Huang, K., Gao, J., Shen, X., Lin, C. and Zhang, G. (1997). Chemical composition and microstructure of uroliths and urinary sediment crystals associated with the feeding of high-level cottonseed meal diet to water buffalo calves. *Res. Vet. Sci.*, 62(3): 275-280.

□□□

21

Surgical and Dietary Management of Obstructive Urolithiasis in Small Ruminants

S.K. TIWARI AND DEEPAK KUMAR KASHYAP*
Professor and Head, Department of Veterinary Surgery & Radiology
College of Veterinary Science & A. H. Anjora, Durg (C.G.) – 491001 India

Introduction

Uroliths are concretions of solid mineral and organic compounds that cause diseases through direct trauma to the urinary tract and obstruction of urinary outflow. In this condition of the urinary tract in which insoluble mineral and salt concretion develop and aggregate around a nidus of proteinous material mainly within the bladder or urethra (Belknap and Pugh, 2002). It is a systemic disease and in majority of cases it occurs because of disturbances in one way or other in the uptake, metabolism or excretion of urolith constituents, promoters or inhibitors besides urinary pH. Urolithiasis is the most important disease all over the world and has multi factorial aetiology. In India, its incidence very high in state like M.P., U.P., Bihar, Panjab, Haryana, Tamilnadu, A.P., Orrissa and at Chhattisgarh also (Gera and Nigam, 1979). Renal stones are more common in ruminants and carnivores but rare in pup and horses (Kienzle, 1991). The incidence of urolithiasis is more in male than females due to larger and shorter urethra in females. The urethral process is the most common site of obstruction in sheep and goat. The second site is distal aspect of sigmoid flexure where urethral process is already amputated.

Formation of Calculi (Calculogenesis)

Urinary calculi or uroliths are formed when inorganic acid and organic urinary solutes precipitate out of solution and this precipitate accumulating around a nucleus (nidus). Several factors including like, the concentration of specific solutes in the urine, the provision of a nidus and the tendency to concretion of precipitates.

Diet: Diet influences urinary constituents and pH, which may affect stone nucleation and growth. Deficiency of vitamin A, administration of estrogens and obesity and associated dietary pattern increases urolithasis. Excessive intake of minerals through highly mineralized water or phosphates from heavy concentrate diets. Similarly, Plants having so many constituents like oxalic acid causes formation of calcium carbonate calculi.

pH: Acidic pH due to solubility of some solutes like uric acid, cystine in with pH have little effect on the solubility of silicic acid. Whereas, alkaline pH due to struvite, calcium carbonate and calcium phosphate which are responsible for calculi formation. A high pH (alkaline) facilitates the precipitation of stones in the urine. Fodder eaters animal normally have urine with a high pH. A low urine pH aids in the solubility of phosphate, carbonate and silica compounds.

Amount of solutes, Nutrients and Vitamins : The amount of solute passes to kidney for elimination is influenced by the diet and nutrients like,

Calcium: Calcium carbonate are common in pastured goats particularly on clover-rich pastures or where oxalate-containing plants occur. Oxalates bind calcium, which come in urine, the calcium then bind with carbonate. It is the most common stone found in goats and sheep.

Increasing calcium consumption increases the risk of nephrilithasis and decreasing calcium consumption lowers the risk. High silica diets having high Ca/ P ratio and alkali forming potentials, contribute to silica urolithiasis in sheep and goat.

Oxalate : Majority of urinary calculi contain oxalate and it is increased manifold in case of ruminants grazing oxalate rich pasture.

Phosphate : Phosphorus concentration is directly correlated with calculi formation. Because of sheep fed high grain diets, it is more prone to urolithiasis.

Potassium : High potassium intake results in a decreased calcium excretion so this may potentially increase the risk for stone formation.

Magnesium : It binds with intestinal and urinary oxalate, causing complex between calcium oxalate leads to calculi formation.

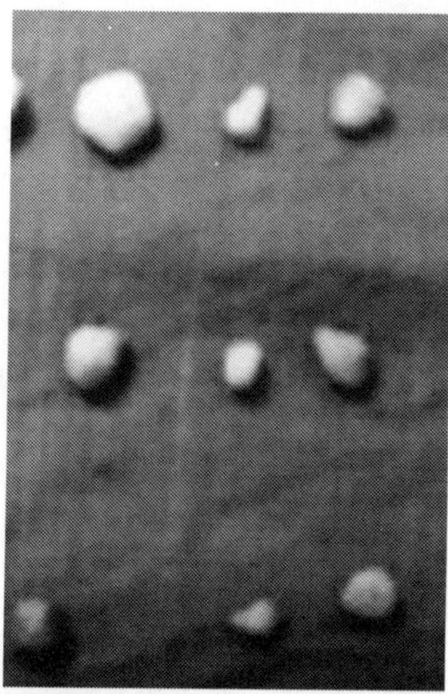

Fig. 1 : Showing the calculi recovered from small ruminants

Protein : Increase intake of protein diet causes nephrolithiasis. Excessive protein leads to increased glomerular filtration rate, calciuria and decreased urinary citrate excretion which are factor for urolithiasis.

Water : Dehdration raises urine specific gravity and uric acid saruration, and decrease urinary pH. Decrease level of water in the body predisposing factor for precipitation.

Vitamin A : Vitamin A deficiency causes desquamation of bladder lining cells. Dead cells act as a nidus on which calculi will begin to form and cause urinary obstruction.

Vitamin C : Excessive consumption of Vitamin C can cause as large amount irritate the bladder and the body compensates after several days and it no longer acidifies the urine.

Clinical Signs

Partial or complete urethral occlusion due to urinary stones lodged in the urethra, blood in the urine, straining and pain to urinate (stranguria), dribbling of urine, urine may dry on the preputial hairs and abdominal pain are common symptoms were seen initially. As the obstruction progresses, the animals shows symptoms like tenesmus, tail twitching, weight shifting, anorexia, colic pain, bloat, depression, and preputial swelling. In goats, there may be increased vocalization and tail twitching. If animal was not treated properly, urethral perforation or urinary bladder rupture occur they will eventually die when the bladder bursts and urine fills the peritoneal cavity leads to uremia.

Diagnosis

Diagnosis was done on the basis of history, Clinical signs and confirmation of the diagnosis can be achieved by deep abdominal palpation in sheep and goats. In this technique, using the fingertips of both hands placed in the flanks, the examiner gently presses each hand toward the midline. A firm, spherical mass can be palpated in the caudal abdomen in obstructed sheep and goats that have an intact bladder. If the bladder is not palpable or ruptured than go for abdominocentesis, transabdominal ultrasonographic examination for confirmation of bladder rupture of the bladder. Abdominocentesis yields voluminous, thin, red or straw colored fluid.

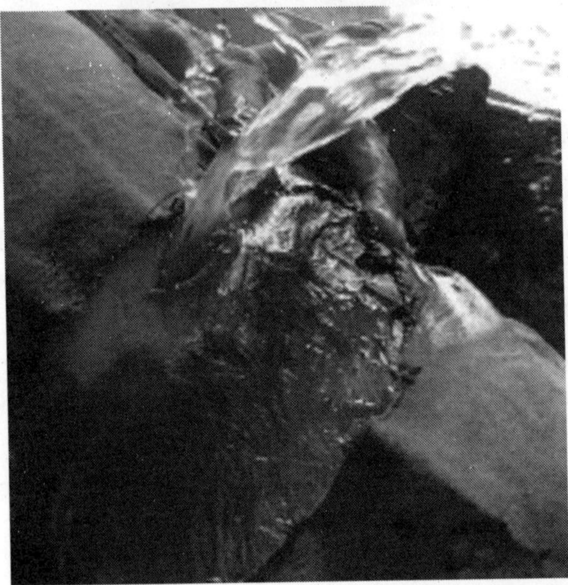

Fig. 2 : Showing the evacuation of straw coloured fluid after abdominocentesis

Surgical Management

Preoperative preparations

It is aimed at correcting the fluid and electrolyte imbalances. Because severely uremic and depressed animals require rehydration and correction of acid-base and electrolyte abnormalities. For this purpose according to degree of fluid loss, Dextrose and Normal saline combination or Normal saline or Ringer's Lactate or combination of fluids are indicated. The volume of fluid administered should be calculated to correct clinical dehydration. Once the animal is rehydrated, fluid therapy may be continued to encourage diuresis.

Animals with early clinical signs of obstructive urolithiasis, may require conservative therapy using tranquilizers and antispasmodics because these drugs helps to relax the retractor penis muscle with straightening of the sigmoid flexure. It should not be used in complicated or advanced cases.

Anaesthesia

Sedation followed by lumbosacral epidural anaesthesia (2% lignocaine HCL;3-4ml) facilitates penile extrusion in all cases of suspected urolithiasis in small ruminants.

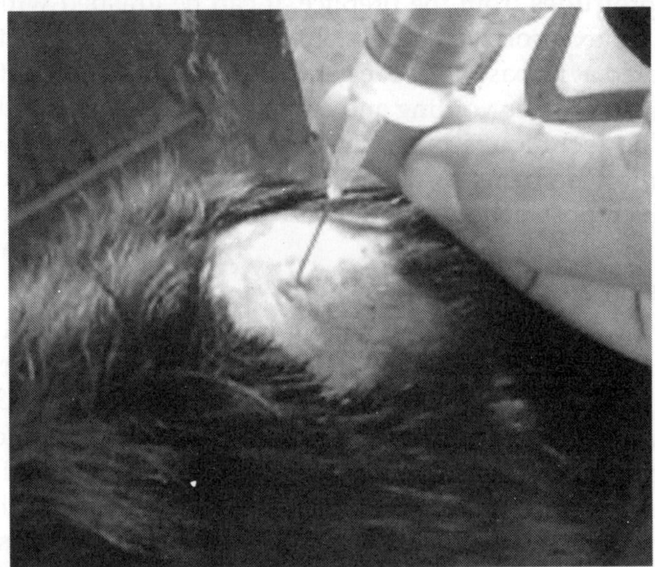

Fig. 3 : Epidural injection of Lignocaine (2%)

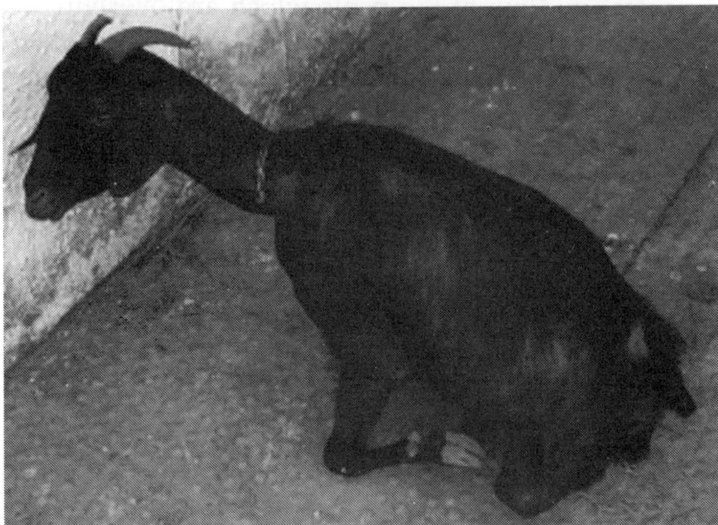

Fig. 4 : Abdomino-pelvic analgesia after Lumbosacral Epidural anaesthesia

Surgical Techniques

1. Urethral process amputation

Uroliths trapped within the urethral process of sheep and goats may be removed by gentle manipulation or by amputation of the urethral process. After proper restraint, tranquilization and/or lumbosacral epidural anaesthesia facilitate penile extrusion. Once animal was sedated, grasp the penis through the skin at the base of the scrotum and force the penis cranially. As the glans protrudes from the prepuce, it can be grasped with gauze, and the penis can be exteriorized completely. If obstructed, the urethral process can be amputated at its base, near the glans of the penis. Immediate restoration of urethral patency, urine voiding and emptying of the distended bladder has been done. The techniques may vary, but the typical procedure requires exteriorization of the penis. Although amputation may be effective in most animals in which obstruction recurs due to the presence of multiple uroliths.

2. Perineal urethrostomy / Penectomy

Perineal urethrostomy and penectomy is mainly used in cases of obstructive urolithiasis in small ruminants. This can be also performed with sedation and local anaesthesia, epidural anaesthesia. Perineal Urethrostomy can be done with regional anesthesia induced by an epidural block, sedation with xylazine hydrochloride, and manual restraint. A 6 cm incision is made on midline in the perineum approximately 4 to 6 cm ventral to the anus (sub-ischial urethrostomy). The penis is elevated to the surgical incision and stay sutures are placed between the perineal fascia overlying the semimembranosus muscle and the tunica albuginea of the penis. A 2 cm incision is made on the caudal and ventral midline of the penis which are overlying the palpable urethral groove. The exposed tunica albuginea is sutured to the subcutaneous tissue adjacent to the skin no. 2-0 and the urethral mucosae is sutured to the skin edges of the surgical wound no. 3-0 or 4-0. Alternatively, the penis may be transected at the ventral aspect of the incision, the proximal stump is exited through the surgical wound, stay sutures are placed circumferentially around the penis from the tunica albuginea to the skin, and the urethral mucosa is sutured to the cut edge of the tunica albuginea. Perineal urethrostomy is indicated in all patients that have already ruptured the penile urethra (Metre and Smith, 1991, Haven *et al.*, 1993, Van, 1987).

3. Urethrotomy

Preoperatively, the calculi are located by palpation or by passage of a flexible catheter into the urethra. Local anaesthetic is injected into the skin and subcutaneous tissue over the site of obstruction. Sometimes, we can also eliminate the obstructing calculus by crushing it through urethral wall, using the clamps or other instruments. The calculus fragments are then passed or drown out of the urethral opening. Otherwise, the urethra is incised over the calculi, all calculi are removed, and the urethra is flushed in both directions to ensure patency. The urethral mucosa and subcutaneous tissue is sutured by absorbable suture catgut size 3-0 or 4-0 and 2-0 respectively. The skin is sutured by the silk no. 2 by interrupted mattress pattern.

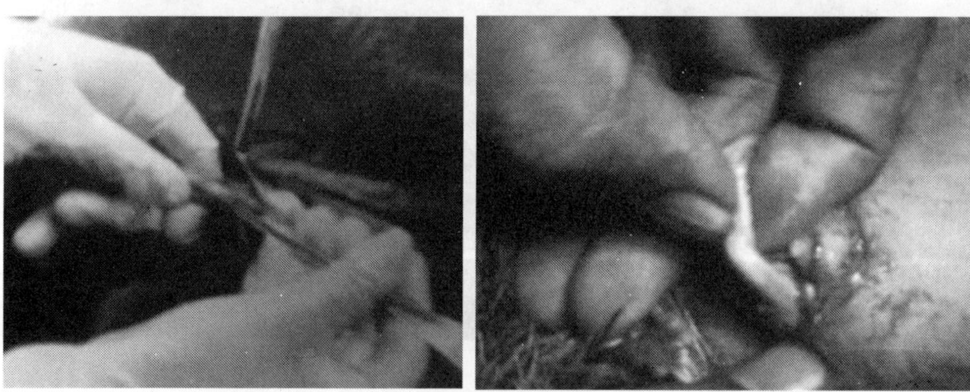

Fig. 5 **Fig. 6**

Showing the lodgement of urethral calculi in small ruminants

4. Cystotomy with urethral hydropropulsion

This can be also performed with sedation and local anaesthesia or epidural anaesthesia. The penis is exteriorized and properly secured to one side of the caudal abdomen. If present, the urethral process is amputated, and a 5-10 French polypropylene catheter is passed retrograde in to the distal urethra. A paramedian approach is performed on the opposite side of the abdomen 1-2 cm. lateral to the prepuce. It is important to place the incision caudal in the abdomen to allow for adequate exteriorization of the bladder. To ensure adequate bladder exposure, the caudal aspect of the laparotomy incision should be located at the level of the rudimentary teats. Once the external sheath of the rectus abdominis is exposed, we enter into the abdominal cavity.

Cystotomy is performed, and calculi are removed from the bladder lumen. A French or rubber catheter is guided in normograde fashion from the bladder into the proximal urethra. Sterile saline solution is flushed into the retrograde catheter to dislodge urolith from the proximal urethra back into the bladder for removal. The cystotomy incision is closed with two layers of absorbable suture in inverting patterns. The abdominal wall is closed by absorbable suture catgut size 2 and subcutaneous tissue 2-0 respectively. The skin is sutured by the silk no. 2 by interrupted mattress pattern.

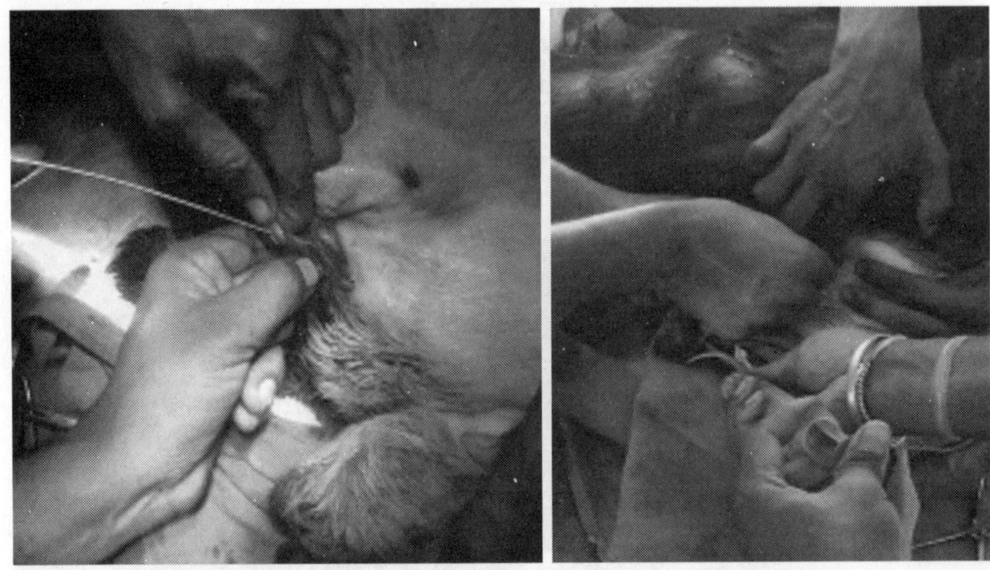

Fig. 7 Fig. 8

Showing the urethral catheterization and hydropropulsion respectively

5. Tube cystotomy

Tube Cystostomy is the treatment of choice for patients for which urethral process amputation is not useful and that have not ruptured the urethra. Although a tube cystostomy may be done with sedation (Xylazine HCl, 0.03 mg/kg, IM) and local lidocaine anaesthesia. This allows optimal aseptic technique and time to perform cystotomy, evacuation of the bladder, thorough lavage and cleaning of the bladder, and placement of the tube cystostomy. The tube cystostomy is maintained until urine is seen dripping from the prepuce for 48 hours. Then, the tube is clamped and urination is monitored. If the animal can urinate, is not painful, and is able to empty the bladder, the tube is removed. If the animal can only partially urinate and continues to retain urine, the tube is left unobstructed for 5 to 7 more days and the process is repeated. On average, remove a tube cystostomy 10 to 14 days after surgery. Prepubic Cystostomy is reserved for patients that have multiple perineal urethrostomies with stricture formation and re-obstruction (Metre and Smith, 1991).

The animal is placed into dorsal recumbency, a 4 cm incision is made on ventral midline immediately cranial to the pubis and the bladder is exited through this incision. The bladder wall is sutured to the linea alba. A 3cm.incision is made into the bladder and the bladder is explored for calculi. If present, then remove it and the bladder mucosa is sutured with absorbable suture material catgut size 3-0 or 4-0 by Lemberts pattern and subcutaneous tissue with 2-0 catgut in continuous pattern. The skin is sutured by the silk no. 2 using interrupted mattress pattern.

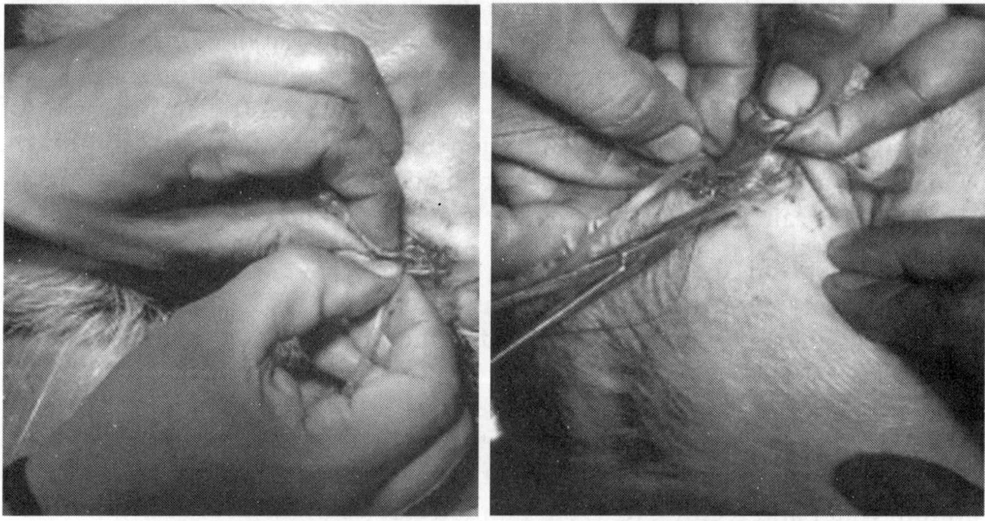

Fig. 9 **Fig. 10**

Showing the insertion of tube while performing tube cystotomy

Post Operative Management

Postoperatively, small animal should be fitted with an Elizabethan collar or muzzle to prevent them from chewing on the catheter. Check the patency of the catheter for urine outflow. The hair around abdomen must be clipped periodically to limit urine scald. Nonetheless, urine scald is a consistent complication of this surgery (May *et al.*, 1998).

Intravenous or oral fluid therapy should be continued for animals that are remain inappetant.

Antibiotic treatment (Streptopenicillin, Ampicillin or Enrofloxacin) must be maintained until at least one week after catheter removal. Sometimes, antibiotic and weak acid solutions, infused directly in to bladder via catheter have been used to control cystitis and promote calculus dissolution.

Non-steroidal anti-inflammatory drugs are administered for post operative pain.

Preventive Measures in Small Ruminants

Regardless of the calculus type involved, dilution of calculogenic ions in the urine is of primary importance in prevention of urolithiasis in small ruminants.

Providing ample of water and balanced diet

Allowing access to pasture or browse may increase dietary water intake. The salt content of the diet can be gradually increased to promote water intake and formation of large volumes of dilute urine. Dilution of calculogenic ions in the urine is of primary importance in prevention of urolithiasis in small ruminants. It is important to impress upon owners the importance of encouraging increased water consumption in ruminants at risk for urolithiasis. Adding sugar-free flavoring to the water may encourage increased intake. The water containers should be regularly and vigorously cleaned to maintain water palatability.

Tank heaters for the winter months. Be sure water is always clean, fresh easily accessible and enough for all individuals.

Feeding frequency and strategies

Provision of a balanced ration in one or two feedings/day induces significant changes in body fluids. Strategic use of concentrate feeds. Ad libitum water and feeding to avoid marked canges in the urine concentration. Provision of Nacl @ 3-5% of daily dry matter intake to stimulate more water intake. For an animal weighing 100 kg and ingesting 2% of its body weight in dry matter per day, this would translate to feeding 60–100 grams of sodium chloride daily. It is extremely important that a reliable source of water be readily accessible at all times for small ruminants on salt-supplemented diets.

As an alternative to salt supplementation, ammonium chloride can be fed at a level of 0.5–1% of dry matter in the diet. At this level, ammonium chloride may induce modest reduction in urine pH, which may render certain calculogenic minerals more soluble in ruminant urine. This salt is unpalatable. For animals fed on an individual basis, molasses should be avoided as a flavoring additive for salted rations, as its high potassium content may diminish the acidifying effect of ammonium chloride. Sugar works well for covering up the flavor of ammonium chloride. Avoidence of calculogenic feeds like Bengal gram, cotton seed meal, sorghum, clovers and other feed suppliments. Ammonium chloride or ammonium sulfate 1 gm/day. Goats eat salt at about 0.5 to 1 ounce per day. Mix 50 pounds of loose trace mineral salt with 2.5 lbs. of ammonium chloride and feed free choice.

Vitamin C is not recommended because large doses irritate the bladder and the body compensates after several days and it no longer acidifies the urine.

Avoidance of early age Castration

Early age of castration is risk factor for development of urethral obstruction whereas incidence is more in castrated one as compare to intact male.

To prevent the disease, male sheep and goats to be used for pets should not be castrated until they are 6 to 12 months old.

Reduction of calculi formation

Phosphatic calculi - Reduction of phosphorus-rich cereal grains and supplements rich in magnesium in the diet might limit formation of phosphate-based calculi. These dietary recommendations should be accompanied by management changes conducive to maximizing water intake. Maintenance of a total ration Ca: P of 2:1 and a dietary Mg level at 0.2-0.3% (DM basis) will prevent phosphatic urolethiasis (Samal *et al.,* 2011).

Bushman *et al* (1965) proved that increases in dietry phosphrus levels generated increases in phosphate ion in the urine of lambs. Soybean products treated with hydrochloric acid have been anecdotally reported to appear more palatable to small ruminants than ammonium chloride salt. The long-term effects of feeding urinary acidifying agents have not been extensively studied in small ruminants. In mature ewes, however, long-term feeding of anionic salts to induce low-grade metabolic acidosis results in a reduction in bone mineral density. Empirically, feeding mature small ruminants grass hay rather than legume hay may reduce the urinary concentration of certain calculogenic minerals.

Calcium uroliths - (Calcium oxalate and Calcium carbonate, low protein, high sodium diet. Water consumption of carbonate): Low calcium, Low oxalate and High (<12% water) to wet food (75% water). When feeding moisture of wet food is not practical, dry food is supplemented (Samal *et al.,* 2011).

Pasture management – Clean all unwanted weeds around the pasture land to prevent accumulation of calculi within the urinary tract. Spray pasture with 2,4-D to kill broadleaf weeds, which tend to be oxalate accumulators.

Allowing only females to graze the pastures as they are less susceptible to develop stones. Avoiding exposure to lush pasture as it promotes lower water consumption, could also help preventing the occurance of urolithiasis (Pattanaik, 2001).

Conclusion

Surgical management of urolithiasis in small ruminants is successful in most of the cases. However, there is high rate of postoperative recurrence of urethral obstruction. The owners of affected animal need to be well informed about this problem prior to surgery.

Dietary/Nutrition management is the best way to prevent urolithiasis. Further experimentations are required to validate the metabolic effects of dietary changes on urolithiasis in small ruminants.

References

Bushman DH, Emerick RJ, Embry LB (1965). Experimentally induced ovine phosphatic urolithiasis: relationships involving dietary calcium, phosphorus, and magnesium, *J Nutr* 87:499–504.

Gera KL, Nigam JM. (1979).Urolithiasis in bovines: A report of 193 clinical cases. *Indian Vet J* 56:417–423.

Haven ML, Bowman KF, Englebert TA (1993). Surgical management of urolithiasis in small ruminants, *Cornell Vet* 83:47–55.

Lipismita, S., Pattanaik, A. K., Mishra, C., Maharana, B. R., Sarangi, L. N. and Baithalu, R. K. (2011). Nutritional stretegies to prevent Urolithiasis in Animals. *Veterinary World*, 4(3):142-144.

May KA, Moll HD, Wallace LM, (1998) Urinary bladder marsupialization for treatment of obstructive urolithiasis in male goats. *Vet Surg*. 27:583–588.

Pattanaik, A. K. (2001). Dietry Implications in Renal Disorders of Farm and Pet Animals, Symposium on *"Nutrition and Dietetics under Clinico-therapeutic Conditions of Pet and Farm Animals"* at IVRI, Izatnagar.

Van Metre DC, House JK, Smith BP, George LW (1996). Treatment of urolithiasis in ruminants: Surgical management and prevention. *Comp Cont Ed Pract Vet* 18: S275–289.

Van Metre DC, Smith BP (1991). Clinical management of urolithiasis in small ruminants, *Proceedings of the Ninth Annual Forum, American College of Veterinary Internal Medicine*, New Orleans, pp 555–557.

Van Weeren PR, Klein WR, Voorhout G. (1987).Urolithiasis in small ruminants. I. A retrospective evaluation of urethrostomy, *Vet Q* 9:76–79.

□□□

22

Physiology of Stress and Its Implications in Poultry

O.P. MISHRA AND ANJALI SINGH
Department of Veterinary Physiology & Biochemistry
College of Veterinary Science & A.H.,Anjora ,Durg(C.G.)

Introduction

Stress has been around since Adam and Eve. Since then, stress is increasing day by day. It is because scientific inventions has increasingly confirmed the crucial role of stress that can play in causing various disorders in our body. Presently stress is a very common term in daily life. Everyone experiences stress at different times in life such as: adult, teens and even kids. But there are things we can minimize and manage the stress that is unavoidable or beyond our control. According to "Oxford Dictionary" the word stress is defined as "a state of affair involving demand on physical or mental energy". Stress is a condition, which can disturb the normal mental and physical health of the body. As per the medical parlance, the word stress can be defined as a disturbance of the body's homeostasis. Psychologists advocate that extreme stress is detrimental to human health but moderate stress proves useful. Homeostasis mechanisms maintaining the constant internal environment in the body thereby keeps the normal physiological function of the animal / birds. A deviation from normal condition is called the stress. Generally the term "Stress" is used to describe the detrimental effects of variety of factors on the health and performance of poultry. Birds have limited body resources for growth, reproduction, response to environmental changes and defense mechanism (Rosales, 1994). Under the stress conditions, there is redistribution of body resources including energy and protein at the cost of decreased growth, reproduction and health (Beck, 1991; Brake, 1987; Gross and Siegel, 1987). Under the long term stress condition or repeated stress, birds became fatigued and weak. These conditions lead to birds starvation and infectious disease (Dohms, 1990; Freeman, 1987). Domestic birds are subjected to frequent stress factors, and therefore it is important to have an effective management program to minimize their effects on the performance and health of the birds, identifying and managing factors that causes stress in birds is a critical part of a successful poultry production. Under this paper physiological mechanisms of stress, common causes of stress, types of stress, effect of stress in poultry (physiological indicator of stress) and future course of stress managemental practices in birds are discussed.

Physiological Mechanism of Stress Regulation

Exposure of birds to stress is an inevitable event in poultry husbandry, when the threshold level of stress is crossed it results in distress to birds. Then the birds show stress syndromes, which are classified into three stages.

1. Stage of alarm reaction (Neurogenic system).
2. Stage of resistance or adaptation (Endocrine system).
3. Stage of exhaustion.

Neurogenic (sympatho- adrenal) system (Short-term regulation of stress): This system consists of sympathetic (post ganglionic) nervous system and adrenal medullary tissue. It controls the rapid response to the animal i.e. fight or flight or alarm (emergency) reaction (Cannon, 1929). This reaction lasts only a short time. It is characterized by increased rates secretion of the catecholamine from the adrenal medulla. These catecholamines prepare the bird for "Fight or Flight" reaction and commanding a rapid release of glucose in blood, depletion of liver glycogen, increased peripheral vasomotor activity, altered ventilation rate and increased neural sensitivity (Selye, 1950; Siegel. 1980). Catecholamines also stimulate the activity of hepatic adenyl cyclase, the enzyme required for the production of cAMP (Robinson and Sutherland, 1971). cAMP regulates the number of energy reaction (physiological processes) and directly increases the formation of antibody (Braun *et al.* 1971).

Effect of short-term stress on the body

- Increase heart rate and blood pressure instantaneously.
- Rapid breathing and the lungs take in more oxygen.
- Blood flow may actually increase 300 to 400% that can prime the muscles, brain and lungs for additional requirements.

- Under this stressing condition spleen releases more red and white blood cells, permitting the blood to transport extra oxygen.
- Fluids are diverted from nonessential locations like mouth and throat. This causes dryness and difficulty in talking. Besides, dryness in throat can cause spasms of the throat muscles and making it difficult to swallow.

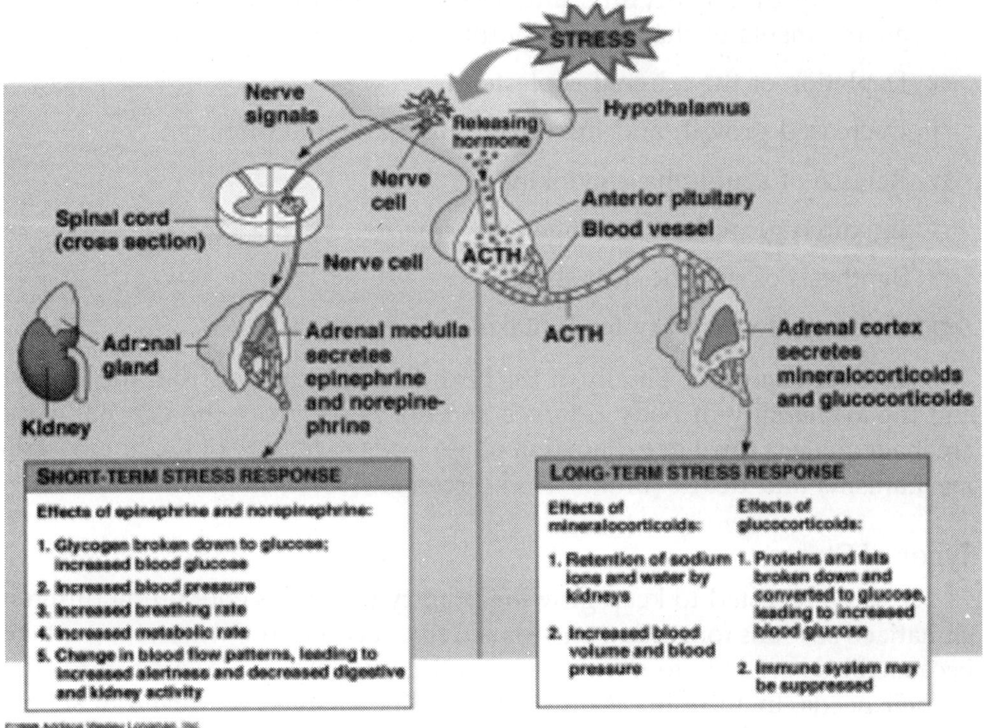

Diagramatic representation of Physiology of Stress

Endrocrine system (Long-term regulation of stress) : Involvement of endocrine system in stress regulation is called the 'stage of resistance'. This system is comprised of hypothalamus-pituitary adrenal axis (HPA). It is characterized by adrenal cortical hypertrophy and increased synthesis and release of adrenal glucocorticoids, known as corticosterone in bird (Siegel, 1971, 1980). Activation of the HPA is a longer-term adjustment by the animal to the surrounding changes. Selye (1936) called it General Adaptation Syndrome (GAS).

The endocrine mechanism of stress regulation is started with the stimulation of hypothalamus and release of ACTH from anterior pituitary, which causes the increase of adrenal cortical steroid secretions. Continuous stimulation to adrenal cortex leads to chronically high levels of corticosteroid hormone. This hormone is responsible for the formation of glucose from body's reserve of carbohydrates, lipid and proteins. Corticosteroids contribute to many of the disease associated with long-term stress, such as, cardiovascular and gastronistestinal disease, hypercholesteraemla, metabolic rearrangements and antibody suppression (Siegel, 1985).

Effect of long-term stress on the body

- Atrophy of the thymus and the bursa of fabrics in young birds, enlargements of the anterior pituitary and the adrenal glands.
- Depletion of the adrenal cholesterol.
- Decreased growth and increased muscle degradation.
- Release of acute-phase cytokines.
- Impaired growth of cartilage and bone.
- Synthesis of specific heat shock
- Decreased voluntary feed intake

Stage of exhaustion : Finally, if the bird does not recover from the stressor and the availability of body reserves and hormones from the adrenal gland are inadequate, a third or exhaustion phase leads to fatigue of the homeostatic mechanisms and death (Brake, 1985; Freeman,1987; Maxwell,1993).

Types of Stress

It was suggested to keep growing poultry in houses containing different climatized sections for resting and for activity (locomotion, water, food intake) because birds are able to choose their optimum temperature area in relation to their needs. In addition, it must be an acknowledged that even in state of the art facilities, there are common sources of stress, which can be grouped under, one or more of the following categories (Freeman, 1987).

Climatic stress (extreme heat and cold, high humidity) (Chancellor and Glick, 1960; Regnier and Kelley, 1981).

- Environmental stress (bright light, wet litter, poor ventilation) (Chancellor and Glick; 1960 Regnier and Kelley, 1981).
- Nutritional stress (shortages of nutrients, feed intake problems) (Ben-Nathan *et al.*, 1981; Gingerich, 1992; Glick *et al.*, 1981).
- Physiological stress (rapid growth, process of maturing sexually) (Freeman, 1987; Mauldin, 1992).
- Physical stress (catching, immobilization, injections, transport (Jones *et al.*, 1988; Gregory *et al.*, 1992).

- Social stress (overcrowding, poor body weight uniformity) (Gross and Siegel, 1981; Craig, 1992; Guhl, 1958).
- Psychological stress (fear, harsh care takers).
- Pathological stress- Exposure to infectious agents is a common source of stress, however challenges may not result in overt disease. When sub-clinical infections due to poor bio-security and sanitation persist, excessive activation of the immune system will result in a condition known as immunological stress. This condition results in a series of changes in nutrient metabolism induced by mediators of the immune response.

In addition to the categories of stress mentioned above, all the possible types of stressors can be broadly classified under two categories (a) avoidable stressors (b) unavoidable stressors Avoidable stressors : Overcrowding, Poor ventilation, Wet litter, Toxins in feed, High ammonia level, Starvation, Dehydration, Poor management condition

Unavoidable stressors : Extreme weather, Handling, Vaccination, Transportation, Debeaking, Lighting, Rapid growth.

Effective stress management involves complete elimination of avoidable stressors and minimizing the load of unavoidable stressors on the birds. High ambient temperature in the tropics, like that of ours in India accompanied by high relative humidity is one of the most important stressor. Birds are more susceptible to high environmental temperature than low environmental temperature due to absence of sweat glands in the feathered body, fatty nature and high body temperature (40.1°C to 41.6°C). The degree of susceptibility to tropical heat stress is higher in broilers than layers. Among broilers males are more susceptible to heat stress than females (Marin, *et al.*, 2002). Good layers housed in cages are more susceptible than poor layers reared on deep litter. High ambient temperatures coupled with high humidity can be devastating to commercial broilers. Heat stress interferes with the broilers comfort and suppresses productive efficiency. Although increased heat is seen as a major problem in poultry production, studies show that it is not only the excessively high temperatures, but also the fluctuation of the temperature.

Physiological response to heat stress

Broilers subject to high environmental temperatures exhibit many behavioral changes which allow them to re-establish heat balance with their surroundings. Broilers rest more during periods of heat stress. Some birds will stand quietly while others simply crouch near walls or waterers. Usually, their wings are spread away from the body to promote cooling by reducing body insulation. Within the bird, blood flow is diverted from certain internal body organs such as the liver, kidneys and intestines to dilated blood vessels of the peripheral tissue (skin) in order to facilitate heat loss.

Hyperventilation or "panting" increases during periods of high environmental temperature. Heat loss through evaporative cooling allows the broiler to dissipate the heat it is generating. However, panting requires increased muscle activity and these results in an increased energy requirement, which is associated with heat stress. Therefore, decreased energy efficiency also accompanies hot weather. Panting would normally expected to occur when the ambient temperature is near or above 30°C.

Relative humidity influences evaporative heat loss through panting. Broilers, as well as other domestic poultry, cannot tolerate high temperature coupled with high relative humidity. Death due to heat exhaustion will occur very quickly, especially in heavier birds, if both temperature and humidity are high. In normal birds, panting will remove approximately 540 calories per gram of water lost by the lungs.

Physiological indicator of stress in poultry Several workers have reviewed the effect of stressors in fowl (Brown 1967, Freeman, 1971, 1976). They found the following indicators of stress in birds:

Atrophy of the thymus and atrophy of the bursa of fabrics in young birds, enlargements of the anterior pituitary and the adrenal glands. Depletion of the adrenal cholesterol. A rise level of plasma corticosterone, insulin or glucagon.

- Increased reliance on glucose as an energy source.
- Hypoglycemia (increased glucose utilization).
- Decreased growth and increased muscle degradation.
- Release of acute-phase cytokines (monokynes and lymphokynes).
- Impaired growth of cartilage and bone.
- Synthesis of specific heat shock proteins.
- Decreased voluntary feed intake (anorexia).
- Increased body temperature.

Changes in the level of plasma metabolites (e.g. glucose, tryglyceride, non-estrified fatty acids and lactate). Epinephrine content in yolk of donor hens also serves as a very good tool to reflect stress load in layer stock. Changes in the numbers of circulating leucocytes profiles (heterophil: lymphocyte ratios and basophil and eosinophil numbers).

- Immunosuppression.
- Excess fat deposition in the abdomen (abdominal fat pad).
- Ascites (water belly) in high producing broilers.

Common causes of stress in birds

Some of the most common causes of stress in poultry as categorized by Rosales (1984) are summarized as follows :

- Poor brooding conditions (low temperatures, cold water)
- Contaminated premises (built-up litter, early exposure to various disease agents)
- High stocking density (limited feeder and dringker space)
- Temperature exteremes (cold and heat)
- Handling, weighing, vaccination, grading and transport (pain, physical damage)
- Beak trimming (handing pain)
- Lack of body weight uniformity (magnified differences in the packing order)
- Rapid growth (Strict nutrient demand)
- Quantitative feed and water restrictions (frustration, hunger)
- Postvaccinal reactions (reduced feed intake, fever)
- Feed quality problems (variation in nutrient content)
- Long or uneven feed distribution (split feeding)
- Sex separate feeding (pressure to restrict body weight gains)
- Harsh caretakers (poor husbandry)
- Inadequate ventilation (deterioration of the air quality)
- Clinical or subclinical diseases (reduced feed intake, fever, pain)
- Poor litter conditions (wet and cold)
- Sexual maturity and onset of egg production (drastic stimulation with feed and light).

Signs of Stress in Birds

- Depression
- Moodiness or irratibility
- Excessive activity
- Feather picking

- Increased pecking
- Increased elimination
- Inactivity or sluggishness
- Lack of desire to socialize
- Abnormal vocalization
- Ruffled feathers
- Sitting at bottom of cage,listlessness

Future Course of Stress Managemental Practices in Birds

Research work in the area of stress physiology should be directed in future in the following directions:

Need good indicator of physiological stress : The physiological indicator of stress such as atrophy of the thymus and bursa of fabrics in young birds, enlargements of the anterior pituitary and the adrenal glands are good indicator of stress but there are inherent problems with their detections. These organs cannot be weighed in live birds and require slaughter of the animal. Therefore, a suitable technique of physiological indicator of stress is currently needed.

- Suitability of the technique : Blood sampling of bird for hormone itself can be associated with techniques themselves. Suitability of technique is also an important factor. Practical problems can be associated with techniques themselves. Some technique may not be suitable for mammalian species but may be suitable for avian species.
- Mechanism of stress : To study the mechanism of stress (climatic and environmental stress) laboratories should be strengthen with some specific facilities like climatic chamber.
- Suitable managemental practices: The production efficiency of poultry is severely affected by various kind of stressors. It has significant effect on economic production of poultry. Appropriate managemental practices can be investigated to reduce the different type of stress in poultry and getting the best returns from them. The research work should begin right from construction of poultry shed, along with feeding, disease control and other managemental options.
- Identification of a physiological cue initiating the vicious cycle of events in birds that are under stress.
- Amelioration of stress in birds at physiological level - Development of a anti-stress kit for birds.

The goal of poultry scientist should be to strike a balance between the hypo-and hyper-stress and to find as much eustress as possible and to minimize distress. While devising strategies for stress control it is necessary to eliminate all avoidable forms of stressors and maintaining unavoidable stressors under control. Thus, the ultimate aim of successful poultry husbandry is not eliminate stress but to maintain it at optimum level for good production efficiency. A targeted multi-disciplinary futuristic approach is advocated so that the problem of stress is well tackled.

Conclusion

Multifarious efforts should be made to develop suitable technology to overcome the problem of follicular atresia as this is one of the main channels responsible for the drop in egg production under stressful conditions.

The goal should be to strike a balance between the hypo and hyper stress and to find as much eustress as possible and to minimize distress. While devising strategies for stress control it is necessary to eliminate all avoidable stressors and to minimize unavoidable stressors.

Ultimate aim should be not to eliminate stress but to maintain it at optimum level for good production efficiency.

Poultry birds are subjected to frequent stress factors, therefore it is important to have effective manage mental program to minimize their effects on performance and health of birds,identifying and managing factors that causes stress in birds is a critical part of successful poultry production.

References

Beck J.R. (1991). *Zootechinica International*, XIV(3): 30.

Ben-Nathan, Drabkin, B.N. and Heller, D. (1981). *Avian Dis.* 25: 214-217.

Brake J.T. (1987). Stress and Modern poultry management. Annuals production highlights. F. Hoffman-La Roche & Co. Ltd. 4002. Basie, Switzerland.

Brake, J.T. (1985). Vineland Update. November. Vineland laboratories, Vineland NJ 08360.

Braun W, Massaki I, Winchurch R and Webb D (1971). *Annals New York Academy of Science* 115:417.

Brown K.I. (1967). Environmental control in poultry production, 101-113, Edit, Carter, T.C. and Oliver & Boyd, Edinburg.

Cannon W.B. (1929). Bodily changes in Pain, Fear and rape: An account of recent research into the function of emotional excitement. IInd ed. Appleton, NY

Chancellor, L. and Glick, B. (1960). *Am.J. Physiol.* 198: 1346-1348.

Craig.J.V. (1992). *Poultry Sci.* 71: 650-657.

Dohms J.E. (1990). Stress: Mechanisms of immune supressions. pp. 22-42 in:proc. 41st North Central Avian Dis. and Poultry immunosuppressive Dis. Symp., Columbus. OH.

Freeman B.M. (1971). *World's Poult. Sci. J.*, 27: 263.

Freeman B.M. (1980). *Research in Vet. Sci.*, 28: 389.

Freeman B.M. (1987). *World's Poult. Sci. J.*, 43: 15.

Gingerich, E.N. (1992). *Avicultura Profesional* 9:144-148.

Glick, B., Day, E.J. and Thompson, D. (1981). *Poultry Sci.* 60:2494-2500.

Gregory, N.G., Wilkins, L.J. Austin , S.D. BNelyovin, C.G. Olvey, D.M. and Tucker, S.A. (1992). *Avian Path.* 21:717-722.

Gross W.B. and Siegle P.B. (1981). *Avian Dis.*, 25: 312.

Gross W.B. and Siegle P.B. (1987). *Avian Dis.*, 27: 972.

Guhl, A.M. (1958). *Animal Behavior* 6: 92-111.

Jagmohan, (2010). Stress in Poultry. Personal Communication.

Jones, R.B., Beuving, G. and Blokhuis, H.J. (1988). *Physiol. and Behavior* 42:249-253.

Marin R.H., Benavi Dex E., Gorica D.A. and Satterlee D.G. (2002). *Poult. Sci.* 81:261-64.

Mauldin, J.M. (1992). *Poultry Sci.* 71: 634-642.

Maxwell, M.H. (1993). *World's Poultry Sci. J.* 49: 34-43.

Regnier, J.A. and Delley, K.W. (1981). *Am. J.Vet. Res.* 42: 294-299.

Robinson G.A. and Sutherland E.W. (1971). New York Academy Sci., 185: 5.

Rosales A.G. (1994). *J. Appl. Poultry Res.* 3: 199.

Selye H. (1936). *Nature*, 7 : 32.

Selye H. (1950). Stress the Physiology and Pathology of exposure to stress. Montreal: Acta Inc.

Selye H. (1976). The stress of life. Me. Graw Hill Book Co., New York.

Siegel H.S. (1971). *World's Poult. Sci.*, 27: 327.

Siegel H.S. (1980). *Bio-Sci.*, 30: 529.

Siegel P.B. (1985). *World's Poult. Sci. J.*, 41: 36.

Tyagi J.S., Moudgal R.P. and Narayan R. (1996). *Ind. J. Anim. Sci.* 11: 375-79.

□□□

23

Current Status of Animal Welfare in India

M. HOQUE
Principal Scientist, Division of Surgery
Indian Veterinary Research Institute, Izatnagar-243 122

Introduction

Animal welfare has been a much concerned and critical subject in scientific, political and public domain in the recent time. However, the concept of animal welfare in our country is as old as our civilisation. It is reflected by the famous quotes of Mahatma Gandhi *"The greatness of a nation and its moral progress can be judged by the way its animals are treated"*. Man has dominion over animals and animal welfare is thus a prerogative of man. The most generally accepted single-sentence definition of animal welfare is: 'the state of an animal as it attempts to cope with its environment' (Fraser and Broom, 1990). In other way, anyone who "owns" an animal, whether on the farm, in the laboratory, in zoos or in the home, has the responsibility to ensure that the animal is fit, healthy, happy and able to achieve normal growth and function. All who are directly concerned with management of animals have a responsibility to promote their welfare through the practice of good husbandry. There is a well-defined and developed concept of the "Five Freedoms", as a comprehensive, practical protocol for assessing the welfare of animals.

The Five Freedoms and Provisions are as folllows:

1. Fredom from thiist, hunger and malnutrition- by ready access to fresh water and a diet to maintain full health and vigour.
2. Freedom from discomfort- by providing a suitable environment including shelter and a comfortable resting area.
3. Freedom from pain, injury and disease- by prevention or rapid diagnosis and treatment.
4. Freedom from fear and distress- by ensuring conditions that avoid mental suffering.
5. Freedom to express normal behaviour- by providing sufficient space, proper facilities and company of the animal's own kind.

Our obligation to animal welfare is reflected in the quotation:

"Kindness and compassion towards all living things is the mark of a civilized society"- Caser Chavez.

More detailed approaches to define the welfare of an animal are revolved around three questions as defined below both in scientific language and common parlance.

Key questions in the assessment of animal welfare

Everyman	Scientific
• Is the animal living a natural life?	• Is the animal living in an environment consistent with that in which the species has evolved and to which it has adopted?
	• Is the animal able to achieve normal growth and function, good health and to sustain fitness in adult life?
• Is the animal fit and healthy?	• Is the animal experiencing a sense of mental satisfaction or, at least, freedom from mental distress?
• Is the animal happy?	

(Webster, 2005)

Animal welfare problems and solutions : Animal welfare issues may be discussed under the following heads:

Welfare of Work Animals- Draught Animals (DAs) like bullocks, horses, camels, elephants, mules and donkeys are still used extensively in our country for ploughing, transportation, carrying loads, lifting water and other allied operations. While at work, in many cases the animals are overworked, underfed, and maltreated. They suffer from injuries and bruises due to whipping and hot iron branding. Even shoeing and castration are done in primitive ways inflicting needless suffering. The implements and carts to which they are hitched are inefficient, crude and painful (Rahaman *et al*, 2005). Public awareness, animal activists and law enforcement authority may alleviate the suffering of the draught animals. Technological improvement in the design of plough, cart and other agricultrural appliances should be done to increase work efficiency and reduce the burden on animals.

Welfare of Production Animals-Animals like cattle, buffalo, sheep, goat, pig, poultry, rabbit etc provide us milk, egg, meat, skin and hide and wool and fur. Transport and handling methods of food animals are primitive and crude. Animals for slaughter are made to walk long distances or transported in overcrowded trucks and trains without proper feed, water and rest. At the slaughter itself animals are handled roughly and animals awaiting their turn watch other animals being sacrificed.

With adoption of intensive husbandry practices, animals are forced to live in close confinement with minimal floor space, which many times does not allow them even to turn ariund, lie down with their legs fully extended or move more than a step forward or backward (Sinha, 1995). High density of animal in an unsanitary enclosure definitely leads to poor health, self-inflicted injuries, cannibalism and many other untoward consequences. Majority of the layer birds are kept crammed into bare wire cages with no room to stretch their wings. Broiler chickens live in even worse condition and are forced to wake up long hours and eat more and more to achieve fast growth rate. They suffer crippling and one out of 100 dies due to heart failure (Butcher, 2002). Birds raised in battery cages under intensive ranging system suffer environmental stressors owing to heat, cold, noises, shortages of feed, water and unhygienic atmosphere. Use of oxytocin in milch animal and anabolic steroid for fattening food animal are also animal welfare issues.

The concept of rural abattoirs should be established to regulate meat hygiene and animal welfare issues. It is important that prompt measures are initiated by Governments to ensure that animal welfare is not compromised in any way. This needs to be done by controlling and regulating the meat trade by way of strictly enforcing the existing rules and regulations during transport and slaughter of animals.

The text of the OIE Guidelines on Animal Welfare, specially with reference to Land Transport and Slaughter of Animals for Human Consumption which has been signed by all the countries of the subcontinent also needs to be strictly implemented by the Governments.

Welfare of Companion Animals-Companion animals appear to be little privileged so far as their welfare aspect is concerned barring a few instances. However, in many cases the animals are confined and isolated; old and infirmed animals are abandoned. The owners may be educated about the welfare aspect so as to avoid such situation. Prevention of killing of stray dogs through inefficient methods has been prevented by the use of alternatives to euthanasia such as animal birth control programmes.

Welfare of Wild and Captive Animals including animals used in entertainment-Wild animal population faces threat due to shrinkage of forest area day by day and their welfare is associated with conservation of forest and santuaries. Poaching and confinement of wild animals for entertainment, cock fighting, show in circuses and zoos where they often meet cruel treatment and early death. Wild animals are frequently kept by different tribal population throughout India for earning a livelihood. Though they are often treated as members of the extended family, cruel treatment during their training is not uncommon(Katti, 1995). Training of dancing bear kept by Kalandar people in Agra region for generations is a classical example. Inhuman use of wild primates and other show animals in various entertainment centers has, however, reduced to significant extent in comparison to the scenario some ten years back because of strict imposition of legal procedures pertaining to animal welfare. Zoo and other animal reservoirs in our country are yet to meet and adopt modern scientific and technical know-how related to feeding, breeding and habitat of wild and zoo animals. Zoo animals are often confined in an artificially created environment, which rarely mimic the natural habitat (Swarup and Ranjan, 2007). In India, legislation has been introduced to ban animals in circuses and it has put an end in the suffering of show animals in this segment though there are problems of their proper rehabilitation.

Welfare of Animals in Experimentation-As man became aware of his surroundings, he acquired knowledge through use of animals that can be evident way back to the great physician Galen (129-200 AD), who used animals to demonstrate that arteries contained blood and not air. Use of experimental animals like rat, mice, hamster, guinea pig, rabbit, cat, dog, monkey, farm animals and bird has been an integral part of biological research. There exists a conflicting views on use of animals in research, ranging from those concerned with animal rights to those who feel it is necessary for propagation of scientific knowledge and welfare of man and animals. All these viewpoints have contributed to the development of ethical principles of animal use in research (Kataria, *et.al.,* 2005).

Judicious use of aninals should be done in research and efforts must be taken to avoid improper experimental design and repetition of experiments. Most of the countries have introduced laws where animals used in experimentation and research have to be cared for properly and experimentation done under strict supervision to avoid unnecessary pain and suffering to these animals. Due to animal welfare movement and regulatory bodies, a number of alternative approaches have been developed, which will either replace or minimize the use of animals in research and development. Animal dissection in school and college curricula has been discontinued. The concept of the 3 R's (Replacement, Reduction and Refinement) first appeared in 1959 in a book entitles, "The Principles of Humane Experimenmtal Techniques" by Russel and Burch (1959) has proven very useful for scientists and review committees in evaluating alternatives to animal experimentation. The authors defined the 3 R's as follows: "Replacement means the substitution for conscious living higher animals of insentient material. Reduction means reduction in the numbers of animals used to obtain information of given amount and precision. Refinement means any decrease in the incidence or severity of inhumane procedures applied to those animals which still have to be used." Alternatives to animals such as computer models have been introduced to avoid unnecessary use of animals in experiments and research. CPCSEA is promoting the development and usage of animal alternatives and Biotech Consortium India Limited (BCIL) has been entrusted to compile a database on potential alternatives to animal experimentation developed world over (Singh, 2005; Singh and Prasad, 2005; Swarup and Ranjan, 2007).

Role of Veterinary profession in animal welfare - The Veterinarian's Oath has been amended recently to clearly identify animal welfare as a priority of the veterinary profession.The newly revised section of the oath reads as follows: 'Being admitted to the profession of veterinary medicine, I solemnly swear to use my scientific knowledge and skills for the benefit of society through the protection of animal health and welfare, the prevention and relief of animal suffering, the conservation of animal resources, the promotion of public health, and the advancement of medical knowledge".

The veterinary profession is committed to promote animal welfare through the art and science of keeping animals fit through attention to good husbandry, hygiene, preventive medicine and prompts treatment of injury and disease. The veterinary graduates need more education on animal welfare as defined by the physical and psychological state of the animal. In veterinary curricula an animal welfare component are being introduced to cater the need of global animal welfare perspectives.

Government Initiative for Animal Welfare

The Constitution of India Article 51-A (g) clearly mentioned: "It shall be the fundamental duty of every citizen of India to protect and improve the Natural Environment including forests, lakes, rivers and wildlife, and to have compassion for all living creatures."

In December1960, India was among the first countries in the world to pass a national act for the protection of animals- The Prevention of Cruelty to Animals Act - 1960 with the object of preventing infliction of unnecessary pain and suffering to animals. However, the violation of the law could not be curved as they lacked strong and effective penalties.

The Animal Welfare Board of India, the first of its kind Animal welfare organization to be established by any Government in the world, was set up in 1962 at Chennai, in accordance with Section 4 of the Prevention of Cruelty to Animals Acts 1960 (No.59 of 1960).The Govt. of India, Ministry of Food and Agriculture constituted the Animal Welfare Board of India on 19 March 1962. The subject of Prevention of Cruelty to Animals was transferred from Ministry of Food and Agriculture to the Ministry of Environment and Forests with effect from 28 March 1990.

Animal Welfare Department(AWD) and Animal Welfare Board of India (AWBI) were established under MoEF which are controlling authority in regard to animal welfare activities in India. The AWD deals with several scheme including provision of shelter houses, provision of ambulence services for animals in distress, animal birth control and immunization of stray dogs, scheme for relief to animals during natural calamities and unforseen circumstances, scheme for scholarship to students for study abroad in animal welfare, assistance to AWBI and CPCSEA. The AWBI assists NGOs involved in animal welfare by providing both technical and financial assistance and also acts as a watchdog for all animal abuse. It hais intensified anti-rabies vaccination and animal birth control(ABC) programme through rahabilitation and adoption of stray dogs to achieve a rabies free India.

National Institute of Animal Welfare (NIAW) has been established under MoEF, GoI at Ballabhgarh, Faridabad, Haryana with the mandate of promoting animal welfare in the country. Objective of the Institute is providing knowledge and training to personnels working with animals in the state veterinary departments, municipal corporations, forensic labs, forestry departments, laboratories, santuaries, animal houses/shelters, pharmaceuticals, diagnostic labs, nominies of AWBI, CPCSEA, SPCA, IAEC, NGOs registered with AWBI, students graduated in Veterinary and Animal Sciences, Fisheries, Wildlife sciences, Biological sciences etc.

Prevention of Cruelty to Animal Act-1960 and amended in 1982 under chapter 4 in our country has the provision for control of experimentation on animals. The act also provides the constitution of Animal Welfare Board to take care of the animals in general, and also provides that the Board constitutes a Committee for the Purpose of Control and Supervision of Experiments on Animals (CPCSEA). CPCSEA is empowered to take care of the legal and ethical aspects of experimental animals being used in research, teaching and development and enact preventive measures whenever there is violation of the law. According to CPCSEA it is now mandatory that every animal facility in the country be registered and all the institutes/universities/industries working on animal experiments have a local Institutional Animal Ethics Committee (IAEC) to monitor the use of animals in experimental work. The mandatory constitution of IAEC has positive impact on ethical use of animals in research.

The new Animal Welfare Act - 2011, proposed by India's Ministry of the Environment and Forests, is poised to replace the Prevention of Cruelty to Animals Act - 1960. It will impose stiffer penalties, and the new act will be easier to enforce, with more precise definitions of what constitutes animal abuse. This will mean less room for guesswork on the part of law enforcement. Overloading a bullock (or ox) cart will now be punishable, as will using force to get an animal to work. In a country where much work is still done by working animals, especially oxen and donkeys, stricter regulation of their working conditions has the potential for greatly alleviating the animals' suffering. The new act specifies that working animals must be provided adequate rest, food, and water. Neglecting animals or keeping them chained may lead to jail term. The new law states that a person in charge of an animal is responsible for seeing that the animal does not suffer, and notes the generally-accepted five freedoms for an animal. The new act will prohibit transport of animals in vehicles that cause injury; pick-up trucks overloaded with goats or cows can often be seen on Indian roads. It will also prohibit the hobbling of legs or tethering on a short chain, or the habitual chaining of any animal. Declawing, defanging, tail-docking and branding are also prohibited. Any form of animal fighting is prohibited. Dynamiting or electrifying streams or lakes is forbidden. Practices designed to improve milk production that are harmful to cows are punishable by a large fine or from two to four years in prison. Breeding and selling of animals will be regulated by the AWBI, which is charged with protecting all Indian animals.

Section V of the draft covers Animal Experimentation, and Section VI covers Performing Animals. Both these sections include much stricter regulations to alleviate the suffering of animals, and they define penalties for infractions.The powers of the AWBI will be expanded to include state Boards, as well as the already-existing national Board.

Governments have taken initiatives to enact laws for the prevention of cruelty to animals, but their efforts are far too limited to be of any significance. Financial constraints and lack of personnel inhibit the implementation of these rules.

In recognition of increasing concern over the issue, World Organization for Animal Health (OIE) has included a chapter in the Terrestrial Animal Health Code on minimal animal welfare standards for trade. They clearly indicated that animal welfare would play an important role in animal husbandry sector and international trade in coming years.

To address the problems of the animal welfare in developing countries like India, it would be inappropriate to adopt international standards implemented in the developed countries. Each developing country should evolve its own standards based on their own individual priorities (Rahaman, 2004).

Role of Non-Government Organisations (NGOs) for Animal Welfare

Animal Welfare Organisations play a key role in the education of the stakeholders in the proper methods of animal welfare and act as pressure groups for the implementation of international standards and guidelines of animal welfare To name a few such organizations are: People for Animals (PFA), Blue Cross, Beauty Without Cruelty (BWC), Centre for Action, Research & Technology for Man, Animal and Nature (CARTMAN), Compassion Unlimited Plus Action (CUPA), InterNICHE, KARUNA, People for the Ethical Treatment of Animals (PETA) and various SPCAs in the country.

Conclusion

Adoption of holistic approach including introduction of more stringent laws, increasing awareness of the people and widening role and responsibility of NGOs and local administration can help improve the animal welfare status. With all these efforts, though the animal suffering has reduced to some extent, still we have to travel a long and difficult journey to contain the "silent suffering'. It is concluded with " *Unseen they suffer, unheard they cry, in agony they linger, in lonliness they die. Is it nothing to you? All ye who pass by"* (Annonymous).

References

Butcher, R. (2002). Stray dog control programme: an international perspective. In Proc. International Seminar on Animal Welfare, Commonwealth Veterinary Assoc. & World Soc. For the Protection of Animal.15-16 February 2002, Bangalore.

Fraser, D, and Broom, D.B. (1990). Farm animal behaviour and welfare. CAB International, Wallingford, Oxon.

Kataria, J.M., Dhama, K. and Mahendran, M. (2005). Cellular and molecular techniques as alternatives to animal use in biological research. 29th ISVS Convention. 9-11 November 2005, IVRI, Iztnagar. Souvenir, pp. 68-74.

Katti, M. (1995). Conflicts or coexistence. *Current Sci.* 69:305-307.

Rahman, S.A. (2004). Animal Welfare: a developing country perspective.Global conference on Animal Welfare: an OIE initiative. Paris, 23-25 February 2004. Proc. Pp 101-118.

Rahman, S.A., Walker, L. and Rickets, W.(2005). *Rev. Sci. Tech. Off. Int. Epiz.* 24:597-612.

Russel, W.M.S. and Burch, R.L. (1959). The principles of humane experimental technique. Methuen & Co. Ltd. London.

Singh, G.R.(2005). Alternatives to animal experiments in teaching and research. 29th ISVS Convention. 9-11 November 2005, IVRI, Iztnagar. Souvenir, pp. 51-52.

Singh, J. and Prasad, G.(2005). Alternatives use of experimental animals in research. 29th ISVS Convention. 9-11 November 2005, IVRI, Iztnagar. Souvenir, pp. 55-67.

Sinha, A. (1995).Whose life is it anyway? A review of some ideas on the issue of animal rights. *Current Sci.* 69:296-301.

Swarup, D. and Ranjan, R. (2007). Animal welfare in India: Issues and strategies. 25th ISVM Convention, 26-28 February 2007, Pantnagar. Abst. pp.29-33.

Webster, J. (2005). Animal Welfare-Limping towards eden. Blackwell Publishing Ltd. Oxford.

□□□

24

Role of Trace Minerals in Immune Function

R. SINGH, S.R. UPADHYAY AND G. MUSTAFA
Division of Veterinary Clinical Medicine & J, Faculty of Veterinary Sciences & A.H.
SKUAST-Jammu, R. S. Pura-181102

Introduction

Much emphasis is placed on balancing the protein, carbohydrate, fiber and fat fractions of dairy diets. However, less attention is focused on the mineral specifications, especially the trace mineral fraction. Trace minerals play key roles in many enzyme systems, functioning of the immune system and consequently impact animal performance. Complex inter-relationships exist between certain micronutrients, immune function and disease resistance in cattle. Several micronutrients have been shown to influence immune responses. The relationship between deficiencies of some micronutrients and disease resistance is less clear. A number of micronutrients have been shown to affect various aspects of immunity in cattle. The interactions between nutritional status, immunology and disease resistance are extremely complex. Despite the apparent involvement of certain micronutrients in the immune system, deficiencies of micronutrients have not always increased the susceptibility of animals to natural or experimentally induced infections. Suttle & Jones (1986, 1989) cautioned against assuming that changes, especially in *in vitro* measures of immune function, are related to decreased disease resistance in the whole animal. They suggested that when micronutrient supplies are limited disease resistance may have priority for nutrients over processes less critical for survival. The purpose of the present paper is to review the effects of trace minerals on immune responses and disease resistance in cattle.

Copper

Copper is considered to have strong effects on the immune system. Copper helps energize the immune system by activating cytochrome-c-oxidase in the mitochondrial electron-transport chain (Failla, 2003). Copper is active in neutrophil production and affects phagocyte killing ability (Linder, 1991). Administration of Cu to Cu-depleted calves increased the ability of isolated peripheral blood granulocytes (primarily neutrophils) to kill ingested *Candida albicans* by over 2-fold (Jones & Suttle, 1981). Neutrophils isolated from calves fed on diets severely deficient in Cu also had impaired ability to kill ingested *C. albicans* compared with calves receiving adequate Cu (Boyne & Arthur, 1981). Neutrophils obtained from calves born to cows fed on a control diet marginally deficient in Cu or the control diet supplemented with 2.5 mg Mo/ kg diet tended to have depressed ability to kill *S. aureus* (Gengelbach *et al.* 1997). Marginal Cu deficiency in dairy heifers also reduced neutrophil killing of *S. aureus* (Torre *et al.* 1996).Compared with Cu-supplemented animals, neutrophils isolated from steers supplemented with 10 mg Mo/kg diet for 8 months had reduced ability to kill *S. aureus* (Xin *et al.* 1991). In rats Cu deficiency also impairs the ability of macrophages to kill yeast cells (Babu & Failla, 1990). The effect of Cu deficiency on macrophage function in cattle has not been studied extensively. Cu deficiency in calves did not affect the ability of macrophages to phagocytize porcine erythrocytes (Gengelbach *et al.* 1997).

Copper is required for antibody development and lymphocyte replication. A number of studies in rats and mice have indicated that both cell-mediated and humoral immunity are greatly depressed by Cu deficiency (Prohaska & Failla, 1993). However, studies in cattle have failed to show consistent effects of Cu deficiency on either cell-mediated or humoral Immune response.

Cu deficiency in calves produced by feeding a diet containing approximately 1 mg Cu/kg diet did not affect *in vitro* mitogen-induced lymphocyte blastogenesis (Stabel *et al.* 1993; Ward *et al.* 1997). In both studies calves were severely deficient in Cu, based on plasma (<0.3mg/l) and liver Cu (< 10mg/kg DM) concentrations, when blastogenic assays were performed. However, in a recent study low Cu status was associated with a reduced response of peripheral-blood lymphocytes to stimulation with T-cell mitogens (PHA and Con A) following weaning and an IBRV challenge (Wright *et al.* 2000). In this study calves were born to dams that received no supplemental Cu or 25 g CuO particles 60-90 d before calving. Calves born to dams that received Cu also received 12.5 g CuO particles 90 d before weaning.

In vivo cell-mediated immunity, assessed by measuring the response to an intradermal injection of PHA, was higher in calves supplemented with 10 mg Cu/kg compared with calves fed on a low-Cu diet (1.1 mg Cu/kg) for 126d (Ward *et al.* 1997). Neither dietary Cu or Mo affected the delayed-type hypersensitivity response to dinitrochlorobenzene in steers (Ward and Spears, 1999).

Limited research suggests that dietary Cu may affect cytokine production in cattle. Mononuclear cells from lactating dairy cows receiving a marginal level of Cu (6-7 mg/kg diet) produced less IFN-γ when stimulated with Con A than cells isolated from cows fed on adequate levels of Cu (Torre *et al.* 1995). IL-2 production by mononuclear cells was not affected by Cu in this study. Production of TNF-α and IL-l by isolated peripheral-blood monocytes following stimulation with *Escherichia coli* lipopolysaccharide was not significantly affected by dietary Cu or Mo (Gengelbach & Spears, 1998). However, TNF-α and IL-l production tended to be lower from monocytes obtained from calves fed on a low-Cu diet supplemented with 5 mg Mo/kg compared with calves receiving adequate Cu. Cu-adequate calves had higher plasma TNF- α concentrations than Cu-deficient calves (Gengelbach *et al.* 1997).

Humoral immune response, also, has not been consistently affected by dietary Cu or Cu antagonists. Antibody production following primary injection of porcine erythrocytes tended to be lower in calves fed on a Cu-deficient diet (1.1 mg Cu/kg) compared with those supplemented with 10 mg Cu/kg diet (Gengelbach & Spears, 1998). Calves fed on the Cu-deficient diet supplemented with 5 mg Mo/kg had a lower primary immune response than Cu-adequate calves. The secondary immune response to porcine erythrocytes also tended to be lower in calves fed on the Cu-deficient diet supplemented with Mo (Gengelbach & Spears, 1998). The addition of 5 mg Cu/kg to a diet marginally deficient in Cu (5 mg/kg) increased antibody responses to ovalbumin administration in growing steers (Ward & Spears, 1999). In other studies, Cu deficiency induced by high dietary Fe or Mo did not consistently affect primary or secondary antibody production in cattle injected with porcine erythrocytes (Gengelbach, 1994; Ward *et al.* 1997). Cu deficiency also did not alter antigen-specific antibody responses in calves inoculated with IBRV and *P. haemotytica* (Stabel *et al.* 1993).

Copper, in combination with zinc, plays a role in superoxide dismutase activity and the removal of oxygen free radicals. It is therefore a key component in the protective mechanism of cellular membranes against superoxide free radical damage. In addition to superoxide dismutase, the copper containing enzyme, ceruloplasmin has been shown to exhibit anti-inflammatory activity, which may prove beneficial when mastitis occurs. Naturally occurring Cu deficiency in lambs grazing improved pastures resulted in increased susceptibility to bacterial infections and greater mortality (Woolliams *et at.* 1986). Disease resistance has been studied experimentally in Cu-deficient cattle by inoculating animals with pathogenic organisms. Clinical signs of respiratory disease following inoculation with IBRV and *P. haemotytica* were similar in Cu-deficient and Cu-adequate calves (Stabel *et al.* 1993). The rectal temperature response to intranasal inoculation with bovine herpesvirus-1 was similar in heifers fed on a diet supplemented with adequate Cu and those fed on the basal diet supplemented with Mo to achieve a dietary Mo:Cu of 2.5:1 (Arthington *et al.* 1996). Workers at the University of Kentucky reported heifers supplemented with 20 ppm copper, from copper sulfate, had lower bacterial counts, SCC and peak rectal temperatures following exposure to an *E. coli* challenge than control animals supplemented with 6 to 7 ppm copper (Scaletti *et al*, 2001). Increasing copper status is therefore a key component in improving mammary health and performance.

Zinc

An array of research in human subjects and laboratory animals has indicated that Zn deficiency reduces immune responses and disease resistance (Chesters, 1997). In cattle surprisingly little research has been carried out to examine the relationship between dietary Zn and immune function. Regarding innate immunity, zinc has a critical role in maintaining the health and integrity of skin due to its role in cellular repair and replacement, all keys to the natural defense mechanisms of the mammary gland, respiratory system and GI tract (Miller *et al.*, 1988; Moynahan, 1981). In addition to improved skin health and integrity, zinc also speeds wound healing (Moynahan, 1981). Superoxide radicals (by-products of somatic cell attacks on bacteria) disrupt cellular membranes and cause cellular damage, leaving the mammary gland more susceptible to infection, scarring, and lost milk production. Cellular membranes in the mammary gland are stabilized against superoxide radicals through the action of superoxide dismutase, which requires zinc for activation (Moynahan, 1981). Zinc is also needed for maintenance of lymphocyte replication and antibody production. Therefore, insufficient zinc status leads to slowed wound healing, impaired immune function, high somatic cell counts and increased incidence of intramammary infection (IMI).

Zinc helps to regulate a wide variety of immune system activities, including T-lymphocytes, CD4, Natural Killer (NK) cells, IL-2, IL-6 and TNF α. Interestingly, IL-2, IL-6 and TNF α are pro-inflammatory mediators produced by monocytes that are directly induced by zinc (Rink and Kirchner, 2000). In addition, zinc apparently possesses antiviral activity. It is known that severe zinc deficiency impairs immune function; however, studies now show that even mild zinc deficiency may impact immune function by decreasing lymphocyte proliferation and in vitro secretion of IL-2 (Pinna *et al.*, 2002). In fact, one animal study found even moderate zinc deficiency increases free radical levels and lipid peroxidation, while decreasing activity of endogenous antioxidant enzymes (Yousef *et al.*, 2002).

Zinc is important in B-cell activity (Kidd *et al.*, 1996), while zinc deficiency has been shown to produce gross atrophy of both the thymus and the T-dependent regions of the spleen (Wirth *et al.*, 1984). Helper T-cell function is also impaired, leading to increased susceptibility to opportunistic infections (Wirth *et al.*, 1984). A genetic disorder (lethal trait A46) of Zn metabolism has been reported in Holstein and Shorthorn calves that results in severe Zn deficiency due to impaired Zn absorption. Calves with lethal trait A46 exhibit thymus atrophy and reduced lymphocyte response to mitogen stimulation (Perryman *et al.* 1989). Cornell University research indicated that cows challenged with *Strep agalactiae* recovered faster when supplemented with additional zinc from zinc methionine as indicated by lower somatic cell counts (Galton, 1989). Research conducted in Germany showed cows fed additional zinc from zinc methionine during the dry period and into early lactation had numerically lower SCC and lower lactate dehydrogenase activity (a measure for mastitis) than control cows (Andersson and Leon, 2000).

Inflammation is a key component of mastitis due to the recruitment of macrophages and neutrophils. Engle *et al.* (1997) reported greater skin swelling response in zinc-adequate calves when compared to marginally zinc-deficient calves. However, the inflammatory response may vary by species or level of dietary antagonists to zinc absorption as Droke and Spears (1993) reported zinc-deficient lambs' response to PHA (a T-cell mitogen) was similar to zinc-adequate animals. In young calves the addition of 150 or 300mg Zn/kg to a control diet containing 65 mg Zn/kg did not affect mitogen-induced blastogenesis, cytotoxicity and IL-2 production by lymphocytes, or phagocytic and bactericidal activity of isolated neutrophils (Kincaid *et al.* 1997). Calves receiving 17 mg Zn/kg diet had a reduced induration response to intradermal injection of PHA compared with Zn-supplemented animals (Engle *et al.*1997). Lambs fed on a semi-purified diet severely deficient in Zn (3.7 mg Zn/kg) showed a reduced blastogenic response to PHA (a T-cell mitogen), but an increased response to PWM (a T-dependent β-cell mitogen; Droke & Spears, 1993). Zn-deficient lambs also had a lower percentage of lymphocytes and a higher percentage of neutrophils in their peripheral blood. The *in vivo* inflammatory response to intradermal PHA administration was similar in Zn-deficient and Zn-adequate lambs. Immune responses in lambs fed on diets marginally deficient in Zn (8.7 mg/kg) did not differ from those observed in lambs fed on adequate Zn (44 mg/kg; Droke & Spears, 1993). Increasing the level of supplemental Zn from 30 to 100 mg/kg diet slightly reduced morbidity from respiratory diseases in newly weaned calves that had been transported (Galyean *et al.* 1995). The addition of Zn as Zn-methionine to a control diet containing approximately 30 mg Zn/kg reduced rectal temperature and increased feed intake in steers after inoculation with IBRV (Chirase *et al.* 1991).

Supplementing cows with zinc methionine reduces SCC by an average of 33% (98,000 cells/mL) while increasing milk production 2.8 lb/d (Kellogg *et al.*, 2004). An additional mode of action for zinc in improving mammary health is related to its role in keratin formation (Moynahan, 1981). Keratin is a wax-like substance secreted into the teat-end orifice or opening. The keratin lining of the teat canal entraps bacteria and prevents their upward movement into the mammary gland through its bactericidal properties. Approximately 40% of the keratin lining in teat canals of Holstein dairy cattle is removed during the milking process, thus requiring continuous regeneration (Bitman *et al.*, 1991).

Cobalt

Limited research indicates that Co deficiency affects neutrophil function and resistance to parasitic infection. Neutrophils isolated from calves deficient in Co had reduced ability to kill C. *albicans* (MacPherson *et al.* 1987; Paterson & MacPherson, 1990). Co-deficient calves had a decreased prepatent period and increased faecal egg output following experimental infection with *Ostertagia ostertagi* (MacPherson *et al.* 1987). Higher faecal egg counts were also observed in Co-deficient lambs after natural infection with gastrointestinal nematodes (Vellema *et al.* 1996).

Selenium

The interaction of selenium and immune function focuses around the selenoprotein, glutathione peroxidase. Glutathione peroxidase inactivates oxygen radicals such as H_20_2 and lipid hydroperoxides thus prevents them from causing cellular damage (Rotruck *et al.* 1973). Selenium appears to be very important as an antioxidant and as a factor in the energy metabolism of phagocytic cells, but the mechanism of its modulation of humoral immunity is not well understood. Research by Reffett *et al.* (1988) indicated that selenium-deficient calves had lower serum IgM concentrations (an antibody produced by B cells) and anti-IBRV titers when challenged with infectious bovine rhinotrachetis virus than selenium-adequate calves. Similarly, polymorphonuclear leukocyte function was reduced in goats (Aziz *et al.*, 1984) and cattle (Gyang *et al.*, 1994) fed selenium-deficient diets as compared to control animals receiving selenium-adequate diets. Research by Maddox *et al.* (1999) and Spears (2000) indicated that bovine mammary endothelial cells grown in selenium-deficient cell culture media exhibited enhanced neutrophil adherence when stimulated with cytokines. These findings suggest selenium may affect neutrophil migration into tissues and subsequent inflammation. Cao *et al.* (1992) reported that Se deficiency in dairy cows resulted in a reduced response of isolated peripheralblood lymphocytes to mitogen stimulation with Con A. They suggested that the impaired response of lymphocytes from Se-deficient cows may be related to altered arachidonic acid oxidation by lymphocytes via the 5-lipooxygenase pathway. Lymphocytes from Se-deficient cows produced less products of arachidonic acid oxidation, specifically 5-hydroxyeicosatetraenoic and leukotriene B4 when stimulated.

Studies have shown that supplementing dairy cattle with adequate levels of selenium will correlate with enhanced glutathione peroxidase activity and optimize host defenses against disease (Sordillo, 2005). Weiss and Hogan (2005) reported that supplementing dairy cattle with adequate levels of selenium (0.3 ppm of dry matter) reduced the prevalence, severity and duration of mastitis as well as SCC. In addition, this report suggested organic forms of selenium have little benefit over inorganic sources, but warrant further investigation.

Chromium

Considerable research has indicated that Cr can affect immune response and disease resistance in cattle. However, responses to supplemental Cr have been highly variable. A number of studies have investigated the effect of dietary Cr on the ability of isolated peripheral lymphocytes to proliferate in response to mitogen stimulation. Lymphocytes from dairy cows supplemented with 0.5 mg Cr as a Cr-amino acid chelate/kg diet from 6 weeks prepartum to 16 weeks post-partum had increased blastogenic responses to concanavalin A (Con A) stimulation (Burton *et al.* 1993).

Addition of Cr to the diet prevented the decrease in blastogenic response that was observed in control cows 2 weeks prepartum. Addition of blood serum from Cr-supplemented cows to cultures of lymphocytes isolated from control cows also increased Con A-induced lymphocyte blastogenesis (Burton *et al.* 1995). In contrast, Cr supplementation (3 mg/d; as a high-Cr yeast) did not affect Con A, phytohaemagglutinin (PHA), or pokeweed *(Phytotacca americana)* mitogen (PWM)-induced blastogenesis of lymphocytes obtained from calves following inoculation with bovine herpesvirus-I (Arthington *et al.* 1997). Other studies in cattle have reported no effect of Cr supplementation (0.4 mglkg; as either a Cr-nicotinic acid complex, high-Cr yeast or CrC13) on PHA or PWM-stimulated lymphocyte blastogenesis (Kegley & Spears, 1995; Kegley *et al.* 1996).

Effects of Cr on cell-mediated immunity have also been evaluated *in vivo* by measuring induration responses following percutaneous application of dinitrochlorobenzene or intradermal injection of PHA. In stressed calves that had been sensitized to dinitrochlorobenzene, Cr supplementation did not affect response to dinitrochlorobenzene application (Moonsie-Shageer & Mowat, 1993; Kegley *et al.* 1997). Addition of 0-4 mg Cr/kg diet (as either $CrCl_3$ or a Cr-nicotinic acid complex) increased inflammatory responses to an intradermal injection of PHA in young calves receiving milk (Kegley *et al.* 1996).

Mononuclear cells from dairy cows supplemented (0.5 mg Cr/kg) with a Cr-amino acid complex produced lower concentrations of interleukin (IL) 2, interferon-γ and tumour necrosis factor (TNF)-α following stimulation with Con A than cells from control cows (Burton *et al.* 1996). However, plasma TNF- α concentrations were not affected by Cr supplementation (high-Cr yeast) in calves before or following inoculation with bovine herpesvirus-I (Arthington *et al.* 1997). There is no evidence to suggest that Cr alters the ability of phagocytic cells to ingest or kill micro-organisms (Arthington *et al.* 1997). Neutrophils isolated from dairy cows supplemented with 0.5 mg Cr/kg diet and control cows had a similar ability to phagocytize fluorescent beads (Chang *et al.* 1996).

Effects of dietary Cr on humoral immunity have been evaluated by measuring specific antibody production following administration of either a foreign protein or a vaccine. Dairy cows supplemented with 0.5 mg Cr/kg diet had greater antibody responses to ovalbumin than control cows (Burton *et al.* 1993). In contrast, the addition of 0-4 mg Cr/kg diet did not affect antibody responses to porcine erythrocyte immunization in stressed cattle (Kegley *et al.* 1997). Supplementing Cr as an amino acid chelate for 6 d before and 28 d following vaccination increased antibody titres to infectious bovine rhinotracheitis virus (IBRV), but not to parainfluenza virus type 3 (Burton *et al.* 1994).

Summary and Conclusions

Balancing rations for today's high performance dairy cattle require that we not only deliver proper amounts of amino acids, energy, carbohydrates and fat, but that we also balance rations to deliver the proper amounts of trace minerals in forms that an animal can utilize. Trace minerals are key components in the normal functionality of the immune system and are therefore critical to maintenance of immune competence for optimal animal performance.

Abbreviations : Con A, concanavalin A; IBRV, infectious bovine rhinotracheitis virus; IL, interleukin; PHA, phytohaemagglutinin; PWM, pokeweed *(Phytolacca americana)* mitogen; TNF, tumour necrosis factor.

References

Andersson R and Leon L. (2000). German dairy study reaf firms Zinpro's benefit in lowering somatic cell counts. *Zinpro Corporation Technical Bulletin*, TB-D-4021.

Arthington JD, Corah LR and Blecha F. (1996). The effect of molybdenum-induced copper deficiency on acute-phase protein concentrations, superoxide dismutase activity, leukocyte numbers, and lymphocyte proliferation in beef heifers inoculated with bovine herpesvirus-l. *Journal of Animal Science* 74: 211-217.

Arthington JD, Corah LR, Minton JE, Elsasser TH and Blecha F. (1997). Supplemental dietary chromium does not influence ACTH, cortisol, or immune responses in young calves inoculated with bovine herpesvirus-l. *Journal of Animal Science* 75: 217-223.

Aziz E.S., Klesium PH and Frandsen J.C. (1984). Effects of selenium on polymorphonuclear leukocyte function in goats. *American Journal of Veterinary Research* 45: 1715-1718.

Babu U. and Failla M.L. (1990). Respiratory burst and Candidacidal activity of peritoneal macrophages are impaired in copperdeficient rats. *Journal of Nutrition* 120: 1692-1697.

Bitman J, Wood D L, Bright S A, Miller R H, Capuco A V, Roche A and Pankey J W. (1991). Lipid composition of teat canal keratin collected before and after milking from Holstein and Jersey cows. *J. Dairy Sci.* 74: 414.

Boyne R and Arthur JR. (1981). Effects of selenium and copper deficiency on neutrophil function in cattle. *Journal of Comparative Pathology* 91: 271-276.

Burton JL, Mallard BA and Mowat DN. (1993). Effects of supplemental chromium on immune responses of periparturient and early lactation dairy cows. *Journal of Animal Science* 71: 1532-1539.

Burton JL, Mallard BA and Mowat DN. (1994). Effects of supplemental chromium on antibody responses of newly weaned feedlot calves to immunization with infectious bovine rhinotracheitis and parainfluenza 3 virus. *Canadian Journal of Veterinary Research* 58: 148-151.

Burton JL, Nonneck BJ, Dubeski PL, Elsasser TH and Mallard BA. (1996). Effects of supplemental chromium on production of cytokines by mitogen-stimulated bovine peripheral blood mononuclear cells. *Journal of Dairy Science* 79: 2237-2246.

Burton JL, Nonnecke BJ, Elsasser TH, Mallard BA, Yang WZ and Mowat DN. (1995). Immunomodulatory activity of blood serum from chromium-supplemented periparturient dairy cows. *Veterinary Immunology and Immunopathology* 49: 29-38.

Cao Y, Maddox JF, Mastro AM, Scholz RW, Hildenbrandt G and Reddy CC. (1992). Selenium deficiency alters the lipoxygenase pathway and mitogenic response in bovine lymphocytes. *Journal of Nutrition* 122: 2121-2127.

Chang X, Mallard BA and Mowat DN. (1996). Effects of chromium on health status, blood neutrophil phagocytosis and in vitro lymphocyte blastogenesis of dairy cows. *Veterinary Immunology and Immunopathology* 52: 37-52.

Chesters JK. (1997). Zinc. In *Handbook of Nutritionally Essential Mineral Elements,* pp. 185-230 [BL O'Dell and RA Sunde, editors]. New York: Marcel Dekker Inc.

Chirase NK, Hutcheson DP and Thompson GB. (1991). Feed intake, rectal temperature, and serum mineral concentrations of feedlot cattle fed zinc oxide or zinc methionine and challenged with infectious bovine rhinotracheitis virus. *Journal of Animal Science* 69: 4137-4145.

Droke EA and Spears JW. (1993). In vitro and in vivo immunological measurements in growing lambs fed diets deficient, marginal or adequate in zinc. *Journal of Nutritional Immunology* 2: 71-90.

Engle TE, Nockels CF, Kimberling CV, Weaber DL and Johnson AB. (1997). Zinc repletion with organic or inorganic forms of zinc and protein turnover in marginally zinc-deficient calves. *Journal of Animal Science* 75: 3074-3081.

Failla ML. (2003). Trace elements and host defense: Recent advances and continuing challenges. *J. Nutr.* 133:1443S.

Galton D. (1989). Effect of Feeding ZINPRO® zinc methionine to Lactating Dairy Cows on Udder Health. Zinpro Corporation Technical Bulletin, TB-D-8911.

Galyean ML, Malcolm-Callis KJ, Gunter SA and Berrie RA. (1995). Effects of zinc source and level and added copper lysine in the receiving diet on performance by growing and finishing steers. *The Professional Animal Scientist* 11: 139-148.

Gengelbach GP and Spears JW. (1998). Effects of dietary copper and molybdenum on copper status, cytokine production, and humoral immune response of calves. *Journal of Dairy Science* 81: 3286-3292.

Gengelbach GP. (1994). Effects of copper deficiency on cellular immunity in cattle. PhD Thesis, North Carolina State University, USA.

Gengelbach GP, Ward JD, Spears JW and Brown TT. (1997). Effects of copper deficiency and copper deficiency coupled with high dietary iron or molybdenum on phagocytic cell function and response of calves to a respiratory disease challenge. *Journal of Animal Science* 75: 1112-1118.

Gyang EO, Stevens JB, Olsen WG, Tsitsamis SD and Usenik E A. (1984). Effects of selenium-vitamin E injection on bovine polymorphonucleated leukocyte phagocytosis and killing of *Staphylococcus aureus*. *Am. J. Vet. Res.* 45: 175.

Jones DG and Suttle NF. (1981). Some effects of copper deficiency on leukocyte function in sheep and cattle. *Research* in *Veterinary Science* 31: 151-156.

Kegley EB and Spears JW. (1995). Immune response, glucose metabolism, and performance of stressed feeder calves fed inorganic or organic chromium. *Journal of Animal Science* 73: 2721-2726.

Kegley EB, Spears JW and Brown TT. (1996). Immune response and disease resistance of calves fed chromium nicotinic acid complex or chromium chloride. *Journal of Dairy Science* 79: 1278-1283.

Kegley EB, Spears JW and Brown TT. (1997). Effect of shipping and chromium supplementation on performance, immune response, and disease resistance of steers. *Journal of Animal Science* 75: 1956-1964.

Kellogg D W, Tomlinson D J, Socha M T and Johnson A B. (2004). Effects of zinc methionine complex on milk production and somatic cell count of dairy cows: twelve-trial summary. *Proc. Anim. Sci.* 20: 295-301.

Kidd MT, Ferket PR and Qureshi MA. (1996). Zinc metabolism with special reference to its role in immunity. *World's Poultry Sci. J.* 52: 309.

Kincaid RL, Chew BP & Cronrath JD. (1997). Zinc oxide and aminoacids as sources of dietary zinc for calves: Effects on uptake and immunity. *Journal of Dairy Science* 80: 1381-1388.

Linder M C. (1991). Biochemistry of Copper. Earl Frieden, ed. Plenum Press, NY, NY.

MacPherson A, Gray D, Mitchell GBB and Taylor CN. (1987). Ostertagia infection and neutrophil function in cobalt-deficient and cobalt-supplemented cattle. *British Veterinary Journal* 143: 348-353.

Maddox JF, Aherne KM, Reddy CC and Sordillo LM. (1999). Increased neutrophil adherence and adhesion molecule mRNA expression in endothelial cells during selenium deficiency. *Journal of Leukocyte Biology* 65: 658-664.

Miller J K, Ramsey N and Madsen F C. (1988). The trace minerals in The Ruminant Animal. D. C. Church, ed. Pp. 342-400. Prentice Hall, Englewood Cliff s, NJ.

Moonsie-Shageer S and Mowat DN. (1993). Effect of level of supplemental chromium on performance, serum constituents, and immune status of stressed feeder calves. *Journal of Animal Science* 71: 232-238.

Moynahan E J. (1981). Acrodermatitis enteropathica and the immunological role of zinc in Safai, B. and R. A. Good, (Eds), Immunodermatology. Plenum Medical Book Co., NY, NY.

Paterson JE and MacPherson A. (1990). The influence of a low cobalt intake on the neutrophil function and severity of Ostertagia infection in cattle. *British Veterinary Journal* 146: 519-530.

Perryman LE, Leach DR, Davis WC, Mickelson WD, Heller SR, Ochs HD, Ellis JA and Brummerstedt E. (1989). Lymphocyte alterations in zinc-deficient calves with lethal trait A46. *Veterinary Immunology and Immunopathology* 21: 239-248.

Pinna K, Kelley D S, Taylor P C, and King J C. (2002). Immune functions are maintained in healthy men with low zinc intake. *J. Nutr.* 132: 2033.

Prohaska JR and Failla ML. (1993). Copper and immunity. In *Human Nutrition - A Comprehensive Treatise,* vol. 8, pp. 309-332 [DM Klurfeld, editor]. New York: Plenum Press.

Reffett JK, Spears JW and Brown TT. (1988). Effect of dietary selenium on the primary and secondary immune response in calves challenged with infectious bovine rhinotracheitis virus. *Journal of Nutrition* 118: 229-235.

Rink L and Kirchner H. (1998). Zinc-altered immune function and cytokine production. Proc. of the Intl. Workshop on Zinc and health: Current status and future directions. Bethesda, MD.

Rotruck JT, Pope AL, Ganther HE, Hafeman DG, Swanson AB and Hoekstra WG. (1973). Selenium: Biochemical role as a component of glutathione peroxidase. *Science* 179: 588-590.

Scaletti RW, Trammell D S, Smith B A and Harmon R J. (2001). Role of Dietary Copper in Altering Response to Intramammary E. Coli Challenge. Proc. of the 2nd International Symposium on Mastitis & Milk Quality, Vancouver, BC, Canada.

Sordillo L M. (2005). Bovine Mammary Immunity and Mastitis Susceptibility: Impact of Oxidant Stress in Transition Cows. Proc. CA ARPAS Conf, Coalinga, CA. October.

Spears J W. (2000). Micronutrients and immune function in cattle. *Proc. Nutr. Soc.* 59:587.

Stabel JR, Spears JW and Brown TT. (1993). Effect of copper deficiency on tissue, blood chraracteristics, and immune function of calves challenged with infectious bovine rhinotracheitis virus and *Pasterurella hemolytica*. *Journal of Animal Science* 71: 1247-1255.

Suttle NF and Jones DG. (1986). Copper and disease resistance in sheep: a rare natural confirmation of interaction between a specific nutrient and infection. *Proceedings of the Nutrition Society* 45: 317-325.

Suttle NF and Jones DG. (1989). Recent developments in trace element metabolism and function: Trace elements, disease resistance and immune responsiveness in ruminants. *Journal of Nutrition* 119: 1055-1061.

Torre PM, Harmon RJ, Hemken RW, Clark TW, Trammell DS and Smith BA. (1996). Mild dietary copper insufficiency depresses blood neutrophil function in dairy cattle. *Journal of Nutritional Immunology* 4: 3-24.

Torre PM, Harmon RJ, Sordillo LM, Boissonneault GA, Hemken RW, Trammell DS and Clark TW. (1995). Modulation of bovine mononuclear cell proliferation and cytokine production by dietary copper insufficiency. *Journal of Nutritional Immunology* 3: 3-20.

Vellema P, Rutten VPMG, Hoek A, Moll L and Wentink GH. (1996). The effect of cobalt supplementation on the immune response in vitamin B12 deficient Texel lambs. *Veterinary Immunology and Immunopathology* 55: 151-161.

Ward JD and Spears JW. (1999). The effects of low-copper diets with or without supplemental molybdenum on specific immune responses of stressed cattle. *Journal of Animal Science* 77: 230-237.

Ward JD, Gengelbach GP and Spears JW. (1997). The effects of copper deficiency with or without high dietary iron or molybdenum on immune function of cattle. *Journal of Animal Science* 75: 1400-1408.

Weiss W P and Hogan J S. (2005). Effect of selenium source on selenium status, neutrophil function, and response to intramammary endotoxin challenge of dairy cows. *J. Dairy Sci.* 88: 4366-4374.

Wirth J J, Fraker P J, and Kierszenbaum F. (1984). Changes in the levels of marker expression by mononuclear phagocytes in zinc deficient mice. *J. Nutr.* 114:1826.

Woolliams C, Suttle NF, Woolliams JA, Jones DG and Wiener G. (1986). Studies on lambs genetically selected for low and high copper status. 1. Differences in mortality. *Animal Production* 43: 293-301.

Wright CL, Spears JW, Brown TT, Lloyd KE and Tiffany ME. (2000). Effects of chromium and copper on performance and immune function of stressed steers. *Journal of Animal Science* 78, Suppl.1(1).

Xin Z, Waterman DF, Hemken RW and Harmon RJ. (1991). Effects of copper status on neutrophil function, superoxide dismutase, and copper distribution in steers. *Journal of Dairy Science* 74: 3078-3085.

Yousef M I, El Hendy H A, El-Demerdash F M and Elagamy E I. (2002). Dietary zinc deficiency induced-changes in the activity of enzymes and the levels of free radicals, lipids and protein electrophoretic behavior in growing rats. *Toxicology*, 175(1-3):223.

□□□

25

Importance of Antioxidant Vitamins on Immunity and Health of Animals

N. PANDA, R.K. SWAIN, H. KAUR AND B. PANIGRAHI
Department of Animal Nutrition, College of Veterinary Science and Animal Husbandry
Orissa University of Agriculture and Technology, Bhubaneswar- 751 003

Introduction

The relation between nutrition and health has long been recognized. Nutritional deficiencies increase morbidity and mortality which can be explained partly by impaired immune responsiveness. The period of last three weeks before and after parturition is termed as transition or per parturient period and is particularly important for health, productive and reproductive performance of dairy animals. Most of the metabolic diseases of dairy cows such as milk fever, ketosis, retained placenta, and displacement of the abomasum, occur within the first 2 weeks of lactation. In addition to metabolic diseases, the majority of infectious diseases experienced by the dairy cow, especially mastitis also develop during this phase which may be due to decreased immunity of the animals.

Host Defense System

When the animal faces an antigenic insult either in the form of bacteria, virus or parasites, the animal's defense system becomes pivotal in the elimination of these harmful organisms. A number of branches of animals host defense system work in synchrony in order to have an effective host defense response.

The defense system of the animal can be divided into 4 different protective systems 1) Specific cellular (cell mediated) immunity 2) Specific non cellular (antibody mediated) immunity 3) non specific cellular immunity (Phagocytes) 4) non specific non cellular (non immunological) (lysozymes, complement, interleukins, transferrin, lactoferrin) (Chew 1996).

The specific immunity is primarily affected by the lymphocytes and phagocytes which is collectively known as leukocytes. The cells are derived from the bone marrow stem cells. There are two main types of lymphocytes T cells and B cells. The lymphocytes are responsible for recognizing the various antigens and each lymphocyte carries a surface receptor with different lymphocytes having different receptors thereby allowing them to recognize a wide range of antigens. The T Cells dedifferentiate in the thymus and function to help B cells to make antibodies, kill virus infected cells, regulate the level of immune response and stimulate the microbicidal and cytotoxic activity of other immune effectors cells. The b cells develop in the bone marrow and differentiate into antibody producing plasma cells. They recognize antigens by their surface immunoglobulin. In order to produce an antibody response, most B cells require the presence of T cell dependant antigen together with help from antigen specific T cells.

Phagocytes (Neutrophils and Macrophages) are primarily responsible for ingesting particles/ pathogens and breaking them down in their phagolysozomes. The main function of PMN is the phagocytosis (engulfing) and subsequent destruction (killing) of foreign materials. The PMN will first migrate (chemotaxis) by chemical gradient toward and adhere tightly the foreign materials to be ingested. The coating of foreign particles (Opsonization) by the immunoglobulin molecules change the negatively charged foreign particles to a positive charge, thereby enabling the negatively charged neutrophils containing specific receptors to both antibody and C3 to bind to these particles. This oxidative bactericidal mechanism of the PMN in protecting the animal is termed as respiratory burst. When the foreign particle is attached to the surface of the PMN, it activates the NADP- oxidase system, resulting in the sequential conversion of a molecule of oxygen to superoxide anion (O_2^-), hydrogen peroxide (H_2O_2), hypochloride ions (OCL^-), hydroxyl radicals (.OH) and singlet oxygen (.O_2). All the radicals are very unstable and especially .OH and .O_2 will react with bacterial lipids to form bactericidal hydroperoxides which kill the bacteria. However, it should be noted that these free radicals when released into the extra cellular environment may be harmful to the immune cells and the surrounding tissues.

These reactive free radicals are generated from normal cellular metabolism can cause oxidation of cellular lipid, DNA and carbohydrates and consequently damage the function of normal cells. In normal conditions excessive oxidative radicals are eliminated by antioxidant systems including non enzymatic components and series of antioxidant enzymes. But during stress and antigenic insult the body's antioxidant system is not enough to neutralize the reactive oxygen species (ROS) produced in the body. Oxidative stress occurs when production of reactive oxygen metabolites (ROM) exceeds the capacity of the antioxidant system of the cell, tissue or body. Certain nutrients act as antioxidants or components of antioxidant enzymes and have a direct effect on oxidative stress. Antioxidants protect cells against the damaging effects of reactive oxygen species by "quenching" the oxygen appetite of free radicals - unstable oxygen molecules that cause damage to cells, DNA and tissues. The antioxidants are serve to stabilize these highly reactive free radicals, thereby maintain the structural integrity of the cells. Therefore antioxidants are very important to the health and production capacity of animals. The supplementation of anti-oxidant nutrients can be useful against oxidative stress and enhances plasma level of fast-acting antioxidants in periparturient dairy cows. Therefore, the concept of preventive approach to manage dairy cow nutrition and production diseases especially mastitis has great potential to assist farmers by providing increased profitability and reassurance regarding the health status of the farm livestock.

Among the antioxidants normally consumed by animals, the antioxidant Vitamins and some trace minerals are particularly importance. These are naturally occurring antioxidant vitamins include carotenoids, Vitamin A, E and vitamin C.

Vitamin A, Carotenoids and Immune Response

Vitamin A (retinol) is important in normal visual function, in differentiation of epithelial cells and immune system. The role of vitamin A in the immune system is not confined to the actions of retinol alone but also includes the actions of carotenoids which may /not be the precursors of Vitamin A.

Among the micronutrients, Vitamin A plays an important role in host defense mechanism. It is essential for the maintenance of integrity of epithelial surfaces, its deficiency cause stratification of cells, followed by sqamous metaplasia and eventually by keratinization. These changes along with desquamation of cells and reduced mucous secretion are wide spread and compromise the physical barriers of the host defense mechanism. Deficiency of Vitamin A impairs DNA synthesis and reduces the turnover of the epithelial cells. It also have an important role in ensuring the normal and optimal functioning of the mucosal surfaces and its deficiency impairs mucosal function in the respiratory, gastrointestinal and genitourinary tracts. There is also impairment of the mucosal immune cell function and alterations in antigen specificity of secretory immunoglobulins produced by the mucosae.

Vitamin A deficiency affects the production of immune cells as it impairs the development of primary lymphoid organs and their cellular proliferation. Daiy cows supplemented with b-carotene had increased lymphocyte proliferation during periparturient period (Daniel *et al,* 1991, Heiraman *et al,* 1990). Neutrophil function is markedly impaired and manifests as impaired chemotaxis and adhesion. The phagocytic activity of neutrophils is also marked depressed in states of vitamin A deficiency. Vitamin A deficiency reduces the numbers of circulating NK cells and imapirs the cytolytic activity of these NK cells and decraese the total lymphocyte and CD4+ lymphocyte counts (Watson *et al,* 1991)

In vitro studies of cell mediated immunity show that responses to mitogenic stimuli such as concavallin A and phytohaemagglutinin are significantly reduced in vitamin A deficiency. And supplementation with Vitamin A for 3 days restores this function. The effects of blood β carotene and vitamin A concentration and lactational status of the cow on the in vitro effects of β carotene on lymphocyte proliferation has been demonstrated. The stimulatory activity of carotenoids on lymphocyte blastogenesis has similarly been seen also in pigs (Hoskinson *et al,* 1989)

Retinoid have also been shown to improve the phagocytic activity of both alveolar and peritoneal macrophages. The normal expression of phagocytic cells associated with the immune response e.g., the production and normal differentiation of B cells and T cells is also responsive to vitamin A status. It appears that Vitamin A modulates the balance between Th1 and Th2 responses. Impaired responses to delayed hypersensitivity (DCH) tests have been noted in vitamin A deficient states. The number of lymphoid cells with surface markers for NK cells and IL-2 and transferrin receptors also was increased substantially in peripheral mononuclear cells in individuals supplemented with β carotene. Similarly β carotene in vitro stimulated human blod mononuclear cells to secrete a novel cytokine and induce hamster macrophages to produce tumor necrosis factor á. Retinoic acid, a metabolite of retinol has been shown to favour the differentiation of activated B lymphocytes to antibody- producing cells which then increase the synthesis and secretion of immunoglobulins, IgM and IgG.

In vitro, b-carotene enhanced the bactericidal activity of bovine blood and mammary PMN isolated from cows during the prepartum period. In the presence of 10^{-8} by 10^{-7} molar b-carotene in vitro, blood and mammary polymorphonuclear leukocytes (PMN) in cows showed enhanced ability to kill S. aureus. Dairy cows supplemented with 300 and 600 mg b-carotene/d had higher killing ability against bacteria in the peripartum period. Work at NDRI showed beneficial effects of b-carotene supplementation on mastitis control and immunity in crossbred cows. Blood PMN from cows supplemented with b-carotene during dry period maintained their phagocytic activity observed with PMN from cows fed only preformed vitamin A (Tjoelker et al, 1990) . Dahlquist and Chew (1985) fed cows with 53,000 IU of supplemental vitamin A/d, 173,000 IU/d or 53,000 IU/day plus 300 mg β-carotene/d starting three weeks before dry-off and continued through the dry period. Cows fed the vitamin A plus β-carotene treatment had fewer new infections during the early dry period (27% of previously uninfected quarters) than cows fed the other treatments (49% for low vitamin A and 50% for the high vitamin A treatments). Oldham et al. (1991) conducted a study using 50,000 IU supplemental vitamin A/d, 170,000 IU/d, and 50,000 IU/d plus 300 mg of β-carotene/d) starting two weeks before dry-off and continuing until the sixth week of lactation. Treatment did not affect new infections during the dry period and at calving or cases of clinical mastitis. Jukola et al. (1996) suggested that plasma concentrations of β-carotene in dairy cows should be >3 mg/L to optimize udder health.

Vitamin E and Selenium

Vitamin E being the major antioxidant in blood reacts with peroxy radicals produced from polyunsaturated fatty acids in membrane phospholipids or lipoproteins to yield a stable lipid hydroperoxide. Through this biochemical reaction vitamin E effectively reduces harmful lipid free radicals and thereby protects tissues from free radical attack. The antioxidant ability of the vitamin E in preventing lipid peroidation is one of the possible mechanism by which vitamin E enhances immune response. Vitamin E is important for both cellular and humoral immune functions. It is reported to enhance the intracellular kill of *E. coli* and *staphylococcus aureus* (major mastitides) by bovine blood neutrophils. Weanling pigs fed a diet deficient in vitamin E and Se had lower mitogen induced lymphocyte proliferative response when cells were incubated with autologous serum. Similarly peripheral lymphocytes obtained from sows fed a diet deficient in vitamin E or vitamin E and Se had reduced mitogen induced proliferation during the immediate prepartum and post partum periods. (Wuryastuti *et al,* 1993). It also modulates prostaglandin release from activated macrophages during infection. Feeding heifers supplemental vitamin E (1g/hd/d) and selenium injection (0.1 mg/kg body weight) 21 days post calving period reduced several measures of mastitis like 1) high somatic cell counts in cow's milk (greater than 2 lakh cells/ ml) by 65% 2) quarter days infected was reduced by 60% 3) Duration of Intra Mammary Infection (IMI) reduced by 45% 4) Clinical mastitis reduced by 35% and 5) IMI at calving also decreased by 40% (Smith *et al.,* 1984). The stimulation index for cell-mediated immunity decreased by 47% in control and 32% in vitamin E supplemented (1000 IU/d) cows during first week of parturition (Rajiv, 2001). Low plasma concentration of a-tocopherol at parturition is considered as a significant risk factor for intramammary infection (IMI) and mastitis during the first week of lactation. Plasma vitamin E concentration in dairy cows and buffaloes is negatively correlated with the rate of intramammary infection (Rajiv, 2001; Panda, 2003). During periparturient period when there is significant decrease in a-tocopherol, the cow/ buffalo's immunity status and neutrophil functions are depressed. That's why 30 to 50% of all clinical mastitis occurs during the first month of lactation. Harjit et al. (2002) suggested that vitamin E @ 1000 IU/cow/d and 1500 IU/buffalo/day should be supplemented to dry pregnant animal at least 30 days before parturition to 30 days of lactation to reduce the incidence of mastitis.

Malbe *et al.* (1995) reported that supplementation of a very low Se diet with 0.2 parts per million (ppm) of Se from selenite or selenized yeast reduced SCC in lactating dairy cows. In a study from New Zealand (Wichtel *et al.*, 1994), mean SCC over an entire lactation was reduced or tended to be reduced when cows were supplemented with 6 to 12 mg of Se/day; however, no difference in clinical mastitis was found between treatments. Erskine *et al.* (1990) found no effects of supplemental Se on mastitis when cows were experimentally challenged with *Staphylococcus aureus*. Weiss *et al.* (1997) reported that feeding 1000 IU/day of supplemental vitamin E during a 60-day dry period to cows with low Se status reduced clinical mastitis during the first week of lactation compared with feeding 100 IU/day. In that same study, feeding 4000 IU of supplemental vitamin E/day during the last 14 days of the dry period further reduced clinical mastitis and reduced new infections at calving. Clinical mastitis incidence during the first week of lactation was 25.0. 16.7, and 3.6% of quarters for cows fed 100 IU/day, 1000 IU/day, or 1000 IU/day during the first 46 days of the dry period followed by 4000 IU/day during the last 14 days of the dry period. An important feature of that study was that cows were fed a low Se diet (0.1 ppm) and had low plasma Se concentrations (0.048 mg/L).

Vitamin E and Se also may guard against peroxidation of arachidonic acid and thereby alter arachidonic metabolism in animals. The mechanism could account for the observed enhanced immune response by maintaining the functional integrity of immune cells.

Vitamin C

Vitamin C (ascorbic acid) is probably the most important water soluble antioxidant in mammals. Most forms of vitamin C are extensively degraded in the rumen, therefore the cow must rely on tissue synthesis of vitamin C. Cows can synthesize vitamin C and it is not considered an essential nutrient for cattle. Chicken also depend upon the renal synthesis of vitamin C. The concentration of ascorbic acid is high in neutrophils and increases as much as

30-fold when the neutrophil is stimulated which probably helps to protect those cells from ROM produced when the cell tries to kill pathogens. Vitamin C supplemented @ of 330 mg/kg reduced mortality and pericarditis in chicks infected with *E. coli*. The amount of vitamin C needed for protective effect increased with higher environmental stress level. Calves supplemented with vitamin C had lower incidence of scouring. Dietary vitamin C supplementation increased concentrations of blood immunoglobulins in dairy calves (Blair and Cummins, 1984). In guinea pigs vitamin C supplementation was shown to be important in maintaining normal and secondary antibody response. Chicks fed 200mg vitamin C/kg of diet during summer stress increased both humoral and cell mediated the immunity and antioxidant status of the birds. (Beura and Panda, 2009). Dietary vitamin C reduces circulating glucocorticoids in chicken (Nockels et al 1973). Santos et al. (2001) reported that plasma ascorbic acid concentrations in dairy cows were not correlated with somatic cell count (SCC). Another experiment evaluated the therapeutic use of ascorbic acid following intramammary challenge with endotoxin (Chaiyotwittayakun *et al.*, 2002) and reported limited effect of vitamin C therapy on clinical signs. Weiss *et al.* (2004) conducted an experiment to examine changes in ascorbic acid status following an intramammary challenge with *E. coli* and observed significant correlations between vitamin C status and clinical signs. Large decreases in vitamin C status were related to longer duration of clinical mastitis and larger decreases in milk production. Current data do not support the use of vitamin C to prevent or help cure mastitis.

Antioxidants and Reproduction

During the peripartum period, there is increased generation of free radicals that overwhelm antioxidant defense mechanism and compromise cellular function. The production of free radicals leads to infertility because steroidogenic enzymes, ovarian steroidogenic tissue, spermatozoa and pre implantation of embryos are sensitive to free radicals damage. Dietary and/ or injectable form of vitamin E supplementation to dairy cows decreased the incidence of retention of placenta, reduced days to first observed estrus and decreased services/conception (Kim et al, 1997). (Kimura et al. (2002) reported that neutrophils from cows with RFM had significantly less killing ability than neutrophils from cows without RFM. Neutrophils from Se-deficient cows have lower killing ability than neutrophils from Se-adequate cows (Hogan *et al.*, 1990). The effect of Se supplementation on RFM is influenced by the vitamin E status of cows. The incidence of RFM for cows that have low vitamin E status often is not influenced by Se supplementation (Harrison *et al.*, 1984). LeBlanc *et al.* (2004) found statistical association between the concentration of tocopherol in serum of periparturient cows and risk of RFM. They found that for every 1 mg/ml unit increase in serum tocopherol concentration (samples taken during the 1 wk before calving), the risk for RFM decreased by 21%. Cows that had a serum tocopherol: cholesterol ratio (ug tocopherol/ml divided by mg of cholesterol/ml) of <2, were three times as likely to have RFM than cows with a ratio >2 and cows with a ratio of <2.5 were twice as likely to have RFM as cows with a ratio >2.5., whereas no associations were found between serum retinol or serum B-carotene and RFM (LeBlanc et al., 2004). Panda et al 2006 found that supplementation of @ 1500 IU from 60 days pre partum to 30 days post partum and 1000 IU from 30 days post partum to 60 days post partum to dairy buffaloes reduced the postpartum estrus interval, days open and services per conception.

It is inferred that appropriate supplementation of antioxidant nutrients (especially vitamin E, Vitamin A and selenium should be practiced so as to increase the immunity and reduce the prevalence of some important health disorders in periparturient dairy animals.

References

Beura, T. K.. (2009). Effect of vitamin E and C on the growth and immunocompetence of broilers during summer . M.V.Sc. Thesis. O.U.A.T., Bhubaneswar.

Blair. L. & Cummins, K.A. (1984). Effect of dietary ascorbic acid on blood immunoglobulin concentration in dairy calves. *J. Dairy Sci.* 67. (suppl.):138

Chaiyotwittayakun, A., R. J. Erskine, P. C. Bartlett, T. H. Herdt, P. M. Sears, and R. J. Harmon. (2002). The effect of ascorbic acid and L-histidine therapy on acute mammary inflammation in dairy cattle. *J. Dairy Sci.* 85:60-67.

Chew, B.P. (1996). Importance of antioxidant vitamins in immunity and health in animals. *Anim. Feed Sci. Techno.* 59:103-114

Heirman, L.R., Chew, B.P. Wong,T.S., Mical,J.J.,and Standaert, F.E. (1990). Effects of dietary b-carotene on lymphocyte function in periparturient dairy cows. *J.dairy Sci.,* 73. (suppl.):166.

Hoskinson, C.D., Chew, B. P. and Wong, T. S. (1989). Effects of b-carotene and Vitamin A on mitogen induced lymphocyte proliferation in pigs *in vivo. Fed. Am. Soc. Exp. Biol. J.,* 3: A663.

Dahlquist, S. P. and Chew, B.P. (1985). Effects of vitamin A and B-carotene on mastitis in dairy cows during the early dry period. *J. Dairy Sci.* 68 (suppl. 1):191 (abstr.).

Daniel, L.R., Chew, B.P., Tanaka, T.S. and Tjoelker, L.W. (1991). b-carotene and vitamin A effects on bovine phagocyte function in vitro during peripartum period. *J. Dairy Sci.,* 74: 124.

Erskine, R.J., R.J. Eberhart, and R.W. Scholz. (1990). Experimentally induced *Staphylococcus aureus* mastitis in selenium-deficient and selenium-supplemented dairy cows. *J. Amer. Vet. Med. Assoc.* 51:1107-1111.

Harjit, K., Chawla, R. Chatterjee, P.N. and Panda, N. (2002). Mastitis control: A nutritional approach. Proc. Technical Symp. on Mastitis and milk quality, 3rd International expo and conference on Dairy and Food Processing Technology, New Delhi, Sept. 4-7, pp 121-127.

Harmon, R.J., and P.M. Torre. (1994). Copper and zinc: do they influence mastitis? Pages 54-65 in Proc. National Mastitis Council, Orlando, FL.

Harrison, J. H., D. D. Hancock, and H. R. Conrad. (1984). Vitamin E and selenium for reproduction of the dairy cow. *J. Dairy Sci.* 67:123-132.

Hogan, J. S., K. L. Smith, W. P. Weiss, D. A. Todhunter, and W. L. Shockey. (1990). Relationships among vitamin E, selenium, and bovine blood neutrophils. *J. Dairy Sci.* 73:2372-2378.

Jukola, E., J. Hakkarainen, H. Saloniemi, and S. Sankari. (1996). Blood selenium, vitamin E, vitamin A, and B-carotene concentrations and udder health, fertility treatments and fertility. *J. Dairy Sci.* 79:838-845.

Kim, H.S., Lee, J.M., Park, S.B., Jeong, S.G., Jung, J.K. and Im, K.S. (1997). Effect of vitamin E and Selenium administration on the performance in dairy cows. Asian-Aust. *J.Anim. Sci.* 10:308-312.

Kimura, K., J. P. Goff, M. E. Kehrli, and T. A. Reinhardt. (2002). Decreased neutrophil function as a cause of retained placenta in dairy cattle. *J. Dairy Sci.* 85:544-550.

LeBlanc, S. J., T. H. Herdt, W. M. Seymour, T. F. Duffield, and K. E. Leslie. (2004). Peripartum serum vitamin E, retinol, and beta-carotene in dairy cattle and their associations with disease. *J. Dairy Sci.* 87:609-619.

Malbe, M., M. Klaassen, W. Fang, V. Myllys, M. Vikerpuur, K. Nyholm, W. Sankari, K. Suoranta, and M. Sandholm. (1995). Comparisons of selenite and selenium yeast feed supplements on Se-incorporation, mastitis, and leukocyte function in Se-deficient dairy cows. *J. Vet. Med.* (Ser. A) 42:111-121.

Nockels, C.F., Lopez, G.A. and Philllips, R.W. (1973). Influence of vitamins A and C on cortcosterone and carbohydrate metabolism in chickens. *Poult. Sci.* 52:1261-1269.

Oldham, E.R., R.J. Eberhart, and L.D. Muller. (1991). Effects of supplemental vitamin A and B-carotene during the dry period and early lactation on udder health. *J. Dairy Sci.* 74:3775-3781.

Panda, N. (2003). Optimisation of vitamin E dose for improved immunity and udder health in Murrah buffaloes. Ph.D. Thesis. NDRI Deemed Univ., NDRI, Karnal.

Panda, N., Kaur, H. and Mohanty, T. K. (2006). Reproductive performance of dairy buffaloes supplemented with varying levels of vitamin E. *Asian-Aust. J.Anim. Sci.* 19:19-25.

Rajiv, (2001). Influence of b-carotene and vitamin E supplementation on udder health and immunocompetence in dairy cattle. Ph.D. Thesis. NDRI Deemed Univ., NDRI, Karnal.

Santos, M. V., F. R. Lima, P. H. M. Rodrigues, S. B. M. Barros, and L. F. L. daFonseca. (2001). Plasma ascorbate concentrations are not correlated with milk somatic cell count and metabolic profile in lactating and dry cows. *J. Dairy Sci.* 84:134-139.

Smith, K. L., Harrison, J. H., Hencock, D. D., Todhunter, D.A. & Conrad, H.R. (1984). Effect of vitamin E and Selenium supplementation on incidence of clinical mastitis and duration of clinical symptoms. *J. Dairy Sci.* 67: 1293-1300.

Tjolker, L.W., Chew, B.P.,Tanaka, T.S. and Daniel, L.R. (1990). Effect of dietary vitamin A and b-carotene on polymorphonuclear leukocyte and lymphocyte function indairy cows during the early dry period. *J. Dairy. Sci.* 73:1017-1022.

Watson, R.R., Prabhala, R. H., Plzia, P.M. and Alberts, D.S. (1991). Effects of b-carotene on lymphocyte subpopulation in elderly human: evidence for a dose- response relationship. *Am. J. Clin.Nutr.* 53:90-94.

Weiss, W.P., J.S. Hogan, D.A. Todhunter, and K.L. Smith. (1997). Effect of vitamin E supplementation in diets with a low concentration of selenium on mammary gland health of dairy cows. *J. Dairy Sci.* 80:1728-1737.

Weiss, W. P., J. S. Hogan, and K. L. Smith. (2004). Changes in vitamin C concentrations in plasma and milk from dairy cows after an intramammary infusion of *Escherichia coli. J. Dairy Sci.* 87:32-37.

Wichtel, J.J., A.L. Craigie, H. Varela-Alvarez, and N.B. Williamson. (1994). The effect of intraruminal selenium pellets on growth rate, lactation, and reproductive efficiency in dairy cattle. *New Zealand Vet. J.* 42:205-210.

Wuryastuti, H., Stowe, H. D., Bull, R.W. and Miller, E.R. (1993). Effects of vitamin E and selenium on immune responses of peripheral blood, colostrum,and milk leukocytes of sows. *J. Anim. Sci.* 71:2464-2472.

□□□

26

Veterinary Nutrition for Animal Welfare in Feed Deficit Situation

J.P. SRIVASTAVA
Ex-University Professor and Chairman, Department of Animal Nutrition, College of Veterinary Sciences and Animal Husbandry
Birsa Agricultural University, Ranchi – 834006, Jharkhad

Introduction

The animal welfare in general are responsible and judged by their health and production, and these are directly related to their state of health. The feeding of animal alone constitute about two third of thye total cost of livestock production.

The importance of feeding can be known through the following lines,

"Who so ever was the Father of a Dieseae, An ill Diet was the Mother"
~ *George Herbert*

There are a number of reasons why animal welfare is an important subject for consideration by livestock owners vis-à-vis their feeding. In most cases, the requirement to optimise animal welfare is not counter to the interests of the livestock producer, since it has been repeatly demonstrated that poor welfare will result in reduced biological and economic out put (Edwards *et al.*, 2006). However, a more powerful force affecting welfare of livestock production has been the growing trend for animal welfare to become a marketing issue. Animal welfare is seen as a matter of great importance by European citizens, which ranked the impoprtance of protecting welfare of farm animals very highly (7.8 on a 1-10 scale) (Eurobarometer, 2007).

The measurement of animal welfare is influenced by the perception of welfare of livestock owners who must provide credence to the out come (Edwards, 2007). Three clearly different perspective on animal welfare have been identified, focusing on natural living, biological function and affective state (Fraser, 2003).

There have been many attempts to provide a scientific definition of animal welfare. The most widely used current definition based upon the 'Five freedoms for animal welfare'. This approach was first formulated by the UK Farm Animal Welfare Council. The Five Freedoms are defined as follows :-

1. Freedom from hunger and thirst.
2. Freedom from thermal and physical discomfort.
3. Freedom from pain, injury and disease.
4. Freedom from fear and stress.
5. Freedom to express normal behaviour.

Farmers to the contrary have a much more positive perception of the current state of farm animal welfare. This has been demonstrated by Te Velde et al. (2002), who explained the opposite perceptions between citizens and farmers based on different interpretation of the components by which perception is determined.

Regarding valued, Te Velde et al. (2002) indicated that both farmers and citizens associate animal welfare with issues such as physical health, an adequate amount of food and drinking water, and sufficient heating and protection. Citizens, however, tend to include two additional values : freedom to move and freedom to fulfill natural desires (Te Velde *et al.*, 2002; Lassen *et al.*, 2006; Marie, 2006). Further more, farmers' norms are clearly related to factors that are important for optimizing production such as fast and efficient growth (Te Velde *et al.*, 2002; Dockes and Kling-Eveillard, 2006; Lassen *et al.*, 2006), which is something they positively relate to animal welfare. Finally, the values and norms of citizens seem to be based on the same set of convictions as those of farmers: animals are meant to serve humen; meat is a substantial part of the human diet; keeping animals and killing them for meat is legitimate; and farmers are there to providev food for the rest of the population (Te Velde *et al.*, 2002).

As a result of the norms expressed by the farmers, no problems were perceived for any of the aspects, since they all relate animal welfare primarily to health. Hence, if an animal eats well, it will grow fast, which means that it is healthy and that the welfare is good (F. Vanhonacker *et al.*, 2008).

Based on the preceeding observations, it could be concluded that the animal welfare is based on proper balanced feeding of the livestock, and vice versa.

This paper will primarily deal feeding of animal in feed deficit situation.

The feeding of livestock for optimum health and production becomes more problematic and cumbersom under deficit situation which further agreevate due to their improper feeding.

The feed deficit situation can broadly be classified and discussed in the following three heads

1. Supply and demand of feed stuffs
2. Under nutrition
3. Mal nutrition

Supply and Demand of Feed Stuffs

The competition between men and animals for the limited land will significantly influence the availability of feeds and fodders for livestock. Further, rapid urbanisation has put pressure on cultivated land being transformed in to real estate. Again, there is a question usually asked and visualized, whom we should feed first - Man or Animals. Obviously men. This hypothesis further reduce the feed and agreevates feed deficit situation. But, however, neither the human beings nor the animals could be ignored in providing an ideal food for their general welfare. The only best solution that could be thought of is to feed animals on those foodstuffs which are not required by human population as far as possible and feasible. Once, Ground nut cake was one of the most demanding protein supplement for animal feeding, now it is not abundantly available in the same volume for animal feeding as it is being used for preparation of protein supplements for human use.

Further, high cost of energy, proteins, minerals and vitamins sources dictate development of new feed resources and new feeding regimes.

Other important factors which influence the crop productivity in the Indian sub-continent are drought & famine, and to a limited extent - periodic floods.

Introduction of high yielding varities strain of crops, further reduces the quantity of crop residues like straw, bhusa and husks for animal feeding.

The gap has further widened due to introduction of exotic blood as a result of cross-breeding programmes for still higher and higher production, which could not be sustained without feeding concentrate feeds.

As such there is a dire necessity to increase the source of supply of concentrate feeds with newer feed resources as livestock feeds, with a view to cut the cost of feeding without lowering the health and performances of the livestock.

The main objective of the feeding is to increase the production efficiency of animals through improvement of efficiency of feed utilization of the existing feed resources, as well as increasing the availability of feed constituents by identifying newer feeds.

To bridge the gigantic gap (roughly - shortage of concentrate 44% ; green fodders 30% and dry roughages 36%), ICAR initiated an AICRP on utilization of agricultural byproducts and industrial waste materials for evolving economic rations for livestock in 1967 at different centres located in various SAUs, Research Institutes and National Institues in the country. These centres were enganged in devising ways and means for incorporation of agro-industrial byproducts in the rations of livestock to develop various economic combinations after identification of incriminating factor(s) and processing to make those suitable for animal feedings. Most of the byproducts have found their way in compounding feed industry for the formulation of balanced rations and in the rations of farm animals by the farmers.

The research findings of the AICRP on Agricultural and agro-industrial byproducts (AIBP) utilization at SAUs, and other research institutes including national institutes could recommend the most of the feeds identified by scientists for animal feeding without affecting health and performances when fed in limited recommended percent in the concentrate mixture (Appendix - I).

The distinction between conventional feeds and non-conventional feed resources (NCFR) various from country to country. What may be classified as NCFR elsewhere may in fact be traditional. In the long term, wider use of NCFR would designate many of these as traditional feeds. Further, more intensive utilization of the available feeds is also necessary in the face of chronic feed deficit situations that occur annually.

Particular attention is drawn to optimum levels of utilization of individual feeds, since in the formulation of practical balanced diets the feeding individual farm animals, one immediate consideration is the technically optimum level of feed which can be used to advantage.

As it may also be perused in Appendix - II, that apart from the beneficial effects, many byproducts/unconventional feedstuffs contain substances that are deleterious to animal health, and are responsible for loering the digestibility of the nutrients, and is associated with poor performances of the animals.

These examples clearly indicate that if byproducts and unconventional feedstuffs are to be effectively utilized in feeding systems, all deleterious components must be removed in order to ensure high performanes in the animals.

This august body may or may not agree with my views that unconventional feedstuffs are not suitable for maintaining good level of production. However, those could be used successfully as scarcity feeds & fodders, and in feed deficit situation to keep the animals alive.

Under Nutrition

In India, majority of our animal population lives on inadequate rations, both quatitatively as well as qualitatively, partly due to scanty availability of feedstuffs in local area and elsewhere, and partly also due to the cost of the feedstuffs and feed supplements.

Inadequacy in dietary nutrient supply penalise animal performances and donot maximise the production of animal products, and between ruminant and non-ruminants.

In actual practice, very few rations are entirely lacking in any of the essential nutrients, a more common feature is partial deficiency in one or more of these. Feeding such rations over a long time produces sub-clinical manifestations of dietary deficiencies, such as slow growth, shy breeding, low production, susceptibility to diseases etc. Since these symptoms are rather non-specific, they are not ordinarily detected.

Where deficiency in nutrients of animal feeds and fodders is due to the absence of certain elements in the soil ; it is rightly said that " Nutrition Starts From Soil".

It would thus be necessary to supplement the ration with missing nutrients from outside sources, or to use a manure, containing the missing element, in proper proportions on the soil holding the fodder crop.

Mal-Nutrition

Although majority of animals in India lives on faulty diets, mal-nutrition is one of the main causes of their degeration. The low production, delayed maturity and heavy mortality are caused mainly due to either inadequate or faulty practices.

In certain areas, some of the elements are present in unusually large quantities which may induce pathological symptoms in local animals. In this case, the problem is to counteract the toxic effect of these subsantnces by adding neutralizing substances to the ration. In all such cases, the pathologists, and the nutritional chemists have got to work side by side in diagnostic work as well as to device methods to combat the problems. As new lands are brought under cultivation, newer problems are bond to arise. Some of the common ailments due to mal-nutrition are presented below.

Fluorosis (Flourine)

In large doses, flourine is toxic to animals and produces pathological symptoms in three to four years time. However, in endemic region it may develop within six to nine months time and even earlier after arrival of cattle. Due to phosphorus deficiency, the animals usually lick the soil which being rich in flourine in such areas, augments the quantity of flourine ingestion. The symptoms are stiffness of gate and lameness. Additional symptoms are anaemia, production of bony growths called exotoses on the long bones and reduction in the strength of the bones.

Goitre (Iodine)

Lack of iodine in the ration causes the disease known an goitre. This disease is however, a zonal problem. The affected animals show an emlargement of a gland called thyroid, situated in the neck so that the neck appears to be highly swollen. Calves born of dams kept on an iodine low ration manifest enlarged thyroid gland and hairlessness.

Molybdenum

Among cattle, particularly calves and cows in milk when grazed on such pasture containing large quantities of molybdenum, develop symptoms of molybdenum poisioning. Such animals are found to suffer from anaemia, diahorrea, with loss of weight and drop in milk yield. An excess of molybdenum apparantly decreases the availability of copper so that such cases may be termes as conditioned copper deficiency.

Selenium

This element has recently been found in large quantities in the grain and fodders grown in certain areas. Cattle consuming such feeds suffer from a disease called alkali disease or blind stagger. The symptoms are loss of hair from the tail and sloughing of hooves and tails.The appetite decreases and the animals show a tendency to stray and to stumble over and bump into objects in their way. In the last stages, paralysis may set in and animals may die with symptoms of pain coupled with respiratory failure.

Besides above, there are other nutritional disprders in animals due to faulty nutrition & otherwise.

Poisonous Plants

Under normal conditions, that is, when the animals are grazed on a bountiful pasture, they usually avoid plants that are toxic in effect, but during period of draught, hungry animals eat in an indiscriminating way resulting in their frequent poisoing. Sometimes, poisonous plants growing in close association under pasture grasses harvested with hay or their seds become mixed with grain, and animals ingesting such feeds may show symptoms of poisioning which may result in death. However, little definite information is available in our country, regarding the occurance of such plants as well as vital statistics of the mortality caused by them.

Cyanogenetic Plants

These plants are so-called because when ingested, they liberate hydrocyanic (prussic) acid which is very potent poison. Plants like, Jowar (Sofghum vulgare), Johnson grass (Sorghum halepanse), Sudan grass (Sorghum vulgare sudanensis), star grasss and bamboo shoots, in their young stages of growth may contain large quantities of hydrocyanic acid. Besides cyanogenetic plants, Kaner (Nerium odorum), Oleander (Nerium abeander) leaves are highly toxic, and ingestion of onle 250 g of these will cause death.

Lantana, a shurb growing on road sides and producing small bright-red flowers, when ingested, may give rise to photo-sensitiveness, blindness and ultimately death.

There are vast field of poisonous plants, and more research are required on the subject.

At times over feeding is responsible for serious situation resulting in death of animals.

Ketosis

Commonly known as acetonaemia or post parturient dyspepsia, is a metabolic disorder usually seen in high-yielding cows within a few days or some weeks after calving. The disease is generally observed in cows which have been usually fattened before calving and are suddenly put after calving on a ration not containing sufficient energy-yielding nutrients.

Bloat

This is a sudden, serious digestive upset that is often the cause of heavy loss. This generally occurs in cattle after they have grazed or given large quantities of green fodders, particularly legumes like berseem and lucerne. The rumen becomes distended with gas causing great pain and often death occurs due to suffocation.

Conclusion

"The final objective in ensuring expanded use of AIBP and NCFR is high performance in animals and of a type that is demonstrated to be economic. With several crop residues, the importance of seeking an economic advantage has been emphasised (Giaever, 1984; Greenhalgh, 1984). The high costs of the pretreatments need to be weighed against the beneficial effects, including the extent of the animal response."

References

Dockes, A.C., Kling-Eveillard, F. (2006). Farmers and advisers representatives of animals and animal welfare. *Livest. Sci.*, 103 (3): 243-249.

Devendra, C., 1989. Potential value of non-conventional feedstuffs for animals in Asia, Paper presented at FFTC-SEARCA seminar on feed grains substitute and non-conventional feedstuffs for livestock and poultry in Asia, 13-17 November, 1985, p 1-25.

Edwards, *et al.* (2006). (cited by Sandra Edwards)

Edwards, (2007). (cited by Sandra Edwards)

Eurobarometer, (2007). (cited by Sandra Edward)

Fraser, (2003). (cited by Sandra Edward)

Edwards, Sandra., (2008). Background to the practicalities of on-farm welfare audits on EW pig farms at the London swine conference.

Filiep Vanhonacker, Wim Verbeke, Els Van Poucke, Frank, A.M. Tuyttens, (2008). Do citizens and farmers interpret the concept of farm animal welfare differently., *Livest. Sci.*, 116: 126-136.

Giaever, H. (1984). The economics of using straw on feed.In straw and other fibrous byproducts on feed, F. Sundstol and E. Owen eds., Elsevier, Amsterdam, The Netherland, p. 558-574.

Greenhalgh, J.F.D. (1984). Upgrading crop and agricultura byproducts for animal production. In Herbivore nutrition in the sub-tropic and tropics. F.M.C. Gilchrist and R.I. Machie eds. The Science Press (Pte.) Ltd., Craightall, South Africa, p. 167-184.

ICAR bulletin (Review series) Principles of feeding farm animals.

ICAR Farm bulletin (New series) no. 23, Nutritional disorders in cattle.

ICAR Proceedings of the AICRP agricultural byproducts workshop – 1977 to 1992.

AICRP on agricultural byproducts, Annual Reports, (1977-1992). Department of Animal Nutrition, College of Veterinary Science and Animal Husbandry, Birsa Agricultural University, Ranchi (Jharkhand State).

Lassen, J., Sandoe, P., Forkman, B. (2006). Happy pigs are dirty? Conflicting perspectives on animal welfare., *Livest. Sci.*, 103(3): 221-230.

Marie, M. (2006). Ethics : The new challenge for animal agriculture., *Livest. Sci.*, 103(3): 203-207.

OIE, (2009). 77th. Annual General Session of the International Committee of the World Organisation for animal health, 24-29n May, 2009, p. 1-10.

Te Velde, H.T., Aarts, N., Van Woerkum, C. (2002). Dealing with ambivalence farmers' & consumers' perceptions of animal welfare in livestock breeding. *J. Agric. Environ. Ethics*, 15(2): 203-219.

□□□

Appendix - I

Recommended Unconventional Feed through AICROP on Agricultural by Products (ICAR Project)

1. Byproducts from sugar industry
   (a) Sugarcane tops (b) Bagasse
   (c) Molasses (d) Press mud
   (e) Condensed molasses soluble/Dried yeast sludge

2. Byproducts from the forests
   I. Leaves of field and tree crops
   (a) Su-babool (Leucaena leucocephala)
   (b) Hada-poda (Richardia brazalensis)
   (c) Jack (Artocarpus integrifolia L.) fruits and leaves
   (d) Sunn-hemp

   II. Inedible plant seeds / cakes
   (a) Babul (Acacia arabica) pods and seeds
   (b) Guar (Cyamposis tetragonaloba) meal

3. Non-edible and other minor oil seed cakes / meals
   (a) Mahua (Madhuca indica)
   (b) Sal (Shorea robusta)
   (c) Karanj (Pongamia glabra)
   (d) Kosum (Schleichera oleosa)
   (e) Neem (Azadiarachta indica)
   (f) Surguja/Niger (Guizotia abyssynica Cass.)
   (g) Rubber (Hevea brasilensis) cake
   (h) Caster bean (Ricinus communis) meal

4. Byproducts of canning and food industry
   (a) Mango (mangifera indica Linn) seed kernel/cake
   (b) Tomato (Lycopersicon esculentum)
   (c) Citrus (Citrus species) peels
   (d) Apple (Malus sylvestris) wastes
   (e) Pine apple (Ananas sativus)

5. Aquatic and sea weeds
   I. Aquatic plant
   (a) Water hyacinth (Echhormia crassepes)

   II. Marine waste and byproducts
   (a) Fish waste (b) Sea weeds
   (c) Unicellular algae

6. Slaughter house byproducts
   (a) Tankage (b) Meat scrab
   (c) Feather meal

7. Use of animal organic and municipal waste
   (a) Cow dung
   (b) Animal urine
   (c) Poultry excreta (Source of Nitrogen)
   (d) Biogas
      (i) Methane for fuel
      (ii) Slurry as manure - which could be used in the feeding of the animals, wholly or partly being rich in microbial protein.

8. Agro-industrial byproducts

   I. Husks and brans
   (a) Rice (*Oryza sativa*)
      1. Rice husk
      2. Rice bran
      3. Rice polish
   (b) Wheat (Triticum aestivum) bran

   II. Conventional oil cakes and meals
   (a) Ground nut (Arachis hypogaea) cake
   (b) Mustard (Brassica species) cake
   (c) Linseed (Linum usitatissimum Linn.) cake
   (d) Cotton (Gossypium species) cake
   (e) Soybean cake
   (f) Til (Sesamum indicum) cake
   (g) Coconut (Cocos nucifera)

   III. Unconventional oil cakes & protein sources
   (a) Sal (Shorea robusta) seed meal
   (b) Mahua (madhuca indica) cake
   (c) Neem (Azadiarachta indica) cake
   (d) Kosum (Schleichera oleosa) cake
   (e) Niger/Surguja (Guizotia abyssynica Cass.) cake
   (f) Karanj (Pongamia glabra) cake
   (g) Caster bean (Ricinus communis) meal
   (h) Rubber (Hevea brasilensis) seed cake

9. Miscellaneous byproducts
   (a) Brewary waste
   (b) Silk worm pupae meal
   (c) Maize gluten feed
   (d) Tapioca waste
   (e) Cassiatora seeds
   (f) Mahua flower and waste from mahua liquor
   (g) Tamarind (Tamarindus indica Linn.) seeds/hulls
   (h) Banana (Musa paradisiacal Linn.) waste

Appendix - II
By products/unconventional Feedstuffs Containing Substances Deleterious to Animal Health

	Feedstuff	Substance
1.	Kosum cake	HCN (Cynogenic glucosides)
2.	Salseed meal Tamarind seed Tree leaves Mango seed kernel	Tannins
3.	Mahua cake/flower	Mowrine
4.	Karanj cake	Karanjin, Pongamine, Pongaglarine
5.	Subabool	Mimosine – Trypsin inhibitor
6.	Neem seed cake	Nimbine
7.	Guar meal	Trypsine inhibitor factor
8.	Water hyacinth	Oxalic acid
9.	Cotton seed	Gossypol
10.	Cocoa pod husks	Theobromin

□□□

27

Biohydrogenation of Unsaturated Fatty Acids by Rumen Microorganisms : Conjugated Linoleic Acid

D.N. KAMRA AND L.C. CHAUDHARY
CAFT in Animal Nutrition, IVRI, Izatnagar-243122 UP

Introduction

The important unsaturated fatty acids (linolenic acid and linoleic acid) are present mainly in green forages and in very low concentrations in ruminant products. The fats of ruminant's origin are more saturated than those of monogastric animals. The consumption of ruminant products is often considered with an increased incidence of heart disease in man and the conversion of PUFA to saturated fatty acids, or biohydrogenation, in ruminants is an important process and this process is carried out by microbes present in the rumen. Recent experimental results suggest that the CLA, a biohydrogenation product of PUFA formed in the rumen, helps in prevention of cancer through conversion to cis-9,trans-11-C18:2 in animal tissues (Knight *et al.*, 2003 and Dang Van *et al.*, 2011).Therefore, decreasing the saturation of fatty acids by rumen microorganisms would help to decrease heart diseases in the human. Other fatty acids in ruminant products also have beneficial effects on human health. The CLA promote health in animals by preventing cancer, decreasing atherosclerosis, increasing lean/fat ratio and improving the immune response (Kritchevsky, 2000; Whigham *et al.*, 2000). Recent experiments suggests that dietary trans-vaccenic acid (TVA, trans-11-C18:1), the biohydrogenation product of the main isomer of CLA formed in the rumen, cis-9, trans-11-C18:2, may be of benefit in the prevention of cancer through endogenous conversion to cis-9, trans-11-C18:2 in mammalian tissues (Lock *et al.,* 2004).

The benefits of CLA were discovered accidentally during a study in which the effect of over cooking of meat was studied. The Ames test, which picks up mutagens and carcinogens, identified a compound which was not related to these compounds and prevented the cancer induced experimentally in mice. The compound was reported as CLA. Researchers are putting lot of efforts in making the human diet healthy by increasing the CLA content of the diet. The main sources of dietary CLA for human beings are meat and milk of ruminant's origin. Hence there is an opportunity to enhance the health promoting properties of these products. The other result of increased CLA formation in the rumen would be expected to be an enhanced immune response in the animal itself, enabling ruminants to deal better with infection. The two main CLA isomer which are beneficial to human heath are cis-9, trans-11 octadecadienoic acid and trans-10, cis- 12 octadecadienoic acid. As the biohydrogenation process is carried out by the anaerobic microbes present in the rumen of the livestock, it affects the composition and quality of ruminant products (Chaudhary *et. al.,* 2004; Mckain *et al.,* 2004 and Wallace *et al.,* 2005). In present paper an attempt has been made summaries the available information on the biohydrogenation of polly unsaturated fatty acids by rumen microbes and the measures how best we can increase the CLA content of the ruminant products specially through dietary manipulation.

Process of CLA Formation in the Animals

The CLA are the intermediates in the conversion of the dienoic acid, linoleic acid to the monoenoic acid, *trans*-vaccenic acid. This conversion takes place by anaerobic bacteria in the rumen. The ruminal bacteria hydrogenate the *trans*-vaccenic acid again to the fully saturated C18:0 (stearic acid) fatty acids. Thus CLA are formed from dietary linoleic acid only as intermediates of the biohydrogenation processes in the rumen. This has been depicted in detail in Fig.1. It has also been shown that the CLA present in milk fat is not derived directly from CLA flowing from the rumen, but is synthesised in mammary tissue from *trans*-vaccenic acid. The enzyme $?^9$- desaturase, forms CLA from *trans*–vaccenic acid in the animal's tissues. The TVA is also formed primarily by ruminal bacteria. It is therefore the total flow of CLA and *trans*–vaccenic acid from the rumen which forms the total pool for CLA deposition in ruminant tissues. Studies (Griinarie and Bauman, 1999 and Knight *et al.,* 2003) have suggested endogenous synthesis as a major source of *cis-9,trans-ll* -18:2 in the milk fat as well as muscle lipids representing 78% and 64% of the total, respectively. The results from different studies suggest that majority of the cis-9,trans-11 CLA in milk fat (70-80%) comes from conversion of vassenic acid by delta 9-desaturase (Bauman *et. al.,* 2003 and Palmquist *et al.,* 2004).

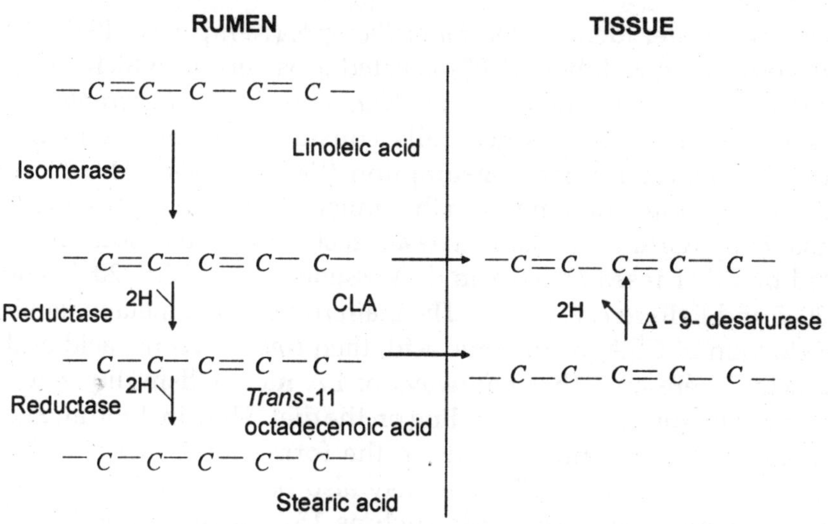

Fig. 1 : Ruminal biohydrogenation of fatty acids (linoleicacid)

Role of Ruminal Bacteria in the Biohydrogenation of PUFAs

The majority of the biohydrogenation of PUFA in the rumen is carried out by the bacterial community. Many ruminal bacteria are inhibited by long chain fatty acids (Sehat *et. al.*, 1998) and gram positive bacteria are more sensitive than gram negative bacteria (Henderson, 1973). PUFAs are toxic but some rumen bacteria are able to saturate the double bonds through biohydrogenation (Polan *et al.*, 1964). Keppler and Tove (1967) study the biohydrogenation fatty acids by *Butyrivibrio* strains and demonstrated that linoleic acid was first converted to *cis*-9, *trans*-11 CLA. The reductases steps were inhibited by oxygen but the LA isomerase could continue to produce *cis*-9, *trans*-11 CLA even if oxygen was present (Hughes *et al.*, 1982). The bacteria involved in the saturation process fall into two distinct groups, depending whether they are able to hydrogenate both the dienoic and the monoenoic acids or only the monoenoic acid. Bacterial species in the type A group is dominated by *B. fibrisolvens* while type B population is mainly *Fusocillus* sp. The type A populations are able to bring down the LA up to CLA while it is type B bacteria, which are producing stearate from PUFA in rumen. This has been depicted in detail in Fig. 2. The *Butyrivbrio fibrisolvens* has greater CLA producing capacity than other ruminal bacteria (Kim *et al.*, 2002). They also reported that growing cells of *B. fibrisolvens* is sensitive to CLA as well as LA.

The *Butyrivibrio fibrisolvens* biohydrogenate the fatty acids and form CLA as intermediates in the process (Kepler *et al.*, 1966). Stearic acid was not formed from LA by *B. fibrisolvens*, however the bacteria responsible for stearate formation were later identified as *Fusocillus* spp. (Kemp *et al.*, 1975). Recently, van de Vossenberg & Joblin (2003) isolated a bacterium which can produce stearate from LA. It was similar to '*Fusocillus*' and close to *Butyrivibrio hungatei*. The *cis*-9, *trans*-11 isomer is generally considered to be the main health-promoting CLA for human consumption (Pariza, 2004). The TVA is also desirable as a product flowing from the rumen because it is converted to CLA in animal boby (Griinari & Bauman *et al.*, 2000). Stearate producers were also reported by other researchers (van de Vossenberg & Joblin, 2003; and Wang *et al.*, 2005 and Pallard *et al.*, 2007). The main route of LA metabolism involves the production of CLA, or rumenic acid, then *trans*-vaccenic acid and finally stearic acid. There are other pathways of LA metabolism, however, which may increase in importance depending on the diet. They include an alternative isomerisation of LA which results in the formation of CLA followed by reduction to *trans*-10-C18:1.The LA may also be hydrated, resulting in the formation of hydroxy fatty acids such as 13-hydroxy, *cis*-9-C18:1. Other unsaturated fatty acids are subject to similar metabolism. Oleic acid has been shown to be metabolised both by biohydrogenation to stearic acid and by hydration to hydroxystearic acid in bacteria isolated from the rumen.The quantitative importance of hydration in comparison to biohydrogenation seems minor (Wallace *et al.*, 2006).

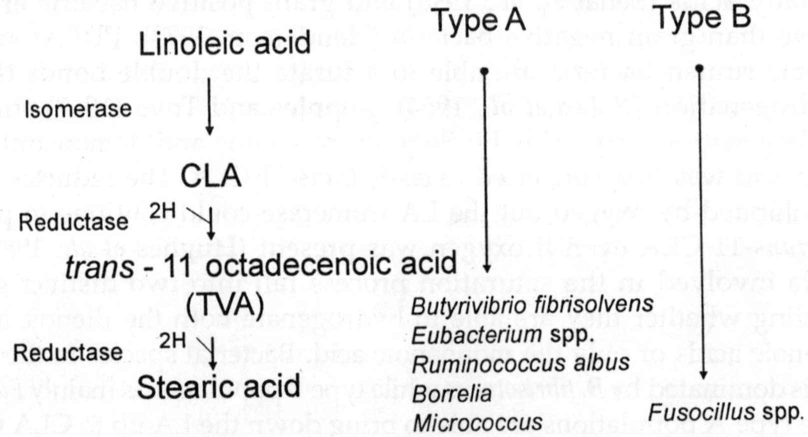

Fig. 2 : Ruminal bacteria responsible for biohydrogenation

Role of Protozoa and Fungi in the Biohydrogenation of PFUs

The fatty acids composition of protozoal cell is different than bacterial cell. The proportion of saturated stearic acid is more in bacterial cell while it is less in protozoal cell. The proportion of CLA and TVA is higher in ciliate protozoa. Klopfenstein *et al.* (1966) reported that in the plasma of defaunated lamb C18:1 fatty acid was higher than faunated animal. Chalupa *et al.* (1967)

observed that higher LA and oleic acid in the milk fat of cow might be due to low number of ciliate protozoa in the rumen. Latham, et. al. (1972) found lipolytic activity in the protozoal fraction of bovine rumen contents and estimated that about 30% of the total activity could be associated with ciliate protozoa. Though the ciliate protozoa are rich in saturated fatty acids the flow of the protozoa from the rumen is less and majority of the protozoa are retained in the rumen. Therefore it seems that contribution of ciliate protozoa in the biohydrogenation of unsaturated fatty acids in the rumen is limited and more research in this direction is required.

Importance of Biohydrogenation in the Rumen

The biohydrogenation of fatty acids in the rumen is one of the activities whish are taken place by rumen microbes. However its roles of in the rumen are not very much clear. It is an important activity in terms of the fatty acids, which are incorporated into meat and milk. Hazlewood and Dawson (1979) suggested that biohydrogenation has an essential role in the utilization of dietary fatty acids by fatty acid auxotrphic bacteria. Lennarz (1966) suggested that function of biohydrogenation in the rumen is disposal of reducing power, essential to bacteria living in the reduce environment. Kemp and Lander (1984) reported that biohydrogenation of PUFA in the rumen is a detoxification mechanisms which is essential for the survival of rumen bacteria as higher accumulation of PUFA is toxic for many rumen bacteria.

Inhibition of Biohydrogenation in the Rumen

It is clear from the literature that biohydrogenation of unsaturated fatty acids in the rumen is an important processes and it affects the fatty composition of ruminant products. By any means if we can control the biohydrogenation process of fatty acids, then there is chance that we may get better livestock product with desired fatty acid composition. Several efforts have been made in this direction to change the composition of ruminant products to get healthier products for human consumption. Dietary manipulation of ruminants diet containing oils rich in unsaturated fatty acids were tried by researchers (Offer, *et al.*, 2001; Loor, *et al.*, 2003; and Wang, *et al.*, 2005). Use of encapsulated oils, to bypass it from ruminal biohydrogenation, fish oil, monensin etc. can be tried to alter the biohydrogenation in the rumen. It is important to learn about this and similar mechanisms if we are to formulate rational mechanisms for modifying biohydrogenation.

Health Benefits of CLA

The different isomers of CLA have been known to exert much beneficial effect in human as well as in animals. The some of the beneficial effects of CLA feeding on animals have been given as follows:

Effect of CLA and Cardio Vascular Disease

Lee *et al.* (1994) reported that rabbits fed on atherogenic diet and supplemented with 0.5g CLA/day for 22 weeks had significantly less triglyceride, plasma LDL cholestrol, and LDL-C/HDI-C ratio than the control animals. Kathirvelan (2007) reported reduced total cholesterol and triglycerides and concluded that antiatherogenic properties of CLA, irrespective of its level in diet. Eder *et al.* (2009) suggested that anti-atherogénic effects observed with CLAs are perhaps mediated not only by CLAs themselves but also by their metabolites. Gebauer *et al.* (2011) concluded from the published results that CLA might have beneficial effects on the heart diseases but its verification in human are essential.

Effect CLA on Cancer

Ip et. al. (1991) reported that experimentally induced mammary tumors were reduced in rats with the administration of CLA. Kathirvelan and Tyagi (2008) reported 37% inhibition of mammary tumor growth in female rats by feeding of CLA enriched ghee. They also concluded that CLA feeding not only inhibited the benign type tumor but malignant tumor as well. Gebauer *et al.* (2011) concluded from the available information that experimental ruminant TFA may beneficially affect risk of CVD and cancer and further research is needed to determine the effects of VA and c9, t11-CLA in humans as well as clarify the isomer-specific effects of CLA.

CLA and Immune System

The CLA feeding has resulted in improvement of immune system of animals Less information is available about effect of CLA on immune and inflammatory responses in animal models (Cook *et al.*, 1993; Cheng *et al.*, 2004 and Kathirvelan, 2007). Albers *et al.* (2003) suggested that the individual isomers of CLA could have different effects on the components of the immune system in human. They also reported that CLA may increase humoral immune response in human. However Yu et al. (2002) showed decrease production of pro-inflammatory products. Kathirvelan (2007) reported that CLA enriched ghee exerted positive response in improving immune system of the animals.

Effect CLA on Diabetes

The CLA feeding has also shown beneficial effect in diabetic cases. Several studies have shown increased blood insulin levels or insulin resistance (DeLany *et al.*, 1999, Tsuboyama *et al.*, 2000 and Roche *et al.*, 2002). Although there were no alterations of blood glucose concentration after glucose tolerance testing, insulin tolerance testing clearly showed a marked insulin resistance in CLA fed female mice (Tsuboyama *et al.*, 2000). In contrast, West et al. (2000) reported no effect of CLA supplementation for 5 weeks on plasma leptin and glucose levels in mice supplemented with 1% CLA.

Improvement of CLA Content of Animal Products

The dietary manipulation of livestock is one of the important strategies to improve the fatty acid composition of the animals. The fatty acid composition of meat, milk and dairy products is highly dependent on the animals' diet (Gahreis *et al.*, 1997 and Kraft *et al.*, 2008). The supplementation of fat especially in protected form alter the fatty acid composition of milk fat. The unsaturated fatty acids, particularly linolenic acid and linoleic acid are present mainly in grasses and in very low concentrations in ruminant products and when the animals consume these fatty acids they goes under biohydrogenation in the rumen with the help of rumen microbes and they convert most of them into saturated form. Thus, if ruminal biohydrogenation of PUFA is controlled, it may be possible to improve the healthiness of ruminant products by increasing their unsaturated fatty acids composition. Recent experimental results suggest that the CLA a biohydrogenation product of PUFA formed in the rumen, helps in prevention of cancer through conversion to *cis*-9,*trans*-11-C18:2 in animal tissues. When ruminants are raised on pasture and green fodder, their meat and milk contain much higher levels of n-3 PUFA and CLA as compared to products from animals raised on stall feeding with concentrates (Kraft *et al.*, 2003, Tyagi *et al.*, 2008).

The dietary factors that provide PUFA substrates results in higher production of CLA and trans-11 18:1 due to dietary supply of plant or fish oils. The second category consists of dietary factors that affect rumen bacteria involved in biohydrogenation, either directly or via changes in rumen environment. Dietary factors that alter milk fat CLA by modifying rumen biohydrogenation generally affect both Group A and Group B bacteria. For example, modifying the forage:concentrate ratio of the diet alters the biohydrogentation of PUFA. The third category includes dietary factors that involve a combination of lipid substrates and modification of rumen biohydrogenation. Say for example feeding of green roughages increases CLA content of animal product. The last is dietary supplements of CLA or trans-11 18:1 fatty acids. These must be in protected form so that its biohydrogenation may not takes place in the rumen (Lock and Garnsworthy, 2003; Flower et.al., 2008; Haung *et. al.*, 2008 and Soressa *et al.*, 2009). Li *et al.*, (2010) concluded that malate and fumarate, as propionate precursors, act as alternative electron sinks and may compete with CH4 generation and bio-hydrogenation of C18:2 in the utilization of metabolic H2. The highest CLA concentration at the early incubation stage was accompanied by reduced propionate proportion. Linoleic acid is also considered one of the potential alternatives to suppress CH4 generation.

It is well known that linoleic acid and linolenic acid are both indirect precursors ofthe CLA isomer cis-9, trans-II but the highest concentration of the isomer is obtained by linolenic acid rich diets (Dhiman *et al.*, 2000). Hence, supplementing the diet with vegetable oils rich in these fatty acids, such as sunflower, soybean, peanut, canola, and linseed increases CLA content in milk as well as meat (Dhiman *et al.*, 1999; Aaes *et al.*, 2004) and thus seems to be an effective strategy for CLA, being much lower than that achieved in milk, as noted later (Raes *et al.*, 2004). Tyagi *et al.* (2006) also reported increase in CLA levels when lactating buffaloes were fed with 30% mustard oil cake in concentrate mixture. The fish oils were shown to be more effective in creasing milk CLA than vegetable oils, although combinations of fish oil and vegetable oils rich in LA were also effective in increasing CLA content (Chilliard *et al.*, 2000, 2001). Abu Ghazaleh (2008) reported slightly lower CLA content when a basal grain diet supplemented with a combination of sunflower oil and fish oil to grazing dairy cows. The various researchers have shown an increased CLA content in milk and meat of ruminant grazed on pasture in comparison to stall fed animals (Loor *et al.*, 2002 Kay *et al.*, 2004, Tyagi *et al.*, 2007). Poulson *et al.* (2004) reported higher CLA content in the muscle of steers raised only on forages compared to steers fed a common high grain feedlot diet. Dang van *et al.* (2011) confirms the hypothesis that ruminal biohydrogenation was more complete with higher diet structure value, leading to higher concentration of stearate and subsequently lower transfer efficiencies of 18:2 n - 6 and 18:3 n - 3 from diet to milk.

The biohydrogenation of PUFA in ruminants is an important activity carried out by anaerobic microbes present in the rumen. The fatty acid composition and quality of ruminant products is greatly influenced by the microbial consortium present in the rumen. Therefore by controlling the biohydrogenation process in the rumen fatty acid profile of the ruminant products can be changed. The CLA content of ruminant product such as milk and meat can be modify up to great extent through dietary manipulation and more and more researches are going on in this direction.

Referances

Abughazaleh, A.A. (2008). Effect of fish oil and sunflower oil supplementation on milk conjugated linoleic acid content for grazing dairy cows. *Anim. Feed Sci. Technol.* 141: 220-232.

Albers, R., Van Der Wielen, R. P., Brink, E. J., Hendriks, H. F., Dorovska-Taran, V. N. and Mohede, I. C. (2003). Effects of cis-9, trans-II and trans-10,cis-12 conjugated linoleic acid (CLA) isomers on immune function in healthy men. *Eur. J. Clin. Nutr.* 57: 595-603.

Bauman, D.E., Corl, B.A., and Peterson, D.G. (2003). The biology of conjugated linoleic acids in ruminants. *Adv. Conjugated Linoleic Acid Res.* 2: 146-173.

Chaudhary, L. C., McKain, N., Richardson, A. J., Barbier, M., Charbonnier, J. and Wallace, R. J. (2004). Screening for *Fusocillus*: factors that affect the detection of ruminal bacteria which form stearic acid from linoleic acid. *Reprod. Nutr. Dev.* 44: 65.

Cheng, W.L., Lii., C.K., Chen., H.V., Lin, T. H. and Liu, K.L. (2004). Contribution of the CLA to the suppression of inflammatory responses through the regulation of NF pathway. *J. Agric. Food Chem.* 52 :71-78.

Chillard, Y, Ferlay, A. and Doreau, M. (2001). Effect of different types offorages, animal fat or marine oils in cow's on milk fat secretion and composition, especially conjugated linoleic acid (CLA) and polyunsaturated fatty acids. *Livestock Prod. Sci.* 70: 31-48.

Chillard, Y., Ferlay, A., Mansbridge, R.A. and Doreau, M. (2000). Ruminant milk fat plasticity: Nutritional control of saturated, polyunsaturated and trans and conjugated fatty acids. *Annual Zootech.* 49: 181-250.

Cook, M.E., Miller, C.C., Park, Y and Pariza, M.W. (1993). Immune modulation by altered nutrient metabolism: Nutronal control of immune-induced growth depression. *Poultry Sci.* 72: 1301-1305.

Dang Van, Q.C., Focant, M., Mignolet, E., Turu, C., Froidmont, E., Larondelle, Y. (2011). Influence of the diet structure on ruminal biohydrogenation and milk fatty acid composition of cows fed extruded linseed. *Anim. Feed Sci.Technol.* doi:10.1016/ j.anifeedsci.2011.05.002.

DeLany, l. P., Blohm, F., Truett, A.A., Scimeca, J.A and West, D.B. (1999). Conjugated linoleic acid rapidly reduces body fat content in mice without affecting energy intake. *American J. Physol.* 276:1172-1179.

Dhiman, T.R., Anand G.R., Satter, L.D. and Pariza, M.W. (1999). Conjugated linoleic acid content of milk from cows fed different diets. *J. Dairy Sci.* 83: 2146-2156.

Dhiman, T.R., Satter, L.D., Pariza, M.W., Galli, M.P., Albright and Tolosa, M.X. (2000). Conjugated linoleic acid content of milk from cows offered diets rich in linoleic and linolenic acid. *J. of Dairy Sci.* 83: 1016-102.

Eder, K., Ringseis, R. (2009). Metabolism and actions of conjugated linoleic acids on atherosclerosis-related even:s in vascular endothelial cells and smooth muscle cells. Molecular Nut. Food Res.

French, P., Stanton, C., Lawless, F., O'Riordan, E.G., Monahan, F.I, Caffrey, PJ. and Moloney, AP. (2001). Fan: acid composition, including conjugated linoleic acid, of intramuscular fat from steers offered grazed grass, gras:; silage, or concentrate-based diets. *J. Anim. Sci.* 78 : 2849-2855.

Gebauer, S.K., Chardigny, J.M., Jakobsen, M.U., Lamarche, B., Lock, A.L., Spencer D., Proctor, S.D. and Baer, D.J. (2011). Effects of ruminant trans fatty acids on cardiovascular disease and cancer: A comprehensive review of epidemiological, clinical, and mechanistic studies. *Adv. Nutr.* 2: 332–354.

Griinari, J.M. & Bauman, D.E. (1999). Biosynthesis of conjugated linoleic acid and its incorporation into meat and milk in ruminants. In Advances in conjugated linoleic acid research, volume 1, pp. 180-200. Edited by M. P. Yurawecz, M. M. Mossoba, J. K. Kramer, M. W. Pariza & G. J. Nelson. Champaign, Illinois: AOCS Press.

Griinari, J. M., Corl, B. A., Lacy, S. H., Chouinard, P. Y., Nurmela, K. V. & Bauman, D. E. (2000). *J. Nutr* 130: 2285-2291.

Henderson, C. (1973). The effects of fatty acids on pure cultures of rumen bacteria. *J. Agric. Sci.* 81: 107-112.

Hughes, P. E., Hunter, W. J. & Tove, S. B. (1982). Biohydrogenation of unsaturated fatty acids. Purification and properties of cis-9,trans-11-octadecadienoate reductase. *J Biol Chem* 257: 3643-3649.

Kathirvalen, C. and Tyagi, A. (2007). Influence of mustard oil/cake feeding on CLA content of buffalo milk. *Indian J. Anim. Nut.* 24: 237-240.

Kathirvalen, C., Tyagi, A and krishnamurthi, P. (2008). Influence of conjugated Linoleic acid ghee feeding on cancer incidences and histopathological changes in 7, 12 dimeth1y benz (a) anthrazene induced mammary gland carcinogenesis in rats. *Vety. Arch.* 78: 511-520.

Kay, J.K, Mackle, T.R., Auldist, M.J., Thompson, N.A. and Bauman, D.E. (2004). Endogenous synthesis of cis- 9, trans-II conjugated linoleic acid in dairy cows fed fresh pasture. *J. Dairy Sci.* 87: 369-378.

Kemp, P. & Lander, D. J. (1984). Hydrogenation in vitro of a-linolenic acid to stearic acid by mixed cultures of pure strains of rumen bacteria. *J Gen Microbiol.* 130, 527-533.

Kemp, P., White, R.W. & Lander, D.J. (1975). The hydrogenation of unsaturated fatty acids by five bacterial isolates from the sheep rumen, including a new species. *J Gen Microbiol* 90: 100-114.

Kepler, C. R. & Tove, S. B. (1967). Biohydrogenation of unsaturated fatty acids. *J Biol Chem* 242: 5686-5692.

Kepler, C. R., Hirons, K. P., McNeill, J. J. & Tove, S. B. (1966). Biohydrogenation of unsaturated fatty acids. *J Biol. Chem* 241: 1350-1354.

Kim, Y. J., Liu, R. H., Rychlik, J. L. & Russell, J. B. (2002). The enrichment of a ruminal bacterium (*Megasphaera elsdenii* YJ-4) that produces the trans-10, cis-12 isomer of conjugated linoleic acid. *J Appl Microbiol* 92 : 976-982.

Klopfenstein, T. J., Purser, D. B. and Tyznik, W. J. (1966). Effects of defaunation on feed digestibility, rumen metabolism and blood metabolites. *J. Anim. Sci.* 25: 765-773.

Knight, T. W., Knowles, S. and Death, A F. (2003). Factors affecting the variation in fatty acid concentrations in lean-eef from grass-fed cattle in New Zealand and the implications for human health. *New Zealand J. Agrl. Res.* 46: 83-95.

Kraft, J., Collomb, M., Mackel, P., Sieber, R. and Jahreis, G. (2003). Differences in CLA isomer distribution of cow's milk lipids. *Lipids*, 38: 657-664.

Kraft, J., Kramer, J.KG., Schoene, F., Chambers, J.R. and Jahreis, G. (2008). Extensive analysis of long-chain IJOlyunsaturated fatty acids, CLA, trans-18: 1 isomers, and plasmalogenic lipids in different retail beef types. *J. Agric. Food Chem.* 56: 4775-4782.

Kritchevsky, D. (2000). Antimutagenic and some other effect of conjugated linoleic acid. *Br J Nutr.* 83: 459-465.

Latham, M.J., Storry, J.E. and Sharpe, M.E. (1972). Effect of low-roughage diets on the microflora and lipid metabolism in the rumen. *Appl. Microbiol.* 24: 871-877.

Lee, K.N., Kritchevsky, D. and Pariza, M.W. (1994). Conjugated linoleic acid and atherosclerosis in rabbits. *Atherosclerosis*, 108: 19-25.

Li, X.Z. Long, R.J. Yan, C.G., Choi S.H, Jin, G.L. Song M.K. (2010). Rumen microbial responses in fermentation characteristics and production of CLA and methane to linoleic acid in associated with malate or fumarate. *Anim. Feed Sci. Technol* 155: 132-139.

Lock, A.L. and Garnsworthy, P.C. (2003). Seasonal variation in milk conjugated linoleic acid and delta 9-desaturase activity in dairy cows. *Liv. Prod. Sci.* 79: 47-59.

Lock, A.L., Corl, B.A., Barbano, D.M., Bauman D.E. and Clement I.P. (2004). The anticarcinogenic effect of trans-11 18:1 is dependent on its conversion to cis-9, trans-11 CLA by Ä9-desaturase in rats. *J. Nutr.* 134: 2698-2704.

Loor, J.J., Hoove, W.H., Miller -Webster, T.J., Herbien, J.H., and Polan, C.E. (2003). Biohydrogenation of unsaturated fatty acids in continuous culture fermenters during digestion of orchardgrass or red clover with three levels of ground corn supplementation. *J. Anim. Sci.* 81: 1611-1627.

Loor, J.J., Bandara, A.B.P.A. and Herbein, J.H. (2002). Characterization of 18: 1 and 18:2 isomers produced microbial biohydrogenation of unsaturated fatty acids from canola and soya bean oil in the rumen of lactating cows. *J. Anim. Physiol. Anim. Nut.* 86: 422-432.

McKain, N., Chaudhary, L.C., Walker, N.D., Pizette, F., Koppova, I., McEwana, N.R., Kopecny, J., Vercoe, P.E. and Wallace, R.J. (2004). Relation between phylogenetic position and fatty acid metabolism of different Butyrivibrio isolates from the rumen. *Reprod. Nutr. Dev.* 44 (suppl.1): S 64.

Pariza, M.W. (2004). Perspective on the safety and effectiveness of conjugated linoleic acid. *Am. J. Clin. Nutr.* 79: 1132S-1136S.

Polan, C. E., McNeill, J. J. & Tove, S. B. (1964). Biohydrogenation of unsaturated fatty acids by rumen bacteria. *J. Bacteriol* 88: 1056-1064.

Raes, K., DeSmet, S. and Demeyer, D. (2004). Effect of dietary fatty acids on incorporation of long chCQil polyunsaturated fatty acids and conjugated linoleic acid in lamb, beef and pork meat: a review. *Anim. Feed Sci. Technol.* 113: 199-221.

Roche, H.M., Noone, E., Sewter, C., Mc Bennett, S., Savage, D., Gibney, M.J., O'Rahilly, S. and Vidal-Puig, A.J. (2002). Isomer-dependent metabolic effects of conjugated linoleic acid: insights from molecular markers sterol regulatory element-binding protein. *Diabetes*, 51: 2037-2044.

Sehat, M., Yurawecz, M.P., Roach, J. E. G., Mossoba, M. M., Kramer, J. K. G., and Ku, Y. (1998). Silver-ion high-performance liquid hromatographic separation and identification of conjugated linoleic acid isomers. *Lipids*. 33: 217-222.

Soressa M. Kitessa, S.A., Andrew Williams, A., Gulati, S., Boghossian, V., Reynolds, J., Pearce, K. I. (2009). Influence of duration of supplementation with ruminally protected linseed oil on the fatty acid composition of feedlot lambs. *Anim. Feed Sci. Technol.* 151: 228–239.

Tsuboyama-Kasaoka, N., Takahashi, M., Tanemura, K., Kim, H.J., Tange, T., Okuyama, H., Kasai, M., Ikemoto, S. and Ezaki, O. (2000). Conjugated linoleic acid supplementation reduces adipose tissue by apoptosis and develops lipodystrophy in mice. *Diabetes*, 49: 1534-1542.

Tyagi A.K., Kewalramani,N., Dhiman,T.R., Kaur, H., Singhal, K.K. and.Kanawajia, S.K. (2006). Conjugated linoleic acid content of milk and milk products from buffaloes fed different fat sources. *Indian J. Anim. Sci.* 76: 742-746.

Tyagi,A., Saluja, M., Kathirvalen, C. and Singhal, K.K. (2008). Enhancement of conjugated linoleic acid and vitamin A and E contents in goat milk through green fodder feeding. *Int. J. Dairy Technol.* 61: 1-8.

van de Vossenberg, J.L. & Joblin, K.N. (2003). Biohydrogenation of C18 unsaturated fatty acids to stearic acid by a strain of *Butyrivibrio hungatei* from the bovine rumen. Lett *Appl Microbiol* 37: 424-428.

Wallace, R.J., Chaudhary, L.C., McKain, N. and Walker, N.D. (2004). Ruminal bacteria on an Atkins diet: metabolic properties of *Eubacterium pyruvativorans. Reprod. Nutr. Dev.* 44 (suppl.1): S82.

Wallace, R.J., L.C. Chaudhary, N. McKain, N.R. McEwan, A.J. Richardson, P.E. Vercoe, N.D. Walker and D. Paillard. (2006). Clostridium proteoclasticum: a ruminal bacterium that forms stearic acid from linoleic acid. *FEMS Microbiol. Lett.* 265: 195-201.

Wang, J.H., Zhu, B.W., Song, M.K. & Choi, Y.J. (2005). Effect of monensin, fish oil or their combination on in vitro fermentation and conjugated linoleic acid (CLA) production by ruminal bacteria. *Anim Feed Sci Technol* 120: 341-349.

West, D.B., Blohm, F.Y., Truett, A.A. and DeLany, J.P. (2000). Conjugated linoleic acid persistently increases total energy expenditure in AKR/J mice without increasing uncoupling protein gene expression. *J. Nutr.* 30: 2471-2477.

Whigham, L.D., Cook, M. E. & Atkinson, R.L. (2000). Conjugated linoleic acid: implications for human health. *Pharmacol. Res.* 42: 503-510.

□□□

28

Emerging Zoonoses and Pathogens of Public Health Significance - An Overview

SANJAY SHAKYA*, K.C.P. SINGH AND SMITA**
*Professor & Head, Department of Veterinary Public Health & Epidemiology
**Dean, College of Veterinary Science & A.H., Anjora, Durg (Chhattisgarh)

Introduction

There has been a remarkable progress in the prevention, control and even eradication of infectious diseases with improved hygiene and development of antimicrobials and vaccines. However, infectious diseases still remain a leading cause of global disease burden with high morbidity and mortality especially in the developing world. Furthermore, there have been threats of new diseases during the past three decades due to the evolution and adaptation of microbes and the re-emergence of old diseases due to the development of antimicrobial resistance and the capacity to spread to new geographic areas. The impact of the emerging and re-emerging diseases in India has been tremendous at socioeconomic and public health levels (Chug 2008). A number of examples from various parts of the world (cutaneous zoonotic leishmaniasis in Manaus, Brazil; Ebola, monkeypox, Rift Valley fever in Africa and the Arabic Peninsula; Crimea Congo haemorrhagic fever in the Middle East; BSE in Europe and the rest of the world; West Nile fever in the United States of America and Canada; paramyxoviruses in Australasia) demonstrate that a wide variety of animal species, both domesticated and wild, act as reservoirs for these pathogens, which may be viruses, bacteria or parasites. These infections have clearly shown that new zoonoses are emerging in both the developed and the developing world. The Office International des Epizooties (OIE) defines an emerging disease as a new infection resulting from the evolution or change of an existing pathogenic agent, a known infection spreading to a new geographic area or population, or a previously unrecognized pathogenic agent or disease diagnosed for the first time (OIE 2004). Emerging and re-emerging zoonoses are infectious diseases that are newly recognized or are newly evolved, or have occurred previously but have more recently shown an increase in incidence or expansion into a new geographic, host or vector range (Bengis *et al.*, 2004).

There are many factors that can lead to the emergence of zoonotic diseases. For example, microbiological factors associated with the agent, the animal hosts/reservoirs and the human victims can result in a new variant of a pathogen that can jump the species barrier. Environmental changes resulting from environmental degradation, human and animal demography, changes in farming densities and practices, including climatic variations and change, can also play a major role. Social, behavioral and cultural risk factors such as food habits, religious beliefs, risk perception and management patterns can also encourage the emergence of zoonoses, as can economic factors such as economic growth or economic hardship. Several of these examples underline the importance of the anthropogenic risk factors for zoonoses emergence. Their capacity to occur very unexpectedly in new places and new animal species underscores the need for stronger international cooperation in ensuring better local, regional and global networks for communicable disease surveillance, which must be integrated across the human and animal health sectors. The major emerging zoonoses reported are listed below.

1. Influenza

The 2009 flu pandemic was an influenza pandemic, and the second of the two pandemics involving H1N1 influenza virus (the first of them was the 1918 flu pandemic), albeit in a new version. First described in April 2009, the virus appeared to be a new strain of H1N1 which resulted when a previous triple reassortment of bird, swine and human flu viruses further combined with a Eurasian pig flu virus, leading to the term "swine flu" to be used for this pandemic. Unlike most strains of influenza, H1N1 does not disproportionately infect adults older than 60 years; this was an unusual and characteristic feature of the H1N1 pandemic. Even in the case of previously very healthy persons, a small percentage will develop pneumonia or acute respiratory distress syndrome. This manifests itself as increased breathing difficulty and typically occurs 3-6 days after initial onset of flu symptoms. Initially coined an "outbreak", the stint began in the state of Veracruz, Mexico, with evidence that there had been an ongoing epidemic for months before it was officially recognized as such. The Mexican government closed most of

Mexico City's public and private facilities in an attempt to contain the spread of the virus; however, it continued to spread globally, and clinics in some areas were overwhelmed by infected people. In June, the World Health Organization (WHO) and US Centers for Disease Control (CDC) stopped counting cases and declared the outbreak a pandemic. (Margret,2009)

The pandemic began to taper off in November 2009, and by May 2010, the number of cases was in steep decline. On 10 August 2010, the Director-General of the World Health Organization, announced the end of the H1N1 pandemic,(WHO,2010) and announced that the H1N1 influenza event has moved into the post-pandemic period. According to the latest WHO statistics (July 2010), the virus has killed more than 18,000 people since it appeared in April 2009, however they state that the total mortality (including deaths unconfirmed or unreported) from the H1N1 strain is "unquestionably higher". Critics claimed the WHO had exaggerated the danger, spreading "fear and confusion" rather than "immediate information". The WHO began an investigation to determine whether it had "frightened people unnecessarily". A flu followup study done in September 2010 found that "the risk of most serious complications was not elevated in adults or children."

2009 flu pandemic in India is the outbreak of swine flu in various parts of India. Soon after the outbreak of H1N1 virus in the United States and Mexico in March, the Government of India started screening people coming from the affected countries at airports for swine flu symptoms. The first case of the flu in India was found on the Hyderabad airport on 13 May, when a man traveling from US to India was found H1N1 positive. Subsequently, more confirmed cases were reported and as the rate of transmission of the flu increased in the beginning of August, with the first death due to swine flu in India in Pune, panic began to spread. The first death was a 14-year-old girl. On 8th and 9 August a 43-year-old man in Ahmedabad, Gujarat, a 42-year-old teacher in Pune and a 53-year-old woman in Mumbai died. On August 10 a 53-year-old doctor in Pune and a 4-year-old in Chennai died. On august 11th a 7-year-old girl in Vadodara, Gujarat died. On August 13, a 26-year-old woman became Bangalore's first victim of swine flu. An eleven-month-old boy, a 75-year-old woman and a 37 year old woman died taking the toll in Pune, severely hit by the virus, to 15 and across the country, to 24.A lady having a young daughter of 5 yrs died near Mumbai in Khopoli on August 14. On August 16, three people died at different hospitals in Bangalore, according to the reports As of March 12, 2010, 1404 confirmed deaths from H1N1 influenza have been reported, and at least 29,904 laboratory-confirmed cases of H1N1 have been reported.

2. SARS

Nearly three years ago, the world experienced another newly emerging microbe – a previously unknown coronavirus – that caused severe acute respiratory syndrome (SARS). Fortunately, the morbidity and mortality associated with the SARS outbreak were not as great as what we observe every year with influenza. The SARS outbreak turned out to be a classic study in epidemiology with regard to tracking the point source, the spread, and the containment. SARS first appeared in Guangdong Province in China. It was not reported to authorities until it emerged in Hong Kong, when an index case, who traveled from Guangdong to Hong Kong, stayed at the Metropole hotel and infected at least 14 people. Those individuals did some traveling throughout the world. Within months anepidemic that temporarily transfixed the world and did extraordinary economic damage in Canada, China, and Hong Kong, and other countries. There were 8,098 reported cases and 774 deaths. SARS taught us an important lesson. Academic scientists, public health officials, and pharmaceutical companies acted together in a way that was unprecedented, leading to the development of promising vaccine candidates in record time. The new microbe was identified in March 2003 and was rapidly sequenced; a vaccine was developed by the following March. In December 2004, a clinical trial of the SARS vaccine began. This likely was the fastest time frame in the history of biomedical research from the identification of a previously unknown microbe to the beginning of a clinical trial. Such rapid progress could not have occurred 30 to 40 years ago. Thus, as microbes continue to emerge, we continue to develop technological advances that will, hopefully, keep us one step ahead of our microbial foes.(Anthony,2005)

3. Buffalopox

Buffalopox is an important contagious viral malady of buffaloes of all ages, occurring in epidemic proportions in countries including India, where buffaloes are reared. The Joint Expert Committee on Zoonosis declared buffalopox as one of the important zoonotic diseases. The committee also emphasized that the mode of transmission of buffalopox to human subjects and other epidemiological features appear similar to cowpox (Singh *et al.*, 2007). Human beings including smallpox-vaccinees contract infection upon close contact with buffalopox virus infected animals, but the extent of disease is greater in non-immunized individuals. The appearance of gross lesions in human beings maintaining close proximity with pox-affected buffaloes, attendants and milkers has been reported from time to time. The lesions are mainly confined to the hands, forehead, face, buttocks and legs. Occasionally, lymphadenopathy has also been recorded. Human-to-human transmission has not been reported. However, after detailed analysis of a 1996 buffalopox outbreak in Maharashtra, opined that (i) the detection of antibodies in 70% of in-contact persons and 17% of individuals who had no history of contact either with infected buffaloes or humans is a public health concern, (ii) the detection of antibodies in these humans could be an indication of subclinical infection which might lead to exposure of the general population to BPXV, and (iii) the virus, after repeated passage in humans, may acquire virulence as is evident from the comparison of BPXV strains of the Maharashtra outbreak and the reference strain (BP4) isolated 40 years ago. Milking of affected animals is one of the major modes of spread. Accordingly, 28% of milkers were affected, including children aged 8 and 11 years, in a Dhulia district outbreak in 1976. This led to a detailed survey of 30 families (n=240; milkmen: 56; morbid: 36) having buffalopox cases in six villages, in which buffalopox attacks had affected up to 69.7% of the milkmen. It was further noted that out of 39 persons who developed lesions, 23% had primary vaccination while 64.1% had both primary and booster vaccination.

4. Plague

Plague is an ancient disease which caused three pandemics since the 6th century but the global transmission has been low in recent years. It is a bacterial zoonosis with rodents being the principle reservoir. The black rat (*Rattus rattus*) and oriental rat flea (*Xenopsylla cheopis*) are notorious reservoir and transmitting agent for human plague in India. The changes in rodent ecology has been identified as the risk factor for reemergence of plague. It has caused 12 million deaths in India since the first recorded case in 1896 in Bombay . After the last laboratory-confirmed case was reported in 1966 in Karnataka, there was a lull for almost three decades till two outbreaks were reported during August-October in 1994, an outbreak of pneumonic plague in Surat, Gujarat and the second outbreak of bubonic plague in Beed, Maharashtra. There were a total of 54 deaths (52 in Surat) and 876 seropositive cases; 596 in Maharashtra, 151 in Gujarat, 68 in Delhi, 50 in Karnataka, 10 in Uttar Pradesh and 1 in Madhya Pradesh. An outbreak of16 confirmed cases of pneumonic plague seen during 2002in Himachal Pradesh. A previous outbreak of 22 similar but unconfirmed cases was reported in this region during 1983. An outbreak of bubonic plague was reported in Uttaranchal in 2004. The control measures require early clinical suspicion, prompt laboratory diagnosis, strict isolation of patients of pneumonic plague, appropriate antibiotic therapy and case contact management. A vaccine is available for persons who have repeated contact with the pathogen. The best plague prevention strategy is an aggressive rodent population control.

5. Leptospirosis

Leptospirosis is an emerging global public health problem. The disease is caused by *Leptospira interrogans* naturally seen in rodents. These parasitise kidneys and are excreted in rat urine. Man and cattle are incidental hosts. They get infected by contact with water or soil contaminated with rat urine. The farm workers, sewer workers, fishermen and miners are at high risk of infection. Due to difficult laboratory diagnosis and a lack of awareness, the real magnitude of the disease remains unknown. International Leptospirosis Society conducted three recent worldwide surveys and estimate about half a million severe cases of the disease worldwide annually. The disease was first described in Andaman Islands, India in 1931. They reported 60 cases confirmed by serology and isolated the causative agent in 26. The 1980s witnessed a sudden increase in leptospirosis and seroepidemiologic and clinical studies show that the disease is endemic in Andaman Islands and southern states of India. The seroprevalence is reported to be high (52.7%) among high-risk population of these Islands and 19.8% and 9.3% in Madras and Bangalore respectively. *L interrogans* serovar valbuzzi of serogroup Grippolyphosa is the causative agent in human patients and rodents. Outbreaks were reported from Mysore, Gujarat, Nagpur and Andamans in 1997. There was a severe outbreak in Mumbai in May 2000 and Kerala in August 2000, causing significant mortality. An outbreak of leptospirosis was also reported in 102 cases in Mumbai following prolonged water logging due to heavy rainfall during July, 2002. Leptospirosis is widespread in animals in other regions as well- West Bengal, Bihar, Punjab, Haryana and Andhra Pradesh and has been reported to be a common cause of acute renal failure in southIndia (WHO 2006).

6. Brucellosis

Brucellosis affects primarily the livestock and is transmitted to humans by ingestion, close contact, inhalation or accidental inoculation. The prevalence of brucellosis in different geographical areas varies with standards of personal and environmental hygiene, animal husbandry practices, species of the causative agent and local methods of food processing. *Brucella melitensis* is the prevalent species seen in man and causes a more severe form of disease. Dogs are carriers of *Brucella canis* which can be transmitted to humans.India has an enormous cattle wealth. The disease has been repeatedly reported in the animals in India. However, very few human studies have been undertaken. It is estimated that the true incidence is 25 times higher than the reported cases due to under diagnosis. Seroprevalence of 17.39% in field veterinarians and abattoir workers has been reported (Thakur and Thapliyal, 2002). Seropositive cases were seen in 28 of 414 (7.0%) patients of pyrexia of unknown origin (PUO) in Varanasi (Sen *et al* 2002) and 28 of 3532 (0.8%) patients of PUO in Kashmir (Kadri *et al* 2000). The studies clearly show a high prevalence of the disease in various parts of India (Smits and Kadri 2005). Vaccination with *B. abortus* 19BA, and hygienic measures can protect the persons who are at occupational risk.

7. Foodborne and Waterborne Diseases

Foodborne microbial diseases account for 20 million cases annually in the world and their incidence is increasing. Nearly half of all known foodborne pathogens have been discovered during the past 25 years.

a) Enterohaemorrhagic Escherichia coli

It causes no signs of illness in its natural host, cattle and sheep, but has a low infectious dose in humans where it causes haemorrhagic colitis and haemolytic uraemic syndrome. It was first described in 1982 associated with consumption of undercooked beef. Ground beef is the most common vehicle for its transmission but can occur in vegetarian and non-beefeating communities, through exposure to fruits, vegetables or water contaminated by bovine or infected human feces. The manure-contaminated irrigation was the source of the largest recorded outbreak affecting more than 7000 children who had consumed contaminated sprouts in Japan. Isolation of Enterohaemorrhagic *Escherichia coli* (EHEC) in beef, cattle stools and in human patients of diarrhoea have been reported in India. Non-O157 EHEC were reported in 1.4% of stools from cases of bloody diarrhoea in Kolkata (Ministry of Health and Welfare 2006). EHEC O157 sorbitol phenotype have been isolated from the Ganges River, Varanasi.The detection of potentially pathogenic O157:H7 in river water is alarming. Some antibiotics enhance EHEC toxin production and induce verotoxin-phages which enhance environmental stability.

b) Vibrio cholera

Cholera is one of the oldest recorded infectious diseases. John Snow first demonstrated the spread of disease by infected water; Pacini in 1854, first described comma shaped bacteria in intestinal contents of cases of cholera and Robert Koch in 1883, showed that cholera was caused by these bacilli, *V cholerae*. The first six pandemics of cholera originated in Bengal and occurred between 1817 to 1923 and the seventh pandemic started in 1961 in Indonesia. These spread to southeast Asia, Middle East, East Africa, Europe and Americas. The last decade of the 20th century witnessed a sharp increase in the global re-emergence of cholera. In September 1992, *V. cholera* O139 Bengal (the first non-O1) appeared in south India. This spread to the rest of India and Bangladesh. Subsequent outbreaks due to this organism were reported in Nepal, Pakistan, southeast Asian countries and Japan. Some cases were also reported on the west coast of the United States, England, Germany and Switzerland. The genome of *V. cholerae* is in a state of constant flux, resulting in the reemergence and displacement of serotypes Inaba and Ogawa. The conversion of Ogawa to Inaba serotype occurs at a rate of 10–5 due to mutation in the gene and *in vivo* selection due to immune response during the course of clinical disease.

c) Listeria monocytogenes

Listerosis is an emerging zoonotic disease. It is estimated that *L. monocytogenes* is responsible for 28% deaths due to foodborne illnesses in the United States. The organism is unbiquitous and inherently robust and can thus survive food-processing and refrigeration of contaminated meat and dairy products. Carriage of the pathogen has been reported in feces and genital tract of 5-10% humans. There has been a significant decline in the disease in countries where active surveillance and sale of dairy products and meat have been regulated. In India, very few studies have been done. In 1970s, scientists reported *L monocytogenes* in cervical secretions of 1.3-3% of cases with bad obstetrical history but none of the 125 samples of cerebrospinal fluid obtained from cases of meningitis were positive.

d) Campylobacter spp

Campylobacter spp. are significant zoonotic poultry pathogens and are the leading cause of bacterial gastroenteritis in the world. Poultry carrying the organism remain healthy carriers and transmit by fecal shedding.Around 2.5 million human infections are reported annually in the United States. The disease is more common in children and there is an emergence of fluorquinolone resistance. In developing countries it is reported in childhood diarrhea involving *C. jejuni* in 13.5% of the diarrhoea patients which was more frequent than combined *Salmonella* and *Shigella* infections (4.3%; $P < 0.001$).

8. Drug-resistant Bacteria

Antimicrobial resistance (AMR) in hospitals and community poses a public health problem. The fecal flora and upper respiratory tract commensals constitute the reservoir for resistant genes. Increased travel and movement of food-stuffs are risks for the spread of resistant genes. The existence of multiresistant clones of common pathogens has been identified. *Staphylococcus aureus* is a devastating human pathogen and is now the most frequently identified drug-resistant pathogen. The prevalence of methicillin resistant *S aureus* (MRSA) has been on the increase and varies in different hospitals in India. More recently community-acquired MRSA outbreaks have been reported (lineage USA 400 MW2 and USA 300). Emergence of vancomycin intermediate resistant *S. aureus* (VISA), vancomycin resistant *S. aureus* (VRSA) and vancomycin resistant enterococci (VRE) has led to clinical failures of glycopeptides. The usefulness of penicillin in the management of gonorrhoea is increasingly compromised due to emergence of penicillinase-producing gonococci (PPNG) and chromosomally mediated resistance (CMRNG). Meningococci have repeatedly caused outbreaks and the disease is endemic in Delhi, Haryana, Uttar Pradesh, Rajasthan, Chandigarh, Jammu and Kashmir and West Bengal. Serogroup A has been the causative agent in most cases. It carries a mortality of ~10% and another 11-19%develop sequelae. The organism developed resistance to sulphonamides during 1950s and 1960s. Reduced penicillin susceptibility (MIC >0.25 mg/l) due to altered PBP2 and plasmid-mediated β-lactamase production with consequent treatment failures and higher rates of complications have been reported. Sulphadiazine resistance was reported in an outbreak in Delhi in 1985-6. A study of 96 culture positive cases from Punjab reported all isolates sensitive to penicillin, chloramphenicol, ampicillin and sulphadiazine. In an outbreak in Delhi in early 2005, all isolates were susceptible to penicillin, ampicillin, rifampicin and ceftriaxone. However, all were resistant to cotrimoxazole and two-thirds were non-susceptible to ciprofl oxacin.

Enteric fever is endemic in India. It is under diagnosed due to lack of culture facilities and poor sensitivity and specificity of Widal test. Resistance of *Salmonella typhi* and *S. paratyphi A* to chloramphenicol, ampicillin and cotrimoxazole is widespread. Low level fluorquinolone resistance is now common and leads to treatment failures and higher incidence of relapses. The growing AMR in *Shigella* isolates is worrying as resistance to azithromycin, ceftriaxone and ciprofloxacin has been on the increase. The emergence and high prevalence of extended-spectrum β-lactamases, Amp C β-lactamase and carbapenemases in the hospitals and the community in enteric bacteria and nonfermenters is a cause of concern. These have spread in humans, food-producing- animals and domestic pets. It is estimated that two-thirds of the global antibiotic production is used in animal husbandry for growth-promotion non-therapeutic purposes. The overuse of antibiotics selects the drug-resistant zoonotic pathogens. Humans get exposed to them through meat, vegetables and water contaminated by animal waste.

9. Melioidosis

There is a growing evidence that the disease is an emerging global problem. The causative pathogen, *Burkholderia pseudomallei,* is an environmental saprophyte in rice paddies, wet soil, mud and pooled surface water. It causes suppurative chronic infection characterized by septicemia and focal abscesses in liver, spleen and other viscera. The disease has been documented from Tamilnadu and Karnataka. Lack of adequate healthcare facilities in rural population, low index of clinical suspicion and nonavailability of diagnostic tests probably contribute to the paucity of reports from the Indian subcontinent. Indians may be at a greater risk of disease than Malays and Chinese. The association of the disease with diabetes mellitus is high. The disease in India has been reviewed by Vidyalakshmi *et al.* (2007). The first culture-proven case in India was a child in Maharashtra in 1990. Isolated cases have been reported from Orissa, Assam, West Bengal and Andhra Pradesh. A series of culture-proven 28 patients collected during Dec 1993 to Dec 2002 in Vellore (Jesudason *et al.* 2003) and a cluster of 25 cases during a span of only 14 months from June 2005 to July 2006 in Mangalore have been reported. Given environmental conditions and a large pool of diabetics in India, there is probably an underestimate of the disease.

10. Chronic and Neoplastic Diseases

A number of chronic and neoplastic diseases are now associated with microbial infections. It is estimated that approximately 1 in 6 of all human malignancies are related to microbial agents, the most significant being gastric and hepatocellular carcinoma and cervical cancer. There is a possibility of development and use of vaccines to prevent hepatitis B, human papilloma virus and *Helicobacter pylori* infections. The seroprevalence rate in children varies up to 50%, increases slowly and steadily to ~ 90% in the young adults and remains constant in later years. It has been implicated in the causation of peptic ulcers, gastric carcinoma, lymphoma, bile duct cancer and even vascular disease. The high prevalence of resistance to metronidazole, clarithromycin and amoxicillin has led to failure of eradication of *H. pylori* infection. The resistance shows geographic variation being higher in south than north India. There is also a high rate of reinfections in Indian subjects (60%). There is a global evidence that persistent infection with *Chlamydia pneumoniae* is associated with pathogenesis of coronary artery disease. There have been serological, molecular, immunohistological and electron microscopic studies from India to show its association with coronary artery disease in patients with and without conventional risk factors and patients with calcifi cation in coronary artery atherosclerosis

Risk Factors for the Emergence of Zoonotic Diseases

i. Microbiological risk factors

In the past century, pandemic outbreaks of influenza and AIDS have cost the lives of tens of millions of people. These events were all caused by multiple introductions of animal viruses, influenza A viruses and SIV of birds and non-human primates respectively - into the human population. Besides these introductions causing major pandemics in humans, a large number of other virus infections have spilled over from animal reservoirs to humans or other susceptible species, resulting in considerable morbidity and mortality as "virgin soil" epidemics. The most recent examples in humans are the introduction of SARS coronavirus and influenza A viruses from the animal world, which caused global concern about their potential to be at the origin of new pandemics. Over the last decades there seems to be a dramatic increase in the emergence or re-emergence of virus threats in humans and animals worldwide. A long list of exotic names like Ebola, Lassa, Rift-Valley, Crimea-Congo, Hendra, Nipah and West-Nile is the illustration of names of just some of the places associated with the origin of viruses that crossed the species boundary to humans, with dramatic consequences in the last ten years alone. Similarly, recent mass mortalities among wild aquatic and terrestrial mammals caused by previously known and newly discovered morbiliviruses, as well as outbreaks of hog cholera, foot-and-mouth disease and fowl plague among domestic animals, highlight this trend. Although improved detection and surveillance techniques, as well as increased media attention may have contributed to our perception of an increase in the incidence of outbreaks of virus infections, it is becoming more and more clear that major changes in our modern society increasingly create new opportunities for virus infections to emerge: a complex mix of changes in social environments, medical and agricultural technologies and ecosystems continues to create new niches for viruses to cross species boundaries and to rapidly adapt to new species. In combating this global threat, we should make optimal use of the new tools provided by the unprecedented advances made in the research areas of molecular biology, epidemiology, genomics and bioinformatics. Serious investment in these areas in the future will not only be highly cost-effective but will also save many lives of humans and animals (WHO, 2004).

ii. Environmental, climatic risk factors

Disease ecology, defined as the interplay between pathogens, hosts and environment, including also anthropogenic factors, may hold important clues to the understanding of disease emergence. Disease emergence may be viewed as an evolutionary response to novel environments. Understanding this process requires that we identify the links between environmental change, new forms of disease and microbial adaptation. A strong link between pathogen biology and epidemiological pattern is found for most OIE List A + B diseases. This List has remained curiously static throughout most of the 20th century despite dynamic farming systems, erosion of the genetic diversity of farm animals, and major animal disease control campaigns. Microbial responses to environmental change in animal agriculture and related food chains does result in the generation of new pathogen species but mainly so when placed in a larger timeframe, spanning across centuries or millennia In the short to medium term we mainly distinguish within species adjustments. Animal disease emergence mostly concerns increase in disease incidence, invasion into new areas or changes in the host range, rather than a novel disease agent appearing for the first time. It follows that the analysis of disease emergence may benefit from methods used to study the ecology of invasion. Successful vertebrate invaders are known to rapidly disperse, showing high reproduction rates. Colonisers are flexible, competitive, and fit a broad range of conditions. This compares to the list of pathogens associated with the emergence of zoonotic diseases, counting a relatively high number of small RNA viruses with high mutation rates. We must understand that how disease agents in farm animals may turn either more aggressive or milder depending on the changing conditions in the animal production environment. Ecology may also explain disease seasonality and annual cycles of retraction and expansion, as driven by climatic and geographical factors. In this regard, the phylogeography of pathogens, any prevailing vectors and host animals, coupled with information on the local livestock production structure and landscape mosaic may constitute the basic elements explaining epidemiological patterns in a given area of interest. Climate change alters vector distribution and abundance, migration patterns of birds and other wildlife, and the survival time of pathogens outside the host. In fact, climate change–perhaps more than any other factor – is likely to contribute to the emergence of novel forms of disease and pathogens. A further area of interest is the accelerated livestock production in areas where protein demand increases on an exponential scale. This trend is particularly pronounced in East and Southern Asia and coincides with the development of megacities around which largescale, industrial-type poultry and pig production units develop to secure local supplies of meat and eggs. The contraction and concentration of production in mainly peri-urban environments forms a major risk factor in disease emergence particularly when viewed in conjunction with the centrifugal demographic force causing more widespread and denser rural populations in some Asian countries. Demography, land pressure, economic development and agricultural intensification are all intertwined and may result in imbalances in livestock production structure, both in terms of the distribution of holding sizes as well as in geospatial terms. This translates into a most heterogeneous risk landscape and it may be argued that this development has contributed to the emergence of the 2003/2004 H5N1 HPAI epidemic in Asia.

"Global change" is increasingly used as collective noun for a wide array of issues believed to contribute to disease emergence in humans. The problem here is that the analysis of risk factors at this aggregate level is not always sensible. Still, it remains that the combination of factors such as globalization, increase in trade and traffic, geography, economic and biotechnological developments, urbanization, land use, climate change, and the "livestock revolution" form causal links with the reported increases in the spread of transboundary animal diseases, food safety hazards and other veterinary public health risks. When UN Agencies advocate that the issue of emerging zoonotic diseases is a matter of growing importance, one particular area of concern may be highlighted: the structure of the livestock industry in the Old World. While the Green Revolution enabled crop productivity increases commensurate with the rapid demand for cereals as staple food, livestock sector developments appear less balanced, at least in geographical terms. Bulk volumes of feed are increasingly moved to areas of high demand. With the disconnection of the "land-feedanimal production-processing-distribution" circuitry, it turns out that the highest density of intensive animal farms is now in the proximity of urban centres. Global pork production becomes retracted to a few hotspots. The EU-25 and East Asia increasingly form global epicentres for monogastric production. The ruminant street stretching from South Asia towards the Middle East, Horn of Africa and eastern Mediterranean will count an ever-increasing number of sheep, goats, cattle and buffaloes. In epidemiological terms this transect presents a gradient in disease occurrence from full endemicity for most OIE List A + B diseases in India and Pakistan and also the Horn of Africa, to disease freedom in southern European Mediterranean. Disease ecology shows that disease spread and the emergence of zoonotics are largely the product of human activity and, therefore, of human choices.

iii. Social, behavioural and cultural risk factors

In the field of epidemiology, anthropology is everywhere and nowhere. Everywhere, because most diseases need some behavioural factors in order to be transmitted. Even ecological changes in very remote areas, like the greenhouse effect, can be related to an anthropogenic origin. Nowhere, because anthropologists are rarely included in teams involved in emerging diseases studies, and because epidemiologists sometimes believe that they are able to practice anthropology by themselves. However, anthropology requires specialist training and specific tools that cannot be overlooked. Fortunately, the involvement of anthropologists is increasing, as illustrated by the recent Ebola outbreaks in Central Africa, where professional medical anthropologists could be present with virologists during the epidemics. The perspective they brought was useful at every level of the disease, from corpse management to prevention.

Though the concept of emergent disease is recent, it has long been known from historical sources that in the past transmissible diseases have been able to surge suddenly, and to disappear just as suddenly. The real new diseases, as well as re-emerging ones, are many, and no stereotypical anthropological approach can be used, as each agent has its specific mode of transmission.

This mode is often referred to as the natural history of the germ, but it also encompasses much cultural component. In the emergence process of viral infections, several stages occur:

1. accidental event (ancient or recent), like a mutation or a recombination in pre-existing zoonotic viruses,
2. breakage of the species barrier, and a first human infection,
3. phase of amplification (epidemisation) among humans (directly or through a vector),
4. identification of the disease,
5. representation of the disease, of its nature, origins and consequences,
6. strategy of elimination or prevention.

At each stage, behaviour and social factors are more and more involved, and therefore the role of anthropology has increasing weight.

iv. Economic risk factors and impacts

The economic impacts of zoonoses (and their control) include (i) reduction in the level of outputs from animal production (lower productivity), (ii) reduction in (perceived or actual) output quality (e.g. food safety), (iii) waste of inputs to animal production (e.g. feed), (iv) resource costs of disease prevention and control, (v) negative animal welfare effects, (vi) international trade restrictions, (vii) human health costs (human life and quality of life, treatment costs, loss in productive output etc.) and (viii) a range of other possible impacts such as effects on the environment, tourism and rural livelihoods. Some examples of these impacts are given in relation to zoonotic diseases, in particular Bovine Spongiform Encephalopathy (BSE). The concept of optimal disease control is presented using the 'lossexpenditure frontier', where the total costs associated with a disease are minimized. The economic risks associated with emerging zoonoses relate to the potential magnitude of the economic impacts. The problem with the decision-making process concerning emerging zoonoses is that (to greater or lesser extents) it is usually characterised by (i) lack of information on the disease in terms of rates of infection and the links between animal and human cases of the disease (BSE is a prime example of this), (ii) high levels of risk in that these diseases may potentially result in very high economic impacts (e.g. resulting from pandemics of high animal and/or human mortality), (iii) given (i), a high level of uncertainty in that the probabilities of different disease/economic outcomes are unsure (including the effect of disease control measures).

There are a number of economic factors that are likely to have increased the risks faced from emerging zoonoses. These include the increasing demand for animal products (especially in lower/middle income countries experiencing relatively high income growth), the increasing competitiveness of global markets and the drive for low cost production, the intensification of animal production with larger flock/herd sizes, increased trade liberalization and the increased movement of animals and people globally.

Assessment of the economic impacts of emerging zoonoses prior to choice of disease control strategy would be useful information for the response decision-making process.

Prevention and Control of Emerging Zoonotic Diseases

There are a number of control methods and tools currently available at the animal reservoir, vector and human levels that are appropriate for the prevention and control of emerging zoonotic diseases.

a) Domestic animals

For domestic animals, the common methods and tools used in disease control includes vaccination of pets or livestock (e.g. as for rabies control), prophylactic use of antiparasitics (e.g . antitrypanosomals or coccidiostats), proper biosecurity and quarantine (e.g. excluding wildlife from domestic stock, hygienic practices in husbandry and among farm workers), eradication programmes (depopulation), appropriate veterinary care, proper herd health programmes. Other such methods include may be breeding for disease resistance, feed and water control, using best animal husbandry practices, routine disease surveillance, testing animals before entering or leaving a farm.

b) Wild animals

There is currently no international organization dedicated to monitoring, reporting and studying wild animal health on a global scale. International conservation organizations such as the World Conservation Union and other international wildlife organizations should be more involved in the coordinated research as well as the current monitoring, and reporting of wildlife-related health issues to public health authorities. Disease surveillance and control in wild animals should take into consideration a number of conservation issues, particularly the conservation status of the species under investigation. Various methods and tools may be undertaken after careful evaluation of the species involved and its ecology. There include isolating and creating of physical barriers to exclude wild animals from farms or human residences, population control by culling, treating and vaccinating defined populations (e.g. oral rabies vaccination of foxes), limiting wildlife movement, conducting preliminary testing of all live import and exports, exercising care in adopting and translocating wild animals.

c) Vector control

Vector control is an effective tool in the prevention and control of vector-borne zoonotic diseases, for example by, spraying against fleas and mosquitoes during plague and Rift Valley fever outbreaks, respectively; and using tick control in outbreaks of Crimean Congo haemorrhagic fever and Lyme disease. Other effective methods involve environmental management through elimination of vector breeding habitats as well as limiting anthropogenic activities that promote vector breeding, such as land-clearing, unplanned development and the destruction of habitats that support vector predators.

Partnership between animal and public health for control of emerging zoonoses

Veterinary Public Health (VPH) is that component of public health activities devoted to the application of professional veterinary skills, knowledge and resources to the protection and improvement of human health. This includes a wide variety of veterinary involvement in different geographical areas depending on the health and wealth status of such area (WHO, 2004). VPH is dedicated to quality assurance systems using monitoring and surveillance throughout food production chains. It is clear that modern Veterinary Public Health is oriented towards healthy feed – healthy animals – healthy food – healthy humans. It is interesting to note that the ten top successes in the 20th century public health effects have for more than 50% largely been influenced by veterinary sciences. An under estimated area is the preventive measures that may be taken to prevent or control emerging zoonoses. As long as not sufficient data are available about potential emerging zoonoses or even zoonoses at large in terms of social impact, economic costs or disability adjusted life years (DALY'S) the issue will never arrive at the political agenda. There are sufficient examples to suggest that preventive programmes to control zoonotic diseases are considerably contributing to public health at lower costs as compared to letting the actual disease burden get along and treat the patients (e.g. brucellosis, tuberculosis). The contribution of veterinarians to existing public health systems is again dependent on the developmental stage. In third world countries with remote medical and veterinary health centers, if at all existing, it should be reconsidered to link human and animal systems ("one medicine" concept). In western world it should be normal to include veterinarians in community health centers as experts in zoonotic prevention, environmental health, food and water safety issues. In the modern industrialized countries veterinary and medical monitoring and surveillance systems should be linked and data used by either party. Effective communication between public health officials and the general public is vital to controlling zoonotic disease, particularly when human-to-human transmission is involved (e.g. SARS or Nipah virus infection). Important areas of public education include health education, promotion of personal hygiene and sanitary practices, use of physical barriers such as mosquito bednets and insecticide-treated screens, and hygienic food handling. In such areas "life expectancy" will be changed in "health expectancy", where veterinary skills are widely used in collective prevention programmes.

Future Concerns on Emergence of Zoonotic Diseases

The important zoonotic diseases and zoonotic agents in the region includes influenza, rabies, Japanese encephalitis, Hanta virus, echinococcosis, cysticercosis, leptospiroisis, Nipah virus (henipaviruses), schistosomiasis. The risk factor for these diseases are well known. Various problems have been encountered by authorities to control them. Various challenges for these are as follows-

Avian influenza

- Biocontainment of large-scale poultry farms
- Monitoring the health status of animals
- Early detection and notification

Rabies

- Domestic dog population control
- Compulsory vaccination of all dogs
- Public awareness and education

Japanese encephalitis

- Integrated vector control
- Vaccination of high-risk human populations.

Echinococcosis

- Proper management of slaughterhouses and meat markets
- Treatment of dogs with antiparasitics
- Public awareness of personal hygiene practices

Cysticercosis

- Strict inspection of pork
- Proper management of slaughterhouses and meat markets
- Public awareness of food safety (need for thorough cooking of pork) and personal hygiene
- Practices (toilet use, hand-washing)

Leptospirosis

- Rodent control
- Proper agriculture practices (e.g. wearing boots)
- Appropriateness of vaccination for high-risk groups

Nipah virus (henipaviruses)

- Education and awareness of flying foxes as a reservoir and potential source of infection,
- Improve sanitary and hygienic practices (e.g. wash fruit and hands before eating)
- Separation of pig farms from orchards and rainforest habitats
- Biosecurity measures and improve herd health practices on large-scale farms

Schistosomiasis

- Proper management of irrigation systems
- Community case detection and mass treatment
- Understanding the role of domesticated animals and wildlife as reservoir hosts

Infrastructural adjustments conducive to surveillance and monitoring for the emergence of zoonoses can be facilitated. Several actions can be taken at the regional level aimed at improving surveillance, prevention and control of zoonoses. Research efforts should be supported on impact of environmental changes and climatic variability on the emergence of microbes. This cannot be achieved unless there is a national plan to strengthen health system and health research systems including human resource development. Adequate finances would need to be allocated to build and sustain appropriate infrastructure. In October 2007, the Government of India has created a new Department of Health Research (DHR) within the Ministry of Health and Family Welfare, Setting up of this new Department is a reflection of Government's intent of moving research to centre stage of health development. Amongst the allocation of business of this Department is to provide technical support for dealing with epidemics and investigation of outbreaks due to new and exotic agents and development of tools for prevention (Kant, 2008). This step is likely to give authority, direction, and boost to health research in this area. It is expected that DHR would play a conductor's role in orchestrating an effective health research response involving all players in emerging infectious diseases. A chain of laboratories with appropriate biosafety would need to be set up rapidly so that new and exotic agents can be handled confidently without posing threat to people and the environment. The centres of excellence within various Ministries, Departments, Universities, research institutions in the country would need to be networked with strong linkages, based on mutual trust, confidence and respect. It would make more economic sense to share rather than duplicate cost intensive infrastructure.

References

Anthony S. Fauci (2005). Robert H. Ebert Memorial Lecture-Emerging and Re-emerging Infectious Diseases:The Perpetual Challenge. Milbank Memorial Fund ,645 Madison Avenue New York, NY 10022.

Bengis, R.C., Leighton, F.A., Fischer, J.r., Artois, M., Morner, T. and Tate, C.M. (2004). The role of wildlife in emerging and re-emerging zoonoses. *Rev. Sci. Tech. Off. Int. Epiz.* 23(2):497-511.

Chan, Margaret (2009). "World now at the start of 2009 influenza pandemic". World Health Organization. http://www.who.int/mediacentre/news/statements/2009/h1n1_pandemic_phase6_20090611/en/index.html.

Chug, T.D. (2008). Emerging and reemerging bacterial diseases in India. *J. Bio. Sci.* (4): 549-555.

http://www.themedguru.com/20100312/newsfeature/swine-flu-claims-3-more-lives-india-toll-1404-86132777.html

Jesudason M V, Anbarasu A and John T J (2003). Septicemic melioidosis in a tertiary care hospital in south India; *Indian J.Med. Res.* 117: 119–121.

Kumar A, Kanungo R, Bhattacharya S, Badrinath S, Dutta T K and Swaminathan R P (2000). Human anthrax in India: urgent need for effective prevention; *J. Commun. Dis.* 32: 240–246.

Lalit Kant (2008). Combating emerging infectious diseases in India : Orchestrating a symphony. *J. Bio. Sci.* 33(4):425-427.

Ministry of Health and Family Welfare (2006). Food safety India: *Escherichia coli* O157:H7 *http://foodsafetyindia.nic.in/ecolitaq.Htm.*

OIE, (2004). General definitions. Chpater 1.1.1. Terrestrial Animal Health Code, 13th edn. Office International des Epizooties. Paris, 3-11.

Sarada D, Valentina G O and Lalitha M K (1999). Cutaneous anthrax involving the eyelids; *Indian J. Med. Microbiol.* 17: 92–95.

Singh, R.K., Hosamani, M., Balamurugan, V., Bhanuprakash, V., Rasool, J.J. and Yadav, M.P. (2007). Buffalopox : an emerging and re-emerging zoonosis. *Animal Health Research Review* 8(1):105-114.

Tenguria, R.K., Khan, F.N., Quereshi, F. and Pandey, A. (2011). Epidemiiological study of zoonotic tuberculosis complex (ZTBC) *World J. of Sci. & Tech.* 1(3):31-56.

Thakur S D and Thapliyal D C (2002). Seroprevalence of brucellosis in man; *J. Commun. Dis.* 34: 106–109.

Vidyalakshmi K, Shrikala B, Bharathi B and Suchitra U (2007). Melioidosis: an underdiagnosed entity in western coastal India: A clinico-microbiological analysis; *Indian J. Med. Microbiol.* 25: 245–248.

WHO (2004). Report of WHO/FAO/OIE joint consultation on emerging zoonotic diseases Geneva, Switzerland.

WHO/Europe (2010). WHO Director-General declares H1N1 pandemic over". http://www.euro.who.int/en/what-we-do/health-topics/communicable-diseases/influenza/news2/news/2010/08/who-director-general-declares-h1n1-pandemic-over.

World Health Organisation (2006). *Zoonotic diseases of public health importance* (Zoonotic Division, National Institute of Communicable Diseases, New Delhi, India) pp. 34–46.

□□□

29

Feeding of Genetically Modified Crops in Poultry

PRAVEEN KUMAR TYAGI, A.V. ELANGOVAN*, A.B. MANDAL AND A.K. SHRIVASTAV
Central Avian Research Institute, Izatnagar-243 122
* National Institute of Animal Nutrition & Physiology, Bangalore

Introduction

The introduction of genetically modified crops in 1996 for herbicide tolerance has consistently been the dominant trait followed by insect resistance. The number of countries growing biotech crops has increased from 6 in 1996, the first year of commercialization, to 18 in 2003 and 25 in 2008. The top eight countries growing more than one million hectares of biotech crops are; USA (62.5 million hectares), Argentina (21.0), Brazil (15.8), India (7.6), Canada (7.6), China (3.8), Paraguay (2.7), and South Africa (1.8 million hectares). In 2008, 5 million small farmers planted 7.6 million hectares of Bt cotton as cotton being the major biotech crop in India (www.isaaa.org). The major importance of GM crops is their capability to contribute to: 1) Increasing crop productivity; 2) Land-saving technology capable; 3) More efficient use of external inputs: 4) Increasing stability of production and 5) to improve the economic and social benefits.

A transgenic plant is produced by introducing artificially a gene or genes into the plant's genetic makeup using recombinant DNA (rDNA) technology. The inserted genes, trans-genes may come from another plant of the same or a different species, or a completely unrelated kind of organism like bacteria or animals and serves to regulate how they function is also transferred into the host plant. In the similar line, Bt maize and Bt cotton are the most common one developed. The first commercial crop of insect protected field corn hybrids that utilized the "Bt" genetic modification, designated as "Event 176", occurred in 1996. Bt maize varieties may contain a gene from a bacterium (*Bacillus thuringiensis*) found in the soil that causes the transgenic corn to produce an insecticidal protein. The gene being transferred may have its genetic code altered to modify its function, in addition to having different regulatory sequences spliced on to control how it is expressed (switched on or off) in the plant.

Most of these crops are used directly as animal feed such as maize, rice, sorghum etc. or as their byproducts from the processing industries such as meals, bran, cakes, distiller grain, etc. Thus there is need for nutritional and safety assessment of feeds from GMO in origin. The safety and nutritional studies with feeds from GM crops in origin have been reviewed (Aumaitre *et al.* 2002, Chesson and Flachowsky 2003, Clark and Ipharraguerre, 2001 and Flachowsky et al, 2005a, 2007). The different nutritional parameters such as digestibility, feed intake, health and performance of target animal species as well as effects on the quality of food of animal origin were studied. Reproduction was also considered in special studies carried out with quails and laying hens.

Transgenic Maize

Transgenic maize for commercial production currently confers either insect resistance (Bt) or herbicide tolerance (glufosinate) or a combination of these traits. The introduction of transgenic maize is for increase in maize production. The maize line DLL25 (B16) was developed by genetically engineering to express tolerance to glufosinate ammonium, the active ingredient in phosphinothricin herbicides. Glufosinate acts like glutamate, the molecule used by glutamine synthetase to make glutamine, that it blocks the enzyme's usual activity and is also involved in ammonia detoxification. The glufosinate reduces glutamine levels and increases the ammonia concentrations in plant tissues, leading to cell membrane disruption and cessation of photosynthesis resulting in plant withering and death. Glufosinate tolerance results from introduction of a gene encoding the enzyme phosphinothricin-N-acetyltransferase (PAT) isolated from actinomycete, Streptomyces hygroscopicus and it catalyzes the acetylation of phosphinothricin, detoxifying it into an inactive compound. The PAT encoding gene (bar) is introduced into the genome by micro-particle acceleration (biolistic) transformation with the maize line developed having field tolerance to phosphinothricin-containing herbicides, thereby to use this herbicide for weed control in maize cultivation. The animal experiments with

Bt-maize were carried out with beef cattle, sheep, growing and finishing pigs, laying hens, broilers as well as growing and laying quails.

Table 1 : Chemical composition of maize (Reuter et al., 2002a)

Chemical composition, g/kg	Isogenic	Transgenic
Crude protein	115.9	110.6
Ether extract	23.3	23.7
Crude fibre	22.7	20.1
N-free-extracts	824.6	831.4
Starch	720.1	733.5
Lysine	2.6	2.8
Methionine	1.9	1.8
Threonine	4.1	3.9

Table 2 : Chemical composition of Maize (Aulrich *et al.*, 2001)

Chemical composition, g/kg	Isogenic	Transgenic
Crude protein	108.1	98.2
Crude ash	14.6	15.9
Ether extract	54.4	55.9
N-free extracts	800.2	804.6
Starch	709.9	707.8
Total NSP	62.1	64.3
Arabinose	15.0	15.3
Xylose	19.8	20.4
Glucose	19.3	20.3

Transgenic maize and chicken performance

Chesson and Flachowsky (2003) reviewed the use of transgenic plants in poultry nutrition. The nutrient composition of Bt maize fell within the range of variability for the relevant nutrients reported for normal maize (Table 1 & 2). Many studies in poultry were conducted with various lines of insect resistant (Bt) maize and glyphosate-resistant maize and soybeans at incorporation levels (50 to 78% maize or 27% soybean) in broiler and layer diet failed to show differences of any consequence in various production parameters monitored between parental or near isogenic lines. Taylor et al. (2003) studied the broiler performance, when fed diet containing grain from different GM maize varieties (Roundup Ready maize or Roundup Ready maize mixed with insect resistant MON810 maize), non-transgenic or commercial maize and observed similar growth performance in broiler chicken. However,

Piva et al. (2001) observed a higher live weight gain in the broiler fed diet contained insect resistant GM maize (MON810) compared to the control conventional maize group fed diet and they suggested that lower mycotoxin content in the GM maize compared to the conventional maize might have been the reason. The results of the study of Tony *et al.* (2003) showed that there were no significant differences (P>0.05) detected concerning feed intake, digestibility, body weight gain and other performance parameters due to feeding of 740 g iso- or transgenic maize/kg. Egg production performance at the age of 23–30 weeks and hatchability for isogenic or Bt-maize at 500 g maize/kg diet) were not significantly influenced in a 4-generation study with laying hens (Halle et al., 2006). The haematological and biochemical parameters were found to be within physiological range with no significant changes on feeding of genetically modified maize hybrid MON 810, which contains a gene for the insecticide protein Cry1A(b), and a conventional non-modified hybrid (Øehout et al., 2009). The comparison of various studies involving transgenic and isogenic feed ingredients in chicken have been presented in Table 3.

Table 3 : Comparison of transgenic and isogenic feed ingredients in chicken

Transgenic Feed Ingredient	Chemical composition	Performance of broiler / layer	Source
Bt Maize	Similar	Similar	Mireles et al., 2000; Aeschbacher et al., 2001; Aulrich et al., 2001; Gaines et al., 2001; Taylor et al., 2001a; Tony et al., 2003; Halle et al 2006
Bt Maize	Similar	FCR improved in BT group	Brake and Vlachos, 1998
Bt Maize	Similar	Higher gain in BT group	Piva et al., 2001
Herbicide tolerant Maize	Similar	Similar	Sidhu et al., 2000
Herbicide tolerant soybean meal	Similar	Similar	Hammond et al., 1996
Bt Cotton	Similar	Similar	Elangovan et al., 2002; Mandal et al., 2004; Elangovan et al., 2006
Bt Potato	Similar	Similar	Halle et al., 2005
Bt Brinjal	Similar	Similar	Shrivastava et al., 2006
Bt Rice	Similar	Similar	Tyagi et al., 2011
Bt Corn	Similar	Similar	Tyagi et al., 2011

Quails performance and Bt Maize

A series of experiments were conducted (Halle *et al.* 2004, Flachowsky *et al.* 2005b, Halle *et al.* 2006) in quails and hens using genetically modified maize (Bt 176). The results concluded that the feeding of diet containing genetically modified maize (Bt 176) to quails over 10 generations (10 X 12 weeks) and to hens for 4 generations (4 X 31 weeks) did not influence animal health, feed intake, feed efficiency, laying performance, hatchability and quality of meat or eggs.

Fate of ingested maize DNA

Factors of major interest include tracking "foreign" DNA in the animal body if GMO are fed, observing animal health and investigating the quality of foods of animal origin. It has been reported that maize DNA can resist in the gastrointestinal tract without much degradation or absorption and excreted via the faecal matter (Reuter and Aulrich, 2003). Feed-ingested DNA is partially resistant to the mechanical and enzymatic activities of the GIT and is not completely degraded suggesting that the absorption of functional large size DNA is low. The foreign DNA may not be incorporated into host cells beyond the use of the basic nucleotide building blocks as nutrients especially in organs responsible for metabolism as liver and kidney and these will be disappear by time as a normal disposal mechanism. These are in line with those of Doerfler *et al.* (1997) and Beever and Phipps (2001) who reported that the GM construct can be detected in the digestive tract and it resist the mechanism of digestion comparable as DNA derived from isogenic maize.

Laube et al. (2003) reported the blood and tissue samples gave negative results with both maize specific and Bt specific primer-probe-systems. However, in the blood, pectoral and thigh muscles, liver, spleen and kidney samples from trials, the plant DNA fragments (chloroplast gene fragments) were successfully amplified in the samples collected at 0h and 4h after feed withdrawal. Further, no more plant DNA amplification showed in the blood and tissue samples collected at 24h after the last feeding (No amplification after PCR).

However, no residues of recombinant DNA were detected in any organ, milk and eggs obtained from animals fed with feeds containing GMP (Einspanier, *et al.*, 2001, Reuter and Aulrich, 2003, Tony *et al.*, 2003, Flachowsky *et al.*, 2005b, El Sanhoty, 2004, Aulrich *et al.* 2002, Broll *et al.*, 2005).

Quality protein maize

Maize is also an important component of livestock feed especially in developed nations where more than 50% of total maize production goes into livestock feed. The nutritional profile of maize is poor as it is deficient in essential amino acids such as lysine, tryptophan and methionine due to a relatively higher proportion of prolamines in maize storage proteins which are essentially devoid of lysine and tryptophan. One such hybrid commodity cereal, quality protein maize (QPM, Shaktiman-1, white coloured variety), developed in India by Directorate of Maize Research, Pusa, New Delhi by incorporating *opaque*-2 gene into the normal maize by conventional breeding methods which improves the nutritional quality of the maize by increasing the contents of two essential amino acids–lysine and tryptophan. A study was undertaken by Tyagi *et al.* (2007; 2008) to determine whether this QPM had any unexpected effects on poultry as a result of compositional changes in the grain that may have altered its nutritional value before its commercial exploitation as poultry feed. The commercial and quality protein maize samples were analysed to contain crude protein-8.97 and 8.67%, respectively and the amino acid contents indicated the lysine content of QPM to be 0.33%, which was about 57% higher than commercial maize (0.21%). The growth performance of broiler chicks fed diets containing commercial or quality maize with respect to body weight gain, feed intake, feed conversion efficiency, carass quality and protein and energy utilization efficiency did not differ significantly. The results of the layer experiment indicated that although the feeds intake and egg production of the laying hens fed QPM diet increased numerically, it did not differ significantly from the commercial maize based diet. The dietary treatment has no significant effects on egg weight, FCR and egg quality. The overall results of the study indicated that the apparent metabolizable energy (AME) and feeding value of quality protein maize for growing broilers (Tyagi et al, and laying hens were found similar to commercial maize.

Bt-potatoes and Chicken Performance

Two genetically modified lines (Cry5-Bt gene, Bt-potatoes) and a non-genetically modified control line from *Solanum tuberosum* L., var. Spunta, were tested for feeding to broiler chicken (Halle *et al.*, 2005) and observed that the composition of the diets, feed intake, body weight and feed conversion were not significantly affected by the potato line.

Bt cotton

The BT cotton hybrid genetically implanted with a gene drawn from certain soil bacteria (*Bacillus thuringiensis* or BT is capable of resisting the damage from cotton bollworms and all pests of insect family called Lepidoptera. The larval stage of the insect(s) attacks the bolls and when the BT_protein (contained in the gene of plant tissue) is ingested, it sticks to the gut (throat) of the larva and the gut wall breaks down making it impossible to feed. In BT cotton, damage to bolls is minimized and need for insect sprays against the bollworm too are greatly reduced, saving the farmer from use of costly poisonous chemicals. There are no adverse impacts on other (non target) insect pests and so sucking pests of cotton, which attack in early stages, have to be managed as usual. This also means that the BT cotton does not kill non-target beneficial fauna. There is no difference in allergenic potential between BT and non-BT cotton entries also. BT cotton is raised along with few rows of the same hybrid not implanted with BT gene - called non-BT or Refuge Rows - a strategy claimed to prevent resistance building up in the target insects against the toxic principle of BT (Badrinarayanan, 2002).

Bt cotton and chicken performance

Three experiments were conducted at Central Avian Research Institute, Bareilly on Bt cotton feeding to broiler chicken sponsored by Maharashtra Hybrid Seeds Company Ltd. (Mahyco), Mumbai and J.K. Agri Genetics Ltd., Hyderabad. In the first experiment conducted by our group (Elangovan *et al.*, 2002), Bt (Mahyco), parental non-Bt and commercially produced solvent-extracted CSM with low free gossypol levels (<0.02% in meal) was tested at 100 g/kg in a maize-soybean meal based broiler diet replacing SBM and rice bran without additional iron. The second study was carried out to evaluate the nutritional value of diets containing meals of MRC 6301 Bollgard (BG) II F2 hybrid cotton containing Cry-X gene (Cry1Ac and Cry2Ab gene), parental (MRC 6301Non-BG II F2) and commercial lines (NHH 44 F2) of cotton supplied by Mahyco (Mandal *et al.*, 2004). In the third study was to evaluate transgenic Bt cotton hybrid seeds (JKC-738 from J.K.Agri Genetics Ltd., Hyderabad, India) resistant to Lepidopteron insect pests by transforming with Bt-Cry1Ac gene (truncated version) of *Bacillus thuringiensis* on broiler chicken performance, mortality, blood biochemicals and carcass characteristics. (Elangovan *et al.*, 2006). The chemical composition between Bt and non Bt lines were similar with low gossypol content (Table 4 & 5). The growth performance in terms of body weight gain, feed intake and feed conversion efficiency, did not differ significantly either at starting (0-4 wks) or overall (0-7 wks) phases. The carcass traits, blood biochemicals, nutrient utilization as well immune parameters remained statistically similar due to various dietary treatments.

Table 4 : Proximate composition (%) of Cotton seed meal

	CP	EE	CF	Ash	NFE
BT CSM	34.40	0.91	11.12	5.32	48.25
Non BT CSM	33.18	0.50	12.65	5.06	48.61
Comm. CSM	35.17	0.77	16.65	5.07	42.34

Table 5 : Protein and Gossypol content (%) of cotton seed and meal

	Protein		Gossypol, total		Gossypol, free	
	Seeds	CSM	Seeds	CSM	Seeds	CSM
BT Cotton	27.1	34.40	1.23	0.74	1.14	0.02
Non BT Cotton	25.2	33.18	1.52	0.58	1.39	0.02
Comm. Cotton	-	35.17	-	0.72	-	0.03

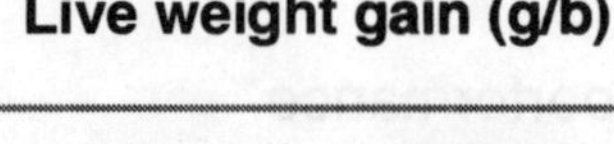

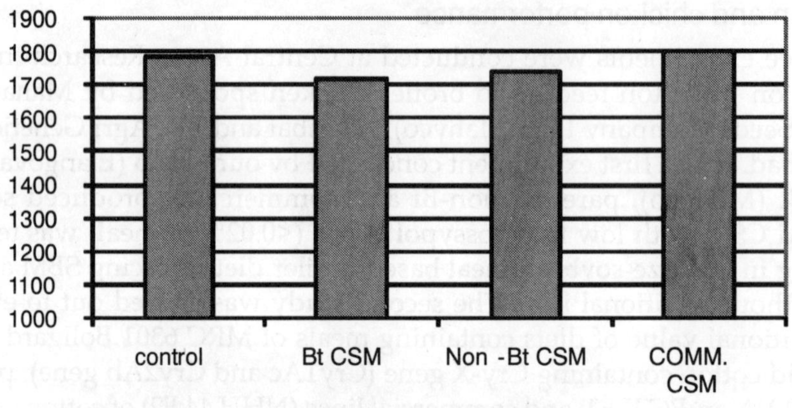

Fig. 1 : Growth performance of broiler fed Bt cotton

Bt Brinjal

Brinjal is one of the most common, popular and principal vegetable crops grown in India. It is very versatile crop adapted to different agro-climatic regions and is grown throughout the year in the country. Damage by insect pests is a major problem in brinjal production in India. The fruit and shoot borer, *Leucinodes orbonalis* (Guen.) (EFSB) is regarded as one of its major insect pest, which attacks all the stages of brinjal crop. In view of this, the Bt brinjal plant developed contains insect resistant *cry1Ac* gene derived from the naturally occurring soil bacterium, *Bacillus thuringiensis* subsp. *kurstaki* (*B.t. k.*) and produces an insect resistant Cry1Ac protein. The Cry1Ac protein produced in Bt brinjal is nearly identical in structure and activity to that found in nature and in commercial *B.t.k.* microbial formulations.

Bt brinjal and chicken performance

Brinjal is not a conventional feed ingredient for poultry and thus there is no literature available on the feeding of Bt or non-Bt brinjal to chicken. A study sponsored by Mayco, Mumbai was conducted at Central Avian Research

Institute, Bareilly in broiler chickens, being model laboratory birds, for bio-safety study including growth performance, nutrient utilization and certain welfare parameters (Shrivastava *et at.*, 2005). The results indicated that addition of dried meals of commercial (non- genetically modified), parental non-Bt and Bt brinjals either at 5% or 10% levels in iso-caloric diets adjusted with all micro-nutrients including amino acids did not exert any adverse effect on growth performance, feed utilization, palatability of feed, blood constituents, humoral and cellular immunity of broiler chickens. The study envisaged that transgenic Bt brinjal is a moderate energy rich feedstuff, which can safely be incorporated up to 10% level in maize-soy based broiler ration.

Table 6 : Chemical composition (%) of transgenic and isogenic Brinjal

Treatments	CP	EE	CF	TA	AIA	Ca	P	Na	K
Commercial	19.32	4.270	19.148	7.052	0.237	0.329	0.350	0.11	2.46
Non Bt	19.34	5.376	17.142	7.272	0.487	0.297	0.329	0.03	2.80
Bt	19.27	5.019	17.909	6.97	0.234	0.283	0.374	0.07	2.95

Table 7 : Amino acid content of Bt brinjal

Amino acid	% of CP
Methionine	1.16
Cystine	1.21
Lysine	3.88
Threonine	2.84
Arginine	4.65
Isolucine	3.28
Leucine	5.27
Valine	3.95
Hisdidine	1.85
Phenylalanine	3.26
Glycine	3.55
Serine	3.30
Proline	5.51
Alanine	3.71
Aspartic acid	9.42
Glutamic acid	11.60

Conclusions

The chemical analyses and performance studies in ruminants, pigs, chicken and quails with genetically modified maize, potatoes, sugar beets and soybeans, demonstrate no significant differences between feeds from transgenic plants of the first generation and their isogenic counterpart. GMP of the second generation is characterized by increased contents of desirable substances (amino acids, vitamins, fatty acids, minerals, enzymes); decreased contents of undesirable substances (mycotoxins, alkaloids, glucosinolates, lignin, phytate) (Flachowshky and Bohme, 2005, Flachowshky *et al.*, 2007). For these GMP crops, feeding studies with the main target species is the most important requisite.

The genetic manipulation has produced a number of new transgenic varieties of commodity crops with desirable features, such as protection against common pests, tolerance to herbicides, and improved nutritional quality characteristics. Trials with poultry, catfish, swine, cattle and sheep have demonstrated that feeds derived from transgenic crop plants are equivalent to conventional crops in safety and feed value. Commercial formulations of such Bt-based products have been registered for use on food crops in the US since 1961. However, questions regarding the digestive fate of DNA and protein from transgenic plants have been raised in regard to human consumption and trade of animal products e.g., meat, milk, and eggs from animals fed transgenic crops. In addition to feed safety assessment, including safety for consumers, animals and environment, nutritional assessment of feeds produced using recombinant DNA techniques is necessary and should be considered as an essential part of safety assessment.

References

Aeschbacher K., Messikommer R., Meile L., Wenke C. (2005). Bt176 corn in poultry nutrition: physiological characteristics and fate of recombinant plant DNA in chickens. *Poultry Sci.* 84: 385-394.

Aulrich, K., Reuter T. and Flachowsky, G. (2002). The fate of foreign DNA in farm animals fed with genetically modified plants, *Proc. Soc. Nutr. Physiol.* 11: 187–188.

Aulrich, K.., Böhme, H., Daenicke, R.,. Halle, I.. and Flachowsky, G. (2001). Genetically modified feeds in animal nutrition. 1st com.: *Bacillus thuringiensis* (Bt) corn in poultry, pig and ruminant nutrition, *Arch. Anim. Nutr.* 54: 183–195.

Aumaitre, A., Aulrich, K.., Chesson, A.., Flachowsky, G. and Piva, G. (2002). New feeds from genetically modified plants: substantial equivalence, nutritional equivalence, digestibility, and safety for animals and the food chain, *Livest. Prod. Sci.* 74: 223–238.

Badrinarayanan, P. (2002). BT cotton technology – Boon or bane. *Agriculture Today*, 38-40.

Beever, D. E., and R. H. Phipps. (2001). The fate of plant DNA and proteins in novel feeds for farm animals. Pages 67–75 in Proc. 24th Congr. Argen. Assoc. Anim. Prod., AAPA. Rafaela, Argentina.

Brake J, Vlachos D. (1998). Evaluation of transgenic event 176 "Bt" corn in broiler chickens. *Poult Sci* 77: 648–653.

Chesson, A. and G. Flachowsky. (2003). Transgenic plants in poultry nutrition. *World's Poultry Science Journal* 59: 201-208.

Doerfler, W. Schubbert R, Heller H, KŠmmer C, Hilger-Eversheim K, Knoblauch M. and Remus R. (1997). Integration of foreign DNA and its consequences in mammalian systems. *Trends in Biotechnology*, 312: 401-406.

El Sanhoty, R.M.E.S., (2004). Quality control for food produced by genetic engineering. Diss., TU Berlin, 155 pp.

Elangovan, A.V., Mandal, A.B. and Johri, T.S. (2002). Comparative Performance of Broilers Fed Diets Containing Processed Meals of BT, Parental Non-BT Line or Commercial Cotton Seeds. *Asian-Australasian Journal of Animal Sciences*, 16: 57-62.

Elangovan, A.V., Tyagi, Praveen K., Shrivastav A.K., Tyagi, Pramod K and Mandal, A.B. (2006). GMO (Bt-Cry1Ac gene) cottonseed meal is similar to non-GMO low free gossypol cottonseed meal for growth performance of broiler chickens. *Animal Feed Science and Technology*. 129: 252–263.

Flachowsky, G. and Böhme, H. (2005a). Proposals for nutritional assessments of feeds from genetically modified plants, *J. Anim. Feed Sci.* 14: 49–70.

Flachowsky, G., Aulrich, K., Böhme, H. and Halle, I. (2007). Studies on feeds from genetically modified plants (GMP) - Contributions to nutritional and safety assessment. *Animal Feed Science and Technology*. 133: 2-30.

Flachowsky, G., Chesson, A. and Aulrich, K. (2005b). Animal nutritional with feeds from genetically modified plants, *Arch. Anim. Nutr.* 59: 1–40.

Gaines A.M., Allee G.L., Ratliff B.W. (2001). Nutritional evaluation of Bt (MON810) and Roundup Ready® corn compared with commercial hybrids in broilers. *Poultry Sci.* 80, Suppl. 1, 51, Abstr. 214.

Halle, I., Aulrichm, K. and Flachowsky, G. (2006). Four generations feeding of GMO-corn to laying hens, *Proc. Soc. Nutr. Physiol.* 15: 114 Abstract.

Halle, I., K. Aulrich and G. Flachowsky, (2004). Four generations of feeding of GMO-corn to breeder quail. (Fütterung von gentechnisch verändertem Mais an Zuchtwachtein über vier Generationen). *Proc. Soc. Nutr. Physiol.* 13:124.

Halle, I., Sanhoty, R.M.E.S. El and Flachowsky, G. (2005). Nutritional assessment of GM-potatoes in broiler feeding, *Proc. Soc. Nutr. Physiol.* 14: 63 Abstract.

Hammond, B.G.; Vicini, J.L.; Hartnell, G.F.; Naylor, M.W.; Knight, C.D.; Robinson, E.H.; Fuchs, R.L. and Padgette, S.R. (1996). The feeding value of soybeans fed to rats, chickens, catfish and dairy cattle is not altered by genetic incorporation of glyphosate tolerance. *Journal of Nutrition*, 126: 717-727.

Laube, I., Spiegelberg, A., Butschke, A., Zagon, J., Schauzu, M., Kroh. and Broll, H. (2003). Methods for the detection of beef and pork in foods using real-time polymerase chain reaction. *Intr. J. Food Sci. and Technol.* 38: 111-118.

Mandal, A.B., Elangovan, A.V., Shrivastav, A.K., Johri, A.K., Kaur, Sarabmeet and Johri, T.S. (2004). Comparison of broiler chicken performance when fed diets containing meals of Bollgard-II Hybrid cotton containing Cry-X gene (Cry1Ac and Cry2Ab gene), parental line or commercial cotton. *British Poultry Science*, 45: 657-63.

Mireles Jr. A., Kim S., Thopson R., Amundsen B. (2000). GMO (Bt) corn is similar in composition and nutrient availability to broilers as non-GMO corn. *Poultry Sci.* 79, 65-66.

Piva, G., M. Morlacchini, A. Pietri, F. Rossi, and A. Prandini, (2001). Growth performance of broilers fed insect-protected (MON 810) or near isogenic control corn. *Poult. Sci.* 80(Suppl. 1):320. Abstract 1324.

Einspanier, R. Klotz, A. Kraft, J., Aulrich, K., Poser, R., Schwägele, F., Jahreis, G. and Flachowsky, G. (2001). The fate of forage plant DNA in farm animals: a collaborative case-study investigating cattle and chicken fed recombinant plant material, *Eur. Food Res. Technol.* 212: 129–134.

Øehout, V., Kadlec1, J., Èítek, J., Hradecká, E.., Hanusová, L., Hosnedlová, B. and Lád., F. (2009). The influence of genetically modified Bt maize MON 810 in feed mixtures on slaughter, haematological and biochemical indices of broiler chickens. *Journal of Animal and Feed Sciences*, 18: 490–498.

Reuter, T. and Aulrich, K. (2003). Investigations on genetically modified maize (Bt-maize) in pig nutrition: fate of feed ingested foreign DNA in pig bodies, *Eur. Food. Res. Technol.* 216: 185–192

Reuter, T. and K. Aulrich, (2003). Investigations on genetically modified maize (Bt-maize) in pig nutrition: Fate of feed ingested foreign DNA in pig bodies. *Eur. Food Res. Technol.* 216:185-192. DOI: 10.1007/s00217-002-0642-7.

Shrivastav A.K., Mandal, A.B., Elangovan A.V., Tyagi Praveen K. and. Tyagi Pramod K. (2005). Technical Bulletin of contract Research project on Impact of feeding insect resistant transgenic Bt brinjal on performance and health of broiler chickens sponsered by Maharashtra Hybrid Seeds Company Ltd. (Mahyco), Mumbai-400 020.

Sidhu, R.S. ; Hammond, B.G.; Fuchs, R.L. (2000). Glyphosate-tolerant corn: The composition and feeding value of grain from glyphosate-tolerant corn is equivalent to that of conventional corn (Zea mays L.). *J. Agri. Food Chem.* 48: 2305-2312.

Taylor, M.L., G.F. Hartnell, S.G. Riordan, M.A. Nemeth, K. Karunanandaa, B. George, and J.D. Astwood, (2003). Comparison of broiler performance when fed diets containing grain from Roundup ready (NK603), YieldGard x Roundup Ready (MON810 x NK603), non-transgenic control, or commercial corn. *Poultry Sci.* 82:443-453.

Tony, M.A., Butschke, A., Broll, A., Zagon, J., Halle, I., Dänicke, S., Schauzu, M., Hafes, H.M. and Flachowsky, G. (2003). Safety assessment of Bt 176 maize on broiler nutrition: degradation of maize-DNA and its metabolic fate, *Arch. Anim. Nutr.* 57: 235–252.

Tyagi, Pramod, K Shrivastav A. K., Mandal, A.B Tyagi and Praveen K. (2011). Evaluation of nutritional value of diets containing Bt. rice grains in broiler chickens. Technical Bulletin of Contract research project between CARI, Izatnagar and M/s Mahyco India Limited Mumbai.

Tyagi K Praveen, Shrivastav A. K., Mandal A. B., Tyagi, K Pramod., Elangovan, A. V. and Deo, C. (2008). The apparent metabolizable energy and feeding value of quality protein maize for broiler chicken. *Indian Journal of Poultry Science*. 43: 169-174.

Tyagi, K Praveen, Shrivastav A. K., Mandal, A.B Tyagi, Pramod K., and Elangovan A.V. (2007). Technical Bulletin "on Nutritional evaluation of quality protein maize for poultry" of Inter institutional collaborative research project between CARI, Izatnagar and Directorate of Maize Research, Pusa, New Delhi.

Tyagi, Praveen K., Shrivastav, A.K., Mandal A.B., Tyagi, Pramod, K, Elangovan, A.V. and Deo, C. (2008). The apparent metabolizable energy and feeding value of quality protein maize for broiler chicken. *Indian Journal of Poultry Science* 43: 169-74.

Tyagi, Praveen K., Shrivastav A.K., Mandal AB., Tyagi Pramod K. and Elangovan AV. (2010). The feeding value of quality protein maize is similar to commercial maize for egg production and quality traits in laying hens. *Indian Journal of Poultry Science*. 45:217-219.

Tyagi, Praveen, K Shrivastav A. K., Mandal, A.B Tyagi and Pramod K. (2011). Comparison of Chicken Performance When Fed Diets Containing MON 89034 x NK603 Corn. Technical Bulletin of Contract research project between CARI, Izatnagar and M/s Monsanto India Limited New Delhi.

□□□

30

Role of Herbal Nutraceuticals in Enhancing Growth Performance, Production & Reproduction in Animals

M.J. SAXENA, K. RAVIKANTH, ANUP KALRA AND SHIVI MAINI
Ayurvet Limited, Village Katha, P.O. Baddi-173 205 , Distt. Solan (H.P.)

Introduction

Ayurveda is the synthesis of Ayur- meaning 'life' and Veda meaning - 'knowledge'. It is the science of life emphasizing mainly on prevention of illnesses and maintenance of health. Health is a dynamic state of wellbeing characterized by a physical, mental and social potential, which satisfies the demands of a life commensurate with age, culture, and personal responsibility. Any deviation from dynamic state of internal milieu or homeostasis is disease. This term 'disease' includes sickness, illness, ill health, and malady. Health Index is directly proportional to optimum health of animal, higher productivity and maximizing profits to farmers, thereby. Ayurveda, the Science of Life, based on strong pillar of positive health, is a holistic approach to total healthcare by means of preventive & curative medicine to maintain complete internal-milieu (dhatusamaya), 'Homeo-stasis' or equilibrium of the various dhatus. It insists on the pro-host approach: "Strengthening the body defense system to fight infection". Ayurvedic therapies incorporate ingredients derived from plant origin. The plant materials have been scientifically evaluated to testify the ancient wisdom blended with modern scientific precision & technology validating their usage for animal & human health care to achieve health, wellness & maximum productivity from livestock. Emergence of the resistent pathogenic strains against antibiotics & deadly chemicals coupled with ever growing concerns of toxicity & environmental contamination has lead to scientific & technological advancement in last few decades, reviving the interest of modern scientist & health care practitioners in herbals. Relevence of science of Ayurveda, as applied to animal health, can be traced back to Mahabharata.

Plant Extracts (phytogenics)

Phytogenics are a group of natural growth promoters (NGPs) derived from herbs, spices or other parts of plants. They are commonly regarded as favorable alternatives to in-feed antibiotics in livestock production. Essential oils represent a concentrated form of phytogenics, containing mainly the active ingredients of the plants. In recent years, the forthcoming ban of in-feed antibiotics, which was implemented in Europe in January 2006, has driven research activities regarding the potential of plant extracts and essential oils as alternatives to antibiotic growth promoters. Plant extracts and/or their active components have shown a large scale of activities: as antimicrobials (phytobiotics), anti-oxidants, digestive stimulators, Immunomoulators, anti-inflammatory, micro flora modifiers, appetizers and performance enhancers (Laurence and Ionesçu, 2004) and are widely used as neutraceuticals for animals.

Potential of herbal nutraceuticals in nutrition on Animals

Animal Nutrition plays very important role in our day to day lives for our health. The same is true for Livestock. Rather it is more important since it directly linked with efficient reproduction & milk production. Any deviation in digestive, reproductive or udder health directly affects the production of animals.

Scientific feeding is aimed towards fulfilling the physiological needs of animals & that is where balanced cattle feeding & compound feeds play a significant role. The Herbaceuticals have been documented for improving the health & milk production when used along with proper feed. Ayurveda, the precious gift from Mother Nature is playing a significant role & likely to play greater role in future along with right nutrition. This would help in improving the overall health & welfare of the mankind. Bioactive molecules derived from nature and referred to as botanicals or herbs or phytogenics which have a history of medicinal use and animal feed applications. In recent years, the ban of in-feed antibiotics, which was implemented in Europe in January 2006, has driven research activities regarding the potential of plant extracts and essential oils as alternatives to antibiotic growth promoters. The potential benefits such as increased feed intake, stimulation of digestion and improved feed efficiency among others have therefore raised the interest among animal nutritionists. However, it is not only in recent years that there were ideas around phytogenics in animal feed. In 1993, Ayurvet Limited took the steps of developing phytogenic/herbal feed additives for animals. Now, 17 years later and backed up by research papers and trials, herbal feed additives are approaching a point where they are a standard ingredient or supplement in modern livestock ruminant and non-ruminant diets. Here we focus upon role of herbal feed additives in animal & poultry nutrition.

Role of Phytogenics and herbal feed additives

Feed additives depending on the specificity of function of additive improve the health, digestibility, productivity, product quality and immunity. It is scientifically established that inclusion of herbal feed additives to ration improves overall growth, performance and productivity of animals, enhances nutrient utilization and feed efficiency, possess immunopotentiating and antioxidant effect, improves gut microflora and also have antimicrobial activity.

Improves gut function

Improvement in gut function is mainly attributed to the possible stimulatory effect of phytogenic substances on digestive secretions, such as digestive enzymes, bile, and mucus. Phytogenic substances from certain herbs viz. *Aegle marmelos, Plantago ovata, Acacia catechu, Corriandrum sativum,* many more herbs and their extracts have also been shown to improve gut microflora and to exert pharmacologic actions within the digestive tract, as evidenced by their gut function modulating efficacy (Satyavati, and Gupta, 1987). Pathogenic bacteria are always present in the gut, but the balance between pathogenic and beneficial bacteria determines whether or not disease will occur. Maintaining a healthy balance between all microflora within the gut is known as eubiosis and can be influenced by bacteria endemic to the microflora (Kolte *et al.,* 2009). In the intestine, bacteria considered beneficial to the gut, including lactic acid forming bacteria like Lactobacillus spp, prevent proliferation of pathogens, such as Salmonella spp., through competitive exclusion for nutrients and for receptor sites on the gut wall. Beneficial bacteria can also produce an adverse environment for pathogenic bacteria to colonise and grow, for example, by the production of short-chain fatty acids which lower the pH and prevent growth of pH sensitive pathogenic bacteria (Kolte *et al.,* 2009). The microflora also have functions in the development of the digestive and immune tissue in the host animal, can produce nutrients that can be used by the host as a nutrient source and also can neutralize some feed toxins and promote an environment in the gut where anti-nutritional factors and toxins are minimised. In the past, manipulation of the microflora to create eubiosis has been achieved by the use of antibiotic feed additives. However, with the severe restriction of antibiotic feed additive use in the EU and increasing consumer concern, alternatives to antibiotic feed additives have been investigated and found to significantly influence this balance also.

Increases feed intake

The stimulatory effect of herbal feed additives on feed intake is due to the claimed improvement in palatability of the diet resulting from the enhanced flavor and odor. The addition of certain herbs viz. *Woodfordia fruticosa, Zingiber officinale, Allium sativum, Trigonella foenum graecum* etc. to poultry and pig ration is also known to improve feed efficiency (Satyavati and Gupta, 1987). Increased palatability of the diets associated with the addition of phytogenics also may be due to their anti-oxidative effects, which might contribute to preserving the desired organoleptic qualities of the diet.

Digestive tonic and growth promoter

Digestion is critical and plays important role in nutrient utilization in monogastrics and fermentation process in ruminants to produce volatile fatty acids and microbial proteins by the action of ruminal microflora. Role of ruminal microflora in digestion of nutrients is vital, so interactions of the normal microbial flora with the host can be manipulated to improve the efficiency of nutrient utilization (Waghmare *et al.*, 2009). Supplementation of certain herbs that have property to modulate the rumen function may be supplementated to animals for efficient cellulose breakdown & digestion, maintenance of normal ruminoreticular functon, intestinal movement, optimum utilization and absorption of nutrients, thus improving feed conversion ratio, productivity and body weight gain in animals. Ruchamax is a potent herbal formulation, which contains 28 different herbs and some minerals. The ingredients of Ruchamax include *Allium sativum, Azadirachta indica, Calotrophis orocera, Centratherum anthelmenticum, Commiphora mukul, Eclipta elba, Embelica ribes, Picorrhiza kurora, Zinziber officinale* and *Piper longum* etc. It is used as an appetizer, restorative, stomachic, digestive tonic & growth promoter product (Bhatt *et al.*, 2009 and Kolte *et al.*, 2009).

Hepato Efficiency Enhancers

Supplementation of certain liver tonic preparations also help to increase the secretion and flow of bile for better digestion and to treat anorexia by maintaining the liver parenchyma in healthy state and regulating liver functions like detoxification of metabolic products, toxic drugs and chemicals and treatment of hepatic dysfunction. The herbal ingredients such as Andrographis paniculata, Eclipta alba, Picrorhiza kurroa, Phyllanthus niruri,

Tephrosia purpurea, Tinospora cardifolia and Boerhavia diffusa (Superliv concentrate premix & Liquid) have been proved to improve feed conversion efficiency, body weight gain and reduce mortality in poultry and swine; owing to their Hepato-protective, Hepato-stimulants and growth promoting properties (Dwivedi *et al.*, 1986).

Another example of polyherbal liver tonic & growth promoter product for cattle is Yakrifit, comprising of herbs namely, *Andrographis paniculata, Eclipta alba, Picrorhiza kurroa, Phyllanthus niruri, Tephrosia purpurea, Tinospora cordifolia* and *Boerhaavia diffusa*, each with documented hepato-protective and hepato-stimulant properties. Yakrifit has earlier been found to counteract hepatopathy and restore liver functions in bovines (Pradhan and Dey, 1996). Polyherbal liver tonic formulations also protects the hepatic parenchyma from various parasitic and liverfluke infestations such as visceral larvae migrants.

Anti-oxidant, Immunomodulator and antistress effect

Various stressors such as high ambient temperature and relative humidity influence the performance of animals & birds by reducing feed intake, feed efficiency, nutrient utilization and feed conversion ratio (Sahin *et al.*, 2003). Various kinds of stressors such as physical, performance, environmental, disease or many more are indicated.

Ayurvedic formulas that treat stress contain herbs with adaptogenic (antistress) effects. Herbs with high antistress & antioxidant activity like amla (*Emblica officinalis*), ashwagandha (*Withania somnifera*), tulsi (*Ocimum sanctum*), Shilajit and many more have proved to be potent oxygen free radical scavenger *in vitro* and *in vivo* models. Medicinal plants or herbs owing immunopotentiating properties can provide an alternative to conventional therapy for a variety of diseases, especially when the host's defense mechanism has to be activated under conditions of impaired immune response (Atal *et al.*, 1996).

Herbs namely *Mangifera indica, Echinacea purpurea, Phyllanthus emblica, Uncaria tomentosa, Withania somnifera, Ocimum sanctum, Tinospora cordifolia, Asparagus racemosus* and many more are scientifically validated to possess antistressor, immunostimulant or immunomodulant and adaptogenic properties. Mangiferin, active constituent of herb Mangifera indica, is a strong inducer of in-vivo and in vitro activation of peritoneal macrophages. Induction of interferon release from macrophages by Mangifera has a potent lymphoproliferative effect on macrophage activation, thus establishing the therapeutic potential of Mangifera as a immunomodulator. Another herb; *Echinacea purpurea* is known to stimulate macrophages, but does not increase resistance to a wide variety of stressors (e.g., physiological stress). However,

Uncaria tomentosa has been shown to stimulate interleukin-1 and interleukin-6 in macrophages, stimulate endothelial cells to produce a lymphocyte proliferating regulating factor, and enhance recovery of leukopenia induced by doxorubicin. Similarly, *Withania somnifera* is well established to augment endogenous antioxidants, maintenance of myocardial antioxidant status, significant restoration of most haematobiochemical and oxidative stress marker parameters by its free radical scavenging activity in addition to potentiating agglutinin antibody titres and complement fixing antibodies (Ziauddin *et al*, 1996). The antioxidant potential of Methanolic extracts of *Ocimum sanctum* as studied by HPLC bases hypoxanthine/xanthine oxidative assay indicated their prime role in free radical elimination, thus combating immunosupression. It can be interpreted that the characteristic dysregulation of stress hormones and neurotransmitters, and the immunosupression thereby can be successfully ameliorated by the botanical adaptogenic remedies including either single herb or combination of different herbs (polyherbal formulation) (Manoharan *et al.*, 2004). An example of such a polyherbal immunomodulator, adaptogenic & antistressor formualation is Stresroak, scientifically validated in amelioration of various kind of stressors eg. production, vaccination, overcrowding, water deprieviation, lead toxicity, cadmium toxicity and to potentiate immune response during different disease conditions eg. Infectious bursal disease & new castles disease, in poultry (Pradhan, 1995 and Sujatha *et al.*, 2010).

Antimicrobial effect

The medicinal or antimicrobial properties of plant-derived substances have been well known for centuries. This property is mainly attributed to the essential oils of these plants namely *Trichyspermum ammi, Cinamonum camphora, Mentha piperita* & many more. *Oregano* and *thyme* are among those which have received a great deal of interest. These plants contain the monoterpenes carvacrol and thymol, respectively, and have demonstrated high efficacy in vitro against several pathogens found in the intestinal tract. This suggests that phytogenic feed additives may be suitable replacements for in-feed antibiotics to improve pig health and growth performance, particularly during the first few weeks post weaning.

Toxin Binder

Aflatoxins have been found to reduce growth and feed efficiency, suppress immune system, reduce antibody titre and cause mortality and morbidity leading to severe economic losses to poultry farmers (Sakhare *et al.*, 2007). Synergistic action of herbal toxin binders (Toxiroak) alongwith liver tonic formulations are scientifically well proven to improve growth, reduce mortality in broiler chickens by better protein and energy utilization by limiting the adverse effects of aflatoxins (Kalorey *et al.*, 2009). In addition to it, other polyherbal toxin binders namely Vilocym and Vilocym Z are popular in poultry industry, among farmers and veterinarians for control of mycotoxicosis.

Natural Methionine

Poultry feeding is one of the most important areas, since feed alone accounts for about 65-70 % cost of the total poultry enterprise. Protein synthesis in chickens is required at a very rapid pace for fast growing broilers and prolific layers and it is necessary that all essential amino acids are available through diet in right proportions. From the nutrition point of view, the amino acids that make up the protein are more important rather than the protein molecule itself. Methionine is required in free as well as conjugated form to perform various metabolic functions. It assists in the breakdown of fats and thereby prevents the build-up of fat in liver and arteries, as well as assisting the digestive system and removing heavy metals from the body since it can be converted to cysteine, which is a precursor to glutathione, which is of prime importance in detoxifying the liver. Its deficiency may manifest in symptoms like fatty liver, retarded growth, reduced feed efficiency, weakness, edema, skin lesions, poor feather condition, decreased egg production, small egg size, immuno-suppression, low carcass yield and disturbances in various metabolic pathways (Ramarao *et al.,* 2003). Improper conversion of methionine can lead to atherosclerosis. Most plants contain very little amounts of Methionine; however, some have significant amounts. High levels of methionine are found in fish, meats, and some other plant seeds. Almost all feed ingredients of plant origin used for compounding poultry ration are deficient in Methionine used and hence DL-methionine is commonly added as supplement in poultry feeds. In the past the requirement of amino acids of chickens used to be met from more than one sources of protein from plant and animal origin.

However, due to increase in prices of quality fish meal and availability of comparatively cheaper Soybean meal, use of all Soya feed started with addition of Methionine as Soybean meal is deficient in Methionine which again is a costly supplement. In poultry ration, just like protein, the vitamins and minerals have equally important role in development of musculature. In the list of vitamins choline (growth promoter) is playing vital role by acting as lipotropic agent, thereby preventing abnormal fatty infiltration in liver, thus ensuring proper metabolism of the body and effective utilization of nutrients (Kanchi *et al.,* 2009). Moreover, it helps in formation of an excitatory neurotransmitter acetylcholine, which is responsible for proper functioning of nervous system and maintains harmony. There is no consistency in the choline content in the natural feed stuffs and also their bioavailability is not predictable. Therefore, in broilers as well layers, choline in combination with chloride (CC) is added as an important feed ingredient.

However, herbal or natural products, which have proven results in various areas of poultry production, can be combined as a mixture and premix can be prepared, which may be used in feed formulations. Supplementation of polyherbal formulations containing ingredient herbs that mimic methionine, choline and biotin like activity, namely Methiorep & Repchol, have scientifically well proven to prevent fatty liver syndrome and to improve overall carcass quality, yield and egg production in broilers (fig. 8) (Kalbande *et al.*, 2009). These herbal amino acid supplements have an added advantage over harmful effects of synthetics, use of which is totally prohibited in organic poultry production (Moritz *et al.*, 2005).

Conclusion

Traditional system of medicines has stood the test of tie for over 4000 years & should not be considered as an alternate to the modern medicine; rather they complement & enhance the production of livestock. Since ancient times, herbs and their products are constantly used for curing illness. However, herbal additives have aroused much scientific interest over the past few years to explore their role as performance enhancers in livestock production. The cited instances in this text are just glimpses from the vast and virgin world of Ayurveda through the clear eye of modern science. It is upto our scientist & industry how best they use this precious gift from Mother Nature for health and welfare of livestock and in turn mankind.

References

Kalbande, V.H., Ravikanth, K., Maini, S. and Rekhe, D.S. (2009). Methionine Supplementation Options in Poultry. *International Journal of Poultry Science.* 8(6): 588-591.

Kanchi, S.N., Kalbande, V.H., Wankhade, S, M., Ghavate, A.M. and Dhok, A.P. (2009). Comparative evaluation of feeding herbal methionine supplement on performance of broilers. 13th Biennial Conference of ANSI (NIANP) Bangalore.

Kolte A.Y, Maini S., Ravikanth, K and Rekhe D.S. (2009). Role of polyherbal formulation in modulating rumen biochemical and growth performance parameters in calves. *Internat. Journal of Veterinary Medicine,* 6 no. 2

Manoharan, S., Ramesh, S., A. Parthiban, A. and Koteswaran, N.D.J. (2004). Effect of poly herbal ingredients of Stresroak on Day old Chick Quality by feeding in parent flocks. *Inter. J. Poult. Sci.,* 3: 773-778.

Moritz, J. S., Parsons, A. S., Buchanan, N. P., Baker, N. J., Jaczynski, J., Gekara, O. J. and Bryan, W. B. (2005). Synthetic methionine and feed restriction effects on performance and meat quality of organically reared broiler chickens. *J. Appl. Poult. Res.* 14: 521–535.

Pardhan, N.R. and Dey, D.K. (1996). Induced hepatopathy in calves and therapeutic efficacy of a herbal liver tonic (AV/LTL/14).*Indian J. of Animal Sci.* 66(12):1238-124.

Pradhan, N.R. (1995). Effects of Stresroak on the performance of broilers. *Ind. J. Poult. Sci.*, 30: 82-84.

Prakash, J., Gupta, S.K. and. Dinda, A.K. (2002). *Withania somnifera* root extract prevent DMBA induced squamous cell carcinoma of skin in Swiss albino mice. *Nutr. Cancer*, 42: 91-97.

Rama Rao, S.V., Panda, A.K., Raju, M.V.L.N., Shyam Sunder, G. and Praharaj, N.K. (2003). Requirement of calcium for commercial broilers and white leghorn layers at low dietary phosphorus levels. *Anim. Feed Sci. Technol.* 106: 199–208.

Sakhare, P.S., Harne, S.D., Kalorey, D.R., Warke, S.R., Bhandarker, A.G. and Kurkure, N.V. (2007). Effect of toxiroak polyherbal feed supplement during induced. aflatoxicosis, ochratoxicosis and combined mycotoxicosis in broilers. *Veterinary Archiv*, 77: 129-138.

Satyavati, G.V. and Gupta, A.K. (1987). Medicinal plants of India. Indian Council of Medical Research, 2: 541.

Sujatha, V., Rastogi, SK., Korde, JP., Maini, S. and Ravikanth K. (2010). Amelioration of heat stress induced disturbances of the antioxidant defense system in broilers. *Journal of Veterinary Medicine and Animal Health.* 2(3): 18-28.

Waghmare, S.P., Kolte, A.Y., Ravikanth, K., Rekhe, D.S. and Maini, S. (2009). Polyherbal Formulation And Rumen Ecology In Calves. *Veterinary Practioner*, 10 (2): 174-178.

Ziauddin, M., Pharsalkar, N., Patki. P., Diswanay, S. and Patwardhan, B. (1996). Studies on the Immunomodulatory effects of *Phyllatus emblica. J. Ethnopharmacol.* 50: 6 9-76.

□□□

31

Various Methods of Crop Residues Improvement and Strategic Supplementation of Deficit Nutrients for Improving Health and Production of Ruminants

PUTAN SINGH
Principal Scientist, Animal Nutrition Division, Indian Veterinary Research Institute
Izatnagar-243 122, UP

Introduction

The major objectives for improving health and productivity in ruminants fed on crop residues or mature pastures are: (1) to supplement nutrients to ensure efficient rumen function and (2) to provide bypass supplements to balance those available from fermentative digestion, and (3) to improve nutritive value of crop residues through urea ammonia treatment and other processes (pelleting and grinding, etc) through developed technologies of IVRI like compressed complete feed blocks (CCFB), urea molasses mineral block (UMMB) and urea ammoniated crop residues and also by developing CCFB for different categories of milk production and medicated CCFB/UMMB for diseased animals. These strategies aim to ensure maximum intake and utilization efficiency of the absorbed nutrients by the healthy and diseased animals.

Upgrading of Straw

The digestibility of straw is about 40 to 50% and the reason for the low digestibility is the lignin which prevents bacteria in the stomach from penetrating it. Thus, if the lignin could be loosened or dislodged then digestibility could at least theoretically be about 90% as the indigestible lignin amount to be about 10%.

Traditional Methods

A. Supplementation

Supplementation with locally available, biologically effective supplements should be a strategy for better utilization of rice straw. Supplements are critical in that they must contain the limiting nutrients in crop residues. In most instances, the limiting nutrient is nitrogenous compounds which can yield ammonia for the bacteria in the rumen. If this is limiting, the speed of digestion will be reduced and leading to a high retention time in the rumen. Supplementing nitrogen can have dramatic results on straw utilization. Supplementation of rice bran, fish meal, locally available oil cakes, urea, mixtures of molasses and urea, mineral and vitamin supplements can be well incorporated into straw-based diets for better responses from ruminants.

B. Pretreatments

A number of methods have been tested which include, treatment with urea/ammonia (NH3), alkali (calcium hydroxide, sodium hydroxide, ammonium hydroxide and sodium carbonate), organic acids (acetic and formic acid) and oxidizing agents (hydrogen peroxide, ozone, sulphur dioxide). The aim of chemical treatment is to increase lignin solubility or decrease the bonds between lignin and cell wall constituents, thereby making cellulose and hemicellulose more susceptible to microbial attack in the rumen. Usually, the small scale farmers depend on urea. The level of inclusion is about 4- 5 kg urea/100 kg of straw. The average daily gain and feed conversion efficiency was improved in buffalo calves fed on urea treated straw compared to control group fed on untreated straw (Dutta *et al.*, 2009).

Microbial treatment methods for improvement of poor quality roughages may prove to be one of the most promising in the future. The main constraint in the process is to find suitable microorganisms which can decompose lignin without degrading too much of the hemicellulose and cellulose. Zadrazil (1984) reviewed that during microbial conversion of poor quality products into feed, *in vitro* digestibility of fungal substrates decreases at the beginning of colonization by white rot fungi and increases afterwards. During incubation, the contents of soluble substances increase.

New Technological Interventions

A. Use of exogenous enzymes

Plant cell wall degrading enzymes stimulate fibre digestion in the rumen. When enzymes are applied to feed prior to consumption, binding the enzyme to the substrate may result in a conformational change that makes the enzymes more resistant to proteolysis. It has been demonstrated that (Morgavi *et al.*, 2000) exogenous fibrolytic enzymes work in synergy with the endogenous rumen microbial enzymes to enhance the digestion of high fibrous feed. Treating feeds with enzymes just prior to feeding may improve digestibility via a number of different mechanisms including, direct hydrolysis, enhanced microbial attachment, changes in gut viscosity, complementary actions with ruminal enzymes, and changes in the site of nutrient digestion. Improvements in palatability and changes in patterns of feed consumption could also occur.

This approach offers exciting possibilities for using enzymes to improve nutrient digestion, utilization and animal productivity and at the same time reduces animal fecal material and pollution. Spraying enzymes onto feeds just before feeding may also provide increased management flexibility for feeding and bypasses any negative interactions that the ensiling process may have on enzyme performance. In addition, use of fibrolytic enzymes would also pave way for effective utilization of paddy straw leading to increased economic benefits for the farmer.

Exogenous fibrolytic enzymes (EFE) have typically been observed to increase the initial rate but not the extent of DM digestion when used in ruminant diets (Varel *et al.*, 1993). However, applying EFE to straw following alkali treatment significantly increased both the rate and extent of DM digestion (Wang *et al.*, 2004).

B. Genetic selection

Genetic improvement of straw quality would be a cheaper and more logical approach. Straw quality *per se* can be improved by 1) breeding or genetic engineering, 2) modification of agronomic practices 3) altering harvesting, threshing and storage methods to optimise straw feeding value. The nutritive value and digestibility of straw vary among varieties of crops and depends on morphological, chemical and environmental factors. This variability presumably could be exploited to improve the nutritional value of the straw of future varieties. These include cell-wall content, lignin and silica contents, leaf to blade ratio, leaf sheath and stem, length of harvested straw, soil fertility and added fertilizer level, soil moisture and degree of senescence of straw at harvest, growth duration, resistance to pest and plant heights.

With wheat straws, greater emphasis is placed on the stem (internodes) fraction than the leaf (sheath and blade) fraction because the stem comprises a much larger proportion of the straw than leaves. In whole rice straw, the proportions of internodes, sheaths and blades tend to be more equal but again more leaf blade material is likely to be lost during harvesting and threshing. The stem contains less ash and protein but more cellulose than the leaves (Doyle *et al.*, 1986). It is found that IVOMD of stem internodes tends to be higher than that of leaf blades and leaf sheaths. Internodes have higher cellulose content than leaves.

Studies on the developing plant varieties can provide important information on the types of manipulation that might be used to improve nutritive value and on the critical time periods during which a plant expresses characteristics important in determining straw quality. During growth, cellulose, hemicellulose and lignin are all being synthesised in the cell wall but the amount of cellulose deposited is greater than that of hemicellulose or lignin until after anthesis and beyond the point of maximum elongation. Synthesis of all three components stopped at the same time, about 4 weeks after anthesis. Between 20 days before anthesis and 30 days after anthesis, the amount of cellulose increased about 3.5 fold, the amount of hemicellulose about 2 fold and the amount of lignin about 5 fold. The pattern in the other stem segments was similar. This shows that manipulations of cell-wall composition to improve feeding value must focus on this period when rapid changes are occurring.

Composition of leaf blade (LB), leaf sheath (LS), and internode (I) of IR36 and IR42 rice plant at harvest

Parameter (%)	IR36			IR42		
	LB	LS	I	LB	LS	I
IVOMD	40	45	51	34	37	50
NDF	67	72	62	70	70	71
Cellulose	30	37	44	31	35	41
Hemicellulose	13	11	11	16	10	11
Lignin	6.2	3.3	3.7	5.5	4.5	7.7

(Roxas, 1984)

Variation in cell contents

The cell contents comprise proteins, peptides and other nitrogen-containing compounds, carbohydrates, fats and minerals. In considerations of straw quality, therefore, the role of the storage carbohydrates is critical: the more storage carbohydrates remaining in straw the higher the digestibility.

This has been expressed by Pearce (1984) as a high correlation between NDS (%) and IVOMD (%). NDS increased rapidly shortly before anthesis and peaked about 4 weeks after anthesis. Subsequently, the amount of NDS in the internode and NDS and organic/dry-matter digestibility declined. Both the amount of NDS and its digestibility approached basal level at the time of grain maturation.

Proteins are efficiently mobilised from senescing plant tissues and, except under conditions of high nitrogen fertilizer application (Roxas et al, 1985), their concentration in straw is low (Darling, 1985). Different plant fractions do not store carbohydrates uniformly. Stems store considerably more than leaf sheaths, which store more than leaf blades. In wheat, the penultimate internode, S2, accumulates most fructans. In wheat, the upper parts of the culm contain larger proportions of NDS than the lower parts, as might be expected from their age, degree of senescence and proximity to photosynthesising leaves in the crop canopy. An understanding of these interactions may identify opportunities for manipulation of carbohydrate reserves so as to achieve high-quality straw for animal production without significant reductions in grain yield and quality.

Current breeding efforts which aim at incorporating resistance to insects, diseases and lodging also lead to improvements in harvest straw quality by reducing straw damage. Duration of growth and nitrogen fertilizer levels also affect protein content of the straw. Early-maturing modern rices have higher grain and possibly, higher straw protein contents than medium-maturing varieties (IRRI, 1985), and tend to have thinner straw and be more susceptible to lodging than medium-maturing rices (IRRI, 1984).

Supplementation Priorities

If supplementation is the goal for cattle grazing low quality forage, priority should first be placed on meeting the protein requirement in order to maximize forage intake and digestion. It is inconsistently proven that protein supplementation for cattle grazing protein deficient forage is extremely effective. In fact, energy supplementation will not be effective if dietary protein is deficient.

Once the producer ensures that the supplementation or feeding program will meet the protein requirement, energy intake should be evaluated. The decision must be made whether the cattle need to maintain body weight and condition, gain weight and condition, or whether they can be allowed to lose some weight and condition. This decision will dictate how much supplemental energy should be provided. Lastly, vitamin and mineral requirements should be compared to expected intake, potential deficiencies identified, and supplemental alternatives evaluated. This is not to say that vitamins and minerals are not important. Priority is given to protein and energy nutrition first because these items are needed in much greater quantities and they have the potential to have much greater impact on animal performance and efficiency of forage utilization.

Protein supplementation

Supplemental protein is extremely important for grazing cattle when forages fail to provide enough protein to meet their nutrient needs. The response to supplementation is high when the CP content of the basal forage is less than 6 to 8% (Kartchner, 1981). Moreover, other factor that necessitate the protein supplements are:

1) Digestibility and availability of forage - as the digestibility of the forage decreases, the availability of the CP to the microbial population and the host animal also decreases (Allden, 1981).
2) Availability of other essential nutrients like energy, vitamins, and minerals, sulfur: nitrogen ratios.
3) Stage of production and growth requirements- Young, growing animals and adults at high production levels are more likely to respond with increased intake and gain when provided protein supplements. Therefore, all the above factors must be considered when predicting performance responses to supplemental protein.

Physical Form of Supplemental Protein

Many protein feed stuffs are available as supplement to roughage diet. The "ideal supplement" is one that best fits the target animal's nutritional needs, easier to handle and present to the target animal and is most economical. They are categorized as follows:

Oil cakes

The most common supplemental protein is derived from oilseed by-products such as soybean meal, cottonseed meal, groundnut cake, sunflower cake, rapeseed meal and copra meal. Although we usually consider these as supplemental protein sources, they also provide significant energy to the diet. However, these feed sources can be expensive at times, and identifying inexpensive alternative native feed sources that provide supplemental protein would be beneficial to ruminant livestock producers. Protein supplementation in the form of groudnut cake, soyabean meal, fish meal (Prakash *et al.*, 1996) or cotton seed cake (Ocen, 1992) increase the DM intake, nutrient utilization, N retention, and thus improves the performance of ruminants fed on rice straw. Among the protein meals, fish meal has been found to be superior in view of greater efficiency of N utilization. The supplemental value of rapeseed and sunflower meals for growing sheep grazing low quality grass pastures was evaluated (Coombe *et al.*, 1987). Sheep receiving no supplement or a urea supplement lost weight, whereas sheep receiving sunflower meal gained weight. Intake of rapeseed meal was low and variable, and resultant sheep performance was also variable and intermediate compared to the performance of control and sunflower meal-supplemented sheep.

Tree foliage

Forage shrubs and trees can be one of the best options to intensify tropical animal production by supplementing traditional low quality crop residues. The legumes species belonging to the genera of Albizzia, *Callandra, Gliricidia, Mimosa, Leucaena, Samanea, Erythrina, Desmanthus, Morus* and *Acacia* are considered as good supplements in ruminant ration. Strategic supplementation of tree legumes is inevitable in small farms because of regular feed shortages. These tree legumes are significant in ruminant nutrition because they

1) Provide high quality and high digestibility biomass resource which is easily available in and around the farm
2) Supplement the nutrients deficient in the diet resulting in enhancement of microbial growth and digestion of cellulosic biomass in the rumen
3) Act as a source of undegradable protein (Table 1)
4) Act as a source of vitamins and minerals to complement deficiencies in the basal fed resource

Table 1 : Rumen degradable nitrogen (RDN), rumen undegradable nitrogen (UDN) and rumen undegradable but available post ruminally (DUN) of some tree forages calculated at a passage rate of 0.05/hours (g/kg DM)

Forage	RDN	UDN	DUN
Acacia catechu	4.8	28.7	16.0
Albizzia stipulata	7.3	28.4	11.6
Artocarpus lakoocha	19.7	11.4	4.6
Bauhinia variegata	16.9	16.1	9.45
Dendrocalamus hamiltonii	11.1	20.6	11.2
Ficus roxburghii	13.2	8.9	2.6
Leucaena leucocephala	14.6	19.1	5.8
Morus alba (mature)	16.3	12.2	5.8

Source: Singh and Makkar, 2000

The leaves of *Leuceana, Erythrina, Desmanthus* and *Morus* are reported to produce beneficial responses like higher ADG and better milk production in ruminants. Majority of tree leaves are rich in nitrogen, sulphur and minerals their supplementation can increase the efficiency of utilization of crop residues by enhancing microbial protein synthesis in the rumen.

Tropical legumes generally are richer in tannins than temperate legumes and therefore should function better as sources of bypass protein. It must be emphasized that when legumes contain a high proportion of protected protein, some other source of rumen fermentable nitrogen will be required, usually urea.

Apart from fresh foliage, the scope of supplementation of dried leaves and hay is under research. Intake and rumen degradation of maize stover in sheep could be improved by supplementing the animals with *Leucaena* hay up to 6 g DM/kg live weight per day (Kimambo *et al.*, 1991). Cassava hay is palatable to ruminants and is proved to be an excellent feed either as the sole diet or as a supplement in diets based on crop residues (eg. urea-treated straws/ sugarcane tops) (Wanapat *et al.*, 1997). Supplementation of cassava hay upto 400g/day in the diet of goats resulted in increased milk yield, probably due to a higher intake of proteins as well as possible effects of bypass protein from the cassava hay Wanapat *et al.* (1997). Supplementation with cassava hay can lower use of concentrate and improve milk yield and milk composition.

Non-Protein Nitrogen

Non-protein nitrogen (NPN) and readily available sources of energy optimize rumen function resulting in increased DMI and improved performance in animals fed diets based on low-quality roughages (Winter and Pigden, 1971). NPN in the form of urea is generally a cheap source of protein. Urea is used directly by rumen microorganisms as a source of nitrogen and is completely ruminally degradable. However, this source of nitrogen is very unpalatable and should be used in moderation. Urea can be used to reduce cost of protein supplement without causing negative effects on performance as long as not more than 25 % of the RDP in the diet is supplied by urea (Woods 1997). Including higher concentrations of urea in protein supplements reduces the supplement palatability and ultimately suppresses intake and animal performance. Moreover, feeding high levels is not cost-effective because much of the urea is not utilized due to the rapid ammonia release rate of urea. This rapid release of ammonia from urea exceeds the rumen microbe's ability to use the ammonia and results in more ammonia being converted back into urea by the liver and excreted. Rapid ammonia release can also cause ammonia toxicity, which can lead to death.

Slow-release NPN

The rate of ammonia release from NPN sources can be influenced both by the physical form of the NPN-containing feed and the specific ammonia-releasing molecule. Various heat and chemical treatment are popular to combine urea with starch from grains and molasses. Biuret is a very safe source of NPN and has an ammonia release curve very similar to soybean meal. The slower release of ammonia also improves the synchronization of nitrogen availability with the slow release of fermentable energy from forages and, potentially, yields more efficient microbial growth in the rumen. Biuret can be utilized at very high levels with forage-based diets and is more cost-effective than feeding natural proteins sources or urea.

The National Dairy Development Board of India has successfully developed and introduced multinutrient blocks based on molasses and urea for dairy buffaloes kept by village smallholders. These blocks-provide micro-organisms rich in sources of fermentable nitrogen, minerals, vitamins, amino-acids and peptides. Rates of consumption of blocks are of the order of 500 g/ animal/day for adult animals fed on rice straw under conditions of complete confinement. UMMB supplementation of straw based diet increase digestibility, feed intake, live weight gain and milk production. Various micro and macrominerals can be incorporated in the blocks to correct the respective deficiencies of the ruminants in developing countries.

Bypass protein

For high producing animals the feeding strategy should also be aimed at supplementation with bypass protein of dietary origin in addition to creating an efficient ecosystem. The source of bypass protein should be an oilseed meal or an animal byproduct meal (supplying protein and fat) and should be given maximum of 30% of the total diet dry matter. The 30% limit is to prevent depression/substitution of the digestible energy of the basal diet. The optimum level and the degree of response to the supplement will depend upon the fermentability of the basal diet.

Effect of supplementation on livestock productivity

Forage intake and digestibility

Feeding supplemental protein improves the amount of forage cattle can consume, plus it can improve the digestibility of the forages consumed. Protein supplementation (185 g/day) in the diet of cross bred calves improves intake of low quality roughage and reduces rate of live mass loss under dry winter condition. Protein supplementation of forages containing more than 9% crude protein will have little effect on digestibility and intake in cattle. When the limiting nutrients are supplied through available supplements, the nutrient digestibility of basal straw can be improved dramatically. This improvement in forage utilization can lead to improved body condition scores, which can in turn lead to improved profit potential of a cattle operation. Table 2 estimates the daily dry matter intake for dry and lactating cows with or without protein supplementation. The value of protein supplementation was slightly enhanced by combining the protein supplement with energy and phosphorus (Van Niekerk and Jacobs, 1985).

Table 2 : Estimated intake of forage with and without supplementation

	Forage intake (% BW,DM basis) of brood cows Dry bred cows	Lactating cows
Low-Quality Forage (<7% CP)		
No supplement	1.5	2.0
Protein Supplement	1.8	2.2
Average-Quality Forage (7-9% CP)		
No supplement	2.0	2.3
Protein Supplement	2.2	2.5
High-Quality Forage (>9% CP)		
No supplement	2.5	2.7
Protein Supplement	2.5	2.7

Supplementation with CP usually improves weight gain and body condition score. An average daily gain of 500 g/day was observed through the supplementation of 500 g cottonseed cake in the ration of HF calves maintained on maize stover (Ocen, 1992). Supplementation of locally available concentrate ingredients and tree foliage has beneficial effect on growth rate of small ruminants. The highest live weight gain and cost benefit ratio was recorded due to *Leucaena* supplementation followed by groundnut cake, Stylo and concentrate. Thus, the supplementation of locally available feed resources to ruminants have wider future application because the technology has ability to improve the production by slight modification of their existing traditional system of management. In addition, nutrient supplementation offers solution to reduce calf mortality during the period of nutritional shortage and may also increase calf performance.

Milk production

Strategic supplementation through locally available feed ingredients is an effective method for improving milk production and digestibility of cereal straws in the crossbred cows. Thomas (1984) and Sutton (1989) mentioned possible beneficial effects on milk yield when supplementing diets with extra CP.

Supplementation Strategies

Although some researchers have suggested that synchrony of release of nitrogen from protein supplements is an important factor for obtaining optimal ruminal digestion of low-quality roughages (Orskov, 1982), most studies conducted under practical conditions do not support this contention. Alternate-day, once-weekly, and daily feeding of protein supplements have yielded similar responses (Huston *et al.*, 1999). Daily CP supplementation is not advantageous over infrequent supplementation. Cows grazing on low quality forage perform equally on daily or infrequent supplementation (Schauer, 2003). Moreover, infrequent supplementation of CP is a managemental alternative to reduce labour costs. In a study by Huston *et al.* (1999), variation in animal weight change was decreased with less-frequent supplementation. This effect was presumably due to less competition for the supplement when greater quantities were provided in a single setting. Research has also suggested that timing of supplementation may influence response to supplementation. Limited data are available, however, relative to timing of supplementation and the performance of cattle grazing low-quality forages.

One strategy of supplementation should be to use the most efficient delivery system to minimize costs and variation of animal intake within a group of cattle. The intake of self fed supplements is dependent on trough space, supplement allowance, supplement form and supplement formulation. Limited trough space generally increases the proportion of non feeders, whereas low levels of competition, as with self-fed supplements, generally increases variation in individual supplement intake (Bowman and Sowell, 1997). By providing a supplement delivery system that optimizes uniformity of consumption and minimizes economic inputs, we can effectively improve beef cattle production systems.

Strategic supplementation of energy

Although protein supplements provide some energy and may stimulate additional energy intake, generally the term "energy supplement" refers to either cereal grains or by-products of the milling industry. In recent years, energy supplements have been classified into either those high in soluble carbohydrate (high in starches and sugars; cereal grains) or those high in structural carbohydrates (high in fiber; soybean hulls, ground nut husk, etc.). Carbohydrates are the main energy yielding substrates for ruminal microbes, however the type of carbohydrate may have a major effect on the rate and extent of fiber digestion.

Energy supply to the rumen can be most efficient when there is a fast NH_3 production. The slower degradation of the fiber may enable better synchrony between energy and NH_3 release. However, the high fiber can lead to substitution effects and use of these feeds as supplements may be more suitable for low fiber basal diets (Poppi and McLennan, 1995). Soluble carbohydrates such as starch or sugar may impede cellulose digestion due to factors such as lowered pH, competition between cellulolytic and non-cellulolytic bacteria for essential nutrients other than energy, or use of alternative energy sources by certain cellulolytic bacteria (Fahey and Berger, 1988). Orskov (1986) found that a small amount of grain (20 to 30% of the diet) produces little or no depression of intake and digestibility of roughages, but a higher level can depress intake to an extent that it is no longer a supplement, but becomes a substitute. In most cases, it is important to insure that the supplement complements the basal diet and does not substitute for it.

Effect of energy supplementation on ruminant productivity

Intake:When choosing an energy supplement, it is important to consider the effect the supplement on the basal diet. The type of carbohydrate has a major effect on the rate and extent of forage digestion (Bowman and Sanson 1996). Intake and digestibility are often depressed when cattle consuming low-quality forages are supplemented with nonstructural carbohydrates such as cereal grains, but low-quality forage intake and utilization has been shown to increase when cattle have been supplemented with fibrous by-product feedstuffs that contain high levels of structural carbohydrates. Some studies have shown an increase in intake when supplementing with structural carbohydrates. However, it was noted that intake does not continue to increase beyond certain levels of supplementation.

Digestibility: Sanson (1993) found that average hay dry matter digestibility for lambs fed supplemental beet pulp was 3.7% greater than for lambs fed supplemental corn. It was concluded that the difference arise as a result of an improved ruminal environment for fiber digestion when beet pulp was fed, which was higher in digestible fiber. However, other studies with corn as a supplement have shown a decrease in forage digestibility. Chase and Hibberd (1987) observed that digestibility of hemicellulose and cellulose decreased linearly as the amount of supplemental corn increased. Additionally, hay and fiber digestibility also decreased as the amount of supplemental corn increased. Supplementation with corn or other concentrate feeds can negatively affect fiber digestion.

Growth performance: Soybean hull based energy supplement was better for body weight gain in pregnant cows compared to soybean meal based protein supplement (Marston *et al.*, 1995). Energy supplemented cows loses less body condition score before calving than protein-supplemented cows, with this advantage continuing throughout the breeding season and until weaning.

Reproductive performance

Energy supplementation has been shown to improve reproductive performance. However, the response appear to be dependent on the timing (pre or postpartum) of supplementation. An early return to estrus following parturition is commonly observed phenomena in high level energy supplemented cows. Pre or post-partum supplements affect different reproductive variables (Wiltbank *et al.* 1962). The level of energy intake in mature cows pre-calving influenced the length of interval from calving to first estrus and the level of energy intake post-calving influenced the conception rate. The postpartum level of energy intake is probably more critical than prepartum level when considering total reproductive performance. However, cows fed energy during gestation had greater pregnancy rates than cows fed protein, but the pregnancy rate was not influenced by postpartum supplementation (Marston *et al.*, 1995).

Supplemental Feeding Program for small ruminants

When forage or browse is limited or of low quality lactating does, does in the last 30 days of gestation and developing/breeding bucks should be fed nearly 500 g/day of a 16% protein commercial feed or homemade mixture (77:20:2.5:0.5 cereal: oilcakes/meal : mineral mixture: limestone). As a general recommendation a complete goat mineral mixture should be offered free choice throughout the year. Low to medium quality forage (> 10% protein) will meet requirements of dry does and non breeding bucks.

In goats nutritional stress appears to be a prime cause of acyclicity (Ndlovu, 1992). It is, therefore, beneficial to supplement the goats maintained on poor nutritional status with those nutrients which have an impact on reproductive performance at the time of stress. Additional nutrient allowance is not needed for pregnant goats grazed on good quality pasture for the purpose of improving kid birth weight. However during lactation it would be advisable to supplement to improve growth and survival rates of kids especially when rain is below the long-term average for the area. Therefore supplementation throughout the reproductive cycle would not be beneficial (Madibela *et al.*, 2002) for well grazed goats.

Rapid rate of foetal growth during the final six weeks of pregnancy imposes a metabolic challenge to the doe, which is met by the mobilization of maternal body tissue and this may result in weight loss of doe, if the dietary supply of nutrients is inadequate (Sibanda *et al.*, 1997). Strategic supplementation of pregnancy allowance during the last month of gestation may be adopted to economize goat production and to minimize reproductive wastage. Optimum period for pregnancy allowance supplementation may depend on intrauterine growth pattern of goat breed; the last month of pregnancy appears to be the most nutritionally sensitive period of gestation for non-descriptive goats found in northern plains of India (Rastogi *et al.*, 2006).

Supplementation of minerals

Cattle will generally obtain enough minerals and vitamins from available forages and grain to survive. But, they do not receive enough minerals and vitamins from forages or grains to optimize digestion and performance. This is because mineral and vitamin content of forages and grains is deficient in certain minerals and varies tremendously depending upon the soil type, weather conditions, time of year, fertilization levels, stage of maturity and storage conditions. Over time, soils can also become depleted in mineral content, resulting in lower mineral levels in forages. Hence, it is needed to provide supplemental minerals and vitamins.

Supplementation strategy

Mineral supplementation for livestock is considered to be the least cost insurance for a better productivity and hence, can be recommended in all types of livestock farming cutting across the economic barrier. The best means of providing minerals to ruminants receiving concentrates would be to combine the minerals with the concentrate diet, including Ca, P, and a trace mineralized salt. Iron may be included if condition deserves for. Sulphur may be added to the premix if non-protein nitrogen is added to the concentrate. The balance of individual minerals is important in this regard to ensure proper absorption and utilization of the minerals.

Animals that primarily depend on pasture have different supplementation needs compared to those receiving concentrates. Free choice mineral mixture or a mineral lick is the preferred option to supplement these animals. A good free choice mineral supplement should have the following characteristic features (McDowell, 1985).

1. Contains a minimum of 6-8% total P. In areas where forages are consistently lower than 0.2% P, mineral supplements with P range 8-10% are preferred.
2. Has a Ca: P ratio not substantially over 2:1
3. Provides a significant proportion (i.e., about 50%) of the trace elements for Co, Cu, I, Mn, Zn and Se if required. Fe is not needed is most circumstances.

4. Sufficiently palatable to allow adequate consumption in relation to requirements.
5. Has an acceptable particle size that will allow adequate mixing without smaller size practice settling out.

Trace mineralized salt is prevalent in organized farming sector. Customized trace mineral premixtures are becoming more common because they are formulated to balance mineral profiles and meet mineral needs depending on the farm condition. Forage testing is recommended for Zn, Cu, Mn and Fe an annual basis to establish herd micro mineral profiles and avoid/ correct mineral imbalance.

Organic minerals

Organic minerals are the supplementation strategy for modern age livestock. The source of minerals in the diet can affect the performance of the animals and the cost-effectiveness of the supplementation program. Organic mineral sources are characterized by the presence of an amino acid or a carbohydrate carrier for the trace mineral that is to be fed to cattle. In a process termed chelation or proteination, the organic carrier molecule is chemically bound to the trace mineral of interest.Organic mineral sources have higher bioavailabilities than inorganic sources of minerals; however, chelated minerals are usually more expensive than inorganic sources.

Requirement

Cattle require different levels of minerals, depending on age, size, sex, physiological state, and level of performance. Nutrient requirements of cattle at different stages of maturity and production are provided in Table 3.

Table 3 : Mineral requirements and maximum tolerable levels for beef cattle

Mineral units	Growing and finishing cattle	Gestating and dry cows	Lactating cows	Maximum tolerable level
Calcium, percent	0.31	0.18	0.27	
Chlorine, percent				
Chromium, ppm				1000.00
Cobalt, ppm	0.10	0.10	0.10	10.00
Copper, ppm	10.00	10.00	10.00	100.00
Iodine, ppm	0.50	0.50	0.50	50.00
Iron, ppm	50.00	50.00	50.00	1000.00
Magnesium, ppm	0.10	0.12	0.20	0.40

Manganese, percent	20.00	40.00	40.00	1000.00
Molybdenum, ppm				5.00
Nickel, ppm				50.00
Phosphorus, percent	0.27	0.18	0.27	
Potassium, percent	0.60	0.60	0.70	3.00
Selenium, ppm	0.10	0.10	0.10	2.00
Sodium, percent	0.07	0.07	0.10	
Sulfur, percent	0.15	0.15	0.15	0.40
Zinc, ppm	30.00	30.00	30.00	500.00

NRC, 1996.

A brief account of the essentiality of individual mineral supplementation is furnished below.

Salt (sodium chloride) : Salt supplementation is always required in ruminates unless the water salinity is very high. Sodium and chlorine are major electrolytes found in body fluids, and there is very little storage. Because of this, cattle will develop deficiencies rapidly and should have constant access to salt or a supplement containing salt.

Phosphorus : Phosphorus is often deficient in forages for lactating cows with superior milking ability. In addition, mature forages are often deficient in phosphorus for most cattle. Phosphorus is high in oilseed meals and also fairly high in grains; so when diets contain substantial amounts of these ingredients, supplementation is usually not needed. Phosphorus is one of the structural components of the skeletal system, and levels build up when cows are grazing lush forages that contain phosphorus at levels above requirements. Some of the phosphorus in bone can be mobilized during early lactation to overcome shortfalls in intake, but prolonged dietary deficiency has been reported to result in depressed reproductive efficiency and milk production.

Calcium : Calcium is usually not deficient in grass forages fed to cattle. In addition, legumes such as alfalfa and clover are high in calcium. Grains and by-product feeds are low in calcium, and diets high in these feed ingredients will need to be supplemented, usually with feed grade limestone or calcium carbonate. Like phosphorus, calcium is a structural part of bone, so temporary shortfalls in the diet can be overcome by the animal mobilizing some of the calcium in bone.

Magnesium : Forages contain adequate magnesium during most of the year, but levels can be very low during times of rapid growth, especially in well-fertilized pastures. The magnesium deficiency may occur during calving seasons and the onset of lactation and when the forage contains high levels of potassium which can interfere with the absorption of magnesium. Supplementation with magnesium oxide is recommended for 30 days prior to calving and during the first three months of lactation.

Sulphur : Sulfur is a component of several amino acids that are the building blocks of protein. Sulfur, other than that fed in the form of protein, is usually needed only when diets contain substantial amounts of nonprotein nitrogen (NPN). In these situations, the ratio of nitrogen to sulfur should be maintained between 10:1 and 15:1. High sulfur levels can interact with copper and molybdenum, which can result in a copper deficiency. It has been shown that the supplementation of poor quality fiber diets with sulphur improved ruminal fiber degradation as well as apparent organic matter digestibility.

Trace Minerals

Zinc : Zinc is a part of many important enzyme systems in the body, and its deficiency leads to depressed feed intake and growth rate, an abnormal hair coat and skin lesions. Zinc is important for male reproduction and immunity. Storage of zinc is minimal, and deficiencies occur rapidly following introduction of animals to a diet severely deficient in zinc. Zinc methionine, an organic form of zinc, has proven to improve performance in cattle.

Copper : Copper is important for adequate growth, reproduction immunity and enzyme function. Unlike zinc, copper is stored in the liver, and levels build up rapidly when animals are fed high levels of copper. Copper oxide should be avoided as a copper source because of its poor bioavailability, which will affect the level of copper required in supplements. High levels of molybdenum, sulfur, iron or zinc in the diet interfere with normal copper absorption and metabolism.

Selenium : The activity of selenium is related to vitamin E, and supplementation with either will help prevent white muscle disease. Marginal selenium deficiency can result in retained placenta, impaired fertility, silent heats and unthrifty weak calves with poor immune response (resulting in high preweaning death losses). Selenium can be provided in mineral mixes or in an injectable form. The maximum level of selenium that can be legally added to a supplement is 3 mg per head per day at its highest intake.

Manganese : Manganese levels in forages vary considerably, depending on the soils on which they are produced. Manganese is a part of several important enzyme systems. A deficiency may result in impaired reproductive performance in both cows and bulls and in the birth of deformed calves.

Cobalt : Cobalt is needed only for the ruminal synthesis of vitamin B12. Cobalt requirements are higher when cattle are fed high-grain diets, because more B12 is required to metabolize the end products of rumen fermentation.

Cobalt may be very deficient in some soils, so including it in trace mineral supplements is a sound practice.

Iron : Iron is a part of hemoglobin which transports oxygen to body tissues. Since most forages contain high levels of iron and because substantial amounts of soil are consumed during grazing, iron is almost never deficient in cattle fed forage-based diets. A more common problem with iron is that it may be excessively high in forages or in drinking water, which can interfere with the absorption of copper and zinc.

Iodine : Iodine makes up part of the thyroid hormones. Iodine is normally included in trace mineral supplements. Added iodine compounds should provide no more than 10 mg of iodine per day.

Mineral supplementation effect on animal productivity

The supplementation of minerals can be recommended for augmenting the productive performance of grazing ruminants. The common reproductive failures in cattle can be successfully managed with mineral supplements. They exert beneficial effects on reproductive performance of indigenous cattle maintained on cereal straw where nutrient imbalances and deficiencies are common. The importance of proper mineral supplementation was demonstrated in the work of Prabowo *et al.* (1984). Lambs fed only chopped napier grass, napier grass plus 100 g/d rice bran, or napier plus rice bran and a complete mineral supplement, gained 8, 37 and 69 g/d, respectively. Feeding minerals increases the rumen microbe population, which is critical to increasing forage digestion. In a study it is demonstrated cattle fed hay had only 39% of the microbial population of cattle fed a full supplement package, while cattle fed minerals and vitamins had 69% of the rumen microbe population. Increased rumen microbe populations can lead to improved forage digestion, which leads to improved body condition scores.

Vitamins

Ruminants are able to meet most of their vitamin requirements through rumen microbial synthesis and dietary supply. Even though, calves are born with minimal stores of vitamins, colostrum feeding satisfy their requirement. The ability to synthesize B vitamins and vitamin K in the rumen develops rapidly when solid feed is introduced into the diet. In ruminants, five classes of vitamins are important. Vitamin A is the most important. Vitamins D, E, K, and some of the B vitamins also are known to be essential. High-quality forages contain large amounts of vitamin A precursors and vitamin E. Vitamin D is synthesized by animal exposure to sunlight and is found in large amounts in sun-cured forages. Supplemental vitamins can be added to the trace mineral salt mixture if needed.

Vitamin A : Liver stores of vitamin A can be depleted when cattle consume a diet of low-quality, mature forage. In that case, supplementation is recommended to prevent potential problems on productive ability of cattle. Supplementing brood cows with vitamin A before (16,000 IU/day) and after (40,000 IU/day) the calving season can increase conception rates by 10 % and decrease calf morbidity by as much as 50 % as compared to a deficient state. Typically, 2 to 4 months of protection can be expected from stored vitamin A. Increasing dietary vitamin A by 5,000 IU per day can double the amount of vitamin A stored in the liver. Supplemental vitamin A is not required when cattle are grazing dormant rangelands, or if the cattle are fed properly cured and stored hay

Vitamin E : Supplementation is recommended for brood cows consuming poor quality forage during late pregnancy through early lactation. During the late stages of pregnancy, vitamin E concentration in the blood tends to decrease below marginal levels. Feeding supplemental vitamin E is an effective method of maintaining proper levels during this period. Neonatal calves must receive dietary vitamin E since placental transfer is very limited. However, it may not be necessary to supply supplemental vitamin E directly to the calf. Feeding an additional 1,000 IU of a-tocopherol (vitamin E) to cattle during the last trimester of pregnancy can increase antibody production and sequestration in the colostrum and increase vitamin E concentration in the colostrum by up to 30 percent. Plasma concentrations of vitamin E in the calf can be maintained above the minimal level by continuing maternal supplementation into the early stages of lactation.

Vitamin D : Sunlight typically stimulates sufficient production of vitamin D in grazing cattle. Vitamin D status is improved more effectively by increasing the animal's exposure to sunlight than by dietary supplementation.

Vitamin K : Ruminal microorganisms generally synthesize and supply vitamin K in amounts adeaquate to meet the ruminant animal's requirements. Supplemental vitamin K usually is justifi ed only when cattle are suspected to have been exposed to vitamin K antagonists. Consumption of a natural vitamin K antagonist (dicumarol) can be a problem if cattle ingest moldy sweet clover forage. Therefore, prevention (avoid feeding moldy sweet clover hay) is a better alternative to supplemental treatments.

B vitamins : Microbial synthesis of the B vitamins in the rumen usually satisfies the ruminant's requirements. Supplementation with B vitamins should not be necessary under normal production situations, especially if cattle consume high-quality forage or are fed supplemental protein and/or energy that improve ruminal digestibility and subsequent microbial synthesis.

Injections of B vitamins seem to be beneficial only to combat overt stress and disease.

Mineral and vitamin supplementation is critical for cattle to achieve the most economical gains possible from the forage and grain they consume. Minerals and vitamins are needed in very small quantities, yet they are a critical part of the overall nutritional package fed to cattle and are the backbone of a successful range cattle program. They play a vital role in nutrient digestion, reproductive performance, the immune system, and in the development of muscle, bones, and teeth. Typically, inadequate intake of essential minerals and vitamins may result in reduced forage intake, inefficient feed utilization, decreased average daily gains, lower reproductive efficiency and poor disease immunity. Supplementing with a balanced mineral and vitamin program enables cattle to obtain more of their needed nutrients from the forages consumed rather than getting needed nutrients from grains or additional supplements.

Multi-nutrient blocks

The type of supplement is important to minimize wastage and to maximize its impact on productivity. Multi-nutrient supplements as blocks, in contrast to liquid or mash supplements hold several advantages, namely, simplicity for transport and management, a more homogeneous intake among animals, reduced need for salt as an intake regulator and less risk in the use of urea as a source of non-protein nitrogen (Ben Salem and Nefzaoui, 2003; Kawas, 2010). Multi-nutrient blocks based on molasses and urea can be hand-crafted by livestock owners. This type of block consist of molasses (25–50%), urea (5–10%), cereal byproducts such as wheat bran or rice bran (15–25%), oil seed meals (10–20%), salt (4–10%), lime (5–10%), and a mixture of a phosphorous source, trace minerals and feed additives (1–5%). The lime will provide more hardness than cement, which has been frequently used to produce blocks in developing countries, and lime is generally 30–40% cheaper (Kawas, 2010). Vitamin A supplement should be added to the protein-mineral mixture during the dry or winter seasons, when low quality forage is available. Two different types of multinutrient lick-blocks can be prepared for wet and dry seasons, respectively, with the following characteristics:

Mineral-protein blocks : This is a low intake block (approximately 0.2–0.3% of body weight) with 30% crude protein or more. The purpose of offering this block is to supplement protein, macro-minerals (calcium, phosphorous, and magnesium), trace minerals (iron, manganese, zinc, copper, iodine, cobalt and selenium), and vitamin A. This supplement can be offered during dry or wet seasons as a reproductive management tool for goats. It is important to consider that during the wet season, forages contain more protein and energy, so it is important to emphasis in mineral supplementation, so that these nutrients can be better utilized. Protein supplementation produces a greater response on DM intake with forages of lower protein content as compared to forages with relatively high protein content.

Protein-energy blocks : These blocks contain minerals, but more energy and less protein (20–25% crude protein) than a mineral-protein block. Intake of this block should be greater (approximately 0.4–0.5% of body weight). This supplement is recommended for the dry season, when availability and quality of forages limit energy intake by goats (Kawas, 2010).

The key to improve the use of crop residues for ruminants is to overcome the barriers to rumen microbial fermentation of lignocellulosics. The two well known factors of rice straw that limit bacterial digestion in the rumen are its high level of ligninification and low content of nitrogen, vitamins and minerals. Therefore, in principle there are two approaches, which should be taken in combination, being straw delignification treatment and nutrient supplementation. Numerous methods of physical, chemical, biological treatment have been worldwide researched and developed. However, to develop any feasible strategies in a particular context, the local physical and socio-economic conditions must be taken into account. The modern technologies like application of exogenous enzymes and plant selection based on varietals and chemical differences provide strong impetus to the ongoing research.

The per unit production potential of Indian livestock is very low. The most important extraneous factor accounting for this is the poor quality feed resources. Forage availability from sources other than crop residues is often scarce, limiting productivity because of imbalance of nutrients and low digestibility of the available feed. Therefore supplemental feeding strategies are inevitable to supply deficient critical nutrients and complement the nutritional attributes of the poor quality roughages. The basic supplemental nutrients are energy from cereals and cereal byproducts, protein from oilseed meals and legume trees, minerals and vitamins. However, nutrient supply should be prioritized according to the physiological stages of the animals. A supplemental feeding program can reduce total cost of production by increasing forage digestion and optimizing the performance. Mutrinutrient blocks are getting popularized in tropical countries reducing feed wastage and increasing the intake. All he supplemental strategies are reported to maximize rumen fermentation and microbial protein synthesis, which in turn contributes to milk production, higher growth rate and profit throughout the grazing season.

References

Allden, W. G. (1981). Energy and protein supplements for grazing livestock. In: F. H. W. Morley (Ed.) Grazing Ruminants. Elsevier Scientific Publishing Co., Amsterdam. pp 289-307.

Ben Salem, H. and Nefzaoui, A. (2003). *Small Ruminant. Res.* 49: 275–288.

Bowman, J.P., and B.F. Sowell. (1997). *J. Anim. Sci.*, 75:543-550.

Bowman, J.G.P. and Sanson, D.W. (1996). Starch- or fiber based energy supplements of grazing ruminants. *Proc. West. Sec. Amer. Soc. Anim. Sci.* 47:118- 135.

Chase, C.C., Jr., and Hibberd, C.A. (1987). *J. Anim. Sci.*, 65:557-566.

Coombe, J.B., Axelsen, A. and Dove, H. (1987). *Aust. J. Exp. Agric.*, 27:513-523.

Dutta, N., Sharma, K., Pattanaik, A.K and Singh, M. (2009). Effect of strategic feeding of urea treated cereal straws supplemented with agricultural byproducts on the performance of growing buffalo calves and heifers. *Animal Nutrition and Feed Technology.* 9(2): 185-193.

Fahey, G,C.and Berger, L.L. (1988). Carbohydrate nutrition of ruminants. In: D.C. Church (ed.). The Ruminant Animal: Digestive Physiology and Nutrition. Prentice-Hall, Englewood Cliffs, NJ. p. 269.

Hibberd, C.A. and Thrift, T.A. (1992). Supplementations of forage-based diets: Are results predictable? *J. Anim. Sci.*, 70:181. (Abstr.).

Huston, F.E., Lippke, H. Forbes, T.D.A., Holloway, J.W. and Machen, R.V. (1999). *J. Anim. Sci.*, 77:3057-3067.

Kartchner, R.J. (1981). *J. Anim. Sci.* 51:432-438.

Kawas, J.R. Andrade-Montemayor, H. Lu, C.D. (2010). Small Ruminant Res. (Article in press).

Kimambo, A.E., Makiwa, A.M., Shem, M.N. (1991). The use of Leucaena leucocephala supplementation to improve the utilisation of maize stover by sheep. Joint Feed Resources Network Workshop on the Complementarity of Feed Resources for Animal Production in Africa, Gaborone (Botswana), 4-8 Mar.

Leng, R.A. (1986). Constraints to ruminant production and concepts to increase productivity from low-digestibility forages. Proceedings of the 5th International Conference on Livestock Production and Diseases in the Tropics held in Kuala Lumpur, Malaysia, 18th - 22nd August, 1986. p. 145.

Madibela, O. R., Mosimanyana, B. M., Boitumelo, W. S. and Pelaelo, T. D. (2002). *S. Afr. J. Anim. Sci.*, 32:14-22.

Marston, T.T., Lusby, D.S., Wettemann, R.P. and Purvis, H.T. (1995). *J. Anim. Sci.*, 73: 657-664.

McDowell, L.R. (1985). Minerals in animal and human nutrition (Tony J Chunha ed.) Academic Press, New York.

Morgavi, D. P., K. A. Beauchemin, V. L. Nsereko, L. M. Rode, A. D.Iwaasa, W. Z. Yang, T. A. McAllister, and Y. Wang. (2000). Synergy between ruminal fibrolytic enzymes and enzymes from*Trichoderma Longibrachiatum*. *Journal of Dairy Science*. 83: 1310–1321.

National Research Council. (1996). Nutrient Requirements of Beef Cattle, seventh revised edition. Washington, D.C.: National Academy Press.

Ndlovu, L.R. (1992). Reproductive performance of indigenous goats in traditionally managed flocks in North-East of Zimbabwe. In: Small Ruminant Research and Development in Africa. Eds. Lebbie, R.B. & Reynolds, S.H.B., Proc. First Biennial Conf. Africa Small Ruminant Network. ILRAD, Nairobi, Kenya, Dec. 1990. ILCA, Nairobi, Kenya. pp. 177-184.

Ocen, W.G. (1992). Performance of cattle given crop residues supplemented with high-quality forages and agro-industrial by-products. LRRD., 4(1).

Orskov, E.R. (1982). Protein Nutrition in Ruminants. pp 41-84. Academic Press, New York.

Orskov, E.R. (1986). Starch digestion and utilization in ruminants. *J. Anim. Sci.,* 63: 1624-1633.

Pearce G R. Beard J and Hilliard E. (1984). Variability in the chemical composition of cereal straws and *in vitro* digestibility with and without sodium hydroxide treatment. *Austalian Journal of Experimental Agriculture and Animal Husbandry 19:* 350-353.

Poppi, D.P.and McLennan, S.R. (1995). Protein and energy utilization by ruminants at pasture. *J. Anim. Sci.,* 73:278-290.

Prabowo, A., J. E. van Eys, I. W. Mathius, M. Rangkuti and W. L. Johnson. (1984). Studies on the mineral nutrition of sheep in West Java, Indonesia. Small Ruminant CRSP Working Paper No. 40, Res. Inst. for Anim. Prod., Bogor (indonesia) and North Carolina State Univ., Raleigh.

Prakash, P., Reddy, D.V., Reddy, R.R. and Krishna, N. (1996). *Anim. Feed Sci. Tech.,* 63: 229-243.

Rastogi, A., Dutta, N. and Sharma, K. (2006). Effect of strategically supplemented pregnancy allowance on nutrient utilization and reproductive performance of goats. LRRD., 18 (11).

Roxas D B, Castillo L S, Obsioma A R, Lapitan R M, Momongan V G and Juliano B O. (1984). Chemical composition and *in vitro* digestibility of straw from different varieties of rice. In: P T Doyle (ed.), *The utilization of fibrous agricultural residues as animal feeds.* Proceedings of the Third Annual Workshop of the Australian-Asian Fibrous Agricultural Residues Research Network, Peradeniya, Sri Lanka, 17-22 April 1983. University of Melbourne, Australia.

Schauer, C. S. D., Bohnert, W., Ganskopp, D. C., Richards, C. J. and Falc, S. J. (2005). Influence of protein supplementation frequency on cows consuming low-quality forage: Performance, grazing behavior, and variation in supplement intake. *J. Anim. Sci.,* 83:1715-1725.

Sibanda, L .M., Ndlovu, L. R. and Bryant, M.J. (1997). *J. Agr. Sci.* 128: 469-477.

Singh, B. and Makkar, H.P.S. (2000). The potential of mulberry tree foliage as an animal feed supplement in India. FAO Electronic Conference on Mulberry for Animal Production, April 2000, Rome, Italy.

Sutton J.D. (1989). *J. Dairy Sci.*, *72*: 2801–2814.

Van Niekerk, B.D.H. and Jacobs, G.A. (1985). *S. Afr. J. Anim. Sci.*, 15: 133 -136

Wanapat, M., Pimpa, O., Petlum, A. and Boontao, U. (1997). Cassava hay: A new strategic feed for ruminants during the dry season. LRRD., 9 (2).

Wang, Y., Spratling, B. M., ZoBell, D. R., Wiedmeier, R. D and T. A. McAllister. (2004). Effect of alkali pretreatment of wheat straw on the efficacy of exogenous fibrolytic enzymes. *Journal of Animal Scence.* 82:198-208.

Wiltbank, J.N., Rowden, W.W., Ingalls, J.E., Gregory, K.E. and Koch, R.M. (1962). *J. Anim. Sci.*, 21:219-225.

Winter, K.A. and Pigden, W.J. (1971). *Can. J. Anim. Sci.*, 51: 777-781.

Woods, B.C. (1997). Effect of inclusion of urea and supplement frequency on intake, digestion, and performance of cattle consuming low-quality, tall grass prairie forage. M.S. Thesis. Kansas State University, Manhattan, Kansas.

Zadrazil, F. (1984). Microbial conversion of lignocellulose into feed. In: Straw and other fibrous by-products. Eds Sundstsl, F., Owen, E. Elsevier, Amsterdam, pp. 276.

□□□

32

Effect of Processing Fibrous Agriculture Residue based Complete Diets on the Performance of Ruminants

Y. RAMANA REDDY, N. NALINI KUMARI, D. SRINIVASA RAO M. VENKATESWARLU AND G.V.N. REDDY

Department of Animal Nutrition, College of Veterinary Science, S.V. Veterinary University, Rajendranagar, Hyderabad, India – 500 030

ABSTARCT

Due to high fibrous nature and low nutrient content of fibrous agriculture residues (FAR), several physical processing methods were employed to improve their utilization in ruminants. Among the physical processing methods, grinding and blending a combination of FAR and concentrate in a certain ratio into mash or pellet was found to be a useful technology for efficient utilization of FAR in ruminants. The dry matter intake, digestibility of DM, OM and CP, nutritive value and nitrogen balance were increased and cell wall constituents digestibility was decreased when FAR based complete diets were processed into mash or pellets. Feeding different FAR based complete feed in pellet form, on an average increased fat corrected milk yield, feed efficiency, fat (%), fat and SNF yield by 30, 24.1, 20.4, 56.5 and 19.6, per cent, respectively but SNF (%) decreased by 8 per cent in lactating cows and buffaloes. Similarly in case of lambs and calves processing of FAR based complete diets into pellets supported an average daily gain of 107 and 669 g, respectively besides improving feed efficiency by 15.7 per cent in both lambs and calves. The impact on nutrient utilization, nutritive value and animal performance was when FAR based complete diets were processed into mash. A complete diet processing unit suitable to rural areas was developed and distributed to research institutions and farmers for transfer of technology from lab to land to improve nutrient use efficiency in animal food chain. But the cost of the machinery, infrastructure required and lack of extension are the main constraints for transfer of this technology.

Introduction

Efficient utilization of fibrous agricultural residues and agro-industrial by-products as animal feed assumed importance due to shortage of dry roughages, concentrates and green fodder to an extent of 19, 62 and 45%, respectively in India (Anon. 2008). Due to cultivation of food and commercial crops, huge quantities of different types of fibrous agricultural residues are produced every year as a renewable resource. In the last 4 decades the availability of fibrous agricultural residues increased by two and a half times contributing to 44% overall feed resource and by the year 2020 its contribution is predicted to reach to 70% of Indian feed budget (Ramachandra *et al.*, 2005). However, these fibrous agricultural residues are rich in fiber and low in nitrogen, minerals and vitamins. Hence, these are not palatable and can not form a sole ration for livestock. Any processing method that improves the nutrient availability from these crop residues will go a long way in bridging the gap between availability and requirement of roughages.

The concept of complete feeds for feeding ruminants is relatively of recent origin in India. In this system, all feed ingredients inclusive of roughages are proportioned, processed and mixed into a uniform blend, supplying adequate nutrients to the animal. The product is fed as a sole source of nutrients. This system ensures the supply of balanced nutrients, controls the ratio of concentrate to roughage, helps in improving utilization of low-grade fibrous agricultural residues, reduces feed wastage and also reduces feeding cost. It also promotes better consumption and avoids refusal of the unpalatable portions of the feedstuffs. Such rations also reduce eating and rumination time and increase resting time.

A more even intake of feed is also associated with less fluctuation in the release of ammonia so that non-protein nitrogen may be more efficiently utilized and may lead to an increase in the general utilization of protein. This system gives good scope for increasing the use of home grown fibrous agricultural residues and by-products. The level of inclusion of different fibrous agricultural residues in complete diets of ruminants is shown in Table 1.The nutrient specifications were given for complete feeds for various classes of ruminants by Owen (1979) and Reddy and Reddy (2003). The roughage portion varies from 30-70 per cent depending upon the physiological status of animals. The roughage content of complete diets is 30-40 per cent for high yielding animals, 40-50 per cent for growing animals and 60-70 per cent for dry animals; whereas the protein content varies from 11-13%. Accordingly the proportion of other ingredients varies. These diets can be processed into mash or pellets. For pelleting of mash feed, traditional steam pelleting or recently developed expander extruder technology can be adopted.

Table 1 : Inclusion levels of different fibrous agriculture residues in complete diets of ruminants

Fibrous agriculture residue	Per cent in complete ration
Sugarcane bagasse	20
Sorghum straw	20-46
Dry mixed grass	30-75
Sunflower straw	30-50
Sunflower heads	33.5-50
Wheat straw	50
Fallen teak leaves	17.5-70
Mango leaves	30-60
Rice straw	40-50
Cotton straw	45

(Reddy and Reddy, 2003)

Processing of Complete Diets

Mash: The different ingredients of the diet are proportioned as per formula into 100 kg batches using appropriate scales. A Hammer mill with 8 mm sieve is used for grinding the ingredients. Through screw conveyor and bucket elevator the ground ingredients are discharged into the hopper fixed on top of the mixer. The ingredients that do not require mixing are directly added to the mixer. Molasses is pumped from the storage tank to a heating tank, where it is heated to 70°C. The heated molasses is sent to the mixer through a dosage tank, as per formula. The micro-ingredients (vitamins and minerals) are made into a premix by mixing them with ground grain or bran and required quantity of the premix is added to mixer directly. Later, all the ingredients are mixed for about 10 minutes and then collected in sacks and stored.

Expander-extruder processing: This is a system, which combines the features of expanding (application of moisture, pressure and temperature to gelatinize the starch portion) and extruding (pressing the feed through constrictions under pressure). The mash containing 12-13 per cent moisture and at room temperature is reconstituted with required quantity of water to get 17-18 per cent moisture in the mixer and then sent to the hopper above the expander-extruder from which it passes through a screw in which it attains 90-95°C by the time it comes out of the die openings. Otherwise, the mash without reconstitution can be sent to hopper and steam is added to get the required moisture while the feed is passing through the screw of expander-extruder. The pellets coming out of the expander-extruder are cooled and collected into sacks.

Effect on Dmi and Nutrient Utilization

Effect of feeding complete diets processed into mash and expander extruded pellets with different fibrous agricultural residues on dry matter intake and nutrient utilization was studied and compared with conventional feeding system by several workers (Table 5). Analysis of 4 to 17 studies revealed that processing of different fibrous agricultural residues into mash and expander extruded pellets improved dry matter intake by 0.29 and 0.32 percentage units in small and large ruminants compared to conventional system of feeding. The digestibility of dry matter (DM), organic matter (OM) and crude protein (CP) was improved by 1.59, 4.12; 2.18, 2.94 and 2.96 and 3.71 percentage units. The impact on digestibility was more with pelleting than grinding (mash) due to application of heat in pelleting process. Heat processing increases starch degradation in the rumen, avoids overloading the ruminant's capacity for small intestine starch digestion and increases total tract starch digestion (Huntington, 1997). Further, heat processing can increase the amount of microbial protein entering the small intestine (Zinn *et al.*, 1998; Theurer *et al.*, 1999) due to increase in amount of ruminally fermentable starch and lowering of protein degradability due to formation of cross linkages between and among peptide chains and with carbohydrates (Reddy *et al.*, 1993) and increasing the digestibility of microbial protein and bypass protein in small intestine. However, digestibility of cell wall constituents such as neutral detergent fiber (NDF), acid detergent fiber (ADF), hemicellulose and cellulose were consistently lower by 1.34, 3.42; 0.73, 6.42; 1.06, 0.69 and 0.78 and 2.41 percentage units in mash and pellet form of fibrous residue based complete diets in comparison to conventional (loose) form of feeding. Reduced fiber digestibility was observed when a severe elevation in the rate of passage is much greater than changes in rate of digestibility. Reducing particle size decreases the filling effects of forage and increases the ruminal passage rate (Allen, 2000) there by affecting the fiber digestibility

The improvement in digestibility of proximate nutrients reflected on nutritive value and nitrogen balance in small and large ruminants. The DCP (%), ME (MJ/kg DM) and nitrogen (N) balance (g/d) values of fibrous agricultural residue based complete diets processed into mash and pellet were improved by 28.55, 2.41 47.78 and 28.55, 7.23 and 83.03 per cent, respectively.

Table 2 : Effect of processing of fibrous agricultural residue based complete diets on DMI and nutrient utilization in ruminants

Parameter	Conventional	Mash	Pellet
DMI (% b. wt.)	2.83 (10)	+0.29 (8)	+0.32 (10)
Digestibility (%)			
DM	58.86 (17)	+1.59 (13)	+4.12 (11)
OM	61.56 (16)	+2.18 (12)	+2.94 (10)
CP	59.87 (17)	+2.96 (13)	+3.71 (11)
CF	56.76 (12)	+1.23 (7)	-0.45 (10)
NDF	55.57 (10)	-1.34 (7)	-3.42 (4)
ADF	51.36 (8)	-0.73 (4)	-6.42 (6)
Hemicellulose	62.09 (8)	-1.06 (4)	-0.69 (6)
Cellulose	52.24 (7)	-0.78 (4)	-2.41 (5)
Nutritive value			
DCP (%)	6.13 (19)	+1.75 (14)	+1.75 (12)
ME (MJ/kg DM)	8.3 (19)	+0.2 (15)	+0.6 (15)
Balance			
Nitrogen balance (g/d)			
Lambs	3.37(5)	4.48(5)	6.65(5)
Calves	24.14(6)	39.26(6)	40.73(4)

Values in parenthesis indicates number of studies considered

(Venkat Reddy *et al.*, 1986; Gowd *et al.*, 1987; Reddy *et al.*, 1994; Madan Mohan *et al.*, 1997; Rao *et al.*, 1997a; Rao *et al.*,1997b; Venkanna *et al.*, 1997; Reddy *et al.*, 2001a; Reddy *et al.*, 2001b; Reddy *et al.*, 2002; Reddy *et al.*, 2003; Nagalakshmi *et al.*, 2004; Nagalakshmi *et al.*, 2006; Ramachandran and Singhal, 2008; Madhavi *et al.* ,2009; Nagalakshmi and Reddy, 2010; Khan *et al.*, 2010).

Effect on Animal Performance

Several studies indicated that, there was an improvement of 7.06-33.70, 0-16.97 and 48.38-53.90 and 8.16-14.33 per cent, respectively in ADG and feed conversion efficiency in growing lambs and crossbred calves fed various fibrous agriculture residues based complete diets in the form of mash and expander extruded complete diets compared to conventional feeding (Table 3). The increased palatability and digestibility of processed rations together with efficient utilization of absorbed nitrogen due to matching supply of energy and minerals may be responsible for increased ADG and feed efficiency in lambs and calves. Zile Sihag *et al.*, (2008) reported that, the straws like gram, soya and black gram can be incorporated up to 60 per cent in pelleted diets to obtain growth from 80-100 g daily in small ruminants.

Table 3 : Effect of feeding processed fibrous agriculture residue based complete diets on growth performance of ruminants

Parameter	Conventional	Mash	Pellet
Lambs[1]			
ADG(g)	72.37	77.48	107.38
FCR	11.65	11.65	10.7
Cost/kg gain (Rs.)	59.03	56.21	47.87
Calves[2]			
ADG(g)	434.78	581.28	669.13
FCR	10.84	9.00	8.29

[1]Each value is the average of six studies
[2] Each value is the average of four studies

(Reddy *et al.*, 1989a; Reddy *et al.*, 1989b; Reddy and Reddy, 1991; Reddy *et al.*, 1994; Reddy *et al.*, 2002; Reddy, 2005; Kirubanath *et al.*, 2003; Ramachandran and Singhal,2008; Madhavi *et al.*, 2010)

Processing of fibrous agricultural residue based complete diets into mash and expander extruded pellets improved milk yield (kg), FCM milk yield (kg), and feed efficiency by 1.90, 8.64; 2.25, 30.00 and 15.64 and 24.17 per cent and decreased SNF (%) by 10.56 and 8.04 per cent over conventional feeding in lactating cows and buffaloes, respectively (Table 4). The fat (%) fat

Table 4 : Performance of lactating animals fed processed fibrous agriculture residue based complete diets

Parameter*	Conventional	Mash	Pellet
Milk yield (kg/d)	5.79	5.90	6.29
FCM yield (kg)	7.1	7.26	9.23
Fat (%)	5.20	4.89	6.26
SNF (%)	10.70	9.57	9.84
Fat yield (g/d)	369.2	355.0	577.8
SNF yield (g/d)	759.7	694.8	908.2
DMI/kg FCM (kg)	2.11	1.78	1.60

*Each value is the average of 5 studies

(Reddy *et al.*, 1988; Reddy *et al.*, 1996; Reddy *et al.*, 2001b; Reddy *et al.*, 2003; Nagalakshmi *et al.*, 2004; Reddy, 2005; Nagalakshmi *et al.*, 2010; Khan *et al.*, 2010)

yield (g/d), and SNF yield (g/d) were increased by 20.39, 56.50 and 19.55 per cent, respectively in lactating cows and buffaloes fed expander extruded pellets of fibrous agricultural residue based complete diets whereas the values were decreased by 5.96, 3.85 and 8.4 per cent, respectively when the complete diets with different crop residues were fed in mash form to lactating cows and buffaloes compared to conventional feeding system. The higher OM and CP digestibility along with higher DMI in buffaloes and cows fed expander extruded complete diets might have resulted in higher fat corrected milk yield, fat (%), fat and SNF yield.

Based on the research findings, a small scale complete feed processing unit which can grind all crop residues was developed under National Agricultural Technology Project (NATP) for use at village level. Twenty four units of small scale complete feed processing units were distributed to different research institutions and farmers in India. This enables the farmers to utilize the crop residues available with them effectively. However, the technology developed is not extensively used due to the factors such as prevailing small holder livestock system, high cost of the machinery (US $ 11000/unit), infrastructure required and lack of extension.

Conclusion

The review of different research studies revealed that fibrous agriculture residues hitherto wasted can be efficiently and economically utilized in the form of complete diets. Feeding of fibrous agricultural residue based complete diets in expander extruded pellets improved dry matter intake, nutrient utilization and performance in ruminants than mash or loose (conventional) form. But the energy cost involved in the processing should be considered from economical point of view while processing fibrous agricultural residue based complete diets into pellets for feeding of ruminants.

References

Allen, M. S. (2000). Effects of diet on short term regulation of feed intake by lactating dairy cattle. *Journal of Dairy Science*, 83: 1598-1624.

Anonymous. (2008). Annual report of National Institute of Animal Nutrition and Physiology (NIANP), Bangalore, India.

Gowd, B. C. S., Reddy, M. R. and Reddy, G. V. N. (1987). Utilization of sunflower heads as roughage source in complete feeds for sheep. *Indian Journal of Animal Nutrition*, 4:28-33.

Huntington, G. B. (1997). Starch utilization by ruminants: from basics to the bunk. *Journal of Animal Science* 75: 852-867.

Kirubanath, K., Reddy, D. N. and Nagalakshmi, D. (2003). Effect of processing cotton straw based complete diet with expander-extruder on performance of crossbred calves. *Asian-Australasian Journal of Animal Science*, 16:1572-1576.

Khan, S.R., Singh, S.K. and Mudgal, V. (2010). Effect of feeding complete rations on the performance of lactating crossbred cows. *Indian Journal of Animal Nutrition*, 27: 261-264.

Madan Mohan, A., Reddy, G.V.N. and Reddy, M. R. (1997). Utilization of sunflower (*Helianthus annuus*) heads as roughage source in complete diets. *Indian Journal of Animal Science*, 67: 1098-1100.

Madhavi, K., Reddy, T. J., Ramana Reddy, Y. and Reddy, G. V. N. (2009). Effect of feeding differently processed neem seed cake (*Azadirachta indica*) based complete diet on intake and nutrient utilization in Nellore sheep. *Indian Journal of Animal Nutrition*, 26: 130-134.

Madhavi, K., Reddy, T. J., Ramana Reddy, Y. and Reddy, G. V. N. (2010). Growth and carcass characteristics of Nellore ram lambs fed on differently processed and detoxified neem (*Azadirachta indica*) seed cake incorporated complete diets. *Animal Nutrition and Feed Technology*, 10: 201-206.

Nagalakshmi, D., Reddy, D. N. and Kishan Kumar, M. (2004). Performance of Murrah buffaloes fed expander pelleted cotton straw based diets. *Animal Nutrition and Feed Technology*, 4: 23-32.

Nagalakshmi, D., Narasimha Reddy, D. and Rajendra Prasad, M. (2006). Evaluation of Sun flower Head based Complete Diet in Lactating cross Bred Cow. *Indian Journal of Dairy Science*, 59: 233-237.

Nagalakshmi, D. and Reddy, D. N. (2010). Effect of feeding expander extruder processed complete diet containing sugarcane bagassse on performance of Murrah buffaloes. *Animal Nutrition and Feed Technology*, 10:1-8.

Owen, J. B. (1979). Complete Diets for Cattle and Sheep 1st eds., Farming Press Limited, Suffolk, England. p. 159.

Ramachandra, K.S., Raju, S. S., Anandan, S. and Angadi, U.B. (2005). Animal feed resources and its impact on livestock production in India. *Indian Dairyman*, 57: 39-47.

Ramachandran, M. and Singhal, K. K. (2008). Cottonseed hulls based complete diets for crossbred calves. Livestock Research for Rural Development 20 (11). Article# 176 http://www.lrrd.org/lrrd20/11/rama20176.htm.

Rao, K. S., Reddy, M. R. and Reddy, G. V. N. (1997a). Utilization of sunflower straw in complete diets of crossbred bulls. *Indian Journal of Animal Nutrition*, 14:123-127.

Rao, K. S., Reddy, M. R. and Reddy, G. V. N. (1997b). Utilization of sunflower heads in complete diets of crossbred bulls. *Indian Journal of Animal Nutrition*, 14:119-122.

Reddy, G. V. N., Reddy, M. R. and Reddy, K.K. (1988). Sunflower straw based complete feed for crossbred cows. *Indian Journal of Animal Nutrition*, 5: 322-324.

Reddy, P. R., Reddy, G. V. N. and Reddy, M. R. (1989a). Utilization of sunflower straw and its heads as sole source of roughage in complete feeds for sheep. *Indian Journal of Animal Sciences*, 59: 128-132.

Reddy, S. K. Reddy, G.V.N. and Reddy, M. R. (1989b). Utilization of wheat straw/berseem hay and poultry droppings in the development of complete feeds for crossbred bulls. *Indian Journal of Animal Sciences*, 59: 981-985.

Reddy, G. V. N. and Reddy, M. R. (1991). Effect of processing cotton seed hulls on nutrient utilization in sheep and goats. *Indian Journal of Animal Nutrition*, 8: 123-126.

Reddy, G. V. N., Reddy, M. R. and Reddy, P. R. (1993). Utilization of certain varieties of sorghum straw by sheep. *Indian Journal of Animal Nutrition*, 10: 173-176.

Reddy, S. K., Reddy, G. V. N. and Reddy, M. R. (1994). Nutrient utilization and growth performance of crossbred heifers fed on fodder based complete diet. *Indian Journal of Animal Sciences*, 64: 862–866.

Reddy, G. V. N., Reddy, M. R. and Das, T. C. (1996). Effects of feeding fodder based complete diet on the production performance of cross bred cows. *Indian Journal of Animal Sciences*, 66: 63-67.

Reddy, G. V. N., Joji Reddy, K. and Nagalakshmi, D. (2001a). Effect of feeding Expander extruder Processed complete Diet containing Maize cobs on Production performance of Buffaloes. *Indian Journal of Animal Nutrition*, 18: 8-14.

Reddy, G. V. N., Joji Reddy, K. and Nagalakshmi, D. (2001b). Nutrient Utilization and rumen fermentation pattern of Sugarcane bagasse based Complete Diets in Buffalo Bulls. *Indian Journal of Animal Nutrition*, 18: 138-145.

Reddy, G. V. N., Reddy, J. K. and Nagalakshmi, D. (2002). Effect of expander extruder processed complete diet containing sugarcane bagasse on growth and nutrient utilization in Ongole bull calves. *Indian Journal of Animal Sciences*, 72: 406–409.

Reddy, G. V. N. (2005). Complete diet system for ruminants. In: Technologies for Enhancing Feed Quality (eds. G.V.N. Reddy, A. R. Reddy, Y. Anjaneyulu and Y. R. Reddy), ANGR Agricultural University press, Hyderabad, India. pp. 14-19.

Reddy, M.R. and Reddy, G.V.N. (2003). Processing of complete diets for ruminants and their effect on animal performance. In: Feed Processing Technology (eds. G.V.N. Reddy, N. Krishna, V.L.K. Prasad, K.J. Reddy and Y.R. Reddy), ANGR Agricultural University press, Hyderabad, India. pp. 168-169.

Theurer, C. B., Huber, J. T., Delagardo-Elorduy, A. and Wanderely, R. (1999). Invited review: summary: summary of steam- flaking corn or sorghum grain for lactating dairy cows. *Journal of Dairy Science*, 82: 1950-1959.

Venkanna, P., Reddy, M. R. and Reddy, G. V. N. (1997). Rumen fermentation pattern on complete diets based on dry mixed grass or cotton seed hulls in crossbred bulls. *Indian Journal off Animal Nutrition*, 14: 245-249.

Venkat Reddy, T., Reddy, M. R. and Reddy, G. V. N. (1986). Utilization of wheat straw and agro-industrial by products in the development of complete feed for sheep. *Indian Journal of Animal Sciences*, 56: 100-104.

Zile, S., Nanda Kishore, S. and Berwal, R. S. (2008). Utilization of pulses straw in complete pelleted feeds for growing lambs. *Indian Journal of Animal Nutrition*, 25: 252-255.

Zinn, R. A., Owens, F. N. and Ware, R. A. (2002). Flaking corn: processing mechanics, quality standards and impacts on energy availability and performance of feed lot cattle. Journal of Animal Sciences, 80: 1145-1156.

□□□

33

Approaches in Diseases Investigation and Outbreak

DINESH CHANDRA AND R. SINGH
Centre for Animal Disease Research and Diagnosis,
Indian Veterinary Research Institute, Izatnagar–243 122 (UP)

Disease investigation– An art

Disease investigation is a multi-disciplinary task requiring the skilled personnel in the area of clinical medicine, epidemiology, laboratory diagnostic (pathology/microbiology/toxicology/Parasitology), and environmental health. Symptoms alone are not enough to diagnose any disease. However, thorough history, clinical (physical and chemical) examination of diseased animals or postmortem of dead animals is needed. In addition, laboratory tests on clinical and morbid samples from such animals are recommended to arrive at conclusive diagnosis. During disease investigation and diagnosis process, many things are learnt with time and practice. The following steps are being suggested for carrying out disease investigation:

Step 1: Preparedness and promptness

After receiving the information (through letter, telegram, telephone, or fax) of a disease in animals population, tentatively diagnosed at field level as: suspected poisoning/ malicious poisoning/ mysterious deaths/ deaths due to unknown reasons, etc, the place should be visited within 24 hour by the disease investigation officers (DIOs or team of experts) along with necessary kits (personal protective equipment, post-mortem kit, transport media, sterile vials and disinfectants, etc). A team of trained veterinarians or experts (usually 2-3 persons) should visit the place after due intimation to the affected party so that someone should be available there to assist the team during the investigation and for collection of samples.

Step 2: Gathering information

After reaching the site of investigation, the information should be collected by having discussions with VO, owners/ farmers, without any bias and prejudice. It would be interesting, if one becomes friendlier and informal with VO/ Farmers/Owners, then factual history of the disease may be extracted and compared. It is sometimes wise to have separate discussion with persons not directly involved and simply acting as an observer. During the discussion, one should also keep asking/ cross questioning, using a set of questionnaire in back of mind, including the date of onset of the disease, details of susceptible animal (age, sex, physiological status, breed, free range, stall fed, total animal population, newly inducted animals, if any, etc), duration of illness, clinical signs, treatment provided, vaccination history, post-mortem lesions, etc. This can also be done through designed proforma to avoid missing any details. The information received is noted down as neatly and completely as possible, because the investigation is often performed under less favourable condition. During questioning, false information may be given knowingly or unknowingly or owner may not cooperate. There may be some dispute or disagreement of opinion among the staff of the farm. Under these circumstances it becomes difficult to obtain correct information. The veterinarian should handle the animal owners with diplomacy and tactfully. He should avoid to use technical terminology as most of the owners/farmers are not able to understand the technical words. It is however, preferred to use local language when asking question to animal attendants. The veterinarian should ask the question in a friendly and cordial atmosphere and should avoid arguments. It has been observed during disease investigation that some animal owners hesitate in revealing accurate history so it is very important to ask them in such a way that they should not feel guilty. In rural areas of developing countries like India, the animals are looked after by the female members of the family. As they are not much educated, they even cannot understand Hindi. Therefore, the use of local language of the area is always advisable by the veterinarian. If the veterinarian is not well versed with local language of that area, he can take the help of his stock assistant/compounder/attendant or any other person from the village who knows both the local and Hindi/English and may act as translator between owner and the animal doctor. Apparently such things are looking minor or of low importance but it may have far reaching effect on confirmatory diagnosis. It should be kept in mind that veterinary should try to separate the owner's observation from his interpretation. Whenever the veterinarian is misled by the anaemnesis, the careful clinical and laboratory examination is essential in such case. If the anaemnesis does not confirm the result of examination, it should be accepted with utmost care/ attention to avoid any misconception.

Note down the animal species population and number of animals being affected and succumbed over a point of time (disease prevalence) or over a period of time (disease incidence) from the record at the facility. Calculate the morbidity rate (%) by dividing the number of affected animals to total number of animals and mortality rate (%) by dividing the dead animals to total number of animals. The case fatality rate (%) is calculated by dividing the number of animals dead due to disease by number of animals affected with same disease. The morbidity, mortality and case fatality rates indicate the nature of etiological agents.

Further, the outdoor and indoor environmental components like contaminated water (high nitrate/ nitrite and fluoride contents in certain areas; water bodies with parasites and pesticides), soil type and topography (leaching, water logging etc), soil composition (like iodine deficiency and Cu, Fe, Zn, etc deficiency or excess in certain areas); quality of fodder/ forage; air quality together with humidity, precipitation and environmental temperature; population density; prevalence of flies, ticks, lice, mites, fauna and flora, etc. are equally important that can adversely affect the animal health and the same should be thoroughly looked during the investigation. The environmental pollutants may cause immune suppression and precipitate other infections, while improper disposal of waste near the animal houses and unhygienic conditions at the farm may build up infectious load. So, every bit of information should be recorded in investigation notebook. Besides, one should also get the information about the kind of management, housing of animals, movement of animals/ humans and other fomites in and out of the facility as these could be the source of infection. Then the probable etiological agent and its source should be traced out using epidemiological methods.

Sometimes, it is observed that team of experts gets influenced by the misleading statements told by the owners or other persons or influenced by the print media hype, NGO's intervention, mass media effect, superstitious beliefs, which most of the time have no scientific. This affects the investigation process. Therefore, it is necessary to collect the information tactfully and diplomatically and try to gather information systematically and scientifically. Team should take the owners in confidence and cross-examine friendly in local language (take help of VO, stockman, attendant or villager) so that they may not hesitate in revealing the facts. The friendly attitude will always repose the confidence in the people in obtaining the information. After collecting the history, the team should sit and logically discuss all these possible variables and by process of exclusion of least possible differential factors, should come out with possible reasons affecting the animal(s).

Step 3: Logical and systematic clinical examination

Once microbes overcome the host, the development of disease follows a set course, whether the disease is acute or chronic: incubation period (entry of the organism to appearance of first clinical sign), prodromal period (relatively of short period exhibited by early anorexia and malaise), clinical period (most acute stage with overt clinical signs) and convalescent period (in this stage body starts regaining pre diseased state followed by complete recovery or carrier state as seen in FMDV). During period of incubation, period of illness and convalescence, the infection spreads. In some diseases like FMD, the convalescent period is very long up to 2 months and carrier state is seen.

At the time of outbreak investigation, animals show different stages of disease development. However, in point source of infection (like parasitic, food borne and water borne infections) many animals exhibit similar stage of clinical signs/ symptoms. DIO should observe and record various stages of clinical development in animals and select the animals exhibiting overt clinical sings for disease identification.

The owners/ farmers often record only dullness, in-appetence and decreased production in animals usually in prodromal and convalescent phase of illness that are not sufficient to identify the disease. So animals exhibiting the most severe clinical illness should be examined clinically for their behavior and general appearance, voice, eating, defecation, urination, mucus discharges, posture, gait, conformation and then for pulse, rectal temperature and respiration. Usually people omit to see the oral mucosa and tongue surfaces and do not go for auscultation and percussion of the body parts right from head to thorax and abdominal areas, thereby loose the diagnosis even the animal is in clinical period.

It is also advisable to examine few typical cases (clinical phase) along with other in-contact animals, which are apparently normal. In some diseases, fever lasts 1-2 days, and then other signs appear. If fever is passed off, it will be a confused state for DIOs who may end up with wrong diagnosis. After recording the history on general aspects, one should ask the owner about total number of animals on the premises, number of animals affected and number of animals dead due to disease to calculate morbidity, mortality and case fatality rates. The DIOs should ask the owner about treatments given to animals and its response. The vaccination and/or other control measures taken by the veterinarian/ owner to contain the disease should be noted. After recording the animal data on present disease, one should see the management aspect of the animals, which includes nutrition, quality of feed and fodder (free from fungus and toxins), pasture grazing or stall-feeding, climate, housing, drainage of water, sources of water supply and ventilation in animal houses.

During the clinical examination, collect EDTA and clotted blood (serum) in sterile tubes, prepare blood smears. Also make smears from aspirates, collect body fluids (pleural, peritoneum, synovial, CSF) depending upon the situation. Collect excisional biopsy or punch (6mm punch) biopsy or and scrapings from skin in 10 % formalin saline and fresh for culture and sensitivity test. In autoimmune skin diseases, 10% tissue is used for immuno-histochemical testing. In case of skin tumor, collect the tumor tissue less than ¼ th inch for better penetration in 1: 9 ratio preservative (10% formalin saline) for IHC for diagnosing infectious diseases.

Step 4: Scientific investigation through systematic necropsy

After clinical examination and recording the history, one should proceed to conduct systematic necropsy of animals and record lesions side by side on the post-mortem proforma in non-technical terms. In some diseases like rabies, incomplete necropsy is required by examining nervous system.

To conduct an effective necropsy it requires consistent procedures, keeping detailed report and photographic records, proper equipment, proper labeling of each sample and experience. Necropsy is enjoyable procedure if persons are wearing personal protective equipment, sharp instruments in kit, tissue holding sterile vials, transport media and other things in order. The description of lesions should be such that it should give the impression, as if carcass is narrating whole story of its death. Remember, systematic necropsy is not only done to know the cause of death of animals, but to provide death certificate of insured animals, to provide reason for death in vetrolegal cases and to fetch materials for laboratory diagnosis. Since pathology is largely an observational science, it should be attempted very carefully and lesions be recorded in simple terms with objectively.

Step 5. Post-mortem (necropsy) examination

After receiving the request proforma (owner or FIR copy) having details of anamnesis, date and time of death, etc.), read out carefully or recollect the clinical history (anamnesis) and other details of the animal (s) (individual / population) before conduction of necropsy. "*Anamnesis is a base line for accurate diagnosis of disease*". Always perform necropsy at a designated place (restricted public access, sheltered from rain and direct sun, away from water sources; on government land); use hygienic methods to shun from flying insects to avoid spread of infection and spillage of body fluids and preferably in broad day light to avoid misinterpretation of colors in lesions. Usually 3 persons (1 necropsist, 2 assistant) are required for necropsy work. Follow the necropsy procedure as per the species described. Follow general statistical rule while carrying out clinical and necropsy examination, particularly when sampling herds or flocks mortality to achieve a 95% probability of detecting infection e.g., if disease is present in 5% of a herd of 500 animals to be 95% confident of finding one positive, assuming that both the sensitivity and specificity of the test is 100%. For laboratory diagnosis always, collect blood/ serum, other body fluids and tissues in different transport media from dead or culled animals. While describing the lesions you see far more in it than when you are merely looking at it. So cultivate the art of description by deliberate practice and describe natural objects clearly, simply and accurately, which will make you better observer. For example, liver shows a single, circumscribed, rounded mass of 2 cm diameter and a thin white capsule enclosing degenerated contents, folded greenish and gelatinous membranous material, with yellow friable material. The surrounding tissue appears normal. From this type of description one can easily make out that, it is a case of probably bile -stained, hydatid cyst of liver. Nevertheless, in many cases the nature of lesions is not very obvious so diagnosis on the gross appearance alone is not possible. So do not get frustrated. In such cases, a discussion of the differential diagnosis is must; so think the reasonable possibilities and weigh the point for and against each of them. So run over the list of main classes of lesions in one's mind remembering this mnemonic: VINDICATE= Vascular disturbances, inflammatory lesion, neoplasm, idiopathic, congenital malformation, autoimmunity, traumatic lesion and endocrine disorder.

Step 6. Post necropsy action

Disposal of the carcass, disinfection of the site and personal protective equipments is utmost importance before leaving the site. Necropsy often tiring due to odd weather or when time runs short to reach the destination in that situation, one should not leave the place before disposal of carcass, cleaning the site and personal belongings. Otherwise, this could be a threat to public and animals.

Step 7. Transportation of materials to laboratory

The morbid samples collected during the clinical and post-mortem examination are transported to the laboratory in shortest possible time. The transport media and ice should be used for maintaining the quality of samples. The samples are subjected to various tests depending upon the facilities available in the laboratories. Some tests are required reference laboratories. Once the disease is confirmed immediately outbreak control measures are taken to prevent the further spread of the infection and its eradication.

Although, based on suspicion of the disease and its dangerous nature, actions are taken before confirmation of the outbreak so that infection is controlled at source soon after the same is confirmed.

Outbreak Management

The epizootics of diseases (infectious and parasitoses) follow a specific course, which are promoted or impaired by ecological, climatic, socio-economic and production condition. The process of outbreak may be checked by carefully directed influence on infectious sources, mode of transmission and susceptible host population. Therefore, it is necessary to protect animal population against epizootics, which have consequences for the economy and human health. Protection against epizootics as well as their control and eradication is achieved by when all conditions, which turn the infectious diseases into real epizootics are sufficiently known like: agent reservoir, mode of transmission, susceptibility of population, analyzing the influence factors like vectors responsible for dynamics of individual epizootics, special geographical, climatic, ecological, socioeconomic, production condition, host specificity, virulence, contagiousness, tenacity of the agent to environment, mode of transmission, possibility of further spreads and potential host population. During disease investigation, all these interactions as well as biotic and abiotic environment factors have to be taken into account.

Depending on the nature and size of the outbreak, each country/state should prepare its own plan of outbreaks management. In case of outbreak suspicion, out break confirmation and later bio-security issues should be taken up rapidly and responsibly, and there should be clear cut systems and protocols developed in advance, so that during outbreak all the team members involved can be clear on their course of action, so that time is not lost in containment of the infection and later its eradication.

For effective outbreak management, logical disease investigation as mentioned above is must. In addition, early recognition of the disease outbreak through rapid and specific diagnostic tests, rapid initiation of control measures and effective communication is critical for containment of the outbreak. For outbreak management one should know the infectious disease cycle namely: the etiological agent, vectors/reservoirs, mode of transmission, pathology and pathogenesis in susceptible host and finally route of escape of etiological agent. The knowledge of microbiology, parasitology, immunology, pharmacology and animal hygiene is also essential. During outbreak management, it is necessary to find out character and extent of an epizootic, to detect the cause and factor responsible for the outbreak and spread of the epizootics, to develop prevention and control (including eradication) strategies and to control the efficacy of anti-epizootic measures.

Disinfection is done to control and contain the infection at source. After that sealing of units and issue of sanitization is done. Then post operation surveillance and freedom from the disease is achieved. While in surveillance zone, restrictions are imposed and sero-surveillance is carried out or vaccination is adopted depending upon the situation. Steps in outbreak management

- Destruction of the agent reservoir and infection at sources (pest and rodent control and culling and slaughter of infected host population).
- Interrupting the transmission process (control of vector population and prohibition of trade or animal movement).
- By modulating the susceptibility of host population (vaccination and optimizing of rearing conditions).

Depending on danger, the prevalence and incidence as well as specific characteristic of the epizootic, following strategies to be adopted for prevention and control:

1. *First Barrier System*: it is essential to have data on international epizootic situation for control of the epizootics.

   a) Prevent import and transit of animals.

   b) Zoosanitary control of animals and animal products crossing frontiers as well as through quarantine and systematic investigation of import.

2. *Second Barrier System*:

   a) Isolation and liquidation of outbreaks by stamping out of in-apparently diseased, infected and latent infections.

   b) Slaughtering (diseased an infected and metaphylactic and prophylactic vaccination of potentially endangered animals).

   c) Eradication of persistent outbreak on the basis of sanitation and control measures like depopulation of whole stock (slaughter or separate unit), permanent diagnostic monitoring and selection of reactors, hygienic measures and vaccination of masses.

3. *Step by step reduction of the prevalence and incidence of epizootics*:

   a) Control of wild life reservoir and immunization of animals.

   b) Hygiene and vaccination

   c) Prompt diagnosis, monitoring, prophylactic and metaphylactic treatment.

d) Slaughtering and liquidation of animals.

e) Pre-expositional vaccination.

4. Interruption of transmission process by

   a) Zoosanitary control of animal movement and general quarantine.

   b) Control of vectors, intermediate host.

5. Obstacles in control of outbreak

   a) Lack of provision for nomadic animal keeping.

   b) Impossibility of imposing restrictions.

   c) Impossibility of prohibiting the exchange of animals and animal products in trade.

   d) Impossibility of controlling the traditional and customary exchange of animals.

   e) Religious prejudices and superstitions.

   f) Numerous wild life populations, agent reservoir which used the same pastures and watery places as domestic animals.

   g) Under developed infrastructure (communication and diagnostics).

   h) Economy does not allow expensive control measures (vaccination of national herd and the compensation of damages by the state.

References

Applied Veterinary Epidemiology. (1989). Edited by Blaha Thomas, Elsevier Science Publishers, Amsterdam, p.343.

Chauhan R.S., Singh R and Singh K.P. (2007). Art of Disease Investigation. IVRI, Izatnagar. pp 82.

Chandra D. and Chauhan R.S. (2006). Mannual of Parasitic Disease Investigation. IVRI, Izatnagar. pp 70.

Martin S.W., Meek A.H. and Willeberg P. (1987). Veterinary Epidemiology, principles and methods. Iowa State University Press.

□□□

34

Canine Dermatitis and its Therapeutical Management

SUSHOVAN ROY* AND MANJU ROY**
*Principal, College of Veterinary sciences & A.H., R.K. Nagar, Agartala, Tripura
**Physiology and Biochemistry Department, College of Veterinary Science & A.H., Anjora, Durg (C.G)

Introduction

The most popular pet world wise is the domestic dogs, *Canis familaris*. Today many scientists agree that all dogs descended from the wolf family alone though earlier it was regarded that dog has originated form wolf, jackal and other members of wolf family. In a word of constant stress and strain, day by day people are getting more and more attached to pets. Pet animals, especially dogs provide unadulterated love and friendship to their masters and family members, a precious something that has become scarce these days. It holds a quite unique position in human society and that's why the most popular pet world wise is the domestic dog.

The skin is a largest organ of the body and, depending on the species and age, may represent 12-24% of an animal's body weight. The skin has many functions, including serving as an enclosing barrier against harmful physiologic and chemical factors and negative effects on bacteria, and it can perceive sensory inputs from the things that it touches such as heat cold, pain and itching. In general these functions are not greatly impeded by most diseases of the skin although failure of the sweating mechanism does seriously interfere with body temperature regulation, and severe burns or other skin diseases may cause fluid and electrolyte loss.

Nothing is more frustrating for either an owner or a veterinarian than a dog that is suffering from a skin disease. And since skin can only respond to disease causing agents in a few selected ways, the appearance of much skin illness will be similar. These responses are redness, blistering, ulcerating, and oozing, thickening and increased pigmentation.

Skin diseases represent a major group of ailments in canines and are caused by various pathogens. Generally bacterial, fungal, allergic, and parasitic and hormonal skin diseases occur in dogs. Less commonly numerous hereditary and immune mediated forms of skin disease also effect dogs. Many skin diseases cause intense itching and this leads to further skin damage from self-mutilation. Rare causes of disease include nutritional deficiencies, viruses and poisons. Skin tumors and cysts are common in older dogs. Dermatologic problems are told to be most commonly encountered and the hardest solved problems by the veterinarians.

Dermatitis is a broad term that refers to inflammatory itching of the skin. It can be chronic or temporary. Dermatitis can be caused by the dog's environment (such as sensitivity to grass), allergies (allergic to flea), bacteria, virus or poor nutrition.

Dog dermatitis is one of the most commonly found infections in canines around the India. The Infection can take form in a number of ways, ranging from inflammed itchy skin t scaly, dry patches. Dog dermatitis is not only unpleasant and gives off a bad odor. It is also acutely uncomfortable and painful for the dog. If the condition is not treated immediately it can escalate and become much more aggravated and cause damage to the dog's health. Many conditions may cause dermatitis like,

1. Irritants and contact dermatitis
2. Atopic dermatitis
3. Seborrheic dermatitis
4. Moist dermatitis (Eczemz)
5. Bacterial dermatitis (pyoderma)
6. Flea allergic dermatitis
7. Hookworm dermatitis
8. Malassezia dermatitis
9. Dermatophytes infection
10. Sarcoptic mange
11. Demodicosis

Irritants and Contact Dermatitis

It is caused by the direct effect of a chemical or irritant on the skin. It is not an uncommon disease of dogs and cats caused by contact with plant or contact with some substances such as acid, fertilizers etc. It occurs in areas where the skin is not well protected by hair such as the feet, chin, nose, the undersurface of the body including scrotum. It may occur after as ingle exposure or repeated exposure. The skin is become rough, scaly and alopecia is common. Excessive scratching damage the skin and causes secondary bacterial infection. Chemicals that can cause irritant dermatitis include acid, alkalies, detergents, soap etc. Neomycin and other topical medicine can produce allergic contact dermatitis. Flea collar dermatitis is an allergic contact dermatitis, control include remove flea collar. Topical and oral corticosteroid can be given to treat irritants and contact dermatitis.

Atopic Dermatitis

Atopic dermatitis is an allergen skin disease of dogs caused by immunological hypersensitivity to common substances in the environment. It is a disease in which there is an inherited tendency to develop IgE antibodies in response to exposure to allergens that are inhaled or absorbed through the skin. It affects about 10% of dog. Susceptible breeds include Golden Retriever, Labrador retriever, Lhasa apso, Dalmatian, Trish setter, boxer etc; although any dog may be affected. Even mixed breeds may suffer. Atrophy normally begins in dogs in 1 to 3 years of age. The dog start to react to wool, house dust, plant fibers with prolonged exposure and multiple allergens, the condition become a year round affair. Dogs scratch undersides of the body, with licking or chewing of the paws. The ear may be reddened and hot to touch with increasing pruritis, alopecia and redness of the ski become evident. The ear flaps are red and inflamed and the canals are filled with a wax that eventually causes bacterial or yeast otitis. The diagnosis can be made base don the history, type of skin lesion, skin scraping, bacterial and fungal culture, skin biopsy etc. For control, the most effective is to avoid the allergen. For treatment, antihistaminic and omega 3 fatty acids are recommended. Corticosteroid like dexamethasone @ 0.01 to 0.2mg/kg can be given to treat atopic dermatitis may suffer of

Seborrheic Dermatitis

Skin disorder that starts around large oil glands, the face, behind ears. It is caused by yeast, called *Pityrosporum avale,* which also causes dandruff. Primary seborrhoea is a genetic condition. It is fairly common skin condition in both humans and dogs. Symptoms develop very slowly and it is characterized by inflammed scalp, greasy, waxy scale and sometimes redden skin rashes, foul odor and dandruff like flakes. Shampoo containing zinc, salicylic acid and sulphur or neem shampoo may help to reduce seborrheic dermatitis. Omega 3 fatty acids, zinc iron biotin, vitamin A, C, E and D and Beta complex are suggested nutritional supplements for seborrheic dermatitis.

Moist Dermatitis

It is normally caused by a bacterial infection. Moist dermatitis is the raw patches on the skin, which can suddenly appear within an hour or two. It can appear any where on a dog's body and rapidly spread. Normally dog bite and scratch at the areas and the area becomes moist, red, raw and may pus forming. Most of the cases of the disease cured with oral and topical antibiotics along with corticosteroid.

Pyoderma

Pyoderma is the medical term used to denote infections of the skin caused by bacteria, defined as a pus producing infection. It is a bacterial infection of the skin and is one of the most common diseases of dogs. It is however relatively rare in cats. The primary bacteria responsible for most canine pyoderma are *Staphylococcus spp*. It is the normal resident of skin, both local and systemic immune response are probably involved in the pathogenesis of pyoderma. The basic and most frequently observed lesion of pyoderma is pustule. Pyoderma is classified as surface, superficial or deep. Surface pyoderma confined to the surface of skin. Two of the most common types are pyotraumatic dermatitis and skin fold dermatitis. Superficial pyoderma, commonly called superficial folliculitis. Systemic antibiotics are appropriate therapy for superficial pyoderma. Deep pyoderma is a serious disease that extends to the dermis. Antibiotic therapy is usually long term.

Flea Allergic Dermatitis

Appears to affect all dogs, regardless of breed or sex. Many dogs and cats develop an allergic reaction to flea saliva, occasionally producing severe skin reactions. Flea normally bites and sucks blood from host to feed themselves. There are over 15 different allergy containing substances or antigens in flea saliva. All of these antigens can produce an allergic reaction if the dogs happens to be sensitive to the substances, Flea continue to bite a host animal long after their hunger is satisfied. Flea allergy dermatitis is a season allergy, since fleas are most active during summer month. One or two fleas can lead to extreme itching. The symptoms of loss of hair at the base of the tail. Common symptoms are hot spots or inflammed sores are common and dog itches intensely. Simple medicated bath, antihistaminic and pyrethroid out door spray are very useful. Single application of selamectin kill 98% flea.

Hook Worm Dermatitis

Hookworm, *Ancylostoma caninum* ca enter through the skin, they can cause hookworm dermatitis. Lesions occur where the hookworm larvae enter the skin. Lesions are usually seen on the feet or areas of the body that come in contact with the ground. These lesions are often itchy causing dogs to lick their feet. Recommended treatment are fenbendazole @50 to 100mg/kg. b.wt. for 3 days and pyrantal palmoate @5mg/kg. b.wt. are the safe for the pups.

Malassezia Dermatitis

Malassezia pachydermatitis also known as pityrosporum pachydermatitis is a saprophytic yeast is a common commensal organism of the healthy dogs. *M. pachydermatis* and Staphylococci play an important role in canine seborrhoeic dermatitis. *M. pachydermatis* is an opportunistic pathogen and produces skin infection depending on host factors and immune suppressive mechanisms. Certain breeds like German shepherd, Dachshunds, Labradors, American cocker spaniels, boxers, spitz etc. are predisposed to this condition. Higher prevalence of the disease is recorded in long haired dogs and those dogs kept indoors. This could be due to the lesser exposure of ultra violet rays of sun, which is deleterious to the yeast organisms. Clinical signs associated with malassezia dermatitis are variable but generally consists of erythema, mild to severe pruritis, yellow to grey scale or greasy wax associated with a yeasty, rancid offensive odor. The lesions are usually first seen on the abdominal skin, but may spread to the entire abdomen and the inguinal region. Dogs with otitis externa typically show head shaking and ear scratching.

Diagnosis is based on history, clinical finding, cytologic techniques, culture and histopathology. Confirm diagnosis is made by demonstrating 1or 2 peanut or foot print shaped unipolar budding yeast organisms. In therapy, generalized and severe cases are usually treated with ketoconazole @ 5 to 10mg/kg b.wt. once or twice daily up to 30 days. Alternately itraconazole can be used @ 5 to 10mg/kg b.wt or terbinafine 2 2.5mg/kg orally daily. Topical therapy for malassezia is affected by shampoos, dips and creams or solutions. Chlohexidine shampoo is superior to ketoconazole and selenium sulfide preparations in the management of malasseziosis.

Dermatophytosis

Dermatophytosis (Ring worm) is a common infectious agent of the dog and cat. It is moore common in young, stary, sick or debilitated dogs. Deramtophytosis is caused by specific types of fungas (Microsporum or trichophyton) that grow in the surface of the skin, nails and hair. *M .canis* causes 70% of the dermatophyte infections in dogs. Infection is aided if the skin surface has been abraded, such as occurs when dogs are groomed or clipped. M. canis is highly contagious. Dermatophytosis tends to occur in dogs that are immuno-compromised, where their immune system is unable to fight off the fungal infections. Some animals may be carriers of the fungus and may infect other dogs that are exposed to them. The most common clinical sign associated with dermatophytosis is circular area of hair loss (alopecia) other clinical signs include scaling, erythema, hyperpigmenattion and itchinose. Dermatophytosis is diagnosed by history and an examination of the skin, using fungal culture. The treatment involves the use of systemic or topical antifungal medications for several weeks. The prognosis generally is good, as most dog will clear the infection over a few months.

Sarcoptic Mange

It is also known as canine scabies, it is a highly contagious infestation of *Sarcoptes scabies canis,* a burrowing mite. Canine scabies can infect all ages and breeds of dogs. The mites usually spend their entire life on a dog. The mites prefer to live on the dog, but will live for several days off of the host in the environment. The mites prefer to live on areas of the skin that have less hair. The symptoms of canine scabies are varied but usually include hair loss and severe itching specially on the elbows, ears, hocks, chest, belly etc. Because of the severe itching and resultant scratching, the skin soon becomes traumatized and variety of sores and infection can develop as a result. The itching seems to be much worse in warm conditions. Trying to make diagnosis of canine scabies can be very frustrating. On average, 20% of the infected dogs will show sarcoptic mites positive in skin scrapping. Therefore, most diagnosis is made on history and response to treatment of scabies.

Ivermectin is one of the most effective treatment against *S. scabei* normally injection is given either weekly or every two weeks in 1 to 4 doses. In most cases treatment is safe and effective. But it is too toxic for collie family of dogs. Selamectin is an ivermectin derivative used for the control of fleas, ticks and sarcoptic mange. This product is probably the best choice for collie or Australian shepherd breeds. Moxedectin is yet another invermectin derivative and milbemyoxime is also has activity against sarcoptic mange. Epinomectin pour on 5% @1ml/10kg b.wt. is also effective. Local application of Annona.squamosa (Sitaphal) leaves is also very effective against sarcoptic mange in dogs.

Demodicosis / Demodectic mange

Demodectic mange in dogs is caused by overpopulation of Demodex canis and if the dog's immune system is unable to keep the mites under control. There are two types of demodectic mange, localized and generalized. Localised consists of 4 spots or lss. Demodectic amnge occurs in localized and generalized forms. Localized may occurs in dogs under 1 year of age. The principal, sign is thinning hair around the eyelids, lips, corners of the mouth, occasionally on the legs. Localized mange usually heals spontaneously in six to eight weeks, otherwise the disease could progress to the generalized form. Dogs with generalized disease develop patches of hair loss on the head, legs and trunk. The skin coat is usually brittle, dry and full of crusts and scabs. There is often very strong unpleasant odor oming from the skin of these dogs. Another form of demodectic mange called pododemodicosis, the mange confined to the paws. Bacterial infections accompany with demodicosis and pododemodecosis also. Several drugs like ivermectin, amitraj, milbemyoxime, herbal medicine have been tried in the treatment of canine demodicosis with varying results.

References

Chatterjee, A. (1989). Skin infection in domestic animals. Maitri. Publication, Kolkata.

Deboer, D.J and Hillier, A. (2001). The ACVC task force on canine atopic dermatitis (XV) fundamental concepts I clinical diagnosis. *Vet. Immune Immunopath.* 81; 271-276.

Griffin, C., Kwochka, K and Mac Donald, J. (1993). Current veterinary Dermatology. Mosby Publication. Linn.MO.

Ihrke, P.I and White, S.D. (1987). Contemporary issues in small animal practice, dermatology, Vol.8, (Nesbitt, G.H. editor) Churchill Living stone, New York.

Roy, S and Roy, M. (2008) Therapeutic evaluation of herbal formulations against canine demodicosis. *Indian Vet. J.* 88: 672-673.

Roy, S., Ghosh, R.C and Sen, S.K. (1992). Therapeutic evaluation of amitraj against demodicosis. *Indian Vet. J.* 67: 463-465.

Roy, S., Roy, M., Ratre, H.K., Patel, J and Tiwari, S.K. (2005). Efficacy of oral ivermectin and erinaplus for the treatment of canine pododemodicosis.

Scott, D., Miller, W and Muller, Cand Kirk's S. Small animal dermatology, W.B. Saunders Co. Philadelphia. PA, 2001.

Stephen, J., Ettinger and Edward C. Fieldman (2004). Text book of vet. Internal medicine, diseases of dogs and cats 5th edn. W.B. Saunders Company.

Wilkinson, G.T and Harvey, R.G. (1994). Small animal dermatology. Volfe, Barcelona, 1-201.

Yathiraj, S. (2005). Diagnosis and therapeutic management of malasseziosis in dogs. Presentedin XXIII annual convention of ISVM at veterinary College, Anjora, Durg, 2 to 4 feb, 2005.

□□□

35

Genomic Selection and its Application for Cattle Improvement

G.K. GAUR AND BHARAT BHUSHAN
Livestock Production and Management Section
Indian Veterinary Research Institute, Izatnagar 243 122 (Uttar Pradesh), India

Genomic Selection

The aim of animal breeding is to change the genetic endowments of the animals and as a result to improve their traits. However, this is not a matter of the genetic manipulation of the animal itself. Genetic programs in dairy cattle have been extremely successful at improving the productivity of dairy cattle populations over the last 50 years. Our traditional approach of using selective breeding (based on sophisticated quantitative selection principles) has been very successful, even though we do not know the exact genes that have increased or decreased in frequency in our populations. We often describe our approach as a "black box" approach, since we do not know exactly what genes have been affected. The use of very effective progeny testing programs and the heavy use of well-proven, elite bulls have indeed been very successful. Several advances have improved the basic approach (e.g., the adoption of contemporary comparisons and later the adoption of the animal model for calculating genetic evaluations), but most of these advances have resulted in incremental improvements in the process. In recent decades, dairy producers and geneticists have recognized the importance of breeding for improved health, reproduction and longevity, so health traits, reproduction and productive life have become a larger part of selection in dairy cattle.

Genomic selection (GS) is a new approach for improving quantitative traits in large breeding populations that uses whole genome molecular markers (high density markers and high throughput genotyping). Genomic prediction combines marker data with phenotypic and pedigree data (when available) in an attempt to increase the accuracy of the prediction of breeding and genotypic values.

For quantitative traits, selection based on marker effects alone has dramatically changed standard practices used in animal breeding. However, in public breeding programs, the benefits of GS have been studied only through computer simulation. Since marker technology is continuously reducing the cost per data point and increasing the number of available markers, genotyping is currently less costly than phenotyping in designed breeding programs. Besides accelerating the selection cycles, GS offers the opportunity to increase the selection gains per unit of time. Therefore, it is believed that alternating progeny field testing with selection based only on markers should increase the genetic gains per unit. However, unresolved questions, such as how much (if any) genetic diversity will be diminished by this combination of phenotypic and GS remain.

Advantages of Genomic Selection

The valuable genomic information has many advantages:

- It predicts genetic merit of young animals with up to double the accuracy of traditional parent averages.
- It has the potential to shorten the generational interval and hence to speed the genetic improvement.
- It enables bull selection program from a much wider genetic pool.
- It provides earlier information about genetic differences between siblings.
- It improves the reliability of current progeny testing results for low-heritability or later-expressed traits, including health and fitness traits.

Genomic breeding value evaluation and selection is now really close to what was once a dream. Even though the cattle's genome has now been decrypted, we know very little about the position and effectiveness of the genes for the majority of the transmission traits. Genomic breeding value evaluation does not work directly on the basis of information about genes, but by using markers.

Single Nucleotide Polymorphism (SNP) Markers

SNP markers are composed of only one genetic letter and there are two different models for every marker in the entire population. Every animal has the genetic information in the form of a double chromosome set; one set from the father and one set from the mother. The result is that every marker for an animal can have three combinations: homozygous option AA, homozygous option BB or heterozygous AB. Heterozygous AB means that the animal received different options from the father and the mother. Many hundreds of thousands of such SNP markers of cattle are known which are shared equally in the entire genome. All chromosomes can now be extracted for all the markers simultaneously through a relatively cheap laboratory method in a one step process. This process is called "typing" or "high-density and high-throughput genotyping". The unit used in the laboratory for testing the markers is called a chip and its numerical value i.e. 10K (in 10K chip), 50K (in 50K chip), 700K (in 700K chip) indicate the number of markers simultaneously tested. A little of the animal's genetic material is used for the typing. The typing's result is n times AA or BB or AB where n is number of markers in chip. As a result of the equal spread of many markers over the entire genome, it is assumed that close to every gene, which influences the production of one of the transmission traits, is one of the markers. This means that the marker is transmitted almost every time, together with the appropriate combination of genes.

The first high-density and high-throughput genotyping assay was the 10K single nucleotide polymorphism (SNP) chip commercialized by Affymetrix (The Bovine HapMap Consortium, 2009). However, the density of SNPs in this panel was insufficient for many genomic studies (including genomic selection (GS) and genome-wide association analyses (GWAS)), which led to the need for a higher density chip. The Illumina BovineSNP50 chip was developed by a consortium of animal scientists using SNP discovery populations in Holstein, Angus and mixed breeds of beef cattle (Van Tassell *et al.*, 2008) and provided much higher density (~50,000 SNPs per animal) than previous high-throughput genotyping assays (Matukumalli *et al.*, 2009). This assay has become the international standard for GS and GWAS in cattle and has even been applied to other species to resolve the evolutionary relationship among the horned ruminants (Decker *et al.*, 2009; MacEachern *et al.*, 2009). While the Illumina BovineSNP50 assay has proven to be extremely useful for many different types of genomic studies, it was realized that even higher density assays are needed to build models for GS with utility across breeds.

A new high-density SNP genotyping chip was introduced in 2010 from Illumina which utilized the same bead technology and single base extension chemistry that was used for the Bovine SNP50K chip. This genotypes approximately 700K SNPs per animal. SNP discovery for the Illumina BovineSNP50 assay was performed using pools of DNA samples from Angus, Holsteins and a group of bulls sampled from the next most important US beef breeds. As a result, there is a bias inherent in the assay towards SNPs that have high minor allele frequency in Angus and Holsteins and the assay performs slightly better for GWAS and GS in these breeds. However, the SNP discovery for the design of the Illumina 700K panels was performed by sequencing a large number of animals from many different breeds (including both *Bos taurus* and *Bos indicus*) to minimize the ascertainment bias in SNP informativeness across breeds.

The end result should be a panel of SNPs that will have high average allele frequencies in almost all cattle breeds but will also contain many loci with low allele frequencies. This is especially important for performing GWAS, since common SNPs cannot be strongly associated with rare or low frequency variants within a population. The larger, more variable panel will contain some SNPs which are at low frequency in the population of interest to facilitate the detection of rare variants within that population. The greatest immediate value of the 700K chips will be the potential for implementing across-breed GS. The real advantage of GS is its ability to simultaneously select for desirable combinations at all loci responsible for genetic variation in a trait using panels of closely linked markers.

Implementation of Genomic Selection

We do not, however, know the different genes and their effects on the performance traits. In order to evaluate an animal's genomic breeding value using its markers, certain advanced tests are necessary. To find out which SNPs, i.e. which markers are connected with which trait, the SNP samples first have to be compared with known (genetic) production traits of selected animals. Animals with known genetic production are daughter proven bulls. From the comparison of the SNP sample with the genetic production of these bulls, it can be determined which SNP has how much influence on the trait. The more reliably proven bulls allocate the SNP to a trait better and indicate the extent of the influence. Proven bulls that are included in this analysis are the so-called "training sample". The training sample/set is thus reference population in which the marker effects are estimated; it contains: (1) phenotypic information from relevant breeding germplasm evaluated over a range of environmental conditions; (2) molecular marker scores; and (3) pedigree information or kinship. Hence, marker effects are estimated based on the training set using certain statistical methods.

The genomic evaluation formulas conveyed from the training sample are then used for the calculation of the genomic breeding values of other (usually younger) animals without their own reliable conventional breeding value information. These animals refer target/validation sample/set and contains the selection candidates (derived from the reference population) that have been genotyped (but not phenotyped) and selected based on marker effects estimated in the training set.

Reliability and Genomic Breeding Values

Genomic selection refers to selection decisions based on genomic breeding values (GEBV). The reliability of genomic breeding values mainly depends on the extent and structure of the training sample as well as the reliability of the daughters' breeding values of the training sample bulls. The genomic formulas can only convey the reliability of the breeding values of younger cows when their genetics (SNP sample) are well-represented via preferably many related animals (sire, dam's sire, paternal half brothers and sisters etc) in the training sample. So the training sample has to be continuously expanded and updated alongside the population development. The reliability of breeding values for younger animals based solely on genomic data (SNP typing).

The direct genomic values (dGW) are calculated from the typings (SNP samples) for all traits. There is also more conventional breeding value information for all animals with known pedigree, namely the pedigree's breeding value. In order that every animal has only one breeding value with maximum information and reliability at a particular time, the direct genomic value is not published but the genomically improved breeding value (gZW) which is a combination of the direct genomical value and the conventional breeding value is given. The weighting is done on the basis of the reliability of both values; i.e. for young animals with only a pedigree breeding value, the direct genomical value counts the most and the unreliable pedigree breeding value can increase the reliability of the genomically improved breeding value ([ZW] gZW) by only 3-5%. Once the conventional breeding value is clearly more reliable from daughter information than from the direct genomic value, it has a higher weighting in the combined gZW. So the combined gZWof daughter proven bulls is usually little different from the purely conventional breeding value.

To calculate/predict GEBV, the entire genome is divided into small segments, their effects are estimated in a reference population, the effects of all loci that contribute to genetic variation are captured and the estimated effects of the segments (the animal carries) are summed across the whole genome.

Statistical Analysis for Estimating Genomic Breeding Values

Statistical analysis of genomic selection experiments aimed to know the effect of all alleles/markers on performance traits (breeding goal traits). We can set up an experiment to estimate the allele effects with 1000-2000 phenotyped and genotyped animals. Classical statistics however encounters the problem of shortage of degree of freedom (more number of markers/ alleles as compared to animals). There are three ways to get around the huge shortage of degree of freedom:

Least Squares (LS) Method: Test all the markers one by one for their statistical significance and set the effects of non-significant markers to zero. Compute the estimates of significant markers simultaneously using LS.

Best Linear Unbiased Prediction (BLUP) Method: Fit the allelic effects as random instead of fixed. The fitting of random effect does not require degree of freedom and thus all allelic effects can be estimated simultaneously. Random effect however requires an estimate of variance of the allelic effect. The method assumes similar variance for all the markers.

Bayesian Estimation Method: This method is similar to BLUP except that the variance of allelic effects is assumed different for every marker and is estimated using a prior distribution for the variance. The prior distribution of variance of marker i (V_{ai}) is assumed as $V_{ai} = 0$ with probability p; $V_{ai} \sim \div^{-2}(v, s)$ with probability (1-p); where p depends on the mutation rate at the marker locus and $\div^{-2}(v, s)$ denotes the inverse-chi squared distribution with v degrees of freedom and scale parameter S.

Marker estimated breeding value (MEBV) or genomic estimated breeding value (GEBV) is predicted by $MEBV_i/GEBV_i = ?M_{ij}$ where M_{ij} is the estimate of the effect of the jth allele/heplotype of animal i.

Application of Genomic Selection for Cattle Improvement

Genomic selection has revolutionized dairy cattle breeding during last several years. Though idea of DNA markers for improving rate of genetic gain in dairy cattle is old by some decades (Smith, 1967; Soller and Beckman, 1983) but adoption of marker-assisted selection by the dairy industry has been limited due to several reasons. For most quantitative traits in dairy cattle, a large number of loci affect the trait with any one locus capturing only a limited proportion of the total genetic variance (Shrimpton and Robertson, 1988; Hayes and Goddard, 2001; Sanna *et al.*, 2008, VanRaden *et al.*, 2009). Furthermore, small gains were only possible with limited number of Markers having high cost of genotyping. Calculation of breeding values using marker information was further a barrier to apply marker-assisted selection.

Sequencing of the bovine genome, which led to the discovery of many thousands of DNA markers in the form of SNP and reduction in cost of genotyping brought revolution in genomic selection. Subsequently, it became possible to make very accurate selection decisions when breeding values were predicted from dense marker data alone (Meuwissen *et al.*, 2001).

Meuwissen *et al.* (2001) demonstrated that accuracies (correlation between true breeding value and EBV) of predicted breeding values from markers alone may be achieved to the level of 0.85. Similarly, Kolbehdari et al. (2006) obtained high correlation between GEBV and true breeding values (0.80) in a simulation study using different heritabilities and evenly or randomly spaced QTLs.

The simulation results suggest that the accuracy of the GEBV for a bull calf at birth may be as high as the accuracy of an EBV of progeny test. Consequently, genomic selection may lead to double rate of genetic gain (Schaeffer, 2006) as compared to 5-19 % improvement in genetic response through marker assisted selection (Boichard *et al.*, 2006). Furthermore, avoiding progeny testing, bull breeding programs may save up to 92% of their costs (Schaeffer, 2006), however, some of these savings may be offset by investment on genotyping. Spelman et al. (2006) reported accuracy of DNA-based BVs as measured by their correlation with progeny test BVs varying from 0.45 to 0.60 for the production traits in validated population of Holstein-Friesian breed. They further predicted that selection based on genomic information will increase the rate of genetic gain in New Zealand by 50-70%. Berry (2007) in Irish Holstein - Friesian dairy cows expected genetic gain through genomic selection @ 0.539 genetic standard deviations per year with accuracy of selection of 0.75 against 0.199 genetic standard deviations per year under the current scheme of progeny testing.

Harris *et al.* (2008) reported reliabilities of GEBV in New Zealand dairy cattle in an experiment performed by the Livestock Improvement Corporation. Their reference population consisted of approximately 4,500 bulls progeny tested by the Livestock Improvement Corporation. The bulls were genotyped for 56,947 SNP using the Illumina Bovine SNP50K chip. After quality checking, 44,146 SNP were retained for analysis. To derive the prediction equations, a wide range of methods were tried including BLUP, Bayes A, Bayes B, least angle regression and Bayesian regression. A polygenic component (additive breeding value) based on pedigree was included in the GEBV. Reliabilities of GEBV for young bulls with no daughter information ranged from 50 to 67% for milk production traits, live BW, fertility, SCC, and longevity, compared with an average 34% for parental average breeding values. Furthermore, Bayesian methods gave slightly greater (2 to 3%) reliabilities than the BLUP approach, whereas the regression methods performed poorly.

Hayes *et al* (2009) reviewed results of genomic selection in Australia. A total of 798 Australian Holstein-Friesian bulls born between 1998 and 2003 and progeny tested by Genetics Australia were genotyped for 56,947 SNP by using the Illumina Bovine SNP50K chip. Samples were screened for the proportion of missing genotypes, and animals with greater than 10% missing genotypes were removed. The phenotypes used were Australian breeding values (ABV) for protein yield, protein percentage, Australian Profit Ranking (APR), and Australian Selection Index (ASI). To reduce the number of SNP to be considered in the prediction equations for computational tractability, the effect of each SNP was tested on each trait.

For each trait, the significant SNP were taken to the next stage. Two methods were used to derive the prediction equations. The first method used was a simple BLUP approach. Second was Bayesian approach (BayesA), which uses the prior knowledge that many SNP are likely to have small individual effects on the trait and only a few will have a moderate to large effect (Meuwissen *et al.*, 2001). Using these predicted SNP effects, the GEBV of the bulls born in 2003 were predicted. These GEBV were then correlated with the current breeding values of these bulls (reliability), which were largely derived from a progeny test.

Records in reference population were 637 and number of SNP used ranged from 3090 to 4369 for different traits. Reliability of genomic breeding values at the time of birth ranged from 0.18 (fertility) to 0.53 (APR) in BLUP method and from 0.14 (fertility) to 0.55 (APR) in Bayesian method. The reliability of the fertility GEBV was substantially lower than the reliability of other traits. This is likely because of the lower heritability of fertility, so more records are required to predict accurate GEBV. The Bayesian method gave small increases in reliability for all traits except fertility, in the order of 2 to 7%.

VanRaden *et al.* (2009) reported reliabilities of GEBV for US and Canadian young bulls. The reference population from which the prediction equations were derived consisted of 3,576 Holstein bulls genotyped for 38,416 SNP with the Illumina Bovine SNP50TM chip. Prediction methods included a method similar to BLUP, which assumed a normal distribution for the marker effects, and a Bayesian method with a heavier tail before allowing for genes of the major effect (similar to BayesA). The parent average or polygenic effect from pedigree was combined with the genomic predictions by selection index to obtain the final GEBV. Averaged across traits, the GEBV had a reliability of 50%, compared with 27% from the parent average alone. Using BLUP rather than the Bayesian approach gave only a slightly (1%) reduced reliability.

Changes in reliability due to the inclusion of genomic data in national genetic evaluations

Trait	Holstein	Jersey	Brown Swiss
Net Merit	+24%	+8%	+9%
Milk Yield	+26%	+6%	+17%
Fat Yield	+32%	+11%	+10%
Protein Yield	+24%	+2%	+14%
Fat Percentage	+50%	+36%	+8%
Protein Percentage	+38%	+29%	+10%
Productive Life	+32%	+7%	+12%

Hayes *et al.* (2009) also reviewed results of genomic selection in Netherlands. Their reference population consisted of 1,583 bulls genotyped with a custom-made SNP chip containing 57,660 SNP, of which 46,529 SNP were used in subsequent analysis. They calculated the accuracy of GEBV by randomly dropping out 5% of the 429 bulls born between 1999 and 2003 from the reference population, calculating GEBV for these bulls, and then correlating them with the actual EBV of the bulls, which included progeny test information. This was repeated 20 times so that each bull was dropped out once and used as a reference bull in the other 19 runs. Their methodology for calculating SNP effects followed the Gibbs sampling scheme proposed by Meuwissen and Goddard (2004), implemented for single SNP rather than haplotypes (Calus *et al.*, 2008). The increase in reliability of GEBV over parent average EBV at the time of birth was 33% (fat percentage), 19% (kilograms of protein), 15% (feet and legs), 13% (udder depth, SCS), and 9% (fertility). They concluded that having a larger number of bulls in their reference population would increase the reliability of GEBV in their selection candidates substantially.

The effect of different breeding structures was investigated by Duthie *et al* (2010). They included selection based on young sires, where no progeny information was available, and selection based on older sires. Genomic information was included in the selection index model and accuracies of genomic estimated breeding values (GEBVs) were predicted based on trait heritability, number of phenotyped animals in the training population, the number of quantitative trait loci (QTL) underlying the trait and the effective population size (Ne). They found that under conventional selection, the economic response was similar between the two breeding structures, however the slightly higher response (5 per cent) when selecting older sires was due to higher accuracy of breeding values due to the availability of phenotypic records on more relatives. It was felt that including genomic information increases the economic response to selection in both breeding structures, however the magnitude of the response in comparison to no GS was higher when selecting younger sires (up to 33 per cent increase) in comparison to the industry average (up to 21 per cent increase) where selection was based on approximately 40 per cent young sires, with a generation interval of less than three, and 60 per cent of older sires.

Summary

Sequencing of the bovine genome, which led to the discovery of many thousands of DNA markers in the form of SNP and reduction in cost of genotyping brought revolution in genomic selection. Genomic selection refers to selection decisions based on genomic breeding values (GEBV). To calculate/ predict GEBV, the entire genome is divided into small segments, their effects are estimated in a reference population, the effects of all loci that contribute to genetic variation are captured and the estimated effects of the segments (the animal carries) are summed across the whole genome. Genomic selection has revolutionized dairy cattle breeding during last several years.

The results suggest that the accuracy of the GEBV for a bull calf at birth may be as high as the accuracy of an EBV of progeny test. Consequently, genomic selection may lead to double rate of genetic gain as compared to 5-19 % improvement in genetic response through marker assisted selection. Furthermore, avoiding progeny testing, bull breeding programs may save up to 92 % of their costs; however, some of these savings may be offset by investment on genotyping.

The genomic selection is being implemented well in USA, New Zealand, Netherlands, Canada, Australia, Germany, Denmark and some other countries for the overall genetic improvement of cattle and the results are encouraging. The increase in reliability of GEBV over parent average EBV at the time of birth ranged from 10 to 50 % for the different traits in various investigations. Genetic gain through genomic selection is expected @ 0.539 genetic standard deviations per year with 0.75 accuracy of selection against 0.199 genetic standard deviations per year under the current scheme of progeny testing.

References

Berry D. (2007). Report on the potential of genomic selection in Irish dairy cattle. Draft Paper I (available on net).

Boichard, D., Fritz., S., Rossignol, M.N., Guillume, F., Colleu, J.J. and Druet. T. (2006). Proceedings of the 8th World Congress on Genetics Applied to Livestock Production (available on net).

Decker, J. E., J. C. Pires, G. C. Conant, S. D. McKay, M. P. Heaton, K. Chen, A. Cooper, J. Vilkki, C. M. Seabury, A. R. Caetano, G. S. Johnson, R. A. Brenneman, O. Hanotte, L.

S. Eggert, P. Wiener, J. J. Kim, K. S. Kim, T. S. Sonstegard, C. P. Van Tassell, H. L. Neibergs, J. C. McEwan, R. Brauning, L. L. Coutinho, M. E. Babar, G. A. Wilson, M. C. McClure, M. M. Rolf, J. Kim, R. D. Schnabel and J. F. Taylor. (2009). Resolving the evolution of extant and extinct ruminants with high-throughput phylogenomics. *Proc. Natl. Acad. Sci.* 106(44):18644-9.

Duthie C, Sawalha R, Navajas E, Roehe R and Roughsedge T. (2010). Economic response that can be achieved from including genomic information to the terminal sire index of beef cattle. Presented to the British Society of Animal Science Annual Conference, April 12 to 14, 2010, Queen's University, Belfast.

Harris, B. L., D. L. Johnson, and R. J. Spelman. (2008). Genomic selection in New Zealand and the implications for national genetic evaluation. Proc. Interbull Meeting, Niagara Falls, Canada (available on net).

Hayes, B. J., and M. E. Goddard. (2001). The distribution of the effects of genes affecting quantitative traits in livestock. *Genet. Sel. Evol.* 33: 209–229.

Hayes, B. J., P. J. Bowman, A. J. Chamberlain and M. E. Goddard. (2009). Invited review: Genomic selection in dairy cattle: Progress and challenges. *J. Dairy Sci.* 92: 433-443.

Kolbehdari, D., Wang, Z., grant, J.R., Murdoch, B., Prasad, A., Xiu, Z., Marques, E., Stothard, P., Moore, S.S. (2009). A whole genome scan approach to map QTL for milk production traits and somatic cell score in Canadian Holstein bulls. *J. Anim. Breed. Genet.* 126(3):216-72.

MacEachern, S., J. McEwan, A. McCulloch, A. Mather, K. Savin, and M. Goddard. (2009). Molecular evolution of the Bovini tribe (Bovidae, Bovinae): is there evidence of rapid.

evolution or reduced selective constraint in Domestic cattle? BMC Genom. 10: 179. Matukumalli, L.K., C.T. Lawley, R.D. Schnabel, J.F. Taylor, M.F. Allan, M.P. Heaton, J. O'Connell, S.S. Moore, T.P.L. Smith, T.S. Sonstegard and C.P. Van Tassell. (2009). Development and characterization of a high density SNP genotyping assay for cattle. PLoS One 4:e5350.

Meuwissen, T. H. E., B. J. Hayes, and M. E. Goddard. (2001). Prediction of total genetic value using genome-wide dense marker maps. *Genetics* 157:1819–1829.

Meuwissen, T. H., and M. E. Goddard. (2004). Mapping multiple QTL using linkage disequilibrium and linkage analysis information and multitrait data. *Genet. Sel. Evol.* 36:261–279.

Sanna, S., A. U. Jackson, R. Nagaraja, C. J. Willer, W. M. Chen, L. L. Bonnycastle, H. Shen, N. Timpson, G. Lettre, G. Usala, P. S. Chines, H. M. Stringham, L. J. Scott, M. Dei, S. Lai, G. Albai, L. Crisponi, S. Naitza, K. F. Doheny, E. W. Pugh, Y. Ben-Shlomo, S. Ebrahim, D. A. Lawlor, R. N. Bergman, R. M. Watanabe, M. Uda, J. Tuomilehto, J. Coresh, J. N. Hirschhorn, A. R. Shuldiner, D. Schlessinger, F. S. Collins, G. Davey Smith, E. Boerwinkle, A. Cao, M. Boehnke, G. R. Abecasis, and K. L. Mohlke. (2008). Common variants in the GDF5-UQCC region are associated with variation in human height. *Nat. Genet.* 40:198–203.

Schaeffer, L. R. (2006). Strategy for applying genome-wide selection in dairy cattle. *J. Anim. Breed. Genet.* 123:218–223.

Shrimpton, A. E., and A. Robertson. (1988). The isolation of polygenic factors controlling bristle score in Drosophila melanogaster. II. Distribution of third chromosome bristle effects within chromosome sections. *Genetics* 118:445–459.

Smith, C. (1967). Improvement of metric traits through specific genetic loci. *Anim. Prod.* 9:349–358.

Soller, M., and J. S. Beckmann. (1983). Genetic polymorphism in variety identification and genetic improvement. *Theor. Appl. Genet.* 67:25–33.

Spelman, R.J., J.Arias., M. Keehan, V. Obolonkin. (2006). Application of genomic information in dairy cattle. Draft Paper (available on net).

VanRaden, P. M., C. P. Van Tassell, G. R. Wiggans, T. S. Sonstegard, R. D. Schnabel, J. F. Taylor, and F. Schenkel. (2009). Invited review: Reliability of genomic predictions for North American Holstein bulls. *J. Dairy Sci.* 92:16–24.

Van Tassell C.P., T.P.L. Smith, L.K. Matukumalli, J.F. Taylor, R.D. Schnabel, C.T. Lawley, C. D. Haudenschild, S. S. Moore, W. C. Warren and T. S. Sonstegard. (2008). Simultaneous SNP discovery and allele frequency estimation by high throughput sequencing of reduced representation genomic libraries. *Nat. Meth.* 5:247-52.

□□□

36

Emerging Challenges and Opportunities in Livestock Production in India

V.B.CHATURVEDI, P.SINGH AND H.C.SINGH
IVRI Izatnagar

Introduction

Accelerating growth of agricultural sector remains a key policy concern in India despite a significant decline in its share in gross domestic product (GDP), which was 48% in 1970/71 to 24% in 2003/04, is decreasing continuously. Rapid growth in livestock production is desirable not only to sustain agricultural growth, but also to reduce rural poverty especially when a majority of the land holdings are small. Fifty-eight percent of rural households have land holding of less than 2 ha and another 32% have no access to land there fore livestock is the only hope. India has a competitive advantage in production of many primary livestock products, but is not competitive in exports of value added products because of high marketing and processing costs and distortions in world markets. Some countries provide huge production and market support to their livestock sectors, while in India such a support is almost non-existent. Nevertheless, to take advantage of expanding global markets, domestic industry has to improve efficiency and food safety and quality standards, which are becoming stringent in the global trade. Research institutions attention on research is required to improve livestock production in proportionate with demand and consumer preferences in limited resources from small holder livestock producers.

Livestock Sector is a Main Base of Indian Agriculture

Importance of agriculture transcends beyond its economic contribution as nearly 72% of Indian population lives in rural areas, and 75% of it depends on agriculture and allied activities for livelihood. Further, more than of 261 million poor in the country, 75% are rural poor and 40% of these belong to farm households and therefore growth in agriculture is critical to the livelihood of millions of rural poor. Ravallion and Datt (1996) have shown that Indian agricultural growth is more pro-poor than the growth of other sectors of the economy. Over the last three decades, India made tremendous progress in food production. However, agricultural growth hardly ever exceeded 3% a year. Keeping in view the pro-poor nature of agricultural growth, the National Agricultural Policy (NAP 2000) targeted a 4% annual growth in agricultural sector by 2020, and emphasized livestock as an important driver of growth. The policy statement concentrated on the need to: (i) evolve a proper livestock breeding policy to increase livestock production and enhance use of draft animals as a source of energy, (ii) generation and dissemination of livestock related technologies to improve animal productivity,(iii) improving marketing, processing and transportation facilities for value addition, (iv) managing grazing lands and rejuvenate pastures, (v) establishing disease-free zones, and (vi) involve co-operatives and private sector in development efforts. Besides, this statement also emphasized bringing up incentives for livestock production at par with crop production. With an enabling policy environment there is a considerable scope to diversify agricultural sector towards livestock activities.

Rapid growth in livestock production is desirable not only to sustain agricultural growth, but also to reduce rural poverty especially when a majority of the land holdings are small. Fifty-eight percent of rural households have land holding of less than 2 ha and another 32% have no access to land. Number of these households may increase due to the further subdivision of land holdings. Livestock are thus an important source of income for smallholders and the landless. Products like milk and eggs are steady source of cash income, and live animals are important natural assets for the poor, which can be easily liquidated for cash during emergency. Small holders and landless together contribute 70% of the country's livestock resources, and are capable of producing at a lower cost because of availability of sufficient labor with them. Evidence shows that small holders obtain nearly half of their income from livestock (Shukla and Brahmankar 1999). Growth in livestock sector is thus more pro-poor than growth in other sub-sectors of agricultural economy.

Besides food production, livestock make important contributions to crop production by supplying draft power, dung and manure. Rapid growth in livestock production is desirable not only to sustain agricultural growth, but also to reduce rural poverty especially when a majority of the land holdings are small. During 1970s livestock were considered an important instrument to counteract adverse effects of land-based green revolution on rural income distribution. The poor were provided credit assistance to build up livestock assets under poverty alleviation programs such as Integrated Rural Development Programme (IRDP). Major support to livestock sector, however, came in the form of 'Operation Flood' program, which was launched in 1970 to link rural milk production with high-demand urban consumption centers through the network of dairy co-operatives. Besides, the dairy industry was protected from cheap imports through licensing, quotas and tariffs. Some important policy initiatives to improve growth and efficiency in livestock production and processing were taken after the initiation of the process of economic reforms in 1991. Entry of private sector into dairy industry was freed from regulations, and the import-substitution policy was given up removing quantitative restrictions on imports and reducing tariff rates.

Processing of livestock products was encouraged by lowering excise duties and corporate taxes. The Agricultural Produce Market Committee Act, that prohibited sale/purchase of agricultural commodities outside state designated markets, has been amended recently to allow private sector to procure produce directly from producers through institutional arrangements like co-operatives, contract farming and producers' associations or by establishing their own markets. The Reserve Bank of India permitted financial institutions to finance contract farming schemes. Nevertheless, there is an apprehension whether smallholder livestock producers can take advantage of the emerging opportunities. Productivity of livestock is low, and smallholders are constrained by a lack of access to markets, capital, inputs, technology and services. Failure to address these constraints may depress domestic production and lead to an import upsurge.

There is also a possibility of emergence of large landholder commercial production systems especially around urban areas to cater to the increasing demand for animal food products there. Smallholders though are efficient even under low-input conditions; economies of scale in production and marketing in commercial production may erode their competitive advantage. Increasing globalization of livestock products markets is an opportunity as well as a threat to India's livestock sector. Global demand for livestock products is increasing and thus offers an opportunity to increase exports. India has a competitive advantage in primary production of many products, but their exports are constrained by low level of processing, distortions in world trade and stringent food safety norms in the international trade. On the other hand, there is an imminent threat of cheap imports especially from the European Union and the United States that heavily protect their livestock industry through subsidies and market support measures. Livestock production is therefore likely to be under significant adjustment pressure in the liberalized economic environment. Whether smallholder livestock producers would be able to expropriate emerging opportunities would depend on their ability to improve efficiency in production, and preparedness of the government and industry to facilitate the adjustment process through policies and investments.

Peculiar Features of Indian Livestock Sector

1. Agricultural growth in general is poverty reducing, but growth in livestock production is more pro-poor than a similar growth in crop production as livestock wealth is more equitably distributed among peoples than cultivable land.
2. Livestock production is growing faster than crop production and contributing towards sustainable agricultural growth. Small-scale livestock producers are constrained by lack of access to markets, credit, inputs, technology and services that deters them from taking advantage of the opportunities resulting from the expanding demand for animal food products in the domestic and global markets.
3. Low level of public investment in the livestock sector is detrimental to the interests of millions of poor livestock producers. Value addition to livestock production is not encouraging and constrains the growth of livestock production, especially amongst small-scale producers; and creation of a conducive policy environment to enable poor households to secure livestock assets, inputs and technology and to improve their access to output markets.
4. It is critical for livestock researchers to understand how livestock systems are changing, whether in the systems in more marginal areas where change is slow or in the rapidly changing systems that are responding to market demand for livestock and livestock products.
5. Rural Indian livestock rearing is a way of living not the enterprise.
6. Livestock rearing is mainly dependent on crop residue. Milk supply has very critical role in human nutrition especially in India as milk is the most important source of protein and calcium, for larger vegetarian population.

Emerging Challenges and Opportunities in Livestock Sector

1. Livestock is an integral part of the socio-economic fabric of rural India since time immemorial, as a source of livelihood and a provider of draft power (energy), manure and fuel. These functions, however, are

changing as economic development is progressing. Rise in income and urbanization is now fuelling rapid growth in demand for animal food products, and the livestock are coming under pressure to produce more. Indian livestock sector responded well to these changes. Over the last three decades livestock production grew faster than crop sector as a whole and made significant contribution to agricultural growth, and is considered as an important sector in poverty alleviation.

2. Though the small farmers have more opportunities in demand-driven livestock production but they have a formidable challenge to improve scale of production, its efficiency and quality to face the competition from large commercial producers in the market place that is going to increase in the near future. The extent to which the small-scale farmers will be benefited from increasing livestock sector growth would depend on how the policies, technologies and institutions responded to their needs.

3. With the increasing income, the share of high-value food products in the food basket of people is increasing. This is what happening in most of the developing countries where sustained rises in per capita income together with urbanization, are resulting in increased demand for animal food products. This rising demand has been accompanied by an increase in domestic supply, and this phenomenon is termed the 'Livestock Revolution'. The factors underlying demand growth have been quite robust in the recent past and are unlikely to subside in the near future giving a further push to the revolution.

4. Most of the developing countries are facing the problems of nutritional insecurity and rural poverty this Livestock Revolution is having capacity in making a significant contribution in improving nutritional security and in reducing their rural poverty.

5. Indian rural poor's have little access to land and thus they have limited opportunities in crop production how ever on the other hand, livestock wealth is more equitably distributed compared to land, and the expanding demand for animal food products generates significant opportunities for the poor to escape poverty through diversifying and intensifying livestock production, by increasing integration of global markets under World Trade Organization creating opportunities for exporting animal food products and earning money.

6. The route to poverty reduction through improving livestock sector, however, is not free from threats as poor livestock producers face numerous constraints in production and marketing. They are constrained by a lack of access to capital, quality inputs, improved technology and

proper support services. They have small-small marketable surpluses and local rural markets are thin and their sales to distant urban markets requires very high transaction costs due to it, poor livestock producers facing very high competition with the large commercial producers and it undermines their economic viability.

7. Global trade of livestock products is dominated by a few developed countries and it is heavily distorted, as some countries of the European Union as well as United States provide a high level of protection to their livestock industry, making it more difficult for developing countries to compete in the global market as well as many developing countries facing the threat of cheap imports.

8. Developing country exports are thwarted by stringent rules of food safety and quality standards. In this situation smallholders will be able to take advantage of these opportunities will depend on how supportive public policy is helping to smallholder livestock production and the extent to which smallholders improve their scale and efficiency of production.Dynamic and fast growing Indian livestock sector is becoming increasingly important regionally, nationally, and internationally, especially for its contribution in alleviating poverty and for its impacts on environmental sustainability.

Suggested Steps for Improving Livestock Sector

1. To achieve sustainable and equitable livestock sector growth in the different systems, it is important that technology, policy and institutional innovations are combined; and specific attention will need to be paid to on how the poor can benefit from the emerging opportunities, which will require targeted and intelligent public-sector research and development interventions.

2. For improving smallholder competitiveness, role of markets, institutions are important, need to identify causes of market failures that prevent smallholders from participating in livestock production and marketing these are credit, insurance, inputs, technology and information and provide solutions.

3. Mapping supply chains for live animals and their products and sub-products and strengthening those chains that benefit most to the producers through public policy.

4. Assessing future demand for animal food products in terms of their quantitative and qualitative requirements, price and other attributes.

5. Evaluating and documenting benefits and costs of alternative institutional models such as contract farming, co-operatives and producers' organizations.

6. Assessing the impact of WTO and Sanitary and Phytosanitary (SPS) regulations on trading livestock products, and their impact on smallholders.

7. Strengthening the role of livestock in poverty alleviation, food security. Environmental protection policies and strategies, risk mitigation, market access, credit, insurance, vulnerability and knowledge management to minimize vulnerability of the poor to risks; and integrating smallholders in the process of industrializing livestock.

8. Improving feeding systems using local feed resources especially through food–feed crop improvement and low-cost feed formulations, reducing the economic losses from animal diseases, conservation and improvement of indigenous livestock breeds, information and knowledge management, particularly for institutional capacity building. Understanding and quantifying livestock's contribution in poverty reduction and changing, policy, institutional and technology options to make livestock sector growth more pro-poor.

Researchable Issues to Address the Future Livestock Development Challenges

1. Feed/fodder is the key issue in livestock/dairy development and research needs to address the issues of a. feed availability constraint as limited land in mixed crop/ livestock systems, need to intensify systems b. focus on dual purpose food/ feed crops c. select for nutritive value crop residues as well as grain yield d. optimize use of locally grown feed and forages e. strategic use of cost effective nutrient supplements.

2. Research needs for addressing the issues of genetics/breeding for livestock/dairy development a. upgrading local breeds by cross breeding for higher producing animals - successful in favorable conditions, but failures elsewhere b. better use of indigenous animal genetic resources c-losing breeds with valuable genetic material d-characterizes breeds with useful traits e. assess species for milk production.

3. Due to the changing scenario it needs new approach in livestock sector to research and knowledge management as well as science based solutions to emerging issues.

4. Monitoring and forecasting the drivers of change from within and beyond livestock in a changing world, challenges forcing for change in production

systems and in the livestock sector due to changing of the demand of livestock products for growing population, improving economic growth and urbanization for milk, meat, eggs, and animal feeds.

5. Uncertainty, instability and volatility in prices, climate change (erratic rainfall, droughts, floods) emergence of new diseases or remerging existing diseases and the supply of feed/ fodder will/may affect future livestock production systems.
6. New innovation for livestock systems approach to change in mindset, involving multiple stakeholders from outset by researchers and new "soft" skills to develop new partnerships and address new problems to deliver research outcomes to lead to development impact.
7. Research on to intensify crop/livestock systems and livestock based adaptation to climate change, control of emerging and zoonotic diseases and improve food/feed safety and market access and conserve tropical livestock breeds and genetic resources.
8. Research for reducing direct losses by developing better disease control practices (e.g India, 10% livestock output by value lost to diseases).
9. Research on zoonotic and other diseases that limit market access, threaten human health and develop cost effective disease surveillance, monitoring and control methods and integrate international, national, provincial and local efforts (eg bird flu).
10. Diagnose causes of environmental impact of livestock production in different regions and systems. Assess consequences of increased demand for livestock products on greenhouse gas emissions from livestock systems.
11. Find ways to intensify livestock production while minimizing impact on people, land, water, air.
12. Identify alternative livelihoods options for poor livestock keepers in marginal areas
13. Research in changing needs new approaches in livestock sector and knowledge management science based solutions to emerging issues to develop creative solutions.

Conclusions

It is critical that livestock researchers should understand how livestock systems are changing, whether in the systems in marginal areas or rapidly changing systems responding to market demand for livestock and livestock products. Within different systems, it is most important that a mixture of technology, policy and institutional innovations be combined for sustainable and equitable livestock sector growth. Beyond broader livestock sector growth, specific attention will be needed for so that poor can be benefited from the emerging opportunities. This will not happen without targeted and proper intelligent public-sector research and development actions. India has a competitive advantage in production of many primary livestock products, but is not competitive in exports of value added products because of high marketing and processing costs and distortions in world markets. Some countries provide huge production and market support to their livestock sectors, while in India such a support is almost non-existent. Thus, there is a need for India to negotiate in WTO for reduction in distortions in world trade as to gain access to world markets. In fact, there exists a considerable potential for India to export livestock food products, mainly dairy products, to the neighbouring countries such as Bangladesh and Sri Lanka, which are deficit in milk production. Nevertheless, to take advantage of expanding global markets, domestic industry has to improve efficiency and food safety and quality standards, which are becoming stringent in the global trade. Increasing investment in research is necessary to improve quantity and quality of Livestock production proportionate with demand growth and consumer preferences. Share of livestock research in agricultural research outlay is less than the contribution of livestock to agricultural gross domestic product, and needs to be stepped up. Further, priorities in livestock research should be objectively assessed with due consideration of efficiency and sustainability of different livestock production systems and their potential impact on the poor livestock keepers.

References

Birthal PS, Joshi PK and Kumar A. (2002). *Priorities for livestock research in India.* Policy Paper 1 . National Centre for Agricultural Economics and Policy Research, New Delhi, India.

Birthal PS, Taneja VK and Thorpe W. (eds). (2006). *Smallholder livestockproduction in India: Opportunities and challenges. Proceedings of an ICAR–ILRI international workshop held at National Agricultural Science Complex, DPS Marg, Pusa, New Delhi 110 012, India, 31 January–1 February 2006.* NCAP (National Centre for Agricultural Economics and Policy Research) – ICAR (Indian Council of Agricultural Research), New Delhi, India, and ILRI (International Livestock Research Institute), Nairobi, Kenya. 126 pp.

Delgado C, Rosegrant M, Steinfeld H, Ehui S and Courbois C. (1999). *Livestock to 2020: The nextfood revolution.* Food, Agriculture, and the Environment Discussion Paper 28. IFPRI (International Food Policy Research Institute), Washington, DC, USA. 72 pp.

Dorward A, Kydd J, Morrison J and Urey I. (2004). Policy agenda for pro-poor agricultural growth. *World Development* 32(1):73–89.

Kurup MPG. (2002). Smallholder dairy production and marketing in India: Constraints and opportunities. In: Rangnekar D and Thorpe W (eds), *Smallholder dairy production and marketing – opportunitiesand constraints: Proceedings of a South–South workshop held at NDDB, Anand, India, 13–16*

Mellor J. (2004). Agricultural growth and poverty reduction: The rapidly increasing role of smallholder livestock. In: Ahuja V (ed), *Livestock and livelihoods: Challenges and opportunities in the merging market environment*. pp. 30–70.

NCAP (National Centre for Agricultural Economics and Policy Research). Institutional learning and change: A review of concepts and principles. NCAP ICAR Policy Brief 21. ICAR (Indian Council of Agricultural Research), New Delhi, India.

Ravallion M and Datt G. (1996). How important to India's poor is the sectoral composition of economic growth? *World Bank Economic Review* 10(1).

Singh P and Muzumdar AB. (1992). Current status of feed and forage management of livestock in India. *Agricultural Situation in India* 47( ):37 –382.

Tanjea VK and Birthal PS. (2004). Role of buffalo in food security in Asia. *Asian Buffalo Magazine* 1(1):4–13.

Warr P. (2003). Poverty and economic growth in India. In: Kalirajan K and Shankar U (eds), *Economicreform and the liberalization of the Indian economy*. Edward Elgar, Cheltenham, UK. pp. 18-209.

World Bank. (1999). India livestock sector review: Enhancing growth and development. World Bank, Washington, DC, USA.

□□□

37

Feeding Strategies of Livestock in Arid Agro-Ecosystem of India

B.K. MATHUR, A.K. MISRA, A.C. MATHUR AND J.P. SINGH
Division of Livestock Production Systems and Rangeland Management
Central Arid Zone Research Institute, Jodhpur - 342 003

Introduction

Indian hot arid zone which is about 12% of total geographical area of the landmass of 0.32 million km² has maximum covering in western Rajasthan i.e. 61% of the total area whereas the other areas in arid region are available in the states of Gujarat, Punjab, Haryana, Andhra Pradesh and Karnataka accounting for 20, 5, 4, 7 and 3% of hot arid area whereas the cold arid area of 8.4 million ha lies in the state of Jammu & Kashmir covering the Leh and Ladakh region. Rainfed agro-ecosystem occupies 68% of India's cultivated area and supports 40% of the human beings and 65% of the livestock population. It produces 44% of food requirements, thus has and will continue to play a critical role in India's agriculture (Singh *et al.*, 2004). Besides their well-established role in agriculture, livestock have crucial role in food security and as risk aversion mechanism for sustaining family, whenever there is crop failure. Any programmes aimed at alleviating poverty through letock production will have to be based on sound knowledge of the situation in small-holder farming systems, including gender issues, in the context of the prevailing socio-economic conditions (Misra *et al.*, 2006).

The hot arid area is characterized by frequent droughts (47% of frequency in the last century) of moderate to severe nature. Due to higher occurrence frequency of droughts in this region of state, the livestock assumes great importance as a drought management measure as agriculture is at the mercy of rainfall pattern which is very uncertain in amount as well as distribution coupled with poor soil condition, higher evapotranspiration and higher wind velocity causing the soil erosion. The hot arid zone of Rajasthan is comprised of 12 districts of the state lying in the western part and these are Barmer, Bikaner, Churu, Hanumangarh, Jaisalmer, Jalor, Jhunjhunu, Jodhpur, Nagaur, Pali, Sriganganagar and Sikar and this arid region of Rajasthan has livestock population of 27.55 million which is about 57% of the total population of the state. Of the total livestock species available in the state sizable number of crossbreed cattle (50.59), indigenous cattle (37.36%), buffaloes (30.66%), sheep (73.31%), goats (49.77) and camel (79.84%) are available in arid zone. Excepting the districts of Hanumangarh and Sriganganagar where the large ruminant production system of cattle and buffalo is dominant having about 54% of total livestock population but in all other districts of arid zone the small ruminants production system accounting from 55% to 77.5% of total livestock population is prevalent. The camels are essentially the animals of arid region having about 80% share of the total population of state (Livestock census, 2003).

Table 1 : Trend in Livestock Population (millions) of Arid and Non arid district of Rajasthan.

S.No	Livestock	Area of Raj.	1997 Census	% of Raj	2003 Census	% of Raj	2007 Census	% of Raj
1	Cattle	Arid districts	4.96	(40.78)	4.12	(37.97)	5.02	(40.46)
		Non Arid districts	7.20		6.73		7.39	
		Total	12.16		10.85		12.41	
2	Buffaloes	Arid districts	3.16	(32.37)	3.20	(30.65)	3.43	(29.77)
		Non Arid districts	6.60		7.24		8.11	
		Total	**9.76**		**10.44**		**11.54**	
3	Sheep	Arid districts	10.46	(73.30)	7.35	(73.5)	7.94	(70.37)
		Non Arid districts	3.82		2.65		3.34	
		Total	14.31		10.00		11.28	
4	Goat	Arid districts	9.53	(56.25)	8.36	(49.76)	11.77	(53.80)
		Non Arid districts	7.41		8.44		10.11	
		Total	**16.94**		**16.80**		**21.88**	
5	Camel	Arid districts	0.53	(70.66)	0.40	(80)	0.35	(82.14)
		Non Arid districts	0.21		0.10			
		Total	0.75		0.5		0.43	
6	Total Livestock (including, horse, pony, etc.)	Arid districts	28.57	(52.56)	27.5	(56.0)	29.08	(50.23)
		Non Arid districts	25.77		21.6		28.81	
		Total	54.35		49.1 **(10.12)****		57.89 **(10.94)****	

** Percentage of Country Livestock Population

According to the 2003 animal census, Rajasthan harbours 49.14 million heads of domestic animals while it was 54.35 million in 1997, thus a decrease of 10.08% between 1997 and 2003 mainly due to drought years. However, as per 2007 census the population again increased to 57.89 million heads, indicating dependence of desert dwellers on animal husbandry .

The harsh climatic conditions prevailing in the arid region, e.g., erratic rains and frequent droughts would suggest that, it is not very suitable for crop farming. Livestock farming has some in built superiority over crop farming as far as growth; stability and resource conservation are concerned. On an average, the region experiences 3 years of drought in every 10 years. The natural forces constituting the soil-climatic complex, which conspire to reduce the crop productivity and cause instability in agricultural production, have much less impact on livestock farming. This is due to differences in the nutritive value of natural vegetation, which mainly sustains livestock.

The superiority of livestock farming for development of arid region is further highlighted by the fact that this region is endowed with some of the best breeds of livestock and drought-hardy perennial grasses. The local breeds of livestock have acquired certain characters to withstand the arid climate, and the characters have been transmitted through generations to make the present hardy breeds of animals. However, due to lack of proper nutrition, genetic potentiality of these animals has not been expressed to its maximum level.

For arid region of Rajasthan the general climatic conditions, topographical features and biotic factors do not encourage agricultural operations in the absence of extractive industry the peasantry has to fall upon animal husbandry as their main occupation. Rearing some of the finest breed of cattle, camel, sheep and goats known for their endurance making much use of the meagre feed resources which are grasses ,herbs, shrubs, tree leaves and cultivated feed and fodder crops.

Though technologies to improve productivity of arid animals in harsh climatic conditions do exist, however, the awareness and rate of adoption in range oriented arid farming systems worldwide is consistently low, because of the existing research and extension set up and related other constraints.

Feeding

Utilization of fibrous crop residues

In India most of the livestock are fed on crop residues, in addition to grazing and then little supplementation, which includes agro industrial by products. Thus in India livestock production is entirely different from the feeding system in vogue in the western countries. The ongoing system of livestock production is due to the adjustment, which the animal husbandry had to make since the country is short of feeds and fodder.

The recent survey carried out by NIANP, Bangalore indicate that there is shortage of 45% of dry roughages, 44% of concentrates and 38% of green fodder). Most of the cattle and buffaloes in India are owned by small farmers and they suffer due to mal-nutrition. Many efforts have been made in the past to augment the feed resources through physical, chemical and biochemical means to enhance the nutritive value of cellulosic wastes and crop by products.

There could be three major strategies for improving animal productivity in the arid region :

Supplementary feeding

Health management

Produce-marketing facilities

Inspite of huge gap existing between availability and demand for dry matter energy and protein at national level for feeding different species of livestock, still in states like Punjab and Haryana cereal straws more specifically rice straw is being burnt in the fields contributing to loss of valuable energy source to the national pool. Under global context wheat straw (25.3%) is the most abundant crop residue followed by rice straw (22.8%), corn stover (15.8%), barley straw (8.3%), sugarcane tops (8.1%) and sugarcane by products (6.3%) as reported by Han and Garett (1986). Asia is producing about 46% of the world supply of crop residues; therefore Asian Animal Nutritionists have paid more attention to improve the nutritive value and utilization of crop residues as animal feed in relation to other regions. Ninety two percent of rice straw and thirty four percent of the wheat straw are produced in Asia.

Feeding system of roughage: fibrous crop residues (FCR) and fibrous agricultural residues (FAR) are subject to various processing methods such as physical, chemical and biological treatments especially in order to their incorporation into ration or complete feed with the aim of enhancing palatability, intake and nutrient utilization with the ultimate objective of improved performance.

Many methods of treatment have been exhaustively investigated before accepting urea ammoniation as the most potential method for field scale application in most of the Asian countries. Urea treatment can be done in different ways, depending on the local conditions and preferences but some rules can be given regarding concentration of urea, duration of treatment, amount of water to be used and way of stacking (Table 3).

Table 2 : Standard conditions for urea ammoniation

Straw	Urea needed/ 100 kg straw	Quantity of water to be added (lit)	Minimum time required for incubation (days)
Wheat straw	3	50	21
Bajra straw	3	40	21
Paddy straw	4	85	10
Maize straw	4	50	14
Jowar straw	4	50	14

Since the temperature of the heap affects the rate of hydrolysis of urea to ammonia, the duration of treatment can be variable depending as the region or season where treatment is done.The type of crop residue used and its initial nutritional quality affects the effectiveness of treatment. Poor quality roughages should higher effect of treatment, probably because high quality straw contains more cell solubles and thus economics of ammoniation reduces.

Normally, fibrous agricultural residues (FAR) have more than 60% dry mater in the form of either cellulose of hemi cellulose. The nutritional characteristics of fibrons agricultural residues is therefore:

Low in energy and protein level

Poor digestibility of DM and low bio availability of energy

Low in calcium, phosphorus and several trace elements

Poor status of carotene level

Low voluntary feed intake

High silica content

Mathur et al 2000 observed that Tharparkar heifers during summer fed with 2.5 percent urea treated wheat straw increases palatability, with increase in water intake and maintained normal blood parameters and sound health. Additionally, there exists a series of reasons which explain the under utilization of fibrous agricultural residues mentioned below, which needs to be considered for exploiting poor quality roughages: -

Availability, annually and seasonally

Geographical distribution of production and use

Transport needs

Storage needs

Alternative uses

Price of other feeds shifts

Availability of other feed stuffs
Need and cost of processing
Physio chemical characteristics of FAR
Managerial capacity of farmer

Utilization of Un-Conventional Feed Resources

Un-conventional feed (UCF) or non conventional feed resources (NCFR) is a relative term and may differ from region to region and time to time in the same country. Non conventional feeds may be grouped according to availability from agro industrial by products and classified as (a) Vegetable protein source (b) Animal protein sources (c) Energy sources and (d) other miscellaneous unconventional feeds. For this purpose, various non-conventional feeds need to be screened for their possible use as regular livestock feed to enhance the nutritional output per unit area. Additional, utilization of agro-industrial by-products also mitigate the problem of disposal of industrial wastes. Inclusion of non-conventional feeds reduces the quantum of concentrate in the diet for optimum animal performance.

In the by-products mentioned above the following characteristics are most important: protein concentration and its biological value quantitative and qualitative composition of amino acids, digestibility, level of energy, fats and carbohydrates, vitamin and mineral content and the amount of fibre and substances that might be hazardous or toxic to the organism. The quantity of by products used as feed depends on the country's resources and the technical equipments used for its preparation preservation and improvement.

Un-Conventional Resource of Desert Region used as Feed are

Tumba (Citrullus colocynthis) Seed Cake - A Cheaper Feed Resource

Tumba plant, an annual creeper, grows naturally in abidance in hot arid areas of the country with minimum possible water availability. It grows and multiply very fast during monsoon season and its fruits; Tumba - are available in the month of October-November. Mature fruits are golden yellow in colour, ball like, 10-12 cm in diameter. The taste of the fruit is very bitter. Tumba seed are rich in fat, having upto 16% oil. The Tumba (Citrullus colocynthis) seed cake (TSC) a by product of the oil extraction industry is nutritionally rich as it contains 16 to 22% CP. Presently, TSC is available in abundance in arid regions and is being used as a fuel for furnances in factories, and its thus wasted.

The studies clearly indicates that in cattle the conventional concentrates can safely be replaced by TSC to the extent of 25%, as a regular ingredient, which constituted guar (*Cymposis tetragonaloba*) korma and oil cakes (mostly til (*Sesamum indicum*) and cotton (*Gossipuim spps.*) seed cake) and also pelleted cattle feeds.

It is observed that the TSC replacement did not affect the palatability and intake of feeds and fodder. There was no significant (1>0.5) difference in milk yield pattern of control and treatment groups, in terms of quantity and quality. TSC feeding to heifers upto calving and onwards did not show any ill effect on different reproductive parameters.

It can, therefore, be inferred that a simple practice of inclusion of TSC in animal feed will definitely lower the cost of animal feeding by 18% to 20% without having any adverse effect on the production, general health and reproductive performance. In addition, it would result in the utilization of locally available non-conventional cheaper protein source, abridging the gape between demand and supply of the scarce protein, thus, benefiting the marginal farmers appreciably (Mathur *et al* 1989, Mathur 1996).

Vilayati Babool (Prosopis juliflora) Pods

Mesquite or Vilayati babool (*Prosopis juliflora)* trees are extensively grown in desert areas, especially to check the shifting of sand dunes. *Prosopis juliflora* provides highly palatable and nutritious pods in large quantities and the flowers produce good quality nectar for honey. Ripe pods which have fallen on the ground are widely consumed by domestic stock and wild ungulates. These are rich in protein and free sugar, which gives them a sweet taste. In Mexico, ripe pods of some *Prosopis* species are ground into coarse flour (Pinot) for human consumption and baked after removing the seeds and pods are also fermented and brewed into a weak beer, because of high carbohydrates and protein contents. Studied pods palatability and its effect on dry matter intake (DMI), water intake, body weight changes, milk yield and blood constituents in goats, sheep and cattle.

Goats : Ten (10) goats in late lactation were divided into two group of 5 each i.e. group I control and group II treatment. Animals of each group were offered weighed quantity of roughage and concentrate on as such basis (consisting of 35% grinded bajara, 40% tumba seed cake and 25% groundnut cake). However, in treatment group 35% bajra in concentrate was replaced by Prosopis juliflora pod powder (PJPP) making ration near about isocaloric. Study showed that PJPP can be used up to 35% in the concentrate of goats (Mathur *et al* 2004). No significant effect was observed on blood parameters and milk yield of goats in late lactation, during extremes of summer in arid zone (Mathur *et. al.,* 2003).

Sheep : A feeding trial was conducted to evaluate the acceptability and palatability of ration comprised of prosopis juliflora pod husk (PJPH) in Marwari sheep. The results of the study indicated that *P. juliflora* pod husk can be used up to 50 percent level in the concentrate along with tumba (*Citrullus colocynthis*) seed cake as low cost ration of the sheep without any adverse effect on animal health (Mathur *et. al.*, 2002).

Cattle : A cheaper and balanced concentrate feed mixture for arid region was tried by simply mixing the locally available ground feed ingredients including *Prosopis juliflora* pods, Tumba (*Citrullus colocynthis*) seed cake, mineral mixture etc. To reduce cost of cattle production initiated feeding trial on lactating Tharparkar cattle of this cheaper concentrate mixture for one year on Tharparkar cattle, at Research cum Demonstration Unit of Tharparkar cattle, KVK, CAZRI, Jodhpur. Farmer accepts this process technology very easily and is possible at livestock owner's doorstep. Since in India livestock keepers are feeding concentrate to their productive animals without engaging labour towards its preparation, which otherwise is practiced in developed countries having organized dairy farms. Since, with each process step of feed preparation cost/energy is involved and ultimately feed become highly costly and livestock owner in India do not follow it due to unaffordable labour cost involved and cost benefit ratio(B:C). During the present scenario when all the food and feed ingredients are at very high price, the cost of cheaper concentrate formulated is less by Rupees 200/=(Rupees two hundred only)/100 kg concentrate.

The acceptability and palatability of formulated concentrate mixture having *Prosopis juliflora* pods was high with no ill effect on health, increases milk and the cost of cattle production reduces significantly. (Mathur *et. al.*, 2009).

Mustard (*Brasssica juncea*) Seed Cake and its Effect on Production Performance of Tharparkar Cattle

Mustard (*Brasssica juncea*) crop is grown for oil in Western Rajasthan, however mustard seed cake is not incorporated in ration of cattle in arid zone. A comparative study was conducted to understand the effect of feeding mustard seed cake in lactating Tharparkar cattle. Experiment was conducted using eight (8) Tharparkar cows divided into two equal groups of four each, forming control (T_1) replacing 25% concentrate by water soaked. Til seed cake (41.4% CP), and treatment (T_2) water soaked mustard seed cake (32.90% CP). The cake and water optimum ratio worked out was 1:3 and 1:2 for Til and mustard seed cake respectively. Til seed cake mixed ration was well acceptable and palatable to cattle from very first day where as mustard seed cake containing ration for the first fortnight, was less acceptable (25 to 30% left) their after cattle developed taste and accepted it. The hemoglobin and blood biochemistry viz glucose, total portion, albumin and urea showed non-significant differences, however MSC fed group showed higher values for globulin and cholesterol. Study revealed higher acceptability, palatability and milk yield of cows in which concentrate was replaced on weight basis by til seed cake in comparison to mustard seed cake fed group, however non significant difference on reproductive health parameters was observed. (Mathur *et al* 2004).

Prosopis cineraria v/s Colophospermum mopane Leaves

Twelve (12) lactating Marwari goats were divided into 3 groups of 4 each namely T_1, T_2 and T_3. T1 and T_2 groups were stall fed for about five week while T_3 group was sent for grazing. Animals of T_1 and T_2 groups were offered balanced diet as per requirement comprising of concentrate feed and *C. ciliaris* as roughage. Additional T_1 group W.S offered with *P cineraria* leaves while T2 group replaced by *C. mopane* leaves. It was observed that T_1 group the palatability of P cineraria was 95% of the quantity offered while in T_2 group it was in reducing trend with 5% to 15% from first and fifth week of trial. The final body weights after V week of trial for T_1, T_2 and T_3 group was 31.95±1.099, 32.40 ±1.982; and 28.4 ±1.699 , kg respectively. Animals of T_1 and T_2 group maintained their body weight while the grazing group showed in average group weight. T_1 and T_2 group consumed the concentrate offered equally, however *Cenchrus ciliaris* grass kutter consumption was higher in T_1 group (1.65 to 1.94 kg/day/group) as compared to T_2 group (1.41 to 1.72 kg/day/group). Water intake in groups T_2 and T_3 ranged from 7.40 to 10.62 and 6.14 to 9.0 liters/day. The total milk yield on an average / animal for a period of 45 days in T_1, T_2 and T_3 was 28.07., 22.53 and 19.73 litres respectively. The milk yield was 19.74% higher in *P. cineraria* fed group (T_1) than *C. mopane* fed group (T_2), and 29.71% more than T_3 group maintained exclusively on grazing. Thus it was observed that the palatability of dry *Colophospermum mopane* leaves was low and decreased with progress of feeding from 15 to 5% from 1st to 5th week and the traditional local *P. cineraria* leaves were better source of supplementation even in the dry form supporting the milk yield of goats (Mathur *et. al.*, 2006). Although sole feeding of fresh *C. mopane* leaves is not possible in goats but it can very well be fed as a part of complete rations at 35-40% of whole ration (Patil *et. al.*, 2007).

Lani (Salsola baryosma)

Salty shrub Lani (*Salsola baryosma*) of arid region available at vegetative stage can be a good source of fodder to animals. Shoots consists of mainly fleshy stem, since leaves are very minute, consisting not more than 5- 7% of the total biomass. The acceptability and palatability of fresh cut shoots showed that Lani is palatable to goats (*Mathur et. al.*, 2007). Thus Lani is found to be a palatable feed of arid region and its feeding has no detrimental effect on health and growth of the goats.

Lana (Haloxylon salicornicum) Seeds

Lana (*Haloxylon salicornicum*) salty weed available in the arid region produces seeds. The seeds of *H. salicornicum* with perianth are rich source of nutrients and contains: Dry matter-93.40,Crude protein- 18.19,Crude fibre – 13.89,Ether extract – 1.80 ,ADF- 35.91,NDF-71.08 and Ash- 24.70 percent. Lana seeds are found to be good source of protein in the concentrate part of lactating cows replacing about 25% of the conventional sesamum cake (Anonymous, 2007) and in camel, replacing concentrate mixture showed good palatability and digestibility (Mathur *et. al.,* 2009).

Effect of Lani (Salsola baryosma) feeding on dry matter and water intake (per day / group) in goats

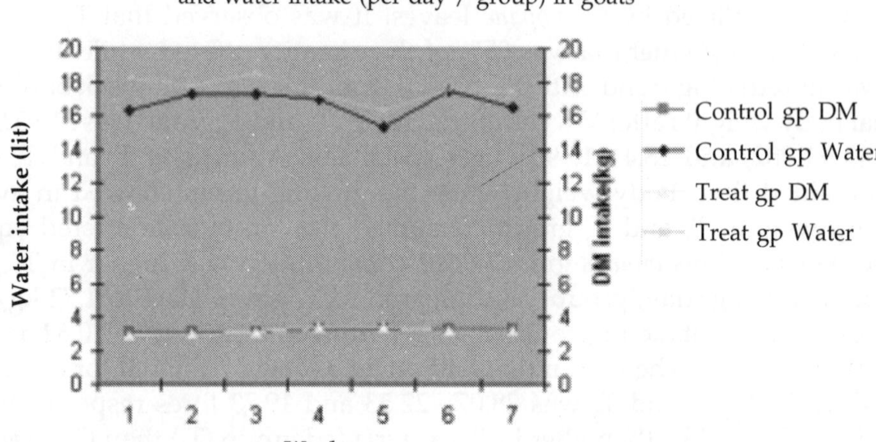

Hardwickia binata

H. binata is available in plenty in the arid region having rainfall above 300 mm. the study showed that the fresh leaves are palatable to goats and sole feeding supports the body weight growth of growing kids (Patil *et. al.,* 2009).

Thornless Cactus (Opuntia ficus indica)

A new fodder source *Opuntia ficus* indica- a thornless cactus introduced in Indian arid region was found to have the fodder value as maintenance feed and was observed to reduce the water requirement if fed along with the dry roughages in goats, sheep and growing cattle. In addition its high mineral content may reduce the mineral requirement, as arid animals are suffering from mineral imbalances (*Mathur et. al.,* 2009).

Cactus (Opantia ficus indica) cladodes were having DM 08.00%, with total ash 26.55% composed of AIA 02.50 and ASA 24. Cacti is rich in minerals particularly Calcium. The mineral rich cactus (Opuntia ficus indica) cladodes have good acceptability, palatability and dry matter intake with higher body weight gain in cattle.

Monsoonal Weeds

The monsoonal weeds available in the rocky and sandy habitat of arid region have a distinct relative preference index for grazing sheep and goats and it was studied to be in the order of 1. Kanti (*Tribulus terristris*), 2. Kagio (*Tetrapogon tenellus*), 3. Santo (*Trianthema protulacastrum*), 4. Lolaru (*Digeria muricata*), 5. Bekario (*Indigofera cordifolia*), and 6. Gangan (*Grewia tanax*) for varieties tested in the region. (Patil *et. al.*, 2005).

Feeding of Mineral Mixtures and Common Salt

Feeding managers of animals should have mineral bricks and common salt, so that deficiency of minerals and common salt may not occur. Calcium, phosphorus, copper and magnesium was significantly low in livestock of villages in arid zone of western Rajasthan. Pica in cattle, buffaloes, camels and goats in this area is another problem related to mineral deficiencies (Mathur *et. al.*, 2005, Mathur *et. al.*, 2009). Milk fever in this area occurs mainly due to calcium deficiency only within one week post-parturient having sufficient level of magnesium. The infertile cattle bears a history of under fed with malnutrition, and per rectum examination of genitalia revealed hypoplastic and / or smooth ovaries and persistent corpus luteum was very common, and they responds to mineral mixture -vitamin supplementation. There is need of area specific mineral mixture supplementation.

Analysis of potentials and problems of livestock production in arid agro-ecosystem of India

On the basis of above discussion, it may be concluded that sustainable development in arid region can only be achieved through optimum utilization of its natural resources. There is tremendous scope of increasing milk production and productivity of indigenous breeds by improving nutrient availability from locally available feed and fodder resources. Availability of key inputs and veterinary services needs to be strengthened and improved to enable the arid farmers for livestock development. A favourable policy environment in terms of access to micro-credit and assured market will have to be provided and socio-economic and technical constraints needs to be addressed. Animal health camps and on-farm trials need to be conducted to create awareness among farmers regarding the adoption of better husbandry practices (Misra *et al*, 2010).

Extension activities in India focuses in the provisions of services e.g., inputs like seed, fertilizer, A.E., feeding material etc., to record vocal appreciation rather than adaptation. Mostly, provision of knowledge appears to receive insufficient attention/contribution. The ultimate decision to adopt a particular technology depends to a a great extent on the farmer's perceptions about the technology, their socio-economic situation and need for the technology.

Feeding management of livestock during drought can be summarized as follow

1. Preparation of ration with urea-molasses for immediate feeding
2. Urea treatment of straw
3. Use of urea molasses mineral blocks
4. Providing vitamin "A" doses
5. Cheaper and balanced concentrate for lactating animals
6. Addition of leguminous crop by products
7. Chopping of straw
8. Mineral mixture-area specific, and common salt
9. Deworming

Health aspect

During the feeding trials conducted for evaluation of above arid unconventional feeds, experimental animals were regularly examined by veterinarian for ill effect of feeding if any on general health and physiological health by collecting and examining blood at regular intervals. Animals were found hale and healthy during feeding trials.

Future research and development needs

1. Agricultural production in arid region is basically based on animal husbandry, hence agriculture policy should be readjusted. Greater emphasis is to be given on livestock farming rather than crop farming in arid region.
2. Establishment of fodder banks at district/town levels and veterinary firstaid facilities with pedigreed males can ensure tremendous increase in livestock productivity.
3. Establishment of perennial components in pasture lands and planing of fodder trees will be helpful.
4. Sustainable integrated farming system models should be developed for different situations to balance livestock, environment and human needs.

5. Educating the people is necessary
6. Land use should be according to its capacity, with priority to agro forestry, pasture development and agro- horticulture.
7. Rainfed farming should be banned in non- irrigated areas receiving upto 150mm precipitation annually. Instead, the farmers should be encouraged, educated and financed to grow endemic, nutritive and highly productive grasses.
8. Low- producing males should be castrated and selection of genetically superior animals within local breeds may be ensured for future breeding programmes.
9. Conservation of local biodiversity is necessary through need based policies and programmes.
10. Use locally available suitable alternate feed resources, e.g., agroindustrial feeds and value addition, to bridge the gap between demand and supply of feed, and avoid competition between livestock and human beings.

References

Administrative Bulletin (2008-09). Directorate of Animal Husbandry, Govt. of Rajasthan Jaipur, Rajasthan.

Annual Report (2008). Central Arid Zone Research Institute, Jodhpur

Anonymous (2007). Feeding Lana (*Haloxylon salicornicum*) and Saji (*Haloxylon recurvum*) to Lactating Rathi Cattle. *Annual Report*, CAZRI 2007, pp.101-102.

Balak Ram (2003). Impact of human activities on land use changes in arid Rajasthan: Retrospect and prospects. (in) Human Impact on Desert environment, pp 44-59. Pratap Narain, Kathju, S., Amal Kar, Singh, M.P. and Praveen-Kumar (Eds). Scientific Publishers, Jodhpur, India.

Census of Livestock (2003). Goverment of Rajasthan, Jaipur.

Census of Livestock (2007). Goverment of Rajasthan, Jaipur.

Chakrawarti Singh and Rollefson, I.K. (2005). Sheep pastoralism in Rajasthan-Still a viable livelihood option? Workshop report, LPPS, Sadri, Dist.-Pali, Rajasthan.

Dutta, T., Taneja, V.K. and Singh, A. (1995). Effect of climatic variables on average daily milk production in crossbred cattle. *Indian Journal of Animal Sciences*, 65(a) : 1004-1007.

Gahlot, A.K. (2005). Animal health management in drought prone area. Seminar on "Sustainable livestock production in arid region", March 22-23, 2005.College of Veterinary and Animal Science, Bikaner (Raj.).

Kaushish, S.K., Bohra, H.C., Mathur, B.K. and Patel, A.K. (1998). In: Fifty Years of Arid Zone Research in India. (eds.). Faroda, A.S. and Manjeet Singh pp.393-426.

Mathur B.K., Singh J.P.,.Rathore V.S,.Singh N.P and.Beniwal, R.K. (2011).Utilization of hot desert shrub: Lana (Haloxylon salicornicum) seeds as feed resource in arid zone. *Indian Journal of Small Ruminants.* 17(2) issue.

Mathur, A.C., Mathur, B.K., Kaushish, S.K. and Patel, A.K. (2001). Effect of package of improved nutritional management practices on true anoestrous cases in buffaloes in rural arid Rajasthan. Paper presented at Ann Conv & National Symposium on 'Fertility management of farm animals under adverse agroclimatic conditions' 6-8 Oct 2001, Jodhpur (India) Souvenir & Abstracts p 39.

Mathur, B. K. and Bohra, H.C. (1993). Nutritive value of *Prosopis juliflora* leaves and pods. Presented at the workshop on potential of *Prosopis* spp. for Arid and Semi Arid Regions of India, Jodhpur. Jodhpur: Central Arid Zone Research Institute, November 22-23, 1993.

Mathur, B.K, Bhati, T.K and Tewari, J.C. (2006b). Comparative palatability of *Prosopis cineraria* v/s *Colophospermum mopane* leaves in lactating Marwari goat in arid region. In: National Symposium on "Livelihood Security and Diversified Farming Systems in Arid Region". January 14-16, 2006. Organized by Arid Zone Research Association of India, CAZRI, Jodhpur. No.3-2, pp.51-52.

Mathur, B.K, Mathur, A.C., Bohra, H.C. and Sharma, B.K. (2006a). Mineral Status in Anestrous Cattle and Buffaloes of Arid Region of Rajasthan. In: XII Animal Nutrition Conference on "Technology Interventions in Animal Nutrition for Rural Prosperity", January 7-9, 2006. Organized by ANSI and ICAR, at Anand Agricultural University, Anand.pp.78.

Mathur, B.K, Patil, N.V., Mathur, A.C. and Patel, A.K. (2005). Impaction of Rumen of desert buck due to Polythene bags- a case study. *Livestock International* 10(5): 17-20.

Mathur, B.K. (1996). Effect of replacement of cotton (*Gossypium* spp.) seed cake from Tumba (*Citrullus colocynthus*) seed cake and sun dried poultry droppings on the performance of sheep. Ph.D. thesis submitted to Rajasthan Agriculture University, Bikaner, Rajasthan.

Mathur, B.K. (2003). Livestock: human need for sustainability in arid environment. In : Human Impact on Desert Environment. (Eds. Pratap Narain, S. Kathju, Amal Kar, M. P. Singh and Praveen- Kumar). Arid Zone Research Association of India and Scientific Publishers (India), Jodhpur, India. pp. 506-514.

Mathur, B.K., Abichandani, R.K. and Patel, A.K. (1999). Higher incidences of twinning in Marwari goats by supplementary feeding in hot arid region. In "Proceedings IX Animal Nutrition Conference", 2-4th December 1999. Acharya N.G. Ranga Agricultural University, Rajendra Nagar, Hyderabad. *Abstract No.* 237., p 144.

Mathur, B.K., Harsh, L.N., Mathur, A.C., Kushwaha, H.L., Bohra, H.C., Prajapat, Dinesh and Tiwari, J.C. (2009). Acceptability and Palatability of a Easily Processed, Balanced and Cheaper Concentrate Mixture Containing *Prosopis juliflora* Pods in Lactating Tharparkar Cattle. In: *"International Conference on Nurturing Arid zones for People and the Environment: Issues and Agenda for the 21st Century"*. Proceedings (Abstracts) of AZCONF 2009, 24-28 November, CAZRI, Jodhpur. pp.242.

Mathur, B.K., Mittal, J.P. and Prasad, S. (1989). Effect of tumba cake (*Citrullus colocynthis*) feeding on cattle production in arid region. *Indian Journal of Animal Sciences* 59: 1464-1465.

Mathur, B.K., Patel A.K., Mathur, A.C., Abichandani, K.K. and Kaushish, S.K. (2000). Wheat straw (untreated treated) consumption by tharparkar heifers during summer under stall fed conditions in "Third Biennial Conference of Animal Nutrition Association" on "Livestock feeding strategies in the new millennium", Nov. 7-9, 2000. CCSHAU., Hissar. No. 282.p.206.

Mathur, B.K., Patel, A.K. and Kaushish, S.K. (2000). Utilization of tumba (*Citrullus colocynthis*) seed cake of desert for goat production. *Indian Journal of Animal Sciences.* 70 (4): 431-433.

Mathur, B.K., Patil, N.V., Mathur, A.C., Bohra, H.C., Bohra, R.C. and Sharma, K.L. (2009). Comparative Mineral Status of Jodhpur District Villagers' Cattle v/s Institute Farm Managed Tharparkar Cattle in Hot Arid Zone. *Proceedings of Animal Nutrition World Conference*, 14-17 Feb., New Delhi, India. pp.61.

Mathur, B.K., Singh J.P., Beniwal, R.K. and Singh, N.P. (2007). Utilization of salty shrub-Lani (*Salsola baryosma*) of arid region as drought feed for goats.FR-55. In: *International Tropical Animal Nutrition Conference*, October 4-7, 2007 NDRI, Karnal. pp.33.

Mathur, B.K., Singh J.P., Sani , Nirmala, Pathak, K.M.L., Rathore, V.S., Kiraroo, B.D., Lukha, Arjun and Beniwal, R.K. (2009). Blood Biochemical & Mineral Profile of Camel Maintained on Different Feeding Regimen in Hot Arid Region of India. In: *"Diversification of Animal Nutrition Research in the Changing Scenario", volume II. Proceedings (Abstract Papers) of 13th Biennial conference of Animal Nutrition Society of India,17-19 December 2009,Banglore.*No.RNPE-134.pp-80.

Mathur, B.K., Siyak, S.R. and Paharia, S. (2002). In corporation of *Prosopis juliflora* Pod husk as Ingredient of low cost ration for sheep in arid region. *Current Agriculture* 26:1-2, 95-98.

Mathur, B.K., Siyak S.R. and Bohra, H. C. (2003). Feeding of Vilayati babool (*Prosopis juliflora*) pods powder to Marwari Goats in Arid Region. *Current Agriculture.* 27(1-2): 57-59.

Misra, A.K.(2006). Integration of livestock in land use diversification.Land Use Diversification for Sustainable Rainfed Areas Agriculture.pp 277-99.(Eds). Sharma K.D and Soni B.Atlantic Publishers and Distributors. New Delhi.

Misra, A.K., Rama Rao, C.A and Ravishankar, K. (2010). Analysis of potentials and problems of dairy production in rainfed agro-ecosystem of India. *Indian Journal of Animal Sciences.* 80(11): 68-75.

Patil,N.V,.Mathur,B.K,.KhanM.S,.Bohra,H.C,.Patel,A.K,.Patidar,M,.Rohilla,P.P,.Saha, D.K Chand Khem,,.Mathur, A.C,.Kachhawaha, S,.Kaushish, S.K, Karim, S.A,,.Shinde, A.K,.Pathak, K.M.L and Lal, Champak. (2009). Improvement of livestock Productivity in Arid Region.Published in "Trends in Arid Zone Research in India.(Editors: Amal Kar, B.K.Garg, M.P.Singh and S.Kathju)pp.180-209. Evergreen Printers, Jodhpur, 481p.

Narain, P., Sharma, K.D., Rao, A.S., Singh, D.V., Mathur, B.K. and Ahuja, Usha Rani (2000). Strategy to combat Drought and Famine in the Indian Arid Zone. Central Arid Zone Research Institute, Jodhpur, 65 p.

Patidar, M., Mathur, B.K., Rajora, M.P. and Mathur, D. (2008). Effect of grass – legume strip cropping and fertility levels on yield and quality of fodder in silvipastoral system under hot arid condition. *Indian Journal of Agricultural Sciences* 78: 394-398.

Patil, N.V, Mathur, B.K, Bohra, H.C. and Patel, A.K. (2005). Relative preference index for arid forages for goat and sheep. National Seminar on "Conservation, Processing and Utilization of Monsoon Herbage for Augmenting Animal Production", December 17-18, 2005. Organized by Indian Society for Sheep and Goat Production and Utilization, at RRS, CSWRI, Bikaner.pp.190.

Patil,N.V.,Mathur,B.K.,Patel,A.K and Bohra,R.C (2011).Nutritional evaluation of Colophospermum mopane as Fodder. *Indian Veterinary Journal*, 88(1) :87-88.

Singh,H.P,Sharma,K.D,Reddy,G.S and Sharma, K.L.(2004). Dryland agriculture in India.Challenges and Strategies for Dryland Agriculture.pp.67-92. *CSSA Special Publication no.*32.Madison,USA.

Singh,J.P.,Mathur,B.K and Rathore,V.S.(2009).Fodder potential of Lana (Haloxylon salicornicum) in hot arid region. *Range Management & Agroforestry* 30(1)34-37

Venkatateswarlu, J., Aantharam, K., Purohit, M.L., Khan, M.S., Bohra, H.C., Singh, K.C. and Mathur, B.K. (1992). Forage 2000 AD The scenario for arid Rajasthan, CAZRI, Jodhpur 32p.

□□□

38

Exogenous Fibrolytic Enzymes as Feed Additives in Ruminants

D. NAGALAKSHMI AND T. VIJAY BHASKER
Department of Animal Nutrition, College of Veterinary Science, Rajendranagar
Hyderabad- 500 030

ABSTRACT

Ruminant animals have a diverse and sophisticated microbial ecosystem for digesting fibrous feedstuffs. Plant cell walls are complex and chemical properties of cell wall compounds and the cross-linked matrix of polysaccharides, lignin and phenolic compounds limits digestion of cell wall polysaccharides by ruminal microbes. Exogenous fibrolytic enzymes (EFE) have successfully used in monogastric animal productions. Recently, use of EFE in ruminants for improving fibre digestion and animal performance has gathered interests of Animal Nutritionsists across the world. The possible mode of action of EFE is complex and could be through their effections on feed prior to consumption, or through enhancement of digestion in rumen by direct hydrolysis or synergism with ruminal micro-organisms and/or increase in post ruminal digestion of fibre and nutrient absorption in small intestine. To date, animal responses to EFE supplements have varied greatly due to differences in enzyme source, application method and types of diets and species. To increase the efficacy of EFE for ruminants future research is required in developing substrate specific cocktail enzymes having proper ratio of individual enzyme activities relative to targeted feed and should be supplemented at optimum dose rate with most appropriate method of enzyme supplementation.

Introduction

Structural polysaccharides such as cellulose, hemicellulose and pectin are the major component of ruminant diets and are the primary source of energy in forage-based diets. The degradation and metabolism of structural carbohydrates is accomplished through synchronous activities of the multitude of microbial enzymes present in the rumen. The insolubility, complex network formed by structural carbohydrate and lignin restricts the efficient utilization of forages and recalcitrant cereal straws by ruminants. Manipulation of ruminal metabolism to maximize the efficiency with which plant cell wall materials are degraded has become an important goal in modern livestock production.

Composition of plant cell wall

Plant cell walls in majority consists of cellulose, hemicellulase and pectins which, are composed primarily of sugars viz., rhamnose, arabinose, xylose, mannose, galactose, glucose, fucose, galacturonic acid and glucuronic acid, arranged as polysaccharides with varying compositions and structures and complexed with hydroxycinnamic acids, lignin, protein, ions and water (McNeil *et al.*, 1984). Cellulose is the most abundant polysaccharide in cell wall accounting for 20 to 30% of dry weight of most plant primary cell wall and consists of linear chains of β-1,4 linked glucose units. Hemicellulose mostly comprises of xylans with backbone of β -1,4 linked xylose residues and attachment of various side chains (acetic acid, arabinose, coumaric acid, ferulic acid, glucuronic acid, 4-O-methylglucuronic acid) to xylose residues. Xylan polymers are also cross-linked to other hemicellulose backbones or to lignin through ferulic acid or 4-O-methylglucuronic acid residues. Xylan backbone also binds strongly to cellulose and interlocks with other xylan polymers, forming an extensive network of cross-links between cellulose microfibrils. Pectin exists in the primary cell wall and its primary structure is a backbone of α-1,4-linked residues of D-galacturonate. The rhamnogalacturonan backbone is interspersed with either rhamnose or galacturonic acid residues substituted with methyl esters groups or sugar side chains. Polysaccharides, hydroxycinnamic acids, lignin, protein and ions are intermolecularly cross-linked through various ionic, hydrogen and covalent bonds to form a three-dimensional matrix that entraps polysaccharide within the cell wall polysaccharides, therefore requiring both hydrolytic enzymes and those capable of cleaving the bonds within the cross-linked matrix.

The plant cell walls are degraded by a combination of bacteria, fungi and protozoa, with bacteria and fungi contributing approximately 80% of the degradative activity and protozoa 20% (Dijkstra and Tamminga, 1995). These micro-organisms produces enzymes that could degrade plant cell wall polymers (cellulases, xylanases, β-glucanases, pectinases), amylases, proteases, phytases and also that degrade specific toxins (eg. Tannases). Efficient digestion of complex substrates in the rumen requires the co-ordinated activities of these enzymes and also, the contact between these enzymes with their feed substrates necessary for their hydrolysis. Though ruminants have a powerful and sophisticated microbial ecosystem to digest fibrous feedstuffs, the ingested cell wall polysaccharides are rarely completely degraded by the ruminal microflora. There is a need to bridge the gap between actual digestibility of feed that occurs *in vivo* and the potential digestibility of feed that would be possible if conditions were ideal (Beauchemin *et al.*, 2003). The digestion of fibre from forages could be enhanced by several biotechnological tools like ionophores, directly fed microbials and enzymes.

Exogenous fibrolytic enzymes

The use of feed enzymes in the monogastric animal production industry has increased dramatically in recent years. The use of exogenous fibrolytic enzymes (EFE) first attracted the attention of ruminant nutritionists over 40 years ago (Burroughs *et al.*, 1960) and with positive responses on nutrient digestion and animal performance (Beauchemin *et al.*, 1995; Schingoethe *et al.*, 1999), the use of EFE in ruminants is being considered. Many of the early enzyme products were poorly characterized, animal responses were variable and no effort was made to design these products specifically for ruminants. Most commercially available enzymatic products that have been tested as food additives for ruminants were not designed specifically for this purpose. Instead enzymatic preparations containing cellulases and xylanases destined for use in food, pulp, paper, textile, fuel and other chemical industries have been used for ruminant studies and hence the results were not encouraging and controversial (Beauchemin *et al.*, 2003). But recently, interest in use of these enzymes increased due to higher feed costs, advancement in technology in production of enzymes resulting in availability of more active and better defined enzyme products and thus reduction in enzyme costs. The EFE that could be used for ruminants are given in Table 1 and are predominantly xylanases, cellulases, pectinases and β-glucanases. Fibre-degrading enzyme activities are generally determined by measuring the rate of release of reducing sugars from pure substrates, with enzyme units expressed as the quantity of reducing sugars released per unit of time per unit of enzyme.

Mode of action of EFE

The goal of exogenous enzyme supplementation is to improve the efficiency of feed utilization in ruminants and reduce waste production. The mode of action of EFE in ruminants is exceedingly complex and continues to be a major focus of the research presently being conducted with these additives.

The EFE alters feed utilization in ruminants either through their effects on the feed prior to consumption, or through their enhancement of digestion in the rumen and/or in the post-ruminal digestive tract.

Table 1: Enzymatic complexes capable of hydrolyzing plant cell walls

Cellulases
Cellulase – EC 3.2.1.4
Cellulose 1,4- β -cellobiosidase – EC 3.2.1.91
Glucan 1,4- β -glucosidase – EC 3.2.1.74
β -Glucosidase- EC 3.2.1.21
Hemicellulases
Endo-1,4- β -xylanase- EC3.2.1.8
Xylan-1,4- β -xylosidase- EC 3.2.1.37
α -N-Arabinofuranosidase- EC 3.2.1.55
Acetylesterase- EC 3.1.1.6
β -mannosidase- EC 3.2.1.25
α -D-glucuronidase- EC 3.2.1.139
α -D-galactosidase- EC 3.2.1.22
Acetyl xylan esterases- EC 3.1.1.72
Ferulic acid esterase- EC 3.1.1.73
Ligninases
Laccase – EC 1.10.3.2
Manganese peroxidase- EC 1.11.1.13
Lignin peroxidase- EC 1.11.1.14
Pectinases
Pectinesterase- EC 3.1.1.11
Pectin lyase- EC 4.2.2.2
Pectate disaccharidelyase- EC 4.2.2.9
Polygalacturonase- EC 3.2.1.15
Galacturan 1,4-α-galacturonidase- EC 3.2.1.67

Preconsumption effects

The EFE can release reducing-sugars from feedstuffs prior to consumption (Beauchemin and Rode, 1996) arising partially from solubilization of neutral detergent fibre (NDF) and acid detergent fibre (ADF) (Gwayumba and Christensen, 1997). The degree of sugar release depends on both the type of feed and the type of enzyme. These enzymes are more effective when applied to dry forage like hay compared to wet forage (Beauchemin *et al.*, 1998) and moisture of 6-10% is sufficient to enable hydrolysis and release of sugars.

Ruminal effects

Limitations to plant cell wall digestion in the rumen could result from insufficient quantities or types of enzyme production by the ruminal microbes, from an inability of degradative enzyme(s) to interact with the target substrates, or from conditions in the rumen not being optimal for enzyme activity (e.g. low ruminal pH).

Direct hydrolysis

The EFE remains active in the rumen and improves digestion through the direct hydrolysis of ingested feed. Hristov *et al.* (2000) reported an increase in ruminal xylanase and cellulase activities with EFE supplementation. Several researchers have shown that exogenous enzymes could enhance fibre degradation by ruminal microorganisms *in vitro* and *in situ* (Table 2).

Synergism with ruminal microorganisms

Supplementing EFE enhances fibre digestion in the rumen by working synergistically with ruminal microbes. The EFE contain enzymatic activities that are normally being limiting for digestion of plant cell walls by ruminal microorganisms. Enzyme extracts from *Aspergillus oryzae* increased the number of ruminal bacteria (Newbold *et al.*, 1992) and worked synergistically with extracts from ruminal microorganisms to enhance release of soluble sugars from hay (Newbold, 1995). The extent of cross-linking by *p*-coumaryl and feruloyl groups to arabinoxylans is one factor that limits the digestion of plant cell walls (Hatfield, 1993). *A. oryzae* has been shown to produce an esterase capable of breaking the ester bridges formed between ferulic and *p*-coumaric acids and arabinoxylan (Tenkanen *et al.*, 1991) and these activities could function synergistically with ruminal microorganisms (Varel *et al.*, 1993).

Hydrolysis of cellulose and hemicellulose is accomplished either by free enzymes or by cellusomal structures comprising multiple enzymes bound non-covalently to form an organized complex (Teeri, 1997). Aerobic fungi, the principal commercial source of exogenous enzymes, hydrolyse plant cell walls by means of free enzymes, whereas hydrolysis of plant cell walls by *Clostridium* spp. and the anaerobic ruminal fungi involves cellulosomal structures (Beguin *et al.*, 1998; Ljungdahl *et al.*, 1998). Cellulosomes plays a role in adhesion of microbial cells to their substrates and attachment of ruminal bacteria to cellulose (Pell and Schofield, 1993) which is absolutely essential for efficient digestion of forages and cereal grains in the rumen (McAllister and Cheng, 1996). Treating lucerne cubes with exogenous enzymes prior to consumption increased bacterial colonization and *in situ* DM disappearance of forage between 3 h and 24 h of ruminal incubation with increase in digestibility of fibre in the rumen and total gastrointestinal tract (Yang *et al.*, 1999). The low fibre in diets of fattening animals compromises the fibre digestion due to fall in pH below 6.2, which is the optimum pH for the functioning of fibrolytic enzymes produced by ruminal micro-organisms (Matte and Forsberg, 1992). In contrast, the pH optima of fibrolytic enzymes produced by aerobic fungi ranges from 4.0 to 6.0 (Muzakhar *et al.*, 1998) and thus EFE enzymes could make a significant contribution to ruminal fibre digestion in fattening animals fed high concentrate diet and thus improve performance (Iwaasa *et al.*, 1997).

Digesta flow

The EFE have been shown to enhance the rate of passage of particulate matter from the rumen. The increase in passage rate could be associated with a faster rate of particle size reduction in the rumen and a corresponding increase in feed intake (Mertens *et al.*, 1984).

Post-ruminal effects

Exogenous enzymes not only heighten fibrolytic activity in the rumen, but also in the small intestine (Hristov *et al.*, 2000). The EFE supplementation increased the xylanase and cellulose activities by 30% in duodenum and by 2-5% in small intestine (Hristov *et al.*, 1998). Increased xylanase activity and nutrient absorption in the small intestine is associated with a decline in intestinal viscosity when fed high grain diets. Beauchemin *et al.* (1999) reported increase in nitrogen and energy retentions due to improvement in the digestibility and absorption of fibre and starch in the lower tract in cows fed barley grain diets.

Exogenous enzymes could work synergistically with the microbes even in the large intestine. The xylanase activity in the faeces increased linearly with increasing levels of enzyme supplementation (Hristov *et al.*, 2000). This heightened fibrolytic activity may have important ramifications with regard to the rate at which faecal material decomposes in the environment.

Effect on nutrient digestibility and microbial activity in rumen

The EFE have shown to increase both *in vitro* and *in situ* fibre degradation of forages (Pinos-Rodriguez *et al.*, 2002) although the results were not consistent (Miller *et al.*, 2008). Similarly many *in vivo* studies with EFE supplementation on nutrient digestibility and rumen microbial activities were variable. The variability in the results was due to influence of many factors affecting the efficiency of these enzymes. The most predominant factors are type of forage (Moharrery *et al.*, 2009; Gallardo *et al.*, 2010), harvesting time of forage (Moharrery *et al.*, 2009), particle size/forage length (Zebeli *et al.*, 2008; Carreon *et al.*, 2010). The results of the in-vitro studies, in addition to above factors were also affected by pH during incubation (Ali Marquez *et al.*,

2009) and microbial population in ruminal fluid/rumen inoculum (Calabro *et al.*, 2008). The other factors attributable to inconsistencies are difference in enzyme type and preparation activities.

Wallace et al (2001) reported positive correlation between cellulase activity and gas production from grass silage and corn silage, but high xylanase acitivy did not increase gas production when glucanase activity was low. Ranilla et al (2008) investigated the effect of xylanase and cellulase on *in vitro* rumen fermentation of alfalfa hay, grass hay and barley straw and observed that *in vitro* fermentation of substrates was higher at short (5 and 10h), but not at long (24h) incubation times and the effects depended on both dose and presence of NDF components in the substrate. Addition of fungal enzyme preparation containing 32 IU/ml of ferulic acid esterase enzyme activity enhanced *in vitro* digestion and ruminal *in situ* degradation of Bermuda grass hay, but pattern and extent of improvement was forage specific (Krueger *et al.*, 2008). The potentially degradable fraction and degradation rate of NDF and ADF of alfalfa hay increased quadratically ($P<0.05$) with supplementation of EFE (xylanase and cellulose from *A. niger* and *Trichoderma viridae*) from 1 to 3g/kg DM, but no effect was observed for corn silage, corn stover, elephant grass, guinea grass and oat straw (Gallardo *et al.*, 2010). Similarly, supplementing mixture (13,000 units cellulose and 2100 IU xylanase/g) at rate of 0-7.5g/kg of either wheat or paddy straw increased cumulative gas production and *in vitro* dry matter (DM) and organic matter (OM) digestibility (Tang *et al.*, 2008).

Most of the studies on supplementation of EFE to forage diets in dairy cows have revealed increase in microbial protein synthesis and rumen fermentation pattern (Hirstov *et al.*, 2007) and apparent digestibilities (Rode *et al.*, 1999; Yang *et al.*, 2000; Knowlton *et al.*, 2002; Chandra Shekhar *et al.*, 2010; Raman Malik *et al.*, 2010). Supplementing EFE (7.1 unit cellulose, 2.3 units xylanase and 61.5 units a amylase/g) at rate of 40g/d to cows increased digestibilities of all nutrients, ammonia nitrogen and total short chain fatty acids in rumen (Gado *et al.*, 2009). The DM intake, digestibilities of NDF and ADF in beef steers increased with spraying of enzyme (cellulose and xylanase) to Bermuda grass immediately after harvesting (Krueger *et al.*, 2008).

Pinos-Rodriguez *et al.* (2002) reported a positive impact on intake, ruminal digestibilities and nitrogen balance in lambs fed alfalfa or rye-grass with EFE supplementation. On other hand addition of EFE mixture (fermentation extracts and soluble from *Aspergillus niger* and *Trichoderma longibachiatum*) did not affect apparent fore stomach or whole tract digestion of guinea grass hay cut at either 35 or 90d of growth in sheep (Avellaneda *et al.*, 2009).

Similarly, no affect on nutrient digestibilities was observed in sheep with addition of EFE to total mixed rations (TMR) (Reddish and Kung, 2007).

Effect of EFE on growth performance

Evidence that exogenous enzymes could improve average daily gain and feed efficiency in beef cattle was recorded by Burroughs *et al.* (1960). When given diets of ground maize, oat silage or lucerne hay treated with an enzyme cocktail containing amylolytic, proteolytic and cellulolytic activities, cattle gained 6.8-24.0% more weight and feed efficiencies improved by 6-21.2%, relative to cattle fed untreated control diets. Leatherwood *et al.* (1960) added a fungal enzyme to a grain supplement for calves fed a lucerne hay-based diet and found no improvement in average daily gain or feed efficiency. Application of different levels (0.25-4.0 litre/tone) of a mixture of xylanase and cellulase products increased daily gains of steers fed lucerne hay or timothy hay cubes by 30 and 36%, respectively, but had no effect on average daily gain when applied to barley silage (Beauchemin *et al.*, 1995). When this same mixture was applied to a 95% grain diet, feed efficiency of cattle fed barley was improved by 11% but performance of cattle fed maize was unaffected (Beauchemin and Rode, 1996). Application of a different mix of fungal enzymes at rates up to 5.0 litre /tone, however increased the final weight and average daily gain of feedlot cattle fed diets based on lucerne silage based diets (Michal *et al.*, 1996) or barley silage (McAllister *et al.*, 1999). Cruywagen and van Zyl (2008) reported that enzyme cocktail derived from ABO 374 fungal strain improved lamb performance on low forage diet. The feed intake, growth rate, feed efficiency, carcass characteristics and meat quality in sheep fed wheat straw or corn stover based diets supplemented with fibrozyme was similar to those fed costly barseem hay based diets (Gad *et al.*, 2011). While, fibrozyme supplementation had no affect on growth performance and carcass characteristics in beef steers (Eun *et al.*, 2009) and in lambs (Almaraz *et al.*, 2010).

Effect of EFE on milk production

The effect of exogenous enzymes on milk production in dairy cows was first examined in mid 1990's (Chen *et al.*, 1995; Lewis *et al.*, 1995). Studies on enzyme supplementation to dairy cow diets have shown increased milk yields of 7-15% (Beauchemin *et al.*, 1999; Lewis *et al.*, 1999; Rode *et al.*, 1999; Schingoethe *et al.*, 1999; Yang *et al.*, 2000), probably due to increased digestibility (Yang *et al.*, 1999; Tricarico *et al.*, 2005), as well as alteration of acetic/propionic acid ratio in rumen (Rode *et al.*, 1999; Giraldo *et al.*, 2008), which increased energy available for milk production (Lewis *et al.*, 1999; Yang *et al.*, 1999). Soliman (2006) reported 23% higher milk production in cows fed peanut hay ensiled with EFE for 45 days and a similar increase in milk yield was observed when fed TMR supplemented with EFE (Gado *et al.*, 2009), but no affect on milk composition was observed. Spraying enzyme preparations on to maize silage in a 50% concentrate diet increased milk production by 2.5 kg /day without altering milk composition (Kung, 1996). As in the studies using beef cattle, production responses by dairy cattle to exogenous enzymes have been variable. Application of enzyme mixtures on to sorghum grain did not improve milk production by Holstein cows (Chen *et al.*, 1995). Similarly, milk responses to EFE depended on the method of application to barley based diets (Beauchemin *et al.*, 1999). Applying a cellulase/xylanase mixture to diets containing 45-50% concentrate and lucerne silage, lucerne hay or a mixture of lucerne silage, maize silage and lucerne hay also failed to increase milk yield (Luchini *et al.*, 1997; Nussio *et al.*, 1997). The positive effect of fibrolytic enzymes on milk production were highly dependent on the level of enzyme applied (Sanchez *et al.*, 1996). Increasing the amount of enzyme applied to Lucerne cubes from 1g/kg to 2g/kg increased milk production from 23.7kg/ d to 24.6 kg/d (Yang *et al.*, 1999). Yang *et al.* (2000) added an enzyme mixture (Biovance Technol, Ohama) to the concentrate, and cows in early lactation produced 2kg/d (5.9%) more milk. However, there was no response when the same enzyme was added to the TMR. Reddish and Kung (2007) observed no effect of EFE containing xylanase and cellulose mixed as dry supplement to TMR on feed intake, milk production and composition in lactating cows.

Steps to improve the effect of EFE in Ruminants

1. *Choice of enzymes should be substrate specific in the targeted feeds*: Not all exogenous enzymes are equally effective at digesting complex substrates such as hay, greens, straws and grain. In straw, the major barriers to microbial digestion are apparently silica, wax and cutin (Bae *et al.*, 1997), whereas in unprocessed grain the pericarp dictates the extent of grain digestion (Wang *et al.*, 1998). Enzyme preparations that digest the structural components limiting the extent of feed digestion in the rumen would be expected to be more efficacious than preparations that just increase the rate of feed degradation in the rumen. Many enzyme preparations are currently in use, with no attempt being made to define the types or activities of the enzymes they contain. Such random employment of enzymes on feeds, without consideration for specific substrate targets, will only discourage or delay adoption of exogenous enzymes for more standard use in the animal production industry. The EFE powder preparation increased both *in vitro* and *in sacco* fibre degradation of alfalfa hay but same EFE could not influence the fibre degradation of corn silage, corn stover, elephant grass, guinea grass and oat straw (Gallardo *et al.*, 2010). Eun and Beauchemin (2008)

reported good potential to increase forage digestibility by ruminants using feed enzyme additives that are formulated to supply appropriate enzymic activities, which dependent on the forage substrate.

2. *Determining the proper ratio of individual enzyme activities relative to the targeted feed in order to maximize their positive effects on animal performance:* Many enzyme preparations are currently in use, with no attempt being made to define the types or activities of the enzymes they contain. Ultimately, enzyme cocktails should be designed specifically to overcome the constraints limiting digestion of a particular type of feed. Component enzymes in such cocktails might vary even for given forage, targeting particular maturity levels and structural barriers. Yang and Xie (2010) reported that the effective fibrolytic activity combination for corn stalks required to reach highest release of reducing sugars were 418-1385 IU xylanase, 111-567 IU carboxymethyl cellulose, 347-376 IU endoglucanase and 2.0 IU ferulic acid esterase per g NDF substrate. For Bahia grass hay, highest DM disappearance was observed for enzyme cocktail having 2g cellulose, 2g xylanase and 0-1g ferulic acid esterase per 100g of substrate (Krueger and Adesogan, 2008). Recent developments in biotechnology made it feasible to engineer such enzyme cocktails containing xylanase, cellulase and b-glucanase activities, but we presently lack the technology for specific production of many other potentially important enzymes (e.g. cutinase, ferulic acid esterase, acetylxylan esterase, arabinofuranosidase).

3. *Identify the optimum dose rates on the targeted feed ingredients/feeds*: Under dosage of enzymes will not be sufficient in digesting complex substrates in straws. Also over treatment of feeds with enzymes may result in blocking sites that may otherwise be available for microbial enzymatic digestion or may prevent attachment by rumen microbes. Giraldo *et al.* (2007) reported that a dose lower than 80 enzymatic units per g substrate was sufficient for *in vitro* ruminal degradation. Similarly Jalilvand *et al.* (2008) supplementation of Natuzyme at rate of 3g per kg DM of forage was sufficient for enhancing forage digestion, while higher levels (6 or 9g/kg DM) adversely affected the fermentation rate of forage. The optimum dose rate for EFE (xylanase and endoglucanase) for alfalfa hay or corn silage was 1.4mg/g forage DM compared to 0.7 or 2.1mg/g DM (Eun *et al.*, 2007).

4. *Appropriate method of enzyme application to the targeted feed for optimum response*: Method of application also influences production responses; it differs from dry forage, fresh forage and silage (Beauchemin *et al.*, 1995; Feng *et al.*, 1996). Methods of EFE application reported are spraying on to concentrate, forage or TMR, top dressing onto TMR and direct introduction into the rumen. Spraying EFE onto dry feed components

(either forage or concentrate) prior to feeding is most effective for eliciting positive response (Wang and McAllister, 2002). Morgavi *et al.* (2000b) observed that spraying fibrolytic enzymes on to feed prior to *in vitro* fermentation improved digestion but direct addition of enzymes into the fermentation media did not illicit a positive response. Beauchemin *et al.* (2004) reported that pretreatment of dry feeds with enzymes applied in a liquid form was important because it created a stable feed-enzyme complex. Several studies have shown that enzymes are less effective if infused directly into the rumen (Lewis *et al.*, 1999; Wang *et al.*, 2001). But ability to feed EFE to ruminants in dry form without spraying them onto feed in a liquid form holds definite advantage for the end user.

5. *Measurement of enzyme activities in the conditions that are representative in the rumen:* Evaluating the activity of EFE and predicting improvement in animal performance is a challenge for future research because temperature, time, substrate concentration, enzyme concentration, product reactions, cofactors and pH, among other factors, have profound effects on enzyme activity. There is a need to develop biological assays that may be more indicative of the value of a given enzyme preparation for ruminants. Specific *in vitro* methods of assessing enzyme activities should be developed that are simulative of rumen conditions. A temperature of approximately 60°C and a pH between 4 and 5 are the optimal conditions for most commercial enzymes (Coughlan, 1985). However, the optimal temperature and pH for assessing enzyme activity are not representative of the conditions in the rumen, which are closer to a pH of 6 to 6.7 and 39°C (Van Soest, 1994).

6. *Lowering enzyme cost*: Once the mechanisms of action and specific targets for degradative exogenous enzymes have been identified, steps can be taken to optimize the application of these preparations. Application concentrations can be minimized by ensuring that the preparations contain the enzyme activities most likely to elicit an improvement in feed utilization. The fermentation medium in production of EFE is one of the important components that determine the final price of the product. The production of enzymes by solid state fermentation is the low cost technology fermentation system that could help in reducing the production cost of EFE. Recently, application of recombinant DNA technology has enabled manufacturers to increase the volume and efficiency of enzyme production, and to create new products (Hodgson, 1994). Genes encoding superior enzymes can be transferred from organisms such as anaerobic bacteria and fungi, typically impractical for commercial production, into well-characterized industrial microbial production hosts (e.g. *Aspergillus* and *Bacillus* spp.).

References

Almaraz, I., Gonzalez, S.S., Pinos-Rodriguez, J.M. and Miranda, L.A. (2010). Effects of exogenous fibrolytic enzymes on *in sacco* and *in vitro* degradation of diets and on growth performance of lambs. *Italian Journal of Animal Sciences*, 9: 6-10.

Avellaneda , J.H. Pinos-Rodr´ýguez , J.M., Gonz´alez , S.S., B´arcenac, R., Hern´andezc, M., Cobos, A., Hern´andez, O. and Montanez, D. (2009). Effects of exogenous fibrolytic enzymes on ruminal fermentation and digestion of Guinea grass hay. *Animal Feed Science and Technology*, 149: 70–77.

Bae, H.D., McAllister, T.A., Kokko, E.G., Leggett, F.L., Yanke, L.J., Jakober, K.D., Ha, J.K., Shin, H.T. and Cheng, K.J. (1997). Effect of silica on the colonization of rice straw by ruminal bacteria. *Animal Feed Science and Technology* 65: 165–181.

Beauchemin, K.A. and Rode, L.M. (1996). Use of feed enzymes in ruminant nutrition. In: Rode, L.M. (ed.) *Animal Science Research and Development – Meeting Future Challenges*. Minister of Supply and Services Canada, Ottawa, Ontario, pp. 103–131.

Beauchemin, K.A., Colombatto, A.D., Morgavi, D.P., Yang, W.Z. and Rode, L.M. (2004). Mode of action of exogenous cell wall degrading enzymes for ruminants. *Canadian Journal of Animal Sciences*, 84: 13-22.

Beauchemin, K.A., Colombatto, D., Morgavi, D.P., Yang, W.Z. (2003). Use of exogenous fibrolytic enzymes to improve feed utilization by ruminants. *Journal of Animal Science*, 81:E37-E47.

Beauchemin, K.A., Rode, L.M. and Sewalt, V.J.H. (1995). Fibrolytic enzymes increase fiber digestibility and growth rate of steers fed dry forages. *Canadian Journal of Animal Science*, 75: 641–644.

Beauchemin, K.A., Rode, L.M., Yang, Z. and McAllister, T.A. (1998). Use of feed enzymes in ruminant nutrition. *Proceedings of the 33rd Pacific Northwest Nutrition Conference*. Vancouver, British Columbia, pp. 121–135.

Beauchemin, K.A., Yang, W.Z. and Rode, L.M. (1999). Effects of grain source and enzyme additive or grain source on site and extent of nutrient digestion in dairy cows. *Journal of Dairy Science*, 82: 378-390.

Beguin, P., Chauvaux, S., Guglielmi, G., Matuschek, M., Leibovitz, E., Chaveroche, M.-K., Miras, I., Alzari, P. and Gounon, P. (1998). The *Clostridium thermocellum* cellulosome: organization and mode of attachment to the cell. *MIE Bioforum, Genetics, Biochemistry and Ecology of Cellulose Degradation*. Suzuka, Japan, p. 107.

Burroughs, W., Woods, W., Ewing, S.A., Greig, J. and Theurer, B. (1960). Enzyme additions to fattening cattle rations. *Journal of Animal Science*, 19: 458-464.

Calabro, S., Moniello, G., Piccolo, V., Bovera, F., Infascelli, F., Tudisco, R. and Cutrignelli, (2008). Rumen fermentation and degradability in buffalo and cattle using the *in vitro* gas production technique. *Journal of Animal Physiology and Animal Nutrition*, 92: 356-362.

Carreon, L., Pinos-Rodriguez, J.M., Barcena, R., Gonzalez, S.S., Mendoza, G. (2010). Influence of fibrolytic enzymes on ruminal disappearance and fermentation in steers fed diets with short and long particle length of forage. *Italian Journal of Animal Science*, 9: 83-87.

Chandra Shekhar, Thakur, S.S. and. Shelke, S.K. (2010). Effect of exogenous fibrolytic enzymes supplementation on milk production and nutrient utilization in Murrah buffaloes. *Tropical Animal Health and Production*, 42: 1465–1470.

Chen, K.H., Huber, J.T., Simas, J., Theurer, C.B., Yu, P., Chan, S.C., Santos, F., Wu, Z., and Swingle, R.S. (1995). Effect of enzyme treatment or steam flaking of sorghum grain on lactation and digestion in dairy cows. *Journal of Dairy Science*, 78: 1721-1727.

Coughlan, M.P. (1985). The properties of fungal and bacterial cellulases with comment on their production and application. *Biotechnology and Genetic Engineering Reviews*, 3: 39-109.

Cruywagen, C.W. and Van Zyl, W.H. (2008). Effects of a fungal enzyme cocktail treatment of high and low forage diets on lamb growth. *Animal Feed Science and Technology*, 145: 151-158.

Diijkstra, J and Tamminga, S. (1995). Simulation of the effects of diet on the contribution of rumen protozoa to degradation of fibre in the rumen. *British Journal of Nutrition*, 74: 617-634.

El-Kady, R.I. Awadalla, I.M. Mohamed, M.I. Fadel, M. and Abd El-Rahman, H.H. (2006). Effect of exogenous enzymes on the growth performance and digestibility of growing buffalo calves. *International Journal of Agricultural Biology*, 8: 354-359.

Eun, J.S. and Beauchemin, K.A. (2008). Relationship between enzymic activities and *in vitro* degradation of alfalfa hay and corn silage. *Animal Feed Science and Technology*, 145: 53-67

Eun, J.S. ZoBell , D. R. Dschaak , C. M. Diaz , D. E. and Tricarico, J. M. (2009). Case Study: Effects of supplementing a fibrolytic feed enzyme on the growth performance and carcass characteristics of beef steers. *The Professional Animal Scientist*, 25: 382–387.

Eun, J.S., Beauchemin, K.A., Schulze, H. (2007). Use of exogenous fibrolytic enzymes to enhance *in vitro* fermentation of alfalfa hay and corn silage. *Journal of Dairy Science*, 90: 1440-1451.

Feng, P., Hunt, C.W., Pritchard, G.T., Julien, W.E. (1996). Effect of enzyme preparations on *in situ* and *in vitro* degradation and *in vivo* digestive characteristics of mature cool-season grass forage in beef steers. *Journal of Animal Science*, 74: 1349-1357.

Gad, S.M., Abdel Gawad, M.H., Sabaawy, E.H. Ali, H.M. and El-Bedawy, T.M. (2011). Effect of fibrozyme and roughage type on growth performance and carcass characteristics of growing Barki sheep. *Indian Journal of Animal Nutrition*, 28: 172-176.

Gado, H.M. Salemb, A.Z.M. Robinson, P.H. Hassan, M. (2009). Influence of exogenous enzymes on nutrient digestibility, extent of ruminal fermentation as well as milk production and composition in dairy cows. *Animal Feed Science and Technology*, 154: 36–46.

Gallardo, I., Barcena, R., Pinos-Rodriguez, J.M., Cobos, M., Carreon, L. and Ortega, M.E. (2010). Influence of exogenous fibrolytic enzymes on *in vitro* and *in sacco* degradation of forages for ruminants. *Italian Journal of Animal Sciences*, 9: 34-38.

Giraldo, L. A. Tejido, M. L. Ranilla, M. J. and Carro, M. D. (2007). Effects of exogenous cellulase supplementation on microbial growth and ruminal fermentation of a high-forage diet in Rusitec fermenters. *Journal of Animal Science*, 85: 1962-1970.

Giraldo, L. A. Tejido, M. L. Ranilla, M. J. and Carro, M. D. (2008). Effects of exogenous fibrolytic enzymes on *in vitro* ruminal fermentation of substrates with different forage:concentrate ratios . *Animal Feed Science and Technology*, 141: 306–325.

Gwayumba, W. and Christensen, D.A. (1997). The effect of fibrolytic enzymes on protein and carbohydrate degradation fractions in forages. *Canadian Journal of Animal Science*, 77: 541–542.

Hatfield, R.D. (1993). Cell wall polysaccharide interactions and degradability. Phenolic constituents of plant cell walls and wall biodegradability. In: Jung, H.G., Buxton, D.R., Hatfield, R.D. and Ralph, J. (eds) *Forage Cell Wall Structure and Digestibility*. American Society of Agronomy, Crop Science Society of America, Soil Science Society of America.

Hodgson, J. (1994). The changing bulk biocatalyst market. *Bio/Technology* 12: 789–790.

Hristov , A.N. Basela, C.E. Melgara, A. Foley , A.E. Roppa, J.K. Hunt, C.W. and Tricarico, J.M. (2008). Effect of exogenous polysaccharide-degrading enzyme preparations on ruminal fermentation and digestibility of nutrients in dairy cows. *Animal Feed Science and Technology*, 145: 182–193.

Hristov, A.N., McAllister, T.A. and Cheng, K.J. (1998). Stability of exogenous polysaccharide-degrading enzyme in the rumen. *Animal Feed Science and Technology*, 76: 165–172.

Hristov, A.N., McAllister, T.A., Cheng, K.J. (2000). Intraruminal supplementation with increasing levels of exogenous polysaccharides-degrading enzymes: effects on nutrient degradation in cattle fed barley grain diet. *Journal of Animal Science*, 78: 477-487.

Iwaasa, A.D., Rode, L.M., Beauchemin, K.A. and Eivemark, S. (1997). Effect of fibrolytic enzymes in barley-based diets on performance of feedlot cattle and *in vitro* gas production. In: *Evolution of the RumenMicrobial Ecosystem, Joint RRI-INRA RumenMicrobiology Symposium*. Aberdeen, Scotland, Poster 39.

Jalilvand, G., Odongo, N.E., López, S., Naserian, A., Valizadeh, R., Eftekhar Shahrodi, F., Kebreab, E., France, J. (2008). Effects of different levels of an enzyme mixture on *in vitro* gas production parameters of contrasting forages. *Animal Feed Science and Technology*, 146: 289-301.

Knowlton, K.F., McKinney, J.M. and Cobb, C. (2002). Effect of a direct-fed fibrolytic enzyme formulation on nutrient intake, partitioning and excretion in early and late lactation Holstein cows. *Journal of Dairy Science*, 85: 3328-3335.

Krueger, N. A. Adesogan, A. T Staples, C. R. Krueger, W. K. Kim, S. C. Littell, R. C. and Sollenberger, L. E. (2008). Effect of method of applying fibrolytic enzymes or ammonia to Bermudagrass hay on feed intake, digestion, and growth of beef steers. *Journal of Animal Science*, 86: 882–889.

Krueger, N.A. and Adesogan, A.T. (2008). Effects of different mixtures of fibrolytic enzymes on digestion and fermentation of bahiagrass hay. *Animal Feed Science and Technology*. 145: 84–94.

Krueger, N.A., Adesogan, A., Staples, C.R., Krueger, W.K., Dean, D.B. and Littell, R.C. (2008). The potential to increase digestibility of tropical grasses with a fungal, ferulic acid esterase enzyme preparation. *Animal Feed Science and Technology*, 145: 95-106.

Kung, L. Jr. (1996). Direct-fed microbial and enzyme feed additives. In: Muirhead, S. (ed.) *Direct-Fed Microbial, Enzyme and Forage Additive Compendium*. The Miller Publishing Company, Minetonka, Minnesota, pp. 15-20.

Kung, L., Jr., Cohen, M.A., Rode, L.M. and Treacher, R.J. (2002). The effect of fibrolytic enzymes sprayed onto forages and fed in a total mixed ratio to lactating dairy cows. *Journal of Dairy Science*, 85: 2396-2402.

Leatherwood, J.M., Mochrie, R.D. and Thomas, W.E. (1960). Some effects of a supplementary cellulose preparation on feed utilization by ruminants. *Journal of Dairy Science*, 43: 1460-1464.

Lewis, G.E. Sanchez, W.K. Hunt, C.W. Guy, M.A. Pritchard, G.T. Swanson, B.I. and Treacher, R.J. (1999). Effect of direct-fed fibrolytic enzymes on the lactational performance of dairy cows. *Journal of Dairy Science*, 82: 611–617.

Ljungdahl, L.G., Blum, D.L., Chen, H., He, Y., Kataeva, I., Li, X. and Ximenes, E.A. (1998). The cellulase/hemicellulase system of the anaerobic fungus *Orpinomyces* and aspects of further cellulase research. *MIE Bioforum, Genetics, Biochemistry and Ecology of Cellulose Degradation*. Suzuka, Japan, p. 19.

Luchini, N.D., Broderick, G.A., Hefner, D.L., Derosa, R., Reynal, S. and Treacher, R. (1997). Production response to treating forage with fibrolytic enzymes prior to feeding to lactating cows. *Journal of Dairy Science* 80 (Suppl. 1), 262.Madison, Wisconsin, 285–313.

Marquez, Mendoza, G., Pinos-Rodriguez, J.M., Zavaleta., Gonzalez, S., Buntinx, S., Loera, O. and Meneses, M. (2009). Effect of fibrolytic enzymes and incubation pH on *in vitro* degradation of NDF extracts of alfalfa and orchardgrass. *Italian Journal of Animal Sciences*, 8: 221-230.

Matte, A. and Forsberg, C.W. (1992). Purification, characterization, and mode of action of endoxylanases 1 and 2 from *Fibrobacter succinogenes* S85. *Applied and Environmental Microbiology*, 58: 157–168.

McAllister, T.A. and Cheng, K.J. (1996). Microbial strategies in the ruminal digestion of cereal grains. *Animal Feed Science and Technology*, 62: 29–36.

McAllister, T.A., Oosting, S.J., Popp, J.D., Mir, Z., Yanke, L.J., Hristov, A.N., Treacher, R.J. and Cheng, K.J. (1999). Effect of exogenous enzymes on digestibility of barley silage and growth performance of feedlot cattle. *Canadian Journal of Animal Science*, 79: 353-360.

McNeil, M., Darvill, A.G., Fry, S.C. and Albersheim, P. (1984). Structure and function of the primary cell wall of plants. *Annual Review of Biochemistry*, 53: 625-663.

Mertens, D.R., Strawn, T.L. and Cardoza, R. (1984). Modelling ruminal particle size reduction: its relationship to particle size description. In: Kennedy, P.M. (ed.) *Techniques in Particle Size Analysis of Feed and Digesta in Ruminants*. Canadian Society of Animal Science Publication No 1, Edmonton, Alberta, pp. 134–141.

Michal, J.J., Johnson, K.A., Treacher, R.J., Gaskins, C.T. and Sears, O. (1996). The impact of direct fed fibrolytic enzymes on the growth rate and feed efficiency of growing beef steers and heifers. *Journal of Animal Science, 74 (Suppl. 1):* 296.

Miller, D.R., Granzin, B.C., Elliott, R. and Norton, B.W. (2008). Effects of an exogenous enzyme, Roxazyme G2 liquid, on milk production in pasture fed dairy cows. *Animal Feed Science and Technology*, 145: 194-208.

Moharrerya, A. Hvelplundb, T. and Weisbjergb, M.R. (2009). Effect of forage type, harvesting time and exogenous enzyme application on degradation characteristics measured using *in vitro* technique. *Animal Feed Science and Technology* 153:178–192

Morgavi, D.P., Newbold, C.J., Beever, D.E. and Wallace, R.J. (2000). Stability and stabilization of potential feed additive enzymes in rumen fluid. *Enzyme Microbiology and Technology*, 26: 171-177.

Muzakhar, K., Hayashii, H., Kawaguchi, T., Sumitani, J. and Arai, M. (1998). Purification and properties of ?-L-arabinofuranosidase and endo-b-D-1,4-galactanase from *Aspergillus niger* KF-267 which liquefied the okara. *MIE Bioforum, Genetics, Biochemistry and Ecology of Cellulose Degradation*. Suzuka, Japan, p. 133.

Newbold, C.J. (1995). Microbial feed additives for ruminants. In: Wallace, R.J. and Chesson, H.C. (eds) *Biotechnology in Animal Feeds and Animal Feeding*. VCH Publishers, New York, pp. 259–278.

Newbold, C.J., Brock, R. and Wallace, R.J. (1992). The effect of *Aspergillus oryzae* fermentation extract on the growth of fungi and ciliate protozoa in the rumen. *Letters in Applied Microbiology* 15: 109–112.

Nussio, L.G., Huber, J.T., Theurer, C.B., Nussio, C.B., Santos, J., Tarazon, M., Lima-Filho, R.O., Riggs, B., Lamoreaux, M. and Treacher, R.J. (1997). Influence of a cellulose/ xylanase complex (C/X) on lactational performance of dairy cows fed alfalfa hay based diets. *Journal of Dairy Science*, 80(Suppl. 1): 220.

Pell, A.N. and Schofield, P. (1993). Microbial adhesion and degradation of plant cell walls. In: Jung, H.G., Buxton, D.R., Hatfield, R.D. and Ralph, J. (eds) *Forage Cell Wall Structure and Digestibility*. American Society of Agronomy, Crop Science Society of America, Soil Science Society of America, Madison, Wisconsin, pp. 397–423.

Pinos Rodriguez, J.M., Moreno, R., Gonzalez, S.S., Robinson, P.H., Mendoza, G. and Alvarez, G. (2008). Effects of exogenous fibrolytic enzymes on ruminal fermentation and digestibilty of total mixed rations fed to lambs. *Animal Feed Science and Technology*, 142: 210–219.

Pinos-Rodrýguez, J. M. Gonzalez, S. S. Mendoza, G. D. Barcena, R. Cobos, M. A. Hernandez, A. and Ortega, M. E. (2002). Effect of exogenous fibrolytic enzyme on ruminal fermentation and digestibility of alfalfa and rye-grass hay fed to lambs. *Journal of Animal Science*, 80: 3016-3020.

Raman Malik and Bandla, S. (2010). Effect of source and dose of probiotics and exogenous fibrolytic enzymes (EFE) on intake, feed efficiency, and growth of male buffalo (*Bubalus bubalis*) calves. *Tropical Animal Health and Production*, 42:1263–1269.

Ranilla, M.J. Tejidoa, M.L. Giraldoa L.A., Tric´arico, J.M. and Carro, M.D. (2008). Effects of an exogenous fibrolytic enzyme preparation on *in vitro* ruminal fermentation of three forages and their isolated cell walls. *Animal Feed Science and Technology*, 145: 109–121.

Reddish, M. A. and Kung Jr, L. (2007). The Effect of Feeding a Dry Enzyme Mixture with Fibrolytic Activity on the Performance of Lactating Cows and Digestibility of a Diet for Sheep. Journal of Dairy Science, 90: 4724–4729.

Rode, L. M., Yang, W. Z. and Beauchemin, K. A. (1999). Fibrolytic Enzyme Supplements for Dairy Cows in Early Lactation. *Journal of Dairy Science*, 82: 2121–2126.

Sanchez, W.K., Hunt, C.W., Guy, M.A., Pritchard, G.T., Swanson, B.I., Warner, T.B. and Higgins, J.M. (1996). Effect of fibrolytic enzymes on lactational performance of dairy cows. *Journal of Dairy Science* 79, Suppl. 1: 183.

Schingoethe, D.J., Stegeman, G.A. and Treacher, R.J. (1999). Response of lactating dairy cows to a cellulose and xylanase enzyme mixture applied to forages at the time of feeding. *Journal of Dairy Science*, 82: 996-1003.

Senthilkumar, S. Valli, C. and Balakrishnan, V. (2007). Evolving specific non starch polysaccharide enzyme mix to paddy straw for enhancing its nutritive value. *Livestock Research for Rural Development* 19(12).

Soliman, M.S. (2006). *Utilization of peanut hay in ruminant feeding*. Ph.D Thesis, Alexandria University, Alexandria, Egypt.

Tang, S.X., Tayo, G.O., Tan, Z.L., Sun, Z.H., Shen, L.X., Zhou, C.S., Xiao, W.J., Ren, G.P., Han, X.F. and Shen, S.B. (2008). Effects of yeast culture and fibrolytic enzyme supplementation on in vitro fermentation characteristics of low-quality cereal straws. *Journal of Animal Science*, 86: 1164-1172.

Teeri, T.T. (1997). Crystalline cellulose degradation: new insight into the function of cellobiohydrolases. *Trends in Biotechnology* 15, 160–167.

Tenkanen, M., Schuseil, J., Puls, J. and Poutanen, K. (1991). Production, purification and characterization of an esterase liberating phenolic acids from lignocellulosics. *Journal of Biotechnology* 18, 69–84.

Titi, H.H. and Tabbaa, M.J. (2004). Efficacy of exogenous cellulase on digestibility in lambs and growth of dairy calves. *Livestock Production Science*, 87: 207–214.

Tricarico, J.M., Johnston, J.D., Dawson, K.A., Hanson, K.C., McLeod, K.W., Harmon, D.L. (2005). The effects of an Aspergillus oryzae extract containing alpha-amylase activity on ruminal fermentation and milk production in lactating Holstein cows. *Animal Science*, 81: 365-374.

Van Soest, P.J. (1994). *Nutritional Ecology of the Ruminant*. 2nd ed. Cornell Univ. Press, Ithaca, NY.

Varel, V.H., Kreikemeier, K.K., Jung, H.G. and Hatfield, R.D. (1993). *In vitro* stimulation of forage fiber degradation by ruminal microorganisms with *Aspergillus oryzae* fermentation extract. *Applied and Environmental Microbiology* 59: 3171–3176.

Wallace, R.J., Wallace, S.J.A, McKain, N., Nsereko, V.L. and Hartnell, G.F. (2001). Influence of supplementary fibrolytic enzymes on the fermentation of corn and grass silages by mixed ruminal microorganisms *in vitro*. *Journal of Animal Science*, 79: 1905-1916.

Wang, Y. and McAllister, T.A. (2002). Rumen microbes, enzymes and feed digestion- A review. *Asian-Australasian Journal of Animal Sciences*, 15: 1659-1676.

Wang, Y., McAllister, T.A., Rode, L.M., Beauchemin, K.A., Morgavi, D.P., Nserki. V. L., Iwaasa, A.D. and Yand, W. (2001). Effects of an exogenous enzyme preparation on microbial protein synthesis, enzyme activity and attachment to feed in the Rumen Simulation Technique (Rusitec). *British Journal of Nutrition*, 85: 325-332.

Wang, Y., McAllister, T.A., Xu, Z.J., Gruber, M.Y., Skadhauge, B., Jende-Strid, B. and Cheng, K.J. (1998). Effects of proanthocyanidins, dehulling and removal of pericarp on digestion of barley grain by ruminal microorganisms. *Journal of the Science of Food andAgriculture* 79: 929–938.

Wang, Y., Spratling, B.M., ZoBell, D.R., Wiedmeier, R.D. and McAllister, T.A. (2004). Effect of alkali pretreatment of wheat straw on the efficacy of exogenous fibrolytic enzymes. *Journal of Animal Science*: 82: 198-208.

Yang, H.J and Xie, C.Y. (2010). Assessment of fibrolytic activities of 18 commercial enzyme products and their abilities to degrade the cell wall fraction of corn stalks in in vitro enzymatic and ruminal batch cultures. *Animal Feed Science and Technology*, 159: 110-121.

Yang, W.S., Beaucheminb, K.A. and Rode, L.M. (2000). A comparison of methods of adding fibrolytic enzymes to lactating cow diets. *Journal of Dairy Science*, 83: 2512-2520.

Yang, W.Z., Beauchemin, K.A. and Rode, L.M. (1999). Effects of enzyme feed additives on extent of digestion and milk production of lactating dairy cows. *Journal of Dairy Science*, 82: 391-403.

Yu, P. McKinnon, J. J. and Christensen, D. A. (2005). Improving the nutritional value of oat hulls for ruminant animals with pretreatment of a multienzyme cocktail: in vitro studies. *Journal of Animal Science*, 83:1133-1141.

Zebeli, Q. Tafaj, M. Junck, B.Ischlager, V.O. Ametaj, B.N. and Drochner, W. (2008). Evaluation of the Response of Ruminal Fermentation and Activities of Nonstarch Polysaccharide-Degrading Enzymes to Particle Length of Corn Silage in Dairy Cows. *Journal of Dairy Science*, 91: 2388–2398.

□□□

39

Bio-Availability of Minerals in Livestock Feeds and Feed Supplements

J.V. RAMANA
Professor and Head, Department of Animal Nutrition, College of Veterinary Science
Sri Venkateswara Veterinary University, Tirupati, Andhra Pradesh, India

Introduction

In order to determine how efficiently an animal utilizes dietary mineral elements, one must know the relative bioavailability of that element from a feed ingredient or complete diet. Chemical analysis of the diet or an individual feed ingredient(s) does not indicate the biological effectiveness of a nutrient. There are many factors that influence the bioavailability of minerals, especially the trace elements. A few include level of mineral intake, chemical form, overall diet digestibility, particle size, interactions with other minerals and nutrients, chelators, inhibitors, physiological state of the animal, water quality, processing conditions to which the individual ingredients or complete diet have been exposed and, of course, the age and species of the animal.

When a trace mineral is ingested its bioavailability is influenced by the specific properties of the mineral as it is in the diet. For example, the valence state of the mineral and its molecular form (inorganic versus organic) are important. Because of these specific properties the mineral may be inclined to form complexes with other components in the gut, which may either hinder or facilitate the mucosal absorption, transport or metabolism of the mineral in the body. It is well known that certain minerals in the inorganic form will compete with other minerals for the necessary binding and absorption sites in the gut.

Knowledge of the bioavailability of trace minerals in feedstuffs and supplemental sources is important for economic feed formulation to support optimal animal performance. Bioavailability should be thought of as an "estimated" value which reflects absorption and utilization of a mineral under of a feedstuff or supplemental compound.

With current technology, determination of bioavailability within its strictest definition is often difficult to impossible for some elements, so acceptable compromises must be made. In other words, there is no one-percentage bioavailability under all conditions.

Natural feedstuffs such as corn, wheat, soybean meal, etc. contain essential trace elements which are required by animals. However, these trace elements are often in a form which renders them unavailable to the animal. Also, even if the elements were totally available, in many cases, they would not be in adequate concentrations to meet the animal's requirement. Therefore, when deficiencies of one or more of the trace mineral elements exist in a diet, they are usually provided to the animal in an inorganic or organic supplemental form. It is advantageous for nutritionists to know the bioavailability of any element in the natural feed ingredient or mineral source used as a dietary supplement. With this knowledge the proper amount of the trace element can be supplied to the animal.

At the present time, more information exists on the utilization of minerals commonly used as supplements than on those in practical dietary ingredients. The term "bioavailability" has been defined as the degree to which an ingested nutrient in a particular source is absorbed in a form that the nutrient is "available" at the tissue level rather than just at the dietary level. Other terms which have been used to express this degree of utilization include "biological availability", "bioactivity", "biopotency" and "bioefficacy" (Ammerman *et al.*, 1995). Bioavailability should not be considered as an inherent property or characteristic of the material being assayed, but, rather, an experimentally determined estimate which reflects the absorption and utilization under conditions of the test (Fairweather-Tait, 1987).

Absorption of Minerals

Before absorption by the absorbing enterocytes from the gastrointestinal tract can take place, the minerals must become available in ionic form (as cations and anions), which is suitable for uptake and transport. In principal, the trans-epithelial transport consists of both, an active trans-cellular component which can be regulated and/or a passive para-cellular component which depends on chemical and electrical gradients existing across the intestinal wall (Nys and Mongin, 1980; Schröder *et al.*, 1996; Jongbloed and Mroz, 1997). The highly-soluble monovalent minerals, such as sodium, potassium, and chlorine can be transported easily. However, the solubility of various other minerals is often low at neutral pH. Their solubility is dependent on the presence of other compounds as they can relatively easy precipitate or form non-absorbable complexes. Well-known complexing food components are phytic acid and oxalic acid (Harland, 1989).

In addition, there are several interactions among various minerals (e.g. calcium and phosphorus; calcium and zinc; copper and zinc; copper, molybdenum and sulphur) which complicate an easy understanding of absorption. Also, viscosity of the chyme in the intestinal tract may negatively affect absorption of minerals.

Methods for Evaluating the Bioavailability of Minerals

There are several factors that affect the bioavailability of minerals. In an excellent review, Guéguen (1961) discussed these factors for phosphorus, but they also apply to a large extent to various other minerals (see also Huyghebaert *et al.*, 1980; Meschy and Guéguen, 1995). These factors, that will only be briefly mentioned here, are as follows:

1. Factors related to the animal (species, sex, age, physiological state, health, differences between individual animals).
2. Factors related to the composition of the diet (amount of mineral intake, ratio between various individual minerals, vitamin levels, protein, fat, fibre and phytate levels).
3. Factors related to the mineral source (fineness, concentration of other minerals, crystallinity, production process, chemical-physical techniques applied, the source of the raw material, the presence as anion or cation, or in some cases in an organic complex).
4. Factors related to the technological treatment that has been applied to the final diet, e.g. mash feed or pelleted diet (DeGroote and Huyghebaert, 1997).

In addition, Jongbloed (1987) showed that even more dietary factors affect mineral digestibility. To give an idea of the complexity of these factors, some results of the research done by Huyghebaert et al. (1980; 1981) on phosphorus can be mentioned. They found that for broilers a sodium/chlorine ratio of 1:3 decreased the availability of phosphorus when compared with a ratio of 1:1. However, at different concentrations of fluorine, the effect of the sodium/ chlorine ratio on phosphorus availability altered completely.

There are two approaches to estimate the bioavailability of minerals for the animal.

1. *In vivo* techniques, which are expensive;
2. *In vitro* techniques, which are relatively cheap.

Another approach is one in between the *in vivo* and *in vitro* techniques, the so-called semi in vivo techniques. These are techniques with cell cultures and tissues. One well-known technique is the Ussing chamber, which has been adopted from rumen absorption studies (Schröder *et al.*, 1995).

Estimation of the bioavailability of minerals from various sources for animals should be closely linked with those biological parameters, that are accurate, distinguishable, easy to execute and relatively inexpensive. They should also lead to tabulated values that can easily be applied in practice, or fit in an existing evaluation system. In order to judge the bioavailability of minerals it is important to know which method and criterion have been used. There are a large variety of methods and criteria used, sometimes leading to large differences. Methods and criteria will be discussed together, because they are often linked to each other.

In vivo Experiments

The following criteria in *in vivo* experiments can be used:

- Animal performance (average daily gain, feed intake, feed conversion ratio, reproduction characteristics);
- Digestion/absorption coefficients;
- Concentrations in several tissues (bone and organs, such as liver, kidneys, muscle, spleen);
- Total mineral content in the animal's body;
- Morphological characteristics in several tissues;
- Blood parameters (concentrations of the minerals, enzyme activities, hormones);
- Concentrations in secretory fluids (bile, pancreatic fluid);
- Concentrations in urine.

Animal performance

Performance as a criterion for assessing the bioavailability of minerals is for several minerals probably the least sensitive response parameter. An effect on performance can only be expected if the animal is fed below its physiological requirement unless a pharmacological effect can be expected (e.g. for copper). Differences in performance can only be noted at large differences in bioavailability or large differences in mineral supply. Broilers are often more sensitive in their performance to differences in mineral supply than other animals, because they have low body reserves of minerals, in contrast to pigs and calves when born.

Digestion/absorption coefficients

Assessing the bioavailability of mineral sources by means of digestion and absorption studies seems to be one of the best direct methods particularly for major minerals. This method is less effective for trace minerals due to the low inclusion levels, the low absorption coefficients and the relatively high endogenous secretion of the specific mineral. Under specific defined conditions, the potential value of products can be measured accurately. However, the problem is that the methods, although they look quite similar, may differ among each other. One large difference may be the basal diet: a more or less practical diet or a synthetic diet (Eeckhout and DePaepe, 1996; BASF, 1996; Pfeffer, 1996). Hence, altered digestibility coefficients may be measured e.g., by a lower faecal endogenous excretion. However, in experimental diets for poultry mostly (semi)-synthetic diets have to be used for assessing phosphorus digestion/absorption due to the fact that broilers are capable of hydrolysing phytate phosphorus with their endogenous enzymes. Otherwise, it may lead to underestimation in digestibility/availability of the phosphorus source under investigation.

A prerequisite for a better harmonization is that the basal diets become more similar among research centres. Methods that are used are the balance technique and the slope ratio technique. Radio-labelled or stable isotopes of major minerals are seldom used, due to their high price. For trace minerals studies, they are used more commonly/frequently. By means of isotopes, excretion can be corrected for endogenous secretion, so that instead of apparent a true digestibility can be obtained.

Concentrations in several tissues

In general, bone parameters are the most commonly used parameters for assessing the bioavailability of calcium, phosphorus, manganese and zinc in mineral sources. A large variety of bone parameters can be used such as fresh bone weight, dry bone weight, fat-free bone weight, bone ash weight, calcium, phosphorus, manganese or zinc content in bone ash, bone density, specific gravity, bone breaking strength, surface of epiphysial plate, and radiological or photometric parameters. Bone ash content and bone breaking strength are most commonly used for calcium and phosphorus, especially for poultry. Several bones can be chosen such as femur, tibia, metatarsals (3rd and 4th), metacarpals (3rd and 4th), tail vertebrae, and toes. The more distal the bones, the more sensitive they are found to be for differences in calcium and phosphorus supply. Because there is a rather large between-animal-variation, quite a large number of observations is necessary. Furthermore, it is an indirect parameter (reference source is generally included), that has to be converted to a direct (tabulated) value. This is one of the disadvantages of using bone parameters, as well as the price of sacrificing the animals. Moreover, the preparation of the bones is very laborious. For calcium, also egg shell strength can be used as a criterion as well as magnesium content in the egg shell or magnesium content in bone.

Some trace minerals may accumulate in specific organs e.g. copper, cobalt, iron, manganese, molybdenum and zinc in the liver, kidney, spleen, or muscle. Furthermore, iodine concentration in thyroids or even thyroid weight can be used as a criterion for the iodine supply. Therefore, for evaluation of particular trace minerals some of these target organs are chosen. For large animals, biopsies can be taken from some organs and tissues. With regard to the liver it has been shown the site of sampling is also of importance (Götze *et al.*, 1978).

Total amount of minerals in the animal body

It seems obvious that the total amount of a mineral that is retained in the animal body is one of the best response parameters for those minerals with a low mineral turnover such as calcium and phosphorus. However, this holds true only if the animals are fed below their mineral requirement. When fed above their mineral requirement, the surplus of the mineral is excreted in the faeces and urine and is, therefore, not retained in the body. This leads to underestimation of the nutritional value of the mineral source, although there are some exceptions such as copper (accretion in the liver) and zinc (accretion in the bones). There are several disadvantages of this method. Sample preparation from a whole body is not an easy task. Furthermore, the amount of the mineral present in the animal body should be doubled at least to obtain a reasonable accurate estimation of value of minerals when using cattle or pigs. Therefore, one should take care that there is a sufficient increase of the amount of mineral in the body. This is much easier when broilers are involved. Accordingly, both accuracy of sampling and amount of increase may result in a substantial variation of the estimated amount of the mineral in the body. Another disadvantage, in the case of large animals, is the price of the animals that have to be sacrificed.

Morphological measurements in various tissues

Some minerals may have an effect on the morphology of tissues because of their interference with tissue formation. For instance manganese has an effect on connective tissue formation. Therefore the perosis severity index has often been taken as a measure for supply of manganese for birds. Furthermore, pancreatic fibrosis or exudative diathesis are used as a criterion for the supply of selenium.

Blood parameters

Blood parameters such as concentration of minerals and activity of specific enzymes may also be used as a criterion for evaluation of the bioavailability of mineral sources. One should realise, however, that there is hormonal regulation to control homeostasis in the extracellular fluid. Therefore, differences in blood levels only occur when the regulatory mechanism is no longer able to maintain the extracellular content of the mineral within the narrow physiological range (Van der Velde *et al.*, 1986). This means that serum mineral levels can only be used at large differences in bioavailability of the mineral sources under investigation. Also, diurnal variation in serum mineral content or enzyme activity may influence the results.

For phosphorus, inorganic phosphorus content of the serum and alkaline phosphatase activity are used as a criterion. Boyd et al. (1981; 1983) showed that for phosphorus, serum alkaline phosphatase activity was highly correlated with bone breaking strength (r=-0.98), although the coefficients of variation for both parameters were high (23%).

For copper, criteria may be blood or serum copper content, superoxide dismutase, cytochrome c oxidase or caeruloplasmin content in the liver. With regard to iron. haemoglobin content in blood or haemoglobin regeneration are well known criteria. The enzymes 5-iodothyronine deiodinase and glutathione peroxidase activity are important parameters for the selenium supply. In ruminants vitamin B_{12} synthesis is an indicator for the supply of cobalt.

Concentrations in secretory fluids

In some cases concentrations of minerals in secretory fluids can be used as a criterion for the supply. This is the case for the content of copper in bile or the zinc content of zinc in pancreatic fluid.

In vitro Techniques

There have been several attempts to derive the bioavailability of minerals from in vitro techniques. So far, this approach has not resulted in satisfactory results, because it is very difficult to simulate the gastric and intestinal conditions properly. Guéguen (1976, 1977) developed the citric acid solubility of phosphorus sources, but came to the conclusion that this method was not accurate enough. Also, several studies at the ID-Lelystad showed that solubility in water and solubility in 2% citric acid were not discriminative enough to rank the phosphorus sources tested (Dellaert *et al.*, 1990; Kemme *et al.*, 1993). With these tests, only inferior sources can be distinguished from good quality sources (Guéguen, 1961; 1976).

Recently, Havenaar et al. (1995) developed a method known as the TNO Intestinal Model (TIM) that simulates gastro-intestinal conditions and claims to be able to accurately simulate absorption conditions including minerals.

Conclusion methods for evaluating the bioavailability of minerals

It appears from literature that there is no single satisfactory method for evaluating the bioavailability of minerals in mineral sources or in raw materials. The method(s) depend on the response parameter(s) as well as the specific mineral in study. For minerals such as calcium and phosphorus, digestibility/ absorbability and bone parameters (bone ash content, bone breaking strength) are the best parameters. The digestibility/absorbability is preferred, because this is a direct method. For several trace minerals other parameters have to be chosen. The next step is to harmonise the methods, formulate the conditions for the experimental set up, and ensure the same response parameters are being measured.

Terms used to express the bioavailability of minerals

In literature, different terms are used to assess and express the nutritive value of minerals for animals e.g., digestibility, absorbability, (bio)availability or even bioefficacy (Partridge, 1980). The term digestibility and absorbability refer to the gastrointestinal tract (feed - faeces). The term (bio)availability, however, is used with several different meanings, and can therefore, be misleading. ARC (1981) defines (bio)availability as the fraction that is retained in the body [feed - (faeces + urine)]. The term (bio)availability is also used in studies assessing the nutritive value of mineral sources, whereby the result is compared with a reference that is assumed to be 100% available (NRC, 1998). In order to define availability in the latter situation, various response parameters that are not directly associated with absorption are used. In addition to absorbability or availability, another distinction can be made between apparent or true, and between ileal and faecal values. However, this will not be discussed further in this paper.

In many cases, however, absolute values, which can differ from one experiment to the other have to be converted to relative values. This is often called the relative bioavailability (RBV).

Absorbability

For minerals that are absorbed from the intestinal tract, the terms absorption and digestion can be used. From the scientific point of view, the term absorbability should only be used as the fraction that is absorbed from the gastrointestinal tract. In this case, digestibility is not the right term when related to minerals, although it is widely used in practice. The term availability should not be used in this case.

Availability

Availability can be used for all other measures not related to disappearance of minerals from the gastrointestinal tract. As in almost all studies the nutritive value of a mineral is related to a reference mineral, the term relative (bio)availability should be used. In addition, it should also be indicated which mineral source is the reference and which response parameter was used.

Factors affecting the bioavailability of mineral sources

Aspects related to the diet are:

- feedstuff composition of the diet
- chemical composition of the diet (proximate analysis and mineral contents)
- vitamin content
- presence of antimicrobial growth promoters or (organic) acids
- chemical composition and purity of the mineral sources tested
- level of supplementation of the minerals tested
- particle size of the mineral source

Aspects related to the animal are:

- animal species, breed and physiological status of the animal
- sex and age
- production (performance) level and type of production

Environmental and management aspects are:

- health status of the animals
- level of feeding expressed as energy level times maintenance requirement for energy
- level of water supply
- feeding method (dry or wet feeding; soaking)
- housing and equipment

Evaluation method

- direct or indirect
- criterion
- reference mineral
- levels of supplementation
- number of replicates
- model used for evaluation (doses-response; linear or non-linear).
- period of feeding the test diet, duration of preliminary and test periods

Organic Mineral Supplements

Inorganic minerals in feed and digestive juices present in chyme as ions interact with available ligands and become bound as various organic complexes or form low solubility salts, which are unabsorbable. It is currently unknown if chelated or complexed mineral supplements dissociate to form free ions at low pH, which are in turn sequestered in a manner similar to inorganic free ions and enter the glycocalyx of the intestinal mucosa for absorption. Alternatively, depending upon stability constants and conditions in the gastrointestinal tract, the organic formsmay be absorbed intact by amino acid or peptide transport pathways, as well as mineral pathways. This may account for the modest increases in availability observed in animal trials. Some of the factors affecting uptake of chelated minerals include the water-lipid partitioning coefficient, site of absorption for the particular mineral and stability of the metal-ligand complex. However, if chelates have strong stability constants, the mineral cannot be released from the ligand for used in metabolism after absorption.

Mineral chelates differ from amino acids in several ways which may affect their ability to be absorbed by amino acid pathways. These included geometry of the molecule, charge density, molecular weight, size binding site affinity, charge of functional group and heterogeneity of amino acids in the complexes. In order to determine the absorptive characteristics of organic minerals, it would be necessary to manufacture the chelates with an intrinsic radiolabel for the element in question, then follow uptake of the element in the living animal which is consuming commercial-type diets in amounts similar to that used under practical conditions. Experiments with simple extrinsinc labeled amino acids in ligated gut sections in purified media cannot truly be relied upon to characterize absorption of these compounds ina living animal. Considering the expense and difficulty of obtaining the necessary information, it is unlikely that scientists will be able to determine the true nature of the absorption of organic chelated and complexed mineral supplements any time in the near future.

Mineral concentrations and relative bioavailabilities of mineral Supplements

Mineral	Supplement	Empirical formula	Mineral concentration (percent)	Relative bioavailability (RV)	Mineral availability (percent of content)
Calcium	Calcium carbonate	$CaCO_3$	38	100.00	38.00
	Bone meal	variable	24	110.00	26.40
	Calcium chloride (dihydrate)	$CaCl_2(H_2O)$	31	125.00	38.75
	Dicalcium phosphate	$Ca_2(PO_4)$	20	110.00	22.00
	Limestone		36	90.00	32.40
	Monocalcium phosphate	$Ca(PO_4)$	17	130.00	22.10
Cobalt	Cobaltous sulfate	$CoSO_4(H_2O)7$	21	100.00	21.00
	Cobaltic oxide	Co_3O_4	73	20.00	14.60
	Cobaltous carbonate	$CoCO_3$	47	110.00	51.70
	Cobaltous oxide	CoO	70	55.00	38.50
Copper	Cupric sulfate	$CuSO_4(H_2O)5$	25	100.00	25.00
	Copper EDTA	variable	variable	95.00	variable
	Copper lysine	variable	variable	100.00	variable
	Cupric chloride (tribasic)	$Cu_2(OH)3$ Cl	58	115.00	66.70
	Cupric oxide	CuO	75	15.00	11.25
	Cupric sulfide	CuS	66	25.00	16.50
	Cuprous acetate	$CuC_2O_2H_3$	51	100.00	51.00
Iodine	Potassium iodide	KI	69	100.00	69.00
	Sodium iodide	NaI	84	100.00	84.00

Mineral	Supplement	Empirical formula	Mineral concentration (percent)	Relative bioavailability (RV)	Mineral availability (percent of ontent)
Iodine	Calcium iodate	Ca(IO)3	64	95.00	60.80
	Diiodosalicyclic acid	$C_7H_4I_2O_3$	65	15.00	9.75
	Ethylenediamine dihydriodine	$C_2H_8N_2$(HI)2	80	105.00	84.00
	Pentacalcium orthoperiodate	$Ca_5(IO_6)_2$	39	100.00	39.00
Iron	Ferrous sulfate heptahydrate	$FeSO_4(H_2O)_7$	20	100.00	20.00
	Ferric citrate	variable	variable	110.00	variable
	Ferric EDTA	variable	variable	95.00	variable
	Ferric phytate	variable	variable	45.00	variable
	Ferrous carbonate	$FeCO_3$	38	10.00	3.80
Magnesium	Magnesium sulfate	$MgSO_4$	20	100.00	20.00
	Magnesium acetate	$MgC_2O_2H_4$	29	110.00	31.90
	Magnesium basic carbonate	$MgCO_3$	31	100.00	31.00
	Magnesium oxide	MgO	55	100.00	55.00
Manganese	Manganese sulfate	$MnSO_4(H_2O)$	30	100.00	30.00
	Manganese carbonate	$MnCO_3$	46	30.00	13.80
	Manganese dioxide	MnO_2	63	35.00	22.05
	Manganese methionine	variable	variable	125.00	variable
	Manganese monoxide	MnO	60	60.00	36.00

Mineral	Supplement	Empirical formula	Mineral concentration (percent)	Relative bioavailability (RV)	Mineral availability (percent of content)
Phosphorus	Sodium phosphate	$NaPO_4$	variable		
	Bone meal	variable	21	100.00	21.00
	Defluorinated phosphate	variable	12	80.00	9.60
	Dicalcium phosphate	$CaHPO_4$	18	85.00	15.30
Selenium	Sodium selenite	Na_2SeO_3	45	100.00	45.00
	Cobalt selenite	variable	variable	105.00	0.00
	Selenomethionine	variable	variable	245.00	0.00
	Selenoyeast	variable	variable	290.00	0.00
Sodium	Sodium chloride	$NaCl$	40	100.00	40.00
	Sodium bicarbonate	$Na(CO_3)_2$	27	95.00	25.65
Zinc	Zinc sulfate	$ZnSO_4(H_2O)$	36	100.00	36.00
	Zinc carbonate	$ZnCO_3$	56	60.00	33.60
	Zinc oxide	ZnO	72	100.00	72.00

Composition of mineral supplements

Supplement	Calcium percent	Phosphorus percent	Sodium percent	Potassium percent	Magnesium percent	Manganese ppm	Iron ppm	Copper ppm	Zinc ppm	Selenium ppm
Bone meal	24.00	12.00	0.46		0.64	30.40	840.00	16.30	424.00	
Calcium carbonate	38.00		0.06	0.06	0.50	279.00	336.00	24.00		0.07
Diamonium phosphate	0.50	20.00	0.04		0.45	500.00	15000.00	80.00	300.00	
Defluorinated phosphate	33.00	18.00	4.50	0.09		220.00	9200.00	22.00	44.00	0.60
Dicalcium phosphate	20.00	18.50	0.08	0.07	0.60	300.00	10000.00	80.00	220.00	0.60
Mono-dicalcium phosphate	16.00	21.00	0.05	0.06	0.50	220.00	7000.00	70.00	210.00	0.60
Mono-ammonium phosphate	0.50	24.00	0.06		0.45	500.00	12000.00	80.00	300.00	
Sodium phosphate		21.80	32.30							
Sodium tripolyphosphate		25.00	31.00				42.00			
Phosphoric acid (75 percent)		23.80					5.00			

Mineral composition of feedstuffs

Feedstuff	Calcium percent	Phosphorus percent	Sodium percent	Potassium percent	Magnesium percent	Manganese ppm	Iron ppm	Copper ppm	Zinc ppm	Selenium ppm
Alfalfa hay	1.40	0.28	0.05	2.43	0.28	30.30	198.00	7.30	18.80	0.41
Corn silage	0.25	0.22	0.01	1.14	0.18	23.50	131.00	4.18	17.70	0.53
Soybean meal	0.25	0.60	0.04	1.97	0.27	27.50	120.00	28.00	60.00	0.1
Corn gluten feed	0.07	0.95	0.26	1.40	0.40	22.10	226.00	6.98	73.30	1.8
Soybean hulls	0.53	0.18	0.03	129.00	0.22	10.00	409.00	17.80	48.00	0.14
Corn	0.30	0.32	0.01	0.44	0.12	7.89	54.50	2.51	24.20	0.6
Barley	0.05	0.35	0.01	0.57	0.12	18.30	59.50	5.30	13.00	1.16

Chelates form a ring structure around the metal ion and have coordinate covalent bonds with the nitrogen (amino) or oxygen (carboxyl) donor groups of amino acids and/or proteinates. Gluconates, fumarates and citrates have only ionicmetal-ligand bonding and are less stable than chelates. All chelates are complexes, but not all complexes are chelates.

The definition of mineral products that are able to be sold as organically-bound mineral compounds is defined by the Association of American Feed Control Officials (AAFCO, 1997).

1. A *Metal Amino Acid Chelate* is the product resulting from the reaction of a soluble metal salt with amino acids with amole ratio of one mole of metal to one to three (preferably two) moles of amino acids to form coordinate covalent bonds. The average weight of the hydrolyzed amino acids must be approximately150 and the resulting molecular weight of the chelate must not exceed 800.
2. A *Metal Amino Acid Complex* is the product resulting from complexing of a soluble metal salt with an amino acid(s).
3. A *Metal (Specific amino acid) Complex* is the product resulting from complexing of a soluble metal salt with a specific amino acid.
4. A *Metal Proteinate* is the product resulting from the chelation of a soluble salt with amino acids and/or partially hydrolyzed protein.
5. A *Metal Polysaccharide Complex* is the product resulting from complexing of a soluble salt with a polysaccharide solution declared as an ingredient as the specific metal complex.

□□□

40

Enzyme Addition in Ruminant Ration

S.V. DESHMUKH AND S.M. WANKHEDE
Department of Animal Nutrition, College of Veterinary Animal Sciences
Parbhani -431402 Maharashtra State

Introduction

Livestock production in developing country like India is constrained because of poor nutrition. Cereal fodder (maize, rice, wheat, sorghum etc) and cereal crop residue are the main sources of feed for ruminants especially during the dry season and winter. It is very well recognized that these crop residues have poor nutritional value because of their low energy, low nitrogen, low minerals and high fibre and acid insoluble ash content. Daily use of concentrate feeds in the ration of ruminants is also limited because the farmers can hardly afford them. The feed shortage problem is made worse by the decreasing availability of land of fodder crop because of rapidly increasing human population, soil degradation, urbanization and effects of climatic variations. Nevertheless over the years, significant improvement has been reported in the digestibility of these roughages through different chemicals such as sodium hydroxide and urea. However, these chemicals pose different problems when used by livestock owners limiting their use by farming community. As an alternate to these chemicals, exogenous feed enzymes is identified as promising alternative to improve the energy availability for ruminants. Commercial enzymes used in the livestock feed industry are products of microbial fermentation. Feed enzymes are produced by fermentation process with the help of seed culture and growth media (Cowan, 1994).

What are feed enzymes for ruminants?

Enzymes are protein molecules and naturally occurring biocatalyst produced by living cells involved in various biochemical processes. In monogastric animals like poultry exogenous enzymes have been used extensively for removing anti nutritional factors from feed ingredients thereby increasing digestibility of nutrients.However, feeding of enzyme to ruminants to improve ruminal digestion had been a questionable issue. The fact being that enzymes are proteineous in nature and are subject to degradation by microbial proteases in the rumen and are inactivated by proteases in the small intestine. These facts have raised the doubt about their ultimate utility in ruminants. However, studies using various enzyme products fed to ruminants have been constantly reported (Bowman *et al.*, 2002 and Colombatto *et al.*, 2003). As per this report, various factors such as type of enzyme and preparation, method of application, quantity of enzyme applied, animal differences and their physiological state have lead to variation of results.

Properties of feed enzyme

Use of feed enzymes in the animal feed has been comparatively recent phenomenon. The industrial enzymes are mainly produced from microorganisms by a process of fermentation and extraction and hence ned to possess desired properties to make them economically viable. Feed enzymes also need to be strong and sturdy to withstand variations in pH and temperatures. They require to have high temperature stability to withstand pelletization process and also have to acquire good keeping quality.The granular form of feed enzyme is found to be more heat stable to withstand pelletization process and it has better shelf life too. The enzyme combinations developed in the west were mainly for wheat and barley, which were inappropriate for Indian diets.Thus in India the concept of use of feed enzymes in ruminant ration is delayed and developed in recent years.Moreover the technology for the production of these enzymes was not well developed in India to produce suitable products for the feed industry. Lastly the feeding and managemental practices are different than western countries therefore the need for external enzyme usage was not felt.

Sources of feed enzyme

Commercially there are several enzyme products available in the market for livestock. Basically all enzyme products have been derived from four bacterial *(Bacillus subtilis, Lactobacillus acidophilus, L. plantarum,* and *Streptococcus faecium,* spp.) and three fungal (*Aspergillus oryzae, Trichoderma reesei,* and *Saccharomyces cerevisiae*) species (Muirhead, 1996). The enzymes are used to speed up the degradative process by which substrates (i.e., feedstuffs) are digested into their chemical components (e.g., simple sugars, amino acids, fatty acids). These chemical compounds are in turn used for growth of cells either by ruminal microbes or by the host animal. Several enzymes are required for complete digestion of complex feeds such as hay or grain (McAllister *et al.,* 2001). The enzymes such as cellulases and xylanses have ability to degrade plant cell walls. (Morgavi *et al.,* 2000a; McAllister *et al.,* 2001). These preparations contain many enzymes, including secondary enzymes such as amylases, proteases or pectinases. The degradation of cellulose and hemicellulose alone requires several enzymes. Therefore the efficacy of enzyme preparation depends upon it's ability to degrade cell wall which may be affected by different proportion and activities of secondary enzymes . Use of combined form of cellulase and xylanase is much more effective than using cellulase alone. Even within a single microbial species, different type and activity of enzymes produced can vary a lot. Enzyme products for ruminants are standardised by the process of blending crude enzyme extracts to obtain specified levels of one or two enzyme activities (McAllister *et al.,* 2001). As there is difference in commercial preparations, the enzyme activity needs to be described when a study is done. Therefore information such as activity rates and enzyme types is to be provided by enzyme manufacturer (ZoBell *et al.,* 2000).

Factors Affecting use of Feed Enzymes

Matching of exogenous enzyme to the feed

For the effective use of feed enzyme specific target needs to be identified because all feed enzymes are not equally effective in digesting complex substrates of feed. Feed enzyme designated to improve the utilization of corn should contain proteases which can digest the protein matrix thereby exposing starch granules to be digested by endogenous ruminal enzyme. In case of straw silica, waxes and cutain are the major barriers for ruminal digestion (Bae et al 1997). In the feed where it is expected to digest the structural component of feed, use of such enzyme which will increase the rate of feed degradation in rumen. Thus the enzyme preparation should be commercially made available with clearly defining the different types and activities of enzyme they contain. Random use of enzyme in feed without consideration of specific substrate target may lead to discouraging results. However, multienzyme preparation can be a better option to overcome the constraints limiting the digestion of a particular type of feed.

Cost effectiveness

Once the specific targets for degradative exogenous enzymes have been identified, the efforts are required to optimize the application of enzyme preparations thereby ensuring that the preparations contain the enzyme activities most to improve feed utilization. In some instances, the activity of crude enzyme preparations may be increased by including specific enzymes most likely to overcome the limitation of feed digestion. Application of recombinant DNA technology has recently enabled manufacturers to increase the volume and efficiency of enzyme production, and to create new products (Ward and Conneely, 1993; Hodgson, 1994). Genes encoding superior enzymes can be transferred from organisms such as anaerobic bacteria and fungi which may impractical for commercial production, into well characterized industrial microbial production hosts (e.g., *Aspergillus* and *Bacillus* spp.). Expression of genes encoding novel enzymes in plants such as canola and potato may be a particularly effective means of lowering the cost of enzyme production (Pen *et al.*, 1993; Van Rooijen and Moloney, 1994).

Level of feed enzyme

Inconsistancies and variation of results associated with the use of exogenous feed enzyme in ruminant ration is due to supplementation with insufficient or excessive enzyme activity. Results of in vivo studies of enzyme addition are typically nonlinear (Beauchemin *et al.*, 1995; Kung *et al.*, 2000), and it is possible to over-supplement. Kung et al. (2000) when offered forage (60% corn silage and 40% lucerne hay; DM basis) treated with increasing levels (0, 1, 2.5 mL/kg of TMR) of an enzyme product to cows reported that low level of enzyme tended ($P < 0.10$) to produce more milk (39.5 kg/d) than those fed the control diet (37.0 kg/d) or those fed the high level of enzyme (36.2 kg/d). These studies demonstrated that low levels of enzyme addition can be more effective than high levels, and the optimal level of enzyme supplementation may depend on the diet. Low levels of enzyme addition may indicate an insufficient supply of enzyme activity. Moderate level of enzyme to ruminant feeds caused some beneficial disruption of the surface structure of the feed either before or after ingestion. When excess enzyme was applied, the beneficial disruption of the feed surface structure may have diminished because the excess exogenous enzyme attached to feed which may have restricted microbial attachment and thus limited digestion of feed (Nsereko *et al.* 2002).

Enzyme-Feed Specificity

Enzyme-feed specificity must be considered for preparation of new feed enzyme for ruminants. As ruminant ration contain different types of fodder and concentrates, in order to have maxiınum benefit, a number of different enzyme sources would need to be used in a typical ration. A middle approach is to use an enzyme that may not be the best on all forages, but is relatively suitable for most feeds. Such generalized approach has been taken for the most part in the development of enzyme products for ruminants.This approach has limited the rate of progress to some extent in terms of bringing effective products to the marketplace. On-farm efficacy of some products may not be same in all situations, contributing to the variability associated with enzyme technology. Because of the relatively high cost of feed enzymes compared to other technologies, livestock producers expect an equally high response in animal productivity. Future research needs a targeted approach where feed enzyme products are formulated for various types of feeds with cost effective approach.

Method of Application of Feed Enzyme

Addition of enzymes in feed

Kopecny et al. (1987) observed no effect on in vitro fibre digestion because cellulase enzyme was rapidly degraded by rumen bacterial proteases. Several studies have suggested that feeding unprotected enzymes may be more beneficial in pre ruminants where rumen microflora is not fully developed. Baran and Kmet (1987) reported that a pectinase-cellulase enzyme additive improved ruminal fermentation in newly weaned lambs but not in adult sheep (with established rumen microflora). Nevertheless recently, there has been renewed interest in the use of enzymes in ruminant diets because some fibrolytic enzymes have been shown to be stable when incubated with protease enzymes. In a study conducted by Hirstov et al. (1998) it was found that fibrolytic enzymes maintained partial activity when added to rumen. However for evaluating enzymes for ruminant diets, integrity of the enzyme is not the only criteria that should be considered as they are required to bind their substrate and catalyze reactions. Zinn and Salinas (1999) reported that a rumen-stable fibrolytic enzyme supplement increased the ruminal digestion of NDF and feed N by 23 and 5 percent respectively. They also reported an improvement in dry matter intake as well as average daily gain in steers supplemented with fibrolytic enzyme. These data suggest that adding enzymes directly (in a dry form) to the diets of ruminants may improve digestion and production.

Spraying of liquid feed enzymes

In the past use of enzymes was restricted to their application on to forages at the time of ensiling. However, this method of application had variable results. Treating feed with enzyme just before feeding is one of the method found to protect or minimize degradation of enzyme by ruminal protease. When exogenous enzymes are applied to feed in this way, binding with substrates causes structural changes which may help to protect these exogenous enzymes from ruminal degradation. Treacher and Hunt (1996) reported that spraying enzymes directly onto feeds, rather than adding at the time of ensiling, enhanced their nutritive values. This approach lead to many possibilities for using enzymes to improve nutrient digestion, utilization, and productivity in ruminants and at the same time reduce animal fecal material and pollution. Spraying enzymes onto feeds just before feeding provides increased management flexibility for feeding the animals and overcomes any negative interactions that the ensiling process may have on enzyme performance. There are number of different reasons for positive effects including, direct hydrolysis, improvements in palatability, changes in gut viscosity, complementary actions with ruminal enzymes, and changes in the site of digestion (Beauchemin and Rode, 1996). Feng et al. (1992) reported that in vitro ruminal fiber digestion was improved by pretreatment of dry grass with fibrolytic enzymes. Lewis et al. (1996) found that spraying of enzymes on grass hay:barley diet resulted in to increased VFA production and NDF digestion. In some instances, enzymes have been applied directly to the grain but in some studies enzymes were applied only to the forage component of the diets prior to mixing into a complete balanced ration. Several studies have reported that addition of high levels of enzymes in the diets resulted in lower milk yields than moderate levels of enzyme treatment (Lewis *et al,* 1999; Beauchemin *et al.*, 1995). Over-treatment of feeds with enzymes may result in blocking sites that may otherwise be available for microbial enzymatic digestion or may prevent attachment by rumen microbes. As far method of application of feed enzyme is concerned more research will be needed in this area.

When to add feed enzyme

Rode *et al.*, (1999) observed that addition of enzyme in the diet of ruminants had improved the performance of ruminants. Moreover; the performance of the animal was found to be greatest when the animal was in the state of negative energy balance. Beauchemin *et al.*, (2000) found that the cows in early lactation receiving supplementary diets with fibrolytic enzyme can enhance milk yield and nutrient digestibility. These results were in accordance with Schingoethe et al. (1999) who observed that cows started receiving the enzyme treated forage during the first 100 days postpartum produced 9 to 15% more milk than cows fed the control diet without fibrolytic enzyme. However, production was not increased when cows were in midlactation.

Responses of feed enzyme

The use of exogenous enzyme for ruminants was first examined in the 1960s, as reviewed by Beauchemin and Rode (1996). Many of these early enzyme products were not well characterized and responses of animals were variable. Due to higher feed costs, in the last decade, researchers have reexamined the potential use of exogenous enzymes for ruminants with better defined enzyme preparations.

Beef Cattle

Several recent studies have reported that the use of exogenous enzyme products in high-forage diets fed to growing cattle (Beauchemin *et al.*, 1995; McAllister *et al.*, 1999; Wang *et al.*, 1999; ZoBell *et al.*, 2000). It is well documented that adding fibrolytic enzymes in the forage based diets can improve fiber digestibility (Beauchemin *et al.*, 1995; Feng *et al.*, 1996), but improved performance of cattle due to increased digestibility of feed may depend on the physiological status of the cattle and the conditions of the experiment. The results of adding fibrolytic enzymes to high-grain diets have been surprisingly more consistent than those for high-forage diets. Addition of enzyme (Xylanase) to a 95% barley-based diet improved feed efficiency by 6 to 12 percent, depending upon the level of enzyme addition (Beauchemin *et al.*, 1997; 1999b; Iwaasa *et al.*, 1997). Increased diet digestibility resulted in to increased feed efficiency (Iwaasa *et al.*, 1997). Similar results were obtained by Krause et al. (1998) who reported a 28 percent increase in ADF digestibility using a similar enzyme product when added to a high-concentrate diet. McAllister et al. (1999) reported use of enzyme in forage (ryegrass silage; 30 percent of the diet) and grain (barley, 70 percent of the diet) based diet has resulted in increased ADG by 10 percent. However, ZoBell et al. (2000) observed no effect when the same enzyme product was added to a high-grain barley-based feedlot finishing diet containing 17 percent forage (DM basis).

Dairy Cattle

Several studies have examined the effects of exogenous enzymes on digestibility and milk production in dairy cows (Beauchemin et al 2000; Lewis *et al.*, 1999; Yang *et al.*, 2000; Kung *et al.*, 2000;Phipps *et al.*, 2000a,b; Bowman, 2001; Sutton *et al.*, 2001). In number of studies and several research documents it was found that the average increase in DMI was 1.0 ± 1.3 kg/d, and the average increase in milk yield was 1.1 ± 1.5 kg/d (3.4% ± 4.7). Thus, when viewed across a variety of enzyme products and experimental conditions, the response is positive, but the variability is also high. Lewis et al. (1999) who treated forage with a cellulase/xylanase mixture and observed that cows in early lactation produced 6.3 kg/d (16%) more milk . However, higher and lower levels of the same enzyme product were less effective. Rode et al. (1999) applied an enzyme product to the concentrate portion of a diet (supplying 1.3 g/kg of TMR on a DM basis) and observed a 3.6 kg/d increase in milk production for cows in early lactation . Yang et al. (2000) added an enzyme mixture to the concentrate, and observed that the cows in early lactation produced 2 kg/d (5.9%) more milk . However, there was no response when the same enzyme was added to the TMR.

Comparative depiction of various studies on effects of supplementing diets fed to cows in early lactation with an enzyme mixture is as below

	Lewis et al., 1999				Rode et al., 1999		Yang et al., 2000		
	Control	Low enzyme	Medium enzyme	High enzyme	Control	Enzyme in conc.	Control	Enzyme in conc.	Enzyme in TMR
DMI, kg/d	24.4^{b}	26.2^{a}	26.2^{a}	26.6^{a}	18.7	19.0	19.4	19.8	20.4
Milk production, kg/d	39.6^{b}	40.8^{b}	45.9^{a}	41.2^{b}	35.9^{f}	39.5^{g}	35.3^{b}	37.4^{a}	35.2^{b}
Milk composition, %									
Fat	3.99^{a}	3.83^{ab}	4.00^{a}	3.75^{b}	3.87^{a}	3.37^{b}	3.34	3.19	3.14
Protein	2.95^{a}	2.87^{b}	2.88^{b}	2.85^{b}	3.24	3.03	3.18	3.13	3.13
Lactose	4.89^{ab}	4.91^{ab}	4.92^{a}	4.81^{b}	4.73^{c}	4.62^{d}	4.65	4.65	4.56
BW change, kg/d	NA	NA	NA	NA	?0.63	?0.60	0.15	0.04	0.14
DM digestibility, %	NA	NA	NA	NA	61.7^{a}	69.1^{b}	63.9^{a}	66.6^{b}	65.7^{ab}
NDF digestibility, %	NA	NA	NA	NA	42.5^{a}	51.0^{b}	42.6		

^{a,b}Means within a study differ ($P < 0.05$).
^{c,d}Means within a study differ ($P < 0.10$).
^{f,g}Means within a study differ ($P = 0.11$).
^{z}Conc = concentrate, TMR = total mixed ration, NA = not available.

It is clear that exogenous enzymes can be effective for ruminants, but it is pretentious to determine all those variable conditions that are most likely to result in positive responses. Using feed enzymes to improve digestion would also reduce faecal material (Kung *et al.*, 2000) as well as supplementing enzyme activity in the faeces.

Commercially Available Feed Enzymes and their Regulatory Status

There are various enzyme formulations available in the market with varied activities. Although these products are standardized, the method of standardization will vary from producer to producer making comparison of different feed enzyme products. The different livestock owners have to look for quality parameters to judge the usage. The parameters would include the type of enzymes present, their activities, production methodology, product form and its free flowing nature for mixability. It is difficult to convert one unit into the other since each unit has its own defination. Because the enzymes used by the feed industry are produced by different microorganisms, the enzyme characteristics as well as the composition of enzymes would be different. However, comparison of enzyme products is difficult except by in vivo testing. Each microorganism produces enzymes with different optimum pH values, different optimum temperature of operation and different affinity for the substrate in feed. It has not yet been possible to develop an in-vitro method that can predict in-vivo performance. All enzyme feed additives are considered as feed additives and are under regulation by the FDA. As of January 1, 1998, the AAFCO Enzyme and Microbial Task Force that includes members of the AAFCO, FDA have put forth guidelines for the use of enzymes in animal feeds. Producers of enzymes must provide the source of the enzyme (organism) along with information on enzyme activity, substrates, reaction products and site of enzymatic activity. Products must also be safe relative to animal, human and environmental concerns. Functionality must be proven via in vitro tests. The therapeutic and production claims are not allowed.

Conclusion

Use of feed enzyme in ruminants depends on cost and the method of application. To have better effect of feed enzyme in ruminant ration various factors such as method of application of feed enzyme, amount of feed enzyme applied, physiological state of the animal etc. must be considered for economical viability of feed enzyme. As our livestock production system is based on usage of fodder and crop residue, lot more research needs to be done to arrive at a concrete conclusion for effective use of exogenous enzyme in ruminant ration. Before application of exogenous feed enzyme in the diet of ruminants as cost-effective tool, future research need must consider feeding and managemental practices which may affect the result.

References

Bae, H. D., McAllister, T. A., Kokko, E. G., Leggett, F. L, Yanke, L. J., Jakober, K. D., Ha, J. K., Shin, H. T. and Cheng, K.J. (1997). Effect of silica on the colonization of rice straw by ruminal bacteria. *Animal Feed Science and Technology* 65: 165-181.

Baran, M., and V. Kmet. (1987). Effect of pectinase on rumen fermentation in sheep and lambs. Arch. Anim. Nutr. Berlin. 7(8): 643.

Bowman, G.R., K.A. Beauchemin, and J.A. Shelford. (2002). The proportion of the diet to which fibrolytic enzymes are added affects nutrient digestion by lactating dairy cows. *J. Dairy Sci.* 85:3420-3429.

Bowman, G.R. (2001). Digestion, ruminal pH, salivation, and feeding behaviour of lactating dairy cows fed a diet supplemented with fibrolytic enzymes. M.S. Thesis, Univ. of British Colombia, Vancouver, Canada.

Beauchemin, K.A., L.M. Rode, M. Maekawa, D.P. Morgavi, and R. Kampen. (2000). Evaluation of a non-starch polysaccharidase feed enzyme in dairy cow diets. *J. Dairy Sci.* 83: 543–553.

Beauchemin, K.A., W.Z. Yang, and L.M. Rode. (1999b). Effects of grain source and enzyme additive on site and extent of nutrient digestion in dairy cows. *J. Dairy Sci.* 82: 378-390.

Beauchemin, K. A., Jones, S. D. M., Rode, L. M. and Sewalt, V. J. H. (1997). Effects of fibrolytic enzyme in corn or barley diets on performance and carcass characteristics of feedlot cattle. *Canadian Journal of Animal Science* 77: 645-653.

Beauchemin, K., A. and L.M. Rode. (1996). Use of feed enzymes in ruminant nutrition. Proc. of the Canadian Society of Animal Science Annual Meeting, Lethbridge, Alberta. Pp 103-140.

Beauchemin, K., A., L.M. Rode, and V.J.H. Sewalt. (1995). Fibrolytic enzymes increase fiber digestibility and growth rate of steers fed dry forages. *Can. J. Anim. Sci.* 75: 641-644.

Colombatto, D., F. L. Mould, M. K. Bhat & E. Owen, (2003). Use of fibrolytic enzymes to improve the nutritive value of ruminant diets: A biochemical and in vitro rumen degradation assessment. *Anim. Feed Sci. Technol.* 107: 201-209.

Cowan, W. D. (1994). Factors affecting the manufacture, distribution, application and overall quality of enzymes in poultry feeds. Pages 175–184 in Joint Proc. 2nd Int. Roundtable on Anim. Feed Biotechnol. – Probiotics, and Workshop on Anim. Feed Enzymes, Ottawa.

Feng, P., C. W. Hunt, G. T. Pritchard, and W. E. Julien. (1996). Effect of enzyme preparations on in situ and in vitro degradation and in vivo digestive characteristics of mature cool-season grass forage in beef steers. *J. Anim. Sci.* 74:1349–1357.

Feng, P., C. W. Hunt, W. E. Julien, K. Dickinson, and T. Moen. (1992). Effect of enzyme addition on in situ and in vitro degradation of mature cool-season grass forage. J. *Anim. Sci.* 70(Suppl. 1):309. (Abstract)

Hirstov, A., T. A. McAllister, and K. J. Cheng. (1998). Effect of dietary or abomasal supplementation of exogenous polysaccharide-degrading enzymes on rumen fermentation and nutrient digestibility. *J. Anim. Sci.* 76: 3146-3156.

Hodgson, J. (1994). The changing bulk biocatalyst market. *Bio/Technology* 12: 789-790.

Hoover, W.H., Kincaid, C.R., Varga, G.A., Thayne, W.V. and Junkins, L.L. Jr. (1984). Effects of solids and liquid flows of fermentation in continuous cultures. IV. pH and dilution rates. *Journal of Animal Science* 58: 692-699.

Iwaasa, A.D., L.M. Rode, K.A. Beauchemin, and S. Eivemark. (1997). Effect of fibrolytic enzymes in barley-based diets on performance of feedlot cattle and in vitro gas production. Joint Rowett Res. Inst. – Inst. Natl. de Recherche Agronomique Rumen Microbiol. Symp., Aberdeen, Scotland, Poster 39.

Kung, L., Jr., R.J. Treacher, GA Nauman, AM. Smagala, K.M. Endres and M.A. Cohen. (2000). The effect of treating forages with fibrolytic enzymes on its *nutritive value* and lactation performance of dairy cows. *J. Dairy Sci.* 83: 115-122.

Kopecny, J., Marounek, M. and Holub, K. (1987). Overenf vhodnosti aplikace celulaz *Trichoderma viride* do krmnych davek prezvykavcu. *Zivocisna vyroba*, 32: 587-592.

Krause, M., K. A. Beauchemin, L. M. Rode, B. I. Farr, and P. Nørgaard. (1998). Fibrolytic enzyme treatment of barley grain and source of forage in high-grain diets fed to growing cattle. *J. Anim. Sci.* 96:1010–1015.

Lewis, G.E., W.K. Sanchez, C.W. Hunt, M.A. Guy, G.T. Pritchard, B.I. Swanson and R.J. Treacher. (1999). Effect of direct-fed fibrolytic enzymes on the lactational performance of dairy cows. *J. Dairy Sci.* 82: 611-617.

Lewis, G.E., C.W. Hunt, W.K. Sanchez, R. Treacher, G.T. Pritchard and P. Feng. (1996). Effect of directfed fibrolytic enzymes on the *digestive* characteristics of a forage-based diet fed to beef steers. *J. Anim. Sci.* 74: 3020-3028.

McAllister, T.A., A.N. Hristov, K.A. Beauchemin, L.M Rode & K.J. Cheng. (2001). Enzymes in ruminant diets. In: Enzymes in farm animal nutrition. Eds. Bedford M.R. & G.G. Partridge. CAB Inter., pp. 273-298.

McAllister, T. A., S. J. Oosting, J. D. Popp, Z. Mir, L. J. Yanke, A. N. Hristov, R. J. Treacher, and K.J. Cheng. (1999). Effect of exogenous enzymes on digestibility of barley silage and growth performance of feedlot cattle. *Can. J. Anim. Sci.* 79: 353–360.

McAllister, T. A., Phillippe, R. C., Rode, L. M. and Cheng, K.J. (1993). Effect of the protein matrix on the digestion of cereal grains by ruminal microorganisms. *Journal of Animal Science* 71: 205-212.

Morgavi, D. P., K. A. Beauchemin, V. L. Nsereko, L. M. Rode, A. D. Iwaasa, W. Z. Yang, T. A. McAllister, and Y. Wang. (2000a). Synergy between ruminal fibrolytic enzymes and enzymes from *Trichoderma Longibrachiatum*. *J. Dairy Sci.* 83: 1310–1321.

Muirhead, S. (1996). *Direct Fed Microbial, Enzyme and Forage Additive Compendium*, 3rd edn. The Miller Publishing Company, Minetonka, Minnesota, 391 pp.

Nsereko, V.L., K.A. Beauchemin, D.P. Morgavi, L.M. Rode, AF. Furtado, T.A. McAllister, AD. Iwassa, W.z. Yang and Y. Wang. (2002). Effect of a fibrolytic enzyme preparation from Trichoderma longibrachiatum on the rumen microbial population of dairy cows. *Can. J. Microbiol.* 48: 14-20.

Pen, J., Verwoerd, T. C., van Paridon, P. A., Beudeker, R. F., van den Elzen, P. J. M., Geerse, K., van der Klis, J. D., Versteegh, H. A. J., van Ooyen, A. J. J. and Hoekema, A. (1993). Phytase-containing transgenic seeds as a novel feed additive for improved phosphorus utilization. *Bio/Technology* 11: 811-814.

Phipps, R. H., J. D. Sutton, D. E. Beever, M. K. Bhat, G. F. Hartnell, J. L. Vicini, and D. L. Hard. (2000a). Evaluation of feed additives in the diet of lactating dairy cows. *J. Dairy Sci.* 83(Suppl. 1):23. (Abstr.)

Phipps, R. H., J. D. Sutton, D. E. Beever, M. K. Bhat, G. F. Hartnell, J. Vicini, and D. L. Hard. (2000b). Effect of cell-wall degrading enzymes and method of application on feed intake and milk production of Holstein-Friesian dairy cows. *J. Dairy Sci.* 83(Suppl. 1):23. (Abstr.)

Rode, L. M., W. Z. Yang, and K. A Beauchemin. (1999). Fibrolytic enzyme supplements for dairy cows in early lactation. *J. Dairy Sci.* 82:2121–2126

Sutton, J.D., R.H. Phipps, D.E. Beever, D.J. Humphries, G.F. Hartnell, and J.L. Vicini. (2001). Comparison of different methods of administration on the effect of fibrolytic enzymes on digestive processes in lactating cows. *J. Dairy Sci.* 84(Suppl. 1):37. (Abstr.)

Treacher, R.J. and C.W. Hunt. (1996). Recent developments in feed enzymes for ruminants. Proc. Pacific Northwest Nutrition Conference. Seattle, WA.

Van Rooijen, G. J. H. and Moloney, M. M. (1994). Plant seed oil-bodies as carriers for foreign proteins. *Bio/Technology* 13: 72-77.

Wang, Y., T.A. McAllister, R.E. Wilde, J. Baah, K.A. Beauchemin, L.M. Rode, J.A. Shelford, and K.J. Cheng. (1999). Effects of monensin, exogenous fibrolytic enzymes and Tween 80 on performance of feedlot cattle. *Can J. Anim. Sci.* 79: 587. (Abstr.)

Ward, P. P. and Conneely, O. M. (1993). Using biotechnology to improve enzyme yields: From DNA to the marketplace. In: C. Wenk and M. Boessinger (eds.) *Enzymes in Animal Nutrition, Proceedings of the 1st Symposium*. Schriftenreihe aus dem Institut für Nutztierwissenschaften Gruppe Ernährung, Kartause Ittingen, Switzerland, pp. 16-21.

Yang, W.Z., K.A. Beauchemin, and L.M. Rode. (2000). A comparison of methods of adding fibrolytic enzymes to lactating cow diets. *J. Dairy Sci.* 83: 2512–2520.

ZoBell, D.R., R.D. Weidmeier, K.C. Olson, and R.J. Treacher. (2000). The effect of an exogenous enzyme treatment on production and carcass characteristics of growing and finishing steers. *Anim. Feed Sci. Technol.* 87: 279–285

Zinn, R.A. and J. Salinas (1999). Influence of fibrozyme on digestive function and growth performance of feed lot steers fed a 78% concentrate growing diet. Pages 313-319 in Proc.15th Annu.Symp.Nottingham University Press. Biotechnology in the feed industry T.P.Lyons and K. A. Jacques.ed.Loughborough Leics UK.

□□□

41

Nutrional Management of Sick Dog

S.P. TIWARI[1], TARINI SAHU, SURENDRA NAIK AND RANJAN GUPTA*

[1]Professor & Head, Department of Animal Nutrition, College of Veterinary Science and Animal Husbandry, Anjora, Durg - 491001 (C.G.)

*Principal Scientist, ICAR, Krishi Bhavan, New Delhi

Introduction

Dogs are the most liked pet animal mainly reared as the companion animals for combating against rising crimes, bomb threats and drug trafficking. Trained dogs are deployed at various vulnerable places along the international border for preventing trans-border crimes, parliament security and international airports. The Alsatians are multipurpose and are 'must' in infantry patrol. Police and Army maintain them for intelligence purposes. They are also good at sniffing out landmines and are trained to walk softly on suspected minefield. The Labrador and Cocker Spaniel are used as sniffing and are used as guide dogs. The Cocker Spaniel is preferred in sniffing operations inside aeroplanes and other cramped places. The Doberman is useful in tracking operations.

Modern day dog has turned into omnivorous with long association with man. Dog can survive on diets made entirely of animal or vegetable origin. Dogs have sharp strong teeth designed for tearing cutting and chewing meat. Dogs need a balance diet i.e. a diet which contains appropriate quantities of all essential nutrients, in addition to being palatable, digestible, safe and of suitable concentration to stay alive and healthy. If the dog will suffer from any illness the dog will need a daily nourishing ration to help him recover from a serious illness.

Special Diets or Modified Diets

Modification in the diet is necessary to feed the patient suffering from different diseases. This is necessary as the metabolism of the individual changing in different diseases with respect to one or more nutrients. For example, carbohydrate utilization is impaired in diabetes mellitus. Hence, (i) modification in the nutrient level (e.g. carbohydrate, fat, protein, vitamins and minerals etc.) is made and modified diets were formulated, (ii) the simplest modification of diets is done into treatment of allergies where the responsible foods are eliminated and (iii) modification in diet consistency is made to suit feeding of critically ill patients (liquid diets). The enteric and parenteral diets used are: (i) modifications in carbohydrate content: high carbohydrate diet is indicated in various liver diseases. Restricted carbohydrate diet is essential in the treatment of diabetes mellitus (ii) modifications in protein content: high protein diets with restriction in other nutrients are prescribed in a variety of diseases such as protein-calorie malnutrition, cirrhosis of liver etc. (iii) modifications in fat content: moderately high fat diet is used in the treatment of severe under nutrition, restricted or low fat may be necessary in the treatment of steatorrhoea and diseases of the liver (iv) modification in vitamin content: increase in the content of vitamins can be easily achieved by the addition of synthetic vitamins, this is essential as most of the therapeutic diets may be partially lacking in one or more vitamins and (v) modification in mineral content: high calcium diet is essential in the treatment of rickets and osteomalacia, while a diet restricted in calcium and phosphate is desirable in renal calculi. Sodium restricted diet is essential in the treatment of cardiac failure. Restriction in salt intake is essential in diseases of kidney (Reddy, 2004).

There are two types of diets; commercial and homemade. The commercial dog foods are of three types: dry, semi moist and canned foods (Purina, 2000).

Dry dog foods: Dry dog food contain moisture 10 to 12%, CP 18 to27%, fat 7 to 15% and carbohydrate 35 to 50%. These diets delivers ME 700-1000 Kcal/kg of the product. Ingredients usually present are cereal grains *e.g.* maize, wheat, oats, barley; cereal by products (e.g. wheat germ meal, maize gluten meal), soybean products (*e.g.* soybean meal, soy grits), animal products (e.g. meat meal, poultry by products), milk products (*e.g.* dried skim milk, dried whey), fats and oils (*e.g.* animal fat) and mineral and vitamin supplements.

Semi moist dog foods: Moisture 25 to 30%, CP 16-25%, fat 5-10% and carbohydrate 25-35%. These diets contain approximately 600-675 kcal ME/kg product. Ingredients usually added are animal products (*e.g.* meat, meat by-products), milk products (*e.g.* dried whey, cheese rind), fats and oils (*e.g.* animal fat), soybean products (*e.g.* soybean meal, soybean flour) and mineral and vitamin supplement.

Canned dog foods: Moisture 74 to 78%, CP 8-15%, fat 2-15%. Canned foods deliver 190-475 kcal ME/kg product. Canned foods commonly formulated to be nutritionally complete. These foods contain meat and/or meat by-products at varying levels. Low level meat based foods are similar in composition to dry foods to which water has been added prior to canning.

Comparison of Dog Food Types

Product characteristics	Dry Food	Semi moist Food	Canned Food
Cost	Low	moderate-high	High
Palatability	Moderate	moderate-high	High
Moisture content	12%	20-25%	74-78%
Metabolizable Kcal/kg	700-1000	600-675	190-475
Complete& Balanced	Yes	Yes	Yes

Recommended nutrient allowance for adult dog (NRC, 1985)

Nutrient	Allowance per 100 kg DM
ME(Kcal)	400
Protein (g)	22
Fat(g)	5.5
Linoleic acid(g)	1.1
Minerals	
Calcium(g)	1.1
Phosphorus(g)	0.9
Ca:P ratio	0.8-1.5:1
Potassium(g)	0.5
Sodium chloride(g)	0.6
Magnesium (mg)	40
Iron(mg)	8.0
Copper(mg)	0.7
Manganese(mg)	0.5
Zinc(mg)	5.0
Iodine(mg)	0.15
Selenium(μg)	10
Vitamins	
A(IU)	500
D(IU)	50
E(IU)	5
Thiamine(mg)	0.1
Riboflavin(mg)	0.25
Pantothenic acid(mg)	1.1
Niacin(mg)	1.2
Pyridoxine(mg)	0.12
Folic acid(mg)	2.2
Vitamin B 12(mg)	2.7
Choline(mg)	125

Signs of Illness: Dull or matted coat, skin itchy or sore, eyes cloudy, red or runny nose, bad breath, diarrhoea or foul smelly odd coloured stool, frequent urination, urinating in the house, vomiting, excessive drinking of water, cough, sneezing, fever, chills and sneezing, pain and fatty lumps.

Cardiac Disease

The goal of nutrition for dogs is to provide adequate calories, protein, fat, vitamins and minerals. Over the years, researchers have discovered that nutrition can play an important role in the management of diseases, including cardiac disease (Freeman, 2000). Most cardiac diseases lead to functional cardiac insufficiency. Causal correlation between nutrition and cardiac diseases are unknown in dogs but there are two reasons for dietetic measures: (i) intake of large amount of food can lead to excessive filling of the stomach and intestine. As a result the diaphragm is kept in a forward direction. Cardiac function, already impaired is further hampered mechanically and (ii) the kidney of animal with cardiac insufficiency tends to retain sodium and water. This give rise to clinical feature of ascites or dropsy. (Anderson, 1984).

Nutritional modulation of specific nutrients

The nutrients most commonly proposed for use in dogs with cardiac disease are:

1. Protein and amino acids

Protein: As early as the 1960s, the restricted protein intake for dogs with congestive heart failure to prevent 'metabolic stresses on the kidneys and liver (Pensinger, 1968) proposed. Unless severe renal dysfunction is present, high-quality protein should be fed to meet canine maintenance requirements (Anderson, 1984).

Taurine: Taurine is an amino acid that is found in high levels in the myocardium. The study showed that Cocker Spaniels supplemented with taurine and carnitine had improvement in clinical parameters and echocardiograph measurements (Bougehold, 1989).

Arginine: Unlike most other species, dogs require dietary arginine, since adequate amounts cannot be synthesised endogenously.

2. Fat

In the past, the major role of fat in diets has been to provide calories and to increase the palatability of diets. Plasma membranes normally contain very low concentrations of omega-3 PUFA, but levels can be increased by a food or supplement enriched in omega-3 PUFA. Dogs with CHF (Congestive Heart

Failure) have been shown to have plasma fatty acid abnormalities, including decreased concentrations of EPA and DHA compared to normal dogs. In one study of dogs with DCM (Dilated Cardiac Myopathy) and CHF, fish oil supplementation at a dose of 25 mg/kg EPA and 18 mg/kg DHA normalised these plasma fatty acid abnormalities (Freeman *et al.*, 1998).

3. Minerals

Sodium : Although healthy animals can easily excrete excess dietary sodium in the urine, this response is blunted in animals with cardiac disease (Boegehold and Kotchen, 1989). When CHF first arises, additional sodium restriction is recommended. This does not necessarily require a therapeutic diet, but it is important to examine each individual diet to make sure it meets this restriction. Diets designed for animals with renal disease are not recommended for most cardiac patients because of the protein restriction, unless severe renal dysfunction is present.

Sodium level in cardiac diet (Anderson, 1984)

Particulars	Na/Kg body weight (mg)	% Na in dry matter of food
Requirement of healthy animals	80	0.4
Recommended Na intake of patients with cardiac insufficiency	8-12	0.04-0.06
Average Na content of:	-	
meat and meat by products,		0.2
cereals		0.02
Diet consisting of:	-	
1/3 meat (30% dry matter),		0.03
2/3 cereals (90% dry matter)		0.017
Contains on average		0.05

Potassium: Furosemide use has been implicated in the development of hypokalaemia due to increased urinary loss of potassium. Hypokalaemia can contribute to arrhythmias directly and by potentiating the arrhythmogenic effects of digitalis toxicosis.

Magnesium: Like potassium, furosemide can cause hypomagnesaemia due to increased magnesium loss in the urine. Hypomagnesaemia can potentiate arrhythmias, decrease myocardial contractility and contribute to muscle weakness.

4. Vitamins

B vitamins: Thiamine deficiency is known to be a cause of cardiomyopathy in people, but there has been little investigation into the role of B vitamins as a cause of disease in dogs. Most commercial therapeutic diets designed for animals with cardiac disease contain increased levels of water soluble vitamins to offset urinary losses (Freeman, 2000).

5. Other nutrients

Carnitine: Carnitine deficiency is associated with primary myocardial disease in a number of dogs, including a family of Boxer dogs (Keene, 1992).

Coenzyme Q10: Coenzyme Q10, like carnitine, is a co-factor in a number of reactions required for energy production and is also a potent antioxidant.

Antioxidants: The major antioxidants include enzymatic antioxidants (e.g. superoxide dismutase, catalase, glutathione peroxidase) and oxidant quenchers (e.g. vitamin C, vitamin E, glutathione and beta-carotene (Freeman, 2000).

Liver Diseases

The liver is one of the largest organs of a dog's body and it plays a major role in the process of metabolism by removing blood toxins from the system. Due to certain reasons like viral or bacterial infections, food poisoning, metal poisoning, congenital abnormalities, and heredity issues, dogs may develop certain liver diseases. Several dog breeds on the other hand, like Doberman pinscher, Bedlington terrier, Miniature Schnauzer, West Highland White terrier, etc., are also at risk of liver diseases, since they are unable to digest certain minerals like copper. Excess hepatic copper has been found in dogs with normal liver histology, dogs with hepatitis, and dogs with end stage cirrhosis. Evidence is accumulating that copper is a cause of liver disease in breeds of dogs other than Bedlington terriers (Thornburg, 2000).

Nutritional Modulation of Specific Nutrients

There are four prime goals of a diet for dog liver disease. These goals include:

1. Proteins

Liver diseases in dogs hinder protein absorption. While a regular diet of a healthy dog should contain at least 25% of protein rich foods. Dog food for the dogs with liver disease should contain only 20% of proteins. While adding protein to the dog food, make sure that it is healthy and high quality protein with least amount of saturated fats and high amount of essential fatty acids like omega 3, for instance, soy protein isolates, dairy products and wheat gluten, you may retain around 30% to 50% of their regular calorie intake as well.

2. Fibres

Both soluble and insoluble fibres should be included in the diet of dog suffering from liver disease. Soluble fibres help in absorption of ammonia and promote the growth of beneficial bacteria that quickens the process of liver cell regeneration. Insoluble fibres, on the other hand, assist the dog's digestive health and prevent issues like constipation; they also bind toxins and promote their removal. Healthy sources of fibres like beets, various vegetables and fruits should be included in the diet while preparing the dog food. Along with fibres, indigestible carbs should also be included.

3. Minerals

While making proper dietary adjustments for the liver disease in dog, one needs to make sure that certain minerals like potassium, sodium and copper are not included in higher amounts. Experts suggest that potassium food sources should be completely avoided. The amount of sodium should also be restricted, especially when the dog is obese or has hypertension. The intake of copper should be restricted amongst the dog breeds. These breeds are likely to develop liver disease due to lack of copper.

4. Vitamins

Including healthy amounts of antioxidants is a must, while planning a diet for dogs with liver diseases. Antioxidants are gained from various vitamins like vitamin A, B complex, C, D, E, K, etc., that are present in fresh vegetables, meat dairy products and fish, and certain herbs like milk thistle.

Best dog food for liver disease: One can either follow healthy food recipe at home or choose certain healthy dog food brand upon confirmation with the veterinarian.

Recipe

Ingredients

- Chicken breast, ¼ cup
- Rice, 3½ cups
- Carrots, 1 cup
- Wheat bran, ½ cup
- Canola oil, 1½ tbsp
- Water, 5 cups

Procedure

Heat up oil in a pan and add chicken breast, wheat bran, rice and carrots to it. Stir well and add 2 cups of water to the mixture. Cover up the pan and let the mixture cook for about 20 minutes. Keep stirring the ingredients occasionally. Check whether the chicken and rice is cooked well and remove the pan from heat. Let the food cool, before serving it to the dog.

Diabetes Mellitus

What is Diabetes in Dogs?

The trigger for the condition of diabetes (also called Diabetes Mellitus) is insulin or the production of it. Insulin controls glucose by preventing extra production from liver and ensuring that excess and unneeded glucose derived from food is put into body stores. In the diabetic dog there is not enough insulin to switch off glucose production by the liver or to efficiently store derived from energy giving foods. The concentration of glucose in the blood then rises. If it goes too high, it is leaked into the urine and expelled from the body. Undetected and untreated diabetes can lead to greater urinary tract infections and cataract.

Nutritional Modulation of Specific Nutrients

The major change you will have to make is to avoid giving the diabetic dog food with sugar and carbohydrates. However, many commercial dog foods contain high amounts of carbohydrates. Carbohydrates are considered a sugar because the body converts it into glucose. When blood sugar level too low, it results in hypoglycaemia, which is a serious condition. Hypoglycaemia happens when blood glucose or blood sugar falls too low, quickly. A diet of strictly dry food is the biggest culprit, but soft-moist dog food can be high in carbs too.

1. Complex carbohydrates

Studies in diabetic dogs indicate that high-fibre diets may also be associated with improved glycaemia control. When comparison was made following long-term feeding of high soluble- fibre diets and high-insoluble-fibre diets for one or two months (Nelson *et al.*, 1991).), a tendency for improved glycaemia control and fewer side effects was seen with the diets containing increased insoluble fibre. Importantly, there seems to be marked variation between the responses of individual diabetic dogs to dietary fibre. In one study (Nelson *et al.*, 1998), significant improvement of all indices of glycaemia control, including lowered daily insulin requirement, was seen in nine of 11 dogs when they were fed a high-fibre diet. The remaining two dogs were found to have improved glycaemia control on the low-fibre diet.

2. Fat

Altered lipid metabolism occurs in dogs with insulin deficiency. Atherosclerosis and arterial disease are not clinical concerns in diabetic dogs. However, it has been known for some time that a large proportion of diabetic dogs have exocrine pancreatic disease (Ling *et al.*, 1977). High-fat diets and hypertriglyceridaemia have been proposed as possible inciting causes of canine pancreatitis (Williams, 1994) and low-fat diets are recommended for dogs with chronic pancreatitis and exocrine pancreatic insufficiency.

3. Protein

The protein composition of the recommended diet for dogs with diabetes is the same as that recommended for the non-diabetic population. However, if microalbuminuria or persistent proteinuria develops, then protein restriction may help slow the progression of diabetic nephropathy in these cases (Karamanos, 1998).

Good foods for diabetic dogs

There are two main choices when developing a diabetic diet, natural foods prepared for the dog or commercial diabetic dog food.

A Natural Diet-A natural diet of homemade and raw foods does not mean table scraps. A natural diet is planned and on purpose and consists of largely unprocessed foods (raw chicken, rice, carrots, etc) that are prepared for the dog. A raw diet is made up of foods that are not cooked.

Some foods included in a homemade diabetic diet would be:

- *Low fat meats:* Choose high-quality meats with little fat like chicken, turkey, fish and eggs.
- *A few fresh vegetables and raw fruits*: Fresh veggies and fruits in moderation (but never grapes or raisins) are high in nutrients and vitamins, and have natural sugars, which are not bad for diabetics like processed and refined sugars are.
- *Some grains*: Certain grains like oats, brown rice and millet are beneficial for diabetic dogs. Used sparingly, these provide fibre which helps control insulin levels.
- *Possibly extra vitamins or minerals*: Vitamin E, for instance, aids in reducing the requirement for insulin.

Foods that should be avoided include

- *Sugar*: Do not feed the food that has sugar in it. Be sure to check that sugar or its other forms (sucrose, fructose, syrup, *etc.*) is not on the list of ingredients.

- *Baked goods*: Eliminate this from dog's diet, including most dog biscuits.
- *Most fats or fatty meat*: Meats with highly saturated fats like beef, ground beef, and pork should not be given. Generally, dog should not be given any foods that have been prepared in fats. A touch of fat is healthy and is already found naturally in meat.
- *An all meat diet*: Over time, this type of diet is harmful because of mineral and other imbalances. Dogs need balance found in grains and vegetables as well.
- *Most dry dog foods*: Most dry dog foods are mainly made up of simple carbohydrates. However, dry diabetic dog foods are generally safe, but still want make sure it is high in protein and vegetables.

Commercial Diabetic Dog Food

While there are some brands of dog food specifically for diabetic dogs, there are not many. Typically veterinarian's advice dog owners to look at 'natural' commercial dog foods (made with natural ingredients) or low-calorie, low-fat food designed to promote weight loss.

Some more popular brands include

- Purina Veterinary Diets DCO (Diabetes) Dog Food
- Solid Gold Natur-Bone (Diabetic Dogs)
- Newman's Own Advanced Dog Food (natural)
- Hills Science Diet (natural)
- Organix Dog Food (natural)

Homemade Diabetic Dog Foods

A diet of homemade natural food can be very beneficial for your dog especially when you are managing a condition like diabetes where nutrition is crucial. When preparing your diabetic dog's food, it is crucial that the diet contains a protein source, a complex carbohydrate source, sufficient vitamins and minerals, and some fat. The guidelines for feeding times and meal size still apply for feeding a diabetic homemade dog food.

Many owners find a balance in good nutrition and time spent cooking by giving their dogs a combination of home-prepared and commercial dog food. Just as with people, a dog with diabetes can have a high quality of life with a balanced lifestyle that includes a good diet of specially formulated diabetic dog foods, medication if necessary and regular exercise.

Chronic Renal Failure

The major principle of dietary management in chronic renal failure is to minimize the build up protein catabolites by restricting dietary protein intake to the animal requirement and providing energy from the nonprotein sources, thus preventing mobilization of animal own tissues (Markwell,1988).

Nutritional Modulation of Specific Nutrients

Provide moderate to high amounts of fat, moderate amount of high quality protein, low phosphorus and lots of fresh, clean, filtered water, juices.

Calories

(i) 1/3 Fat

Start with small amounts and gradually increase, watching for digestive upset + decreasing amount if diarrhoea occurs.

(ii) 1/3 Protein

High quality protein is key, daily protein requirement increases for dogs in CRF. As long as phosphorus is kept low and shouldn't worry about feeding too much protein.

(iii) 1/3 Carbs

While dogs don't have a nutritional need for carbs, may need to feed up to 50% carbs to keep phosphorus low.

Homemade Diet

1. Fat

Meats: Use high fat meat: lamb is very high in fat, pork, dark meat chicken + turkey have more fat than white meat but poultry is still a low-fat meat so leaving skin on is preferable. Beef has less phosphorus than chicken, lamb and turkey are in between.

Eggs: Yolks are high in fat but also high in phosphorus so feed in moderation.

Dairy: Whole-milk yogurt, cottage cheese, ricotta etc. Use dairy products with the most fat when fed but feed in moderation because they are high in phosphorus.

Oils: Coconut oil, fish (body) oil like Salmon oil or EPA oil. Do not use cod liver oil (too high in vitamin D, tough for failing kidneys to process), or polyunsaturated vegetable oils (high in omega-6 fatty acids causing inflammatory reaction, it is harmful for dogs with kidney disease and also not a good source of nutrition like canola oil.

2. Protein

Feed high quality, low phosphorus sources of protein.

Eggs – Having high quality protein but yolks are rich in phosphorus. Cooking egg whites increase their bioavailability.

Meat – Raw or lightly cooked meat is a source of high quality protein.

Various recommendations have been made about the amount of protein that should be offered, from 0.66g/kg body weight/day (Bovee, 1977) to 2.0-2.2g/kg bodyweight/day (Polzin *et al.*, 1981).

3. Low phosphorus

The dog should be fed with low phosphorus not more than ~4.55mg/kg body weight during the advanced kidney failure.

4.55 kg dog: 68-182 mg (up to 272 mg in very early stages)

11.35 kg dog: 170-455 mg (up to 682 mg in very early stages)

22.7 kg dog: 340-900 mg (up to 1364 mg in very early stages)

34 kg dog: 511-1364 mg (up to 2045 in very early stages)

22.72 kg dog: 680-1818 mg (up to 2727 in very early stages)

Foods highest in phosphorus include bones, dairy products, fish (with bones), organ meats, and egg shell. Calcium carbonate as a source of Ca (@100mg/kg bodyweight/day) should be added in the diet of CRF affected dogs and in no case bone meal should be fortified.

Sodium supplementation has been recommended, primarily to compensate for obligatory sodium loss occurring through damaged nephrons. In addition to this, decreased sodium intake may lead to a reduction in the ability to reabsorb bicarbonate (Schmidt and Gavellas, 1977). The following nutrient should be acceptable in the diet of dog during CRF:

Acceptable in large amounts

- Egg Whites, sweet potatoes, cereals like cream of wheat, cream of rice, glutinous rice (sticky), barley, white bread.
- Grains should be cooked and boiling veggies may reduce their phosphorus levels.

Acceptable in moderate amounts

- Higher fat meats (see meats), 20% fat ground beef, pork, lamb +liverwurst, green tripe.

- Winter squash (acorn or butternut), whole grains like brown rice, millet + whole wheat bread.

Acceptable in small amounts only

- *Low-fat meats* (have more phosphorus), turkey, lean beef or skinless chicken breast, organ meats (beef heart, chicken liver, beef liver/kidney), canned fish
- *High phosphorus grains like oatmeal;* dairy products-cottage cheese, whole milk, yogurt, cheddar cheese or whole eggs yolks.

Carbs: Adds calories, it can keep phosphorus levels low.

- *Veggies:* Cooking leaches out phosphorus, potassium and magnesium so vegetables be cooked in without adding water from outside. Boiling does also destroy vitamins, but steaming or boiling removes more phosphorus than baking.

Note: Celery (high sodium), parsley + dandelion greens are diuretics and these may not be good choices for kidney failure patients.

Note: Arthritic dogs should avoid white potatoes, tomatoes, eggplant and peppers

Note: Cabbage is good for ulcers, common in kidney disease.

Some veggie ideas with phosphorus amounts: Asparagus, beets, carrots, cauliflower, celery, dandelion greens.

- *Fruits*: Do not need to be cooked or pureed, they are digestible as is, but note that too much fruit may lead to loose stools.

Colored fruits like papaya + mango are good for dogs with arthritis.

Bananas + pumpkin are high in potassium.

Avoid grapes + raisins which have been linked to kidney failure in some dogs.

- *Grains :* If you do feed grains stick to those low in phosphorus. White rice is lower in phosphorus than brown rice and cream of wheat, cream of rice are low phosphorus alternatives.

Other Restrictions

- *Individual :* If dog has high potassium levels (as seen with advanced kidney disease), try to limit it in their diet, this includes food like: bananas, pumpkin, potatoes, pears, sardines, yogurt, carrots are all high in potassium.

- If potassium levels are low, you will need to supplement diet with potassium salts.
- If dog has high blood pressure limit the amount of sodium in their diet.

Supplement recommended

- Salmon oil- up to 1 gram / 10lbs of body weight daily
- Coenzyme Q10- 15mg/ 10lbs body weight, 3x daily
- Vitamin E- 50 IU daily/ 25 lbs of body weight.
- Vitamin B-complex
- Moderate amounts of vitamin C- 500mg/50lb. Dog
  (Don't use multivitamin/mineral products with phosphorus or vitamin D).

Gastro-Enteric Diseases

This can be arise from many causes including bacteria, viruses, parasites, toxins, dietary factors, neoplasia and a variety of specific conditions such as exocrine pancreatic insufficiency and lactase deficiency (Markwell, 1988). A dietary manipulation is important as primary or supportive treatments in most gastric diseases.

Nutritional Modulation of Specific Nutrients

1. Energy

Chronic gastric diseases associated with chronic vomiting and/or protein-losing gastropathy will predispose to the development of protein-calorie malnutrition. It is therefore important to feed a high energy diet to enable sufficient calorie intake to maintain lean body mass and allow gastric healing.

2. Protein

Protein induces gastric acid secretion by inducing the release of the hormone gastrin from the gastric antrum and duodenum. Reducing dietary protein in the short term may therefore help dogs with gastritis and gastric ulceration, as it will reduce gastric acid secretion. Furthermore, protein is very important for palatability and provides an additional source of calories when feeding a fat-restricted diet. In acute gastritis, a highly digestible, high quality protein should be fed.

3. Fat

High-fat foods delay gastric emptying and thus increase acid secretion via an indirect increase in gastrin secretion. Fat also reduces gastroesophageal sphincter tone and therefore encourages gastroesophageal reflux. Low-fat foods are therefore generally indicated in gastric disease, as they help to reduce acid secretion in gastritis and gastric ulceration, and hasten gastric emptying in functional delayed gastric emptying (pylorospasm). A low-fat diet is also indicated in dogs with concurrent enteritis or pancreatic disease because fat maldigestion and malabsorption is common in these conditions.

4. Carbohydrate and Fibre

Carbohydrate provides the main source of calories in most gastric diseases in which a low-fat diet is indicated. Carbohydrates should therefore be highly digestible and readily available.

Fibres have varying effects on gastric emptying depending on the type:

(i) Soluble fibre delays gastric emptying, thus increasing acid secretion; it is therefore contraindicated in gastritis and most gastric diseases.

(ii) Insoluble fibre may, however, actually speed gastric emptying and have a helpful buffering action while in the stomach; however, more work is necessary to assess its benefits before its use can be generally recommended.

5. Vitamins and Minerals

There are no vitamin requirements specific to gastric disease, but adequate amounts and a good balance of essential vitamins should be included in long-term diets for gastric disease. The most important mineral to consider in gastric disease is potassium, as chronic vomiting often results in hypokalemia. This is particularly seen with concurrent anorexia. Dietary supplementation with potassium may therefore be necessary after checking the patient's potassium status.

Rickets (Osteomalacia)

Rickets is an ailment that occurs in dogs when they are not receiving the correct allocation of nutrients, such as vitamins D, calcium and phosphorus. The major abnormality present is failure of normal mineralization of osteoid and in the young animal of the cartilaginous matrix in the epiphyseal growth plates (Campbell and Griffith, 1984).This is most typically caused by the excessive intake of meat. Left untreated, rickets can result in skeletal abnormalities, such as bowed legs, pelvic deformities and spinal curvature. This disease can be treated by providing correct amount of vitamin D, calcium and phosphorus.

Vomiting

Vomiting is caused by inflammation of the stomach (gastritis), and often happens when dogs eat grass or spoiled food. Uncomplicated gastritis, where the dog is fairly alert and has little or no fever is best treated without drugs. If vomiting continues for more than 24 hours or if at any time dog acts depressed and unresponsive, then follow these steps:

Step 1 Allow no food or water until your dog has gone for at least six hours without vomiting. The digestive tract needs complete rest.

Step 2 Begin giving very small amounts of water at frequent intervals. If there is more vomiting, go back to stage 1 for another six hours. Offer water every 15 minutes or so. Give a

Poodle sized dog one teaspoonful at a time, a German shepherd about two tablespoonfuls. Over a period of several hours, gradually increase the amounts offered, until your dog's thirst is satisfied. After at least 24 hours, you may begin offering small amounts of food.

Step 3 Begin offering small amounts of bland, easy to digest food. Give a poodle-sized dog about one half teaspoonful at a time. A large dog can have as much as a tablespoonful. Over a period of twenty four hours, gradually increase the amounts being fed until your dog's hunger is satisfied.

Step 4 The following day, begin mixing the bland diet half and half with your dog's normal food. Instead of one or two big feedings, divide your dog's normal amount of food into four or five small feedings.

Diarrhoea

Diarrhoea is caused by inflammation of the intestine (enteritis). It may happen at the same time as vomiting, (gastroenteritis) or all by itself. The diet should contain low fibre cereals, low protein and easily digestible protein foods like curd, egg. Oral rehydration therapy is important. The following liquid may be useful to feed (Reddy, 2004).

Urolithiasis / Urinary Stones

Although a number of different types of urolith have been reported in dogs, including those associated with drugs and toxins such as sulphonamides, struvite (magnesium ammonium phosphate hexahydrate) accounts for approximately 40 per cent of canine urolithiasis cases and can be successfully treated with diet alone. Diet is also a central component in the treatment and management of calcium oxalate, urate and cystine uroliths, as well as playing a key role in preventing or reducing the risk of recurrence of virtually all types of urolith encountered (Sturgess, 2009).

Food Ingredients	Quantity
Cooked rice gruel (100g DM)	500ml
Sugar	60g
Cheese (50g DM)	200g
Cream (30gDM)	100g
Maize oil or Safflower oil	15g
Hard cooked egg	100g
Dicalcium phosphate	10g
Potassium chloride	15g
Mineral-Vitamin supplement	as per dose

Note: Above diet should be fed@100ml/kg body weight.

Veterinarian may advise you to have less oxalate (a salt in some foods that binds calcium), regular salt, or animal protein (such as beef or pork), also composed of magnesium ammonium phosphate (struvite) or calcium oxalate. The relative proportion of these two types of urolith has varied between different countries and over time but they account for more than 80% of all canine uroliths (Osborne *et al.,* 2008).

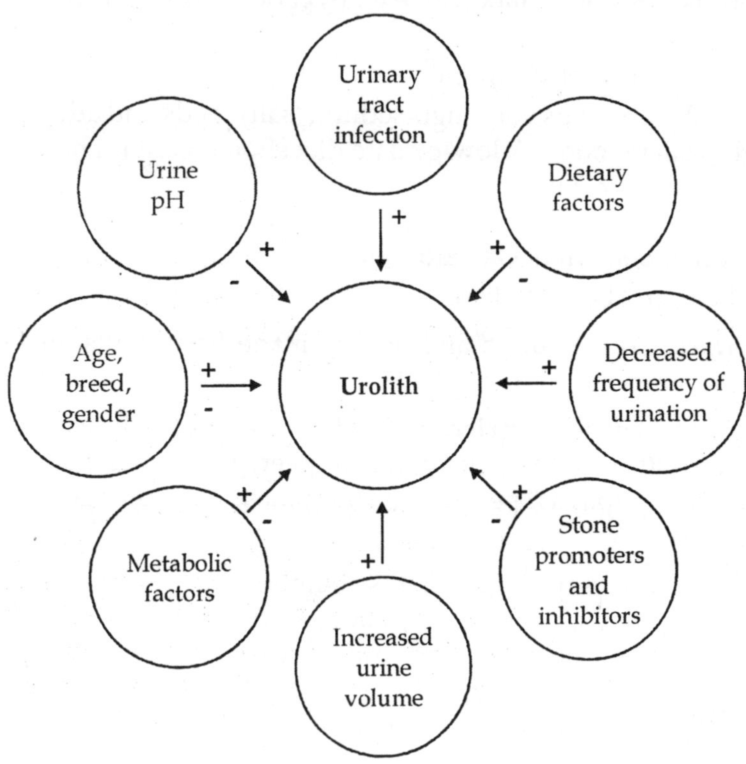

Various factors affect the risk of urolithiasis

Certain risk factors are well characterised for canine struvite urolithiasis. Some of these may be inter-linked, but struvite uroliths occur more commonly (Osborne *et al.*, 2008) in the following category of dogs:

- Middle-age adult dogs - Most commonly between 2-9 years of age (average ~6yrs).
- Certain breeds - e.g., Miniature Schnauzer, Welsh Corgi, Dachshund, Miniature Poodle, Cocker Spaniel, Lhasa Apso and Labradors.
- Alkaline urine - As struvite is very much less soluble in alkaline urine.
- Female dogs - Approximately 70-90% of struvite uroliths occur in females.
- Dogs with urinary tract infections -70% or more of all canine struvite uroliths are associated with a urease producing urinary tract infection. The most common bacteria are *Staphylococcus spp*, *Proteus spp*. and occasionally *Klebsiella spp* or *Pseudomonas spp*. Hydrolysis of urea by urease liberates NH_3 that is a component of struvite (increasing urine saturation) and also raises urine pH (decreasing struvite solubility).
- Abnormalities of metabolism e.g., hyperadrenocorticism.

Nutritional Modulation of Specific Nutrients

This meal plan limits very high-sodium (salt) foods and added salt. It also limits high-oxalate foods. A low-oxalate diet should contain no more than 40 to 50 mg oxalate per day.

1. Foods Low in Sodium or Oxalate

- Food Group Food Choices
  - *Drinks*: Coffee, juices and nectars made from fruits and vegetables recommended in this table.
  - *Fruits*: Apples, apricots (fresh or canned), avocado, bananas, cherries(sweet), grapefruit, red or green grapes, lemon and lime juice, melons, papayas, peaches, pears, pineapples, oranges, strawberries (fresh).
  - *Vegetables*: Asparagus stalks, bamboo shoots, broccoli, cabbage, cauliflower, chicory, corn, cucumbers, endive, kale, lettuce, lima beans, mushrooms, onions, peas, peppers, potatoes, radishes.
  - *Breads, cereals, and grains*: Egg noodles, rye bread, cooked and dry cereals without nuts or

- *Meat/meat replacement$, fish, poultry*: Meat, fish, fresh or frozen poultry (such as chicken or turkey),eggs, egg whites, egg replacements
- *Milk and milk products*: Cottage cheese, ricotta cheese, milk, yogurt.
- *Soup*: Homemade soup made with types vegetables and meats listed in this table.
- *Dessert/sweets*: Cookies, cakes, ice cream, pudding without chocolate or nuts.
- *Fats and oils*: Butter, margarine, cream, oil.
- *Other foods* :Unsalted potato chips, herbs such as garlic, garlic Powder, and onion powder; lemon juice, vinegar

2. Moderate-Oxalate Foods

❑ Food Group Food Choices

- *Drinks*: Fruit and vegetable juices made from fruits and vegetables in this table, rice milk, hot cocoa, tea
- *Fruits*: Blackberries, blueberries, black currants, cherries (sour), fruit cocktail, mangoes, orange peel, prunes, purple plums
- *Vegetables*: Baked beans, carrots, celery, green beans, parsnips, tomatoes, turnips
- *Breads, cereals, and grains* : White bread, cornbread/corn meal , oatmeal
- *Meat/meat replacements, fish, poultry*: Sardines
- *Dessert/sweets*: Chocolate cake
- *Fats and oils*: Macadamia nuts, pistachio nuts, English walnuts

3. Foods Not Recommended High-Oxalate Foods

❑ Food Group Food Choices

- Drinks Chocolate drink mixes, soy milk, instant iced tea, fruit
- Juices of fruits listed in this table
- Fruits Apricots (dried), red currants, figs, kiwi, plums, rhubarb
- Vegetables Beans (wax, dried), beets and beet greens, dark greens of all kinds, kale, okra, tomato paste
- Breads, cereals, and grain Amaranth, barley, white corn flour, fried potatoes, fruitcake, grits,
- Soybean products, sweet potatoes, wheat germ and bran

- Meat/meatreplacements,fish, poultry
- Dried beans, peanut butter, soy burgers
- Dessert/sweets Carob, chocolate
- Fats and oils Nuts (peanuts, almonds, , cashews), nut butters, sesame seeds
- Other foods Poppy seeds

4. High-Sodium Foods

If you eat too much sodium (salt), you may increase the calcium in your urine. That may cause calcium stones to form. Avoid the following foods:

- Salt, salt seasonings, and monosodium glutamate (a seasoning salt added to foods)
- Soy sauce
- Salted crackers and snack foods
- Vegetables prepared in brine (such as pickles, sauerkraut)
- Cured and processed meats (such as cold cuts, smoked fish)

Approximate Nutrition Analysis

Calories: 1,918; Protein: 89g (19% of calories); Carbohydrate: 264g (55% of calories); Fat: 57g (27% of calories); Cholesterol: 357mg; Sodium: 2,542mg; Fibres: 16g.

Dermatosis

Although cutaneous manifestations of nutritional deficiencies of various kinds are well documented in dogs, it is rare to find simple nutritional deficiencies as cause of skin disorders in dogs in clinical practice. Consequently few cases of alopecia, dermstosis, excessive hair shedding and pigmented defects can be cured by nutritional therapy alone.

Nutrition Modulation of Specific Nutrients

1. Energy and Protein

Dogs are rarely fed diets deficient in energy and protein by intention. However, disease causing decreased food consumption or malassimilation of nutrients may induce kwashiorkor-and marasmus-like conditions with effects on coat and skin. By feeding highly palatable and digestible diets, treatment of such diseases are supported (Anderson, 1984).

2. Fat

Cutaneous manifestations of fat deficient diets are documented in young puppies (Hansen and Wiese, 1943). The symptoms of a deficiency of unsaturated fatty acids are quits non- specific. It produces dry hair and dry scaly skin.

3. Minerals

Severe deficiencies of sodium chloride, iodine, magnesium or zinc may, among other symptoms, also affect coat and skin but simple nutritional deficiencies are rare under normal circumstances. The conditions are mostly seen as multiple deficiencies with emaciation for other reasons or with heavily unbalanced diets (Anderson, 1984).

4. Vitamins

Hypervitaminosis A and D may occur by accidental or intentional over supplementation with synthetic products as well as natural sources. Hypervitaminosis A is described to cause pruritus and dry skin with rashes and Hypervitaminosis D to make skin and hair dry and brittle (Mosier, 1978). Deficiency of water-soluble vitamins is unlikely to occur when dogs are fed conventional diets. Most ingredients commonly fed to dogs are good sources of these vitamins and dogs do not have any need for dietary sources of vitamin C. Excessive feeding of meat from certain fishes and raw egg whites will result in deficiencies of thiamine and biotin respectively.

Nutritional Therapy in Canine Dermatology

Good nutritional therapy in canine dermatology means optimal nutrition rather than excessive supplementation of any single nutrient. The most appropriate kind of nutritional therapy is to check the diet for nutritional adequacy and if necessary change it. Indications for parental administration of nutrient are extremely rare. Dietary supplementation as well as parental administration of nutrients will only work when diet lacking a nutrient supplied by the product, have been fed for a long time. Local as well as systemic administration of vitamin A has been tried on almost all disorders of keratinisation but topical irritation and systemic toxicity limits its use (Anderson, 1984).

Zinc Responsive Dermatosis

Zinc responsive dermatosis has quite recently been highlighted in the veterinary literature (Kunkle, 1980). Zinc Deficiencies are believed to commonly affect huskies and northern breeds of dog partly because they evolved to survive on diets containing lots of fish and sea-creatures. The flesh of these animals would have been particularly high in naturally digestible forms of zinc (and also vitamin A which is important for zinc absorption). Often the diets we feed or huskies and sled dogs do not provide enough zinc, or provide it forms that are difficult to digest.

Sled dogs are most likely to be affected by zinc deficiencies during times of stress, hormonal changes such as puberty, or for females, seasons or pregnancy. Zinc deficiency manifests as 'zinc responsive dermatosis' (ZRD) in many dogs. This is a skin condition that primarily affects areas of the face and head, particularly the muzzle, ears and around the eyes where hair-loss occurs and red, scaly patches of skin develop, 50mg of Zinc/Kg diet on dry matter basis is recommended by NRC but even that Zinc level could be considered marginal at high levels of calcium, copper and cobalt, diet s rich in phytates such as soybean meal, high in dietary fibre or low in protein (Sandstead, 1981).

Stress

Stress is a part and parcel of our daily lives, and so it is for our pets. Pets are extremely sensitive to their surroundings and are known to develop emotional bonding with their owners, environment as well as fellow pets. Any change in the environment triggers stress in pets and are also responsible immunity and ill health.

Common stress conditions in dogs

1. *Separations stress-* When the pet is separated from its parents, owners or environment it induces a serious stress.
2. *Climatic stress-* The change in climate induces stress in pets. During the times of changing weather stress is higher compared to extremes of constant temperature.
3. *Confinement stress-* If confined to or tied up the stress is more compared to a freely moving pet.
4. *Change of ownership-* The pet is attached to its owners and in case of ownership change stress sets in.
5. *Emotional stress-* If due to any reason the pet is not given enough attention, stress builds in.
6. *Disease stress-* When diseased the pet is low in energy and mentally depressed that serves as a cause of great stress.
7. *Performance stress-* If the pet is overworked because of any reasons (presentation is shows, training etc) it results in stress.

8. *Travelling stress*- If travelled for long distances in car, flight or any other vehicle stress can trigger.

Tips to Keep Pets Stress Free

- Provide personal care and company to the pet at home.
- Provide regular exercise and find time to play with the pet.
- Don't use corrective measures such as yelling and hitting since they only increase anxiety in pets.
- Don't let the pet 'lounge' around. Be sure to provide enough stimuli to pets by playing and petting them.
- Contrary to popular belief, getting another pet, as company for lonely pet, does not necessarily alleviate boredom.

If the dog is exhibiting behaviour that is anxiety, help from a qualified professional is to be sought as soon as possible.

Several antistress medications are useful since either they work as adaptogenic, mood modifier or reduce the effect of the catabolic activity caused due to stress. Behaviour therapy in conjunction with medication can alleviate stress in pets (Agarwal, 2010).

References

Agarwal, M. (2010). Stress and its management in pets. *Pet Health Bulletin.* 1 (3).

Anderson, R.S. (1984). In: Nutrition and Behaviour in Dogs and Cats.1st Ed.Pergamon Press

Boegehold, M. A., Kotchen, T. A. (1989). Relative contributions of dietary Na+ and Cl- to salt-sensitive hypertension. *Hypertension.* 14: 579–583.

Bovee, K.C. (1977). Diet and Kidney Failure. In The Kal Kan Symposium for the Treatment of Dog and Cat Disease. Kal Kan Foods Inc., 25-28 Vernon, CA90058, U.S.A

Bovee, K.C., Bover, C.R, andBover, H. (1987). Dietary Management of Renal Failure. *Tijdschrift voor Diergeneeskunde.* 112: 825-915.

Campbell, J.R.and Griffith, I.R. (1984). Bones and Muscles. In: Canine Medicine and Therapeutics.2nd Ed.Blackwell. Oxford, 138.

Cobb, M., Mitchell, A. R. (1991). Plasma electrolyte concentrations in dogs receiving diuretic therapy for cardiac failure. *Journal of Small Animal Practice.* 33: 526–529.

Freeman, L.M. (2000). Nutritional modulation of cardiac diseases. Waltham Focus.10 (2).

Hansen, A. E. and Wiese, H.F. (1943). *Proc.Soc.exp.Biol.Med.*52, 205-208.

Karamanos, B. (1998). The dietary management of diabetes. *Dialogue Diabetes Literature Review Service.* 3: 11-15.

Keene, B. W. (1992). L-carnitine deficiency in canine dilated cardiomyopathy. In: Current veterinary therapy XI. Philadelphia: W. B. Saunders Co, 780.

Kunkle, G.A. (1980). In: *Current Veterinary Therapy*, VII.Saunders, Philadelphia.

Ling, G. V., Lowenstein, L. J., Pulley, T.and Kaneko, J. J. (1977). Diabetes mellitus in dogs: A review of initial evaluation, immediate and long-term management, and outcome. *Journal of the American Veterinary Medical Association*. 170: 521-530.

Markwell, P.J. (1988). Clinical Small Animal Nutrition. Dog and Cat Nutrition. 2nd Ed. Pergamon, Oxford, 111.

Mosier, J.E. (1978). *Mod.Vet.Pract.* 59: 105-109.

National Research Council. (1985). Nutrient requirements of dogs. National Academy of Sciences. Washington D.C.

Nelson, R. W., Ihle, S. L., Lewis, L. D. (1991). Effects of dietary fibre supplementation on glycaemia control in dogs with alloxan-induced diabetes mellitus. *American Journal of Veterinary Research*. 52: 2060-2066.

Nelson, R. W., Scott-Montcrieff, C., DeVries, S., Davenport, D.and Neal, L. (1998). Effect of dietary insoluble fibre on control of glycaemia in dogs with naturally acquired diabetes mellitus. *Journal of the American Veterinary Medical Association*. 212: 380–386.

Osborne CA *et al*. (1995). Canine and feline urolithiasis: relationship of etiopathogenesis to treatment and prevention. In: *Canine and Feline Nephrology and Urology*, 798–888.

Osborne CA *et al*. (2008). Analysis of 451,891 canine uroliths, feline uroliths, and feline urethral plugs from 1981 to 2007: perspectives from the Minnesota urolith center. *Vet Clin Small Anim* .39: 183-197.

Pensinger, R. R. (1968). Nutritional management of heart disease. In: Kirk, R. W. ed.*Current veterinary therapy III*. Philadelphia: W. B. Saunders: 229–232.

Polzin, D.J., Osborne, C.A., Hayden, D.W.and Steves, J.B. (1981). *Minn. Vet.J.* 21: 16-29.

Purina, R. (2000). Comparing pet foods. *The Veterinarian*.24 (7): 18.

Reddy, D.V. (2004). In: Applied Nutrition. Oxford and IBH.

Sandstead, H.H. (1981). In: Disorders of Mineral Metabolism.1.Academic Press, 93-157.

Schmidt, R.W. and Gavellas, G. (1977). Bicarbonate reabsorption in experimental renal disease; effect s of proportional reduction of sodium phosphate intake. *Kidney Int.* 12: 393-402.

Sturgess, K. (2009). Dietary management of canine urolithiasis. *In: Practice* 31(7): 306-312.

Thornburg L.P. (2000). Dog liver diseases diet. *Journal of Veterinary Diagnostic*. 12(2).

Williams, D. A. (1994). Diagnosis and management of pancreatitis. *Journal of Small Animal Practice*. 35: 445–454.

□□□

42

Poultry Production in India : Opportunities and Challenges

A.K. PANDA, M.V.L.N. RAJU AND S.V. RAMA RAO
Project Directorate on Poultry, Rajendranagar, Hyderabad

Introduction

Poultry farming was confined to rearing of few chickens and ducks in the back yards till early 1960s and egg and chicken meat production was insignificant. However, during the past four decades, poultry industry in India has transformed itself from the age-old backyard farming into a dynamic agri-based industry. Several breakthroughs in poultry science and technology have led to the development of genetically superior breeds capable of higher production (layer 320-330 eggs; broiler 2.2-2.4 kg at 6 wks). This together with standardized package of practices on nutrition, housing and management, and disease control have contributed to spectacular growth rates in egg (4-6% per annum) and broiler production (10-12% per annum) in India. Consistent with increase in productivity, the annual per capita availability also increased to 49 eggs and 1900g of meat. However, it is far below the recommended consumption of 180 eggs and 10.8 Kg poultry meat per person per annum. Thus to meet the nutritional requirement, the layer and broiler industry has to grow several folds.

Present Scenario

Chicken dominates the poultry production in India. Nearly 95% of the total eggs are produced by chickens. India ranks third in egg production and fifth in chicken meat production in the world (Watt Excutive Guide, 2010). The Poultry Industry with the strength of 227 million layers and 2224 million broilers employs 2 million persons and contributes over Rs. 35, 000 crores to GNP. The poultry industry is concentrated in certain pockets of the country. The state of Andhra Pradesh leads the country in poultry production followed by West Bengal in the east, Maharashtra in the west, Tamilnadu in the south and Punjab in the north. Commercial poultry farms are concentrated more in urban and semi-urban areas although nearly 65% of the population of the country lives in rural areas. Availability of eggs is highly non-uniform in different parts of the country primarily due to wide variation in the production levels. Much of the eggs produced are consumed by the urban population while the rural and tribal areas have little access to the eggs and meat produced from the industrial sources and the availability is very low. In spite of rapid growth, the poultry industry suffered many set backs in recent times due to rising cost of feed, incidence of emerging and reemerging diseases, fluctuating market price of egg and broilers, climate change etc. which need to be addressed to make the poultry sector as a sustainable enterprise.

Feed status

Success on poultry production rests primarily on the quality of the bird employed, comforting environment and provision for good feed, the last being most expensive of all other inputs, deserves befitting attention. Feed accounts for 65-70% of broiler and 75-80% of layer production cost. Under organized sector about 7MMT and 8.5MMT broiler and layer feed are manufactured, respectively. The requirement will be doubled in another 5 years.

Table 1 : Poultry feed requirement (million metric tons, MMT)

	2005	2010	2015
Cereals			
Maize	5.55	9.25	19.79
Others	1.83	2.36	3.05
Total cereals	7.38	11.61	22.84
Protein meals			
Soyabean meal	3.72	4.80	11.35
Ground nut extractions	0.73	0.94	1.22
Others	0.73	0.94	1.22
Total protein meals	5.18	6.68	13.79
Compounded feed			
For layer sector	7.3	9.42	12.20
For broiler sector	4.92	9.91	25.71
Total feed	12.22	19.33	37.91

Source : Chaddha (2005)

The great concern and current sensitivity are feed raw material prices and the resultant feed prices which have gone up significantly. Maize is the popular cereal used in combination with protein meal like soybean meal, which comprises 70-80% of the broiler feed formulation, have touched a historical high in recent times. Production of maize increased from 9.65 million metric tons (MMT) in 1989-90 to 18 MMT in 2009-10 and soybean meal from 3.52 MMT in 1999-2000 to 7 MMT in 2009-10. Average increase in maize availability has been 3.8% per annum which is far below the growth rate of egg or meat production. Thus, there is a need to increase the production of maize and soybean or explores the usefulness of other alternate energy and protein rich feedstuffs to maize and soybean meal, respectively, in poultry diets.

Avenues opened to overcome shortage

In view of the large gap between the demand and availability of feedstuffs for poultry production, a holistic approach is needed to meet the demand of ever growing poultry industry. Some of the approaches in these respects are

- *Identification of newer feed resources :* Since the production of cereals and oil seeds may not increase significantly, the availability of grain and oil seed meal to feed industry is expected to decrease. This would lead to escalation in the cost of feed ingredients and consequently the cost of eggs and meat. To some extent such a situation can be corrected by developing strains that need less feed input. However, feed ingredients that are not related to human consumption and available in plenty should be identified and their suitability should be tested.
- *Utilization of structural carbohydrates and phytate phosphorus :* With the advancement of technology, the reduction in dependency of poultry on the storage plant carbohydrate, protein or other nutrient and to allow them to make greater use of structural carbohydrates and other nutrients to meet the requirement of highly genetic potential stocks. Hence the dimension from research should change from as such providing feed than technologies that utilize feed better. There are many components of feed such as B-glucans, pentosans, mannans, cellulose,lignin and phytic acid which can not be digested by poultry. These non digestible feed ingredients frequently generate digestive stress in poultry with a consequent reduction in nutrient utilization and wet litter problems. These problems could be largely alleviated by use of feed enzymes.
- *Overcoming limitations of Agro-industrial byproducts and unconventional feed stuff :* The influence of agro-industrial byproducts and unconventional feed ingredients on the performance of industrial

commercial layers and broilers needs to be established before they are incorporated into feeds on regular basis. It is also essential to identify suitable easily adoptable and economically viable methodology to inactivate anti-nutritional factors and enhance the nutrient availability. The nutritive value of a variety of maize and soybean meal replacers has been examined and despite their potential, the utilization in practical formulations is negligible due to constraints imposed by several anti-nutritional, technical and socio-economic factors. These constraints need to be resolved by the feed industry utilizing the services of scientists, planners and policy makers.

- *Processing of feeds and their impact on nutritional improvement*-Commercial poultry diets normally involve the admixture of a number of different feed ingredients. Processing is related to the treatment of materials during or immediately following and mixture with the purpose of providing a balanced diet suitable for consumption of poultry. Many incriminating factors of feed are also destroyed due to processing. The loss of nutrient through excreta and the cost of production can be minimized through processing of feed. This process generally involves some degree of grindings of the material which improves uniformity of admixture provides particles of a size perceived to be suited to the target group and may make nutrients more available for digestion in the birds. Subsequently the feed may be subjected to heat treatment or pelleting. The production of crumbles and pellet feeds, especially for broilers are in increasing trend. Steam pelleting and extrusion is much more effective to reduce microbial contamination in feedstuffs.

Marketing

Though, commercial production of eggs and chicken meat on scientific principles has been well standardized, marketing of eggs and broiler meat is not fully organized except few in urban sectors. Eggs are still transported in open condition and in un-refrigerated vehicles. Eggs are sold as commodity in India and purchased by consumers mostly from shop next door for daily needs. Eggs are channeled through wholesale dealers, sub-dealers, retailers etc. in two to three stages, which raises the cost of eggs by 10-15% over the actual sale price at producer's place. Broilers are sold live or slaughtered at the place of sale. Some times the birds are dressed and displayed for sale in the open air with out any concern for hygiene. Similarly eggs are sold in open without consideration for preservation of their quality. Seasonal variations in consumption and demand of eggs and meat pose greatest challenge to the stabilization of prices. The fluctuations at times go to the extent of up to 30-40% in a short period of 3-4 weeks. Thus, there is a need to strengthen the marketing system. Some of the approaches in this direction are

- Development of reliable and stable market chain round the year for marketing of poultry products.
- Facilities for hygienic slaughter and preservation of eggs should be made available at market places in both urban and rural areas.
- Formation of producer co-operatives/ Associations and Rural market yards will help in proper marketing.
- National Egg Coordination Committee, a farmers' cooperative agency has been contributing to the improvement in marketing of eggs. However, more systematized marketing strategy and the State's involvement in minimizing the channels are required for making poultry farming remunerative and cost effective in the years to come.
- Because of the location of farms in semi urban and urban areas that too concentrated in few states, availability of eggs and chicken meat are high in these areas only, but in rural areas and rest of the country the availability is low. Thus, there is a vast scope to tap the rural markets and NE states where availability is low.

Egg and Meat Processing

Trading of chicken in India is primarily done in number and not by weight at the wholesale level. Live and fresh dressed broilers account for the bulk of sales and sale of processed meat is limited (below 5%). However, acceptance of processed chicken is on the rise, particularly in the urban markets. Due to pollution and environmental concerns, slaughtering of birds under unhygienic conditions at open places is being discouraged. Thus, the sale of slaughtered chicken is expected to increase. Hence, there is a need to develop processing facilities. Hence, there is an urgent need of many chicken processing plants in the near future and sale of processed chicken to increase both to cater domestic as well as export markets.

A few plants for processing eggs have been installed using state of the art machinery in some states with an average daily turnover capacity of 0.7-0.8 million eggs. Whole egg powder, yolk powder, egg weight powder, lysozyme etc. are being produced under high standards of operation. Egg powder from India is well accepted in EU, Japan and Far-east. However, to tap the international market there is a need to establish many more egg processing plants. It has been told that India is geographically ideally located to cater to the middle East and far eastern countries for shell eggs. Therefore vast scope exists to increase the export of shell eggs from India to these countries.

Disease management

Another major area that needs attention to sustain the growth of poultry industry is the disease management with special focus on bio-security. Management of diseases in poultry plays an important role for the progress of the industry. Birds in the commercial farms are reared in open sided houses and maintained under optimum management conditions. Birds are reared under veterinary supervision. Vaccination is regularly practiced to protect the bird against diseases. In spite of all the measures, the poultry industry in India suffered a major set back last year due to the out break of Avian Influenza. The industry suffered serious trade losses following downfall in consumption of poultry meat and eggs for about 6 months. However, India is now again free from Avian Influenza.

To minimize the occurrence of disease in poultry the three most important components of disease control are Bio-security, Vaccination and Medication. Bio-security refers to all measures taken to secure prevention of all types of pathogens in poultry farms. Effective bio-security and implementation of successful hygienic procedures are increasingly dependent on Hazard Analysis Critical Control Point approach (HACCP). The principles of HACCP such as hazard analysis, critical control points, critical limits, correction, recording and verification should be strictly followed for analyzing risk assessment and risk management. Vaccination should be practiced regularly following the regulatory procedures.

Priorities for effective disease management in making the poultry industry a sustainable enterprise are

- *Trans-boundary disease* - Many of the diseases which are not endemic to India (Avian influenza, VV+MD) may enter through of germplasm and biologicals. This need strict quarantine measures.
- *Food safety* - There is a worldwide concern to minimize the use of antibiotics in poultry because of disease resistance and antibiotics residues in food chain. In such case suitable alternatives need to be explored, which could be beneficial and cost effective. Many products of such nature like Probiotics, Gut acidifiers, immunomodulators, etc. are available in the market, but need further research.
- *Establishing and strengthening surveillance and monitoring system* - The surveillance and monitoring system should be carried out in established laboratories. There is need to establish a National Avian Disease Laboratory with all modern facilities for surveillance and monitoring of infectious disease in poultry.

- *Diagnoses through genomic approach* - Efforts are needed to develop new diagnostics and biological using genomic approaches for rapid and accurate diagnosis and effective control of poultry disease.

Climate Change

Increasing concentration of green house gases (GHG) in the atmosphere has contributed to an increase in the earth's atmosphere , am occurrence known as global warming (FAO, 2006). The global atmospheric concentrations of GHG have increased markedly as a result of human activities. Livestock agriculture counts 35-40% of methane emission and nearly 70% of nitrous oxide world wide (Steinfeld et al., 2006). Of the total methane emitted in India estimated contribution of cattle is 51%, buffalo 42%, sheep 2%, goat 4.2% and other livestock contributes only 0.6%. Though contribution of poultry farming to global warming is not alarming, poultry production will be affected because of global warming. Climate changes will adversely affect the poultry production and poultry health, because birds can tolerate narrow range of temperature ranges. The increasing proportion of poultry production in tropic and sub-tropical regions make it necessary to reconsider the selection strategy for adapting to high temperature. There is a need to address other issues like housing design, environment control, nutritional management and disease control to cope with new climatic extremes.

Rural Poultry Production

Nearly 65% of India's population is living in rural areas. The fruits of commercial poultry production in India have been limited to the urban and semi-urban areas and the rural poultry sector remained unchanged. Just 25% population living in urban areas consumes about 75-80 % of eggs and poultry meat (Panda et al., 2010). Non-availability of poultry products and low purchasing power of the rural people devoid them of access to the highly nutritious products like egg and meat, thereby, resulting in malnutrition. Free range and small scale semi-commercial back-yard poultry production can be advantageously promoted in rural areas, as the large commercial poultry production continues to be concentrated in urban and peri - urban locations. It can be used as a powerful tool for alleviation of rural poverty, eradication of malnutrition and creation of gainful employment in vast rural areas.

Adopting small scale poultry farming in backyards of rural house holds will enhance the nutritional and economic conditions of these people. A new avenue for poultry exports is also opening up as a result of the growing worldwide trend towards the consumption of eggs and meat from birds reared under free-range conditions. The enormous contributions from the public sectors resulted in development of many chicken varieties suitable for backyard/ rural poultry farming. Project Directorate on Poultry, Hyderabad under the aegis of Indian Council of Agricultural Research has developed two such promising crosses namely Vanaraja and Gramapriya. Vanaraja is a dual purpose bird, while Gramapriya is having good egg production potential. The attractive multicolor feather pattern, adaptability under diversified conditions and production potential in backyards made these birds quite popular in almost all parts of this country. Many institutions are working hard to develop varieties of chicken suitable for rural poultry farming and some of them are given in below.

Table 2 : Birds developed for rural poultry production

Name	Type	Feather pattern	Purpose	Organization
Vanaraja	Breed cross	Multicolour	Dual	PDP, Hyderabad
Gramapriya	Breed cross	Multicolour	Dual	PDP, Hyderabad
Giriraja	Synthetic	Multicolour		UAS Bangalore
Krishna - J	Synthetic	Mixed (Black/ brown)	Egg	JNKVV, Jabalpur
Gramalakshmi	Breed cross	Mixed brown	Egg	KAU, Mannuthy
CARI - Gold	Breed cross	Mixed brown	Dual	CARI, Izatanagar
CARI-Shyama	Breed cross	Mixed black	Dual	CARI, Izatanagar
CARI-Nirbheek	Breed cross	Multi colour	Dual	CARI, Izatanagar
Nicobari	Native cross	White and black	Egg	CARI, Portblair

Conclusions

Inspite of various challenges in the past, the poultry production in India continues to exhibit spectacular growth. With increasing demand for chicken egg and meat, the poultry production in India foresees further expansion and industrialization. There is a need for coexistence of rural and commercial poultry farming for sustaining the growth in poultry production in the country to bridge the gaps in the supply chain of poultry products between rural and urban areas. Adoption of small scale poultry farming in backyards of rural house holds will enhance the nutritional and economic status of the rural people. With the advent of knowledge in different fields of poultry, the authors believe the future challenges will not be a hindrance and thus sees a bright future for poultry production in this country in the years to come.

References

Chadha, R.C. (2005). Indian feed industry scenario vis-à-vis World. Proc. XXIII Annual Conference and Symposium of Indian Poultry Science Association, January, Hyderabad, India: 92–109.

FAO, (2006). Livestock – a major threat to environment; Remedies urgently needed. GEF_UNDP, Asian Development Bank and United Nations Development.

Panda, A.K., U. Raj Kumar, S.K. Bhanja and M.K. Padhi, (2010). Rural Poultry Production - A Tool for Alleviating Poverty and Malnutrition in India. Proceedings of the National Seminar on Animal Resource Development and Poverty Alleviation. OUAT, Bhubaneswar. June 8-9, pp. 33-36.

Steinfled, H., Gerber, P., Wassenar, T.Castle, V., Rosales, M. and de Hann C. (2006). Livestock long shadow; Environmental issues and options. FAO, Rome, Italy.

Vision, (2030). Project Directorate on Poultry (ICAR), Hyderabad, India

Watt Executive Guide (2010). World Poultry Trends.

□□□

43

Dietary Modifications for Addition of Functionality in Meat and Poultry by Conjugated Linoleic Acid Enrichment

V.K. PASWAN, D.P. SINGH AND ALOK JHA
Department of Animal Husbandry & Dairying, Banaras Hindu University, Varanasi

Introduction

Meat is animal flesh which includes the skeletal muscle, associated fat and other organs that is used as food. Although from a strictly nutritional point of view, meat and meat products are optional and non-essential component of a human diet (Millward, 1999); however, these are essential component of the food of people in developed countries (Fernández-Ginés, 2005). Meat is rich source of all the essential nutrients such as proteins, fats, vitamins and minerals and the proportion of all the nutrients is in close proportion to the human body composition. However, there is considerable evidence showing an association between meat consumption and several ill-effects such as cardiovascular diseases, cancer, obesity etc. contributed mainly from the content of fat, saturated fatty acids, and cholesterol in the meat. In spite of all these, meat occupies a pivotal position in the food of human being worldwide and will remain important component of human food in the world.

Consumer now a days are more health conscious. They are more interested and ready to pay for the products which are more beneficial, wholesome and health promoting in order to improve their wellbeing. So, in order to curb the prevalence of chronic diseases and promote health to the consumers, several attempts were made to modify the meat by adding ingredients which are beneficial for the health or by eliminating or reducing components that are harmful. These modifications resulted in development of functional meat, i.e., the meat that influences one or more functions of the consumer in a favourable way, exceeding the effects of normal adequate nutrition; thus; improving their health and well-being and reducing the risk of chronic diseases. The production of functional meat including the poultry meat has a promising scope in the coming future.

Addition of functionality in meat and poultry has been attempted by several ways of nutritional modifications such as enrichment of meat and poultry with PUFAs (n-6 and n-3 fatty acids) with CLAs, ractopamine, antioxidants such as Vitamin E and Selenium, ascorbic acid, â-carotene. The effects of these are well reviewed by Pisulewski (2005) and Aalhus and Dugan (2001). The present paper analyse critically the scope of addition of functionality in meat and poultry meat by enriching them with CLA.

Effect of Conjugated linoleic acid

Several beneficial effects of CLA are reported by several workers which include reduction of risk of cancer, prohibition of arteriosclerosis, fall in plasma cholesterol level, anti-diabetic and anti-adipogenic effects, strengthening of the immune system, metabolism of vitamin A, bone modelling etc. (Fritsche and Steinhart, 1998; Pariza, 1999; Aydin *et al.*, 2001; Crespo and Esteve-Garcia, 2001; Carta *et al.*, 2002; Aletor *et al.*, 2003; Banni *et al.*, 2003; Belury, 2003; Cook *et al.*, 2003; Kritchevsky, 2003; Watkins *et al.*, 2003). In addition, CLA has been reported to improve feed efficiency in rats (Chin *et al.*, 1994) and repartition body fat to lean in mice (Park *et al.*, 1997). In light of above beneficial effects of CLA efforts are being made to increase the consumption of CLA via the natural diet of human being by increasing CLA content in the food ingredients of animal origin such as milk, meat and eggs.

Conjugated linoleic acid is a mixture of positional and geometric isomers of linoleic acid with two conjugated unsaturated double bonds, one in cis and the other in trans configuration at various carbon positions in the fatty acid chain. Although, more than a dozen isomers of CLA have been detected in foods of ruminant origin but the major CLA isomer whose physiological importance is well recognized is cis-9, trans-11 which comprise 80-90% of all the isomers. In ruminants, CLA is synthesized in the rumen from other fatty acids during the process of biohydrogenation of unsaturated fatty acids by some rumen bacteria (Kritchevsky, 2000; Khanal and Dhiman, 2004). Kepler and co-workers (1966) described the formation of CLA as an intermediate compound during the biohydrogenation of linoleic acid to stearic acid in the rumen by *Butyrivibrio fibrisolvens*. Although some CLA is produced in the rumen, the major source in lactating cows is its endogenous synthesis from another fatty acid biohydrogenation intermediate trans-11 transvaccenic acid by the action of enzyme Ä9-desaturase. The endogenous synthesis of CLA by Ä9-desaturase occurs in adipose tissue of muscle and mammary glands. In lactating animals the mammary gland is the main source of formation of CLA (Corl *et al.*, 2001; Griinari and Bauman, 1999). However in meat animals including poultry muscle adipose tissue is the prime organ of CLA synthesis. So the CLA content in the fat of meat is from two source i.e. from exogenous synthesis by microbes of rumen and by endogenous synthesis in the adipose tissue and is a function of rumen outflow of CLA and transvaccenic acid, plus tissue activity of Ä-9 desaturase enzyme. So, conjugated linoleic acid requirements in humans are met mainly by animal-derived products including milk, meat and their products.

Dietary modifications for enhancing CLA in meat

The CLA content in meat is affected by several factors such as dietary manipulation, animal type ie ruminants versus non ruminants, grazing versus stall feeding and other post-harvest related factors. Of all these factors, animal diet appears to affect it the most and has been given due importance in enhancing the CLA content of food products. Although meat and milk from ruminants are the richest source of CLA for humans, it is possible to enhance the CLA content of meat from non-ruminants and poultry by supplementing CLA in their diet. Currently there are two sources of CLA; one is synthetic and produced by alkaline isomerization of linoleic acid enriched vegetable oils. A second novel source is modified tall oil, which is a byproduct of the paper industry (O'Quinn *et al.* 2000). The content of CLA may be increased by 40 times in breast and thigh meat, by feeding CLA enriched diets to broilers (Aletor *et al.*, 2003; Aydin *et al.*, 2001; Sirri *et al.*, 2003; Du & Ahn, 2002). Individual differences among the animals and post harvest regulation investigations of these aspects have identified that dietary manipulations, regulatory processes and animal differences can have significant impact on the CLA content of ruminant fat (Khanal and Olson, 2004).

Enrichment of meat and poultry with conjugated linoleic acid

A number of studies have examined the effects of dietary conjugated linoleic (CLA) isomers on the fatty acid composition of the broiler carcass. These studies were largely aimed at increasing CLA content in broiler tissues as a means to develop functional properties of poultry meat destined for human consumption. Results for study on CLA shows that the CLA isomers are easily absorbed and readily incorporated into adipose tissue and cell mebrane phospholipids in monogastric animals (Kramer *et al.*, 1998). Feeding CLA oils to poultry resulted in its linear deposition in adipose tissue and intramuscular fat in several experiments and the relationship is true even at high concentrations of dietary CLA, ranging from 0-2%.

Aalhus and Dugan (2001) studied the effect of CLA on feed intake, growth rate, carcass composition, pork quality and palatability in feeding trials with pigs. They observed that CLA did not affect growth rate and feed intake however, results for feed conversion efficiency were mixed. In their study, they found fat to lean repartitioning effects of CLA resulting into reduced subcutaneous fat and increased lean meat in commercial pork cuts. However, although CLA reduced subcutaneous fat, it consistently increased levels of loin muscle intramuscular fat i.e. marbling resulting into improved meat palatability. It also increased fat hardness and thus may also be useful in designing pork where fat softness has previously been an obstacle.

Fat to lean repartitioning effects of CLA

Although the CLA content of both dairy and meat products may appear to be unique to the specific products, it is not the case and depends largely on the CLA content of the original milk and meat fats. For meat products, it also depends on the sampling site, e.g., lean versus fatty steak and muscle versus tissue fat. In their study, Aalhus and Dugan (2001) found that fat to lean repartitioning effects of CLA resulting into reduced subcutaneous fat (6.6-6.8%) and increased lean meat (2.3-2.7%) in commercial pork cuts.

Table 1 : Effects of Lipids content in breast and drumstick meat of poultry on various dietary level of CLA (mg/100 g of tissue) (Adopted from Sirri *et al.*, 2003)

Fatty Acids	Breast Meat			Thigh Meat		
	CLA-0%	CLA-2%	CLA-4%	CLA-0%	CLA-2%	CLA-4%
SFA	276.7	244.3	177.8	582.7	596.4	625.2
MUFA	241.4	143.5	176.7	670.1	425.4	462.9
PUFA	333.6	310.5	360	835.1	774.8	852.5
CLA	1.5	32.1	69.5	4.7	95.5	177.4
n-3	27.6	28.5	24.2	64.7	50.8	51.0
n-6	296.9	238.2	258.2	691.9	581.1	579.5
n-6/n-3	10.8	8.4	10.7	10.8	11.4	11.4

Negative impact of Enhancing CLA in meat

Despite all the beneficial effects, some deviations in the quality of CLA enriched meat have been reported. CLA enriched meat is more tough, dark and less red and yellow as confirmed by sensory tests. Colour and flavour of

CLA enriched meat were in favour of the test panel, whereas, texture and juiciness were assessed negatively. The toughness of the meat was due to higher proportion of saturated fatty acids in CLA enriched muscle tissues (Du & Ahn, 2002; Simon *et al.* 2000, Szymczyk *et al.*, 2001; Aletor *et al.* 2003; Siri *et al.*, 2003; Badinga *et al.*, 2003). The increased incorporation of CLA into carcass lipids inevitably led to higher relative concentrations of saturated fatty acids and lower relative concentrations of mono-unsaturated fatty acids in adipose tissue and intramuscular fat, whereas poly-unsaturated fatty acids (including CLA isomers) are not affected. In view of negative effects of saturated fatty acids consumption on human health (WHO/FAO 2003, WHO 2004), this effect could be interpreted as detrimental. However, it has also been indicated that the above changes, in relative proportions of fatty acids in broiler carcass, may reduce the susceptibility of lipids to oxidation, thus increasing their oxidative stability (Aletor *et al.*, 2003). Although the total sum of poly-unsaturated fatty acids in the CLA enriched muscle tissues remain unchanged, the content of essential individual n-6 and n-3 fatty acids are decreased. These negative effects probably are associated with inhibitory action of CLA isomers on Ä9-desaturase activity (Smith *et al.*, 2002), resulting into the low proportion of mono-unsaturated fatty acids in the modified carcass. Similarly, the decrease in concentrations of n-6 and n-3 fatty acids is caused by inhibition of Ä6-desaturase, involved in desaturation of linoleic and á-linolenic acid to their long-chain derivatives (Bretillon *et al.*, 1999).

In several trials, feeding CLA isomers to broilers had negative effects on their production performance, mainly feed intake and growth rate. For instance, Szymczyk and coworkers (2001), reported reduced feed intake and weight gain over the range of dietary CLA levels of 0-1.5%. Du and Ahn (2002) reported non-significant reduction in the body weight of the broilers with the increased levels (from 0 to 4%) of dietary CLA. However, no such changes were observed by Sirri and coworkers (2003) over the same dietary CLA concentrations. Further, the question of sensory quality of CLA-enriched poultry meat should be addressed. According to available evidence, dietary CLA improves oxidative stability of this meat. Dietary CLA increases the content of SFAs and decreases the content of PUFAs in chicken meat and thus improve the lipid and colour stability and reduce the production of volatile compounds in both irradiated and non-irradiated chicken meat, during refrigerated storage (Du *et al.*, 2000).

Conclusion

Addition of functionality in the meat and poultry through CLA enrichment has promising scope due to their health promoting effects to the consumers. CLA enriched functional meat reduce the of risk of cancer, prevent arteriosclerosis, reduce plasma cholesterol level, has anti-diabetic and anti-adipogenic effects and thus prevent obesity, strengthen the immune system, participates in the metabolism of vitamin A, assists in bone modelling etc. Although several factors affect the CLA enrichment of muscles, the dietary modification and strategic supplementation of the ration for CLA enhancement in the meat and poultry has greater impact. CLA isomers are easily absorbed from the diet and readily incorporated into adipose tissue and cell membrane phospholipids in monogastric animals and fairly in ruminants. Despite all the beneficial effects, the question of sensory quality of CLA-enriched meat and poultry should be addressed as the CLA enriched meat is more tough, dark and less red and yellow and fat to lean repartitioning effects are evident.

References

Aalhus, J.L. and Dugan, M.E.R. (2001). Improving Meat Quality through Nutrition. *Advances in Pork Production*. 12: 145.

Aletor V.A., Eder K., Becker K., Paulicks B.R., Roth F.X., Roth-Maier D.A. (2003). The effects of conjugated linoleic acids or an a-glucosidase inhibitor on tissue lipid concentrations and fatty acid composition of broiler chicks fed a low-protein diet. *Poult. Sci.* 82: 796-804.

Aydin R., Pariza M.W., Cook M.E. (2001). The importance of conjugated linoleic acid in animal and human nutrition. 2001, in: Materials of the XV European Symposium on the Quality of Poultry Meat, 9-12 September 2001, Kusudasi, Turkey, pp. 131-138.

Badinga, L., Selberg, K.T., Dinges, A.C., Comer, C.W., Miles, R.D. (2003). Dietary conjugated linoleic acid alters hepatic lipid content and fatty acid composition in broiler chickens. *Poultry Science* 82: 111-116.

Banni, S., C.S.D. Heys and K.W.J. Wahle, (2003). Conjugated linoleic acid as anticancer nutrients: Studies in vivo and cellular mechanisms. In J. Sebedio, W.W. Christie and R. Adolf (ed) *Advances in Conjugated Linoleic Acid Research*, 2: 267-281. AOCS Press.

Belury, M.A, (2003). Conjugated linoleic acids in type 2 diabetes mellitus: implications and potential mechanisms. In J. Sebedio, W.W. Christie and R. Adolf (ed) Advances in Conjugated Linoleic Acid Research, Vol. 2, pp 302-315. AOCS Press, Champaign, IL.

Bretillon, L., J. M. Chardigny, S. Gregoire, O. Berdeaux, and J. L. Sebedio. (1999). Effects of conjugated linoleic acid isomers on the hepatic microsomal desaturation activities in vitro. *Lipids* 34:965–969.

Carta, G., E. Angioni, E. Murru, M.P. Melis, S. Spada and S. Banni, (2002). Modulation of lipid metabolism and vitamin A by conjugated linoleic acid. Prostaglandins Leukot. Essent. *Fatty Acids.*, 67: 187-191.

Chin, S.F., Storkson, J.M., Albright, K.J., Cook, M.E. and Pariza, M.W. (1994). Conjugated linoleic acid is a growth factor for rats as shown by enhanced weight gain and improved feed efficiency. *J. Nutr.* 124: 2344- 2349.

Cook, M.E., D. Butz, G. Li, M. Pariza, L. Whigham and M. Yang, (2003). Conjugated linoleic acid enhances immune responses but protects against the collateral damage of immune events. In J. Sebedio, W.W. Christie and R. Adolf (ed) Advances in Conjugated Linoleic Acid Research, Vol. 2, pp: 283- 291. AOCS, Champaign, IL.

Corl, B.A., L.H. Baumgard, D.A. Dwyer, J.M. Griinari, B.S. Phillips and D.E. Bauman, (2001). The role of delta(9)-desaturase in the production of cis-9, trans- 11 CLA. J. *Nutr. Biochem.*, 12: 622-630.

Crespo N., Esteve-Garcia E. (2003). Dietary fatty acid profile modifies abdominal fat deposition in broiler chickens. *Poult. Sci.* 80: 71-78.

Du, M., Ahn D.U. (2002). Effect of dietary conjugated linoleic acid on the growth rate in live birds and abdominal fat content and quality of broiler meat. *Poult. Sci.* 81: 428-433.

Du, M., Ahn, D.U., Nam, K.C., Sell, J.L. (2000). Influence of dietary conjugated linoleic acid on volatile profiles, color and lipid oxidation of irradiated and raw chicken meat. *Meat Science*, 56: 387- 395.

Fernández-Ginés JM, Fernández-López J, Sayas-Barberá E, PérezÁlvarez JA. (2005). Meat Products as Functional Foods: A Review. *J. of Food Sci.* 2: R37–R43.

Fritsche, J., S. Fritsche, M.B. Soloman, M.M. Mossoba, M.P. Yurawecz, K. Morehouse and Y. Kim, (2000). Quantitative determination of conjugated linoleic acid isomers in beef fat. *Eur. J. Lipid Sci. Tec.*, 102: 667-672.

Griinari, J.M. and D.E. Bauman, (1999). Biosynthesis of conjugated linoleic acid and its incorporation into meat and milk in ruminants. In M.P. Yurawecz, M.M. Mossoba, J.K.G. Kramer, M.W. Pariza and G.J. Nelson (ed) Advances in Conjugated Linoleic Acid Research. Vol. I., pp: 180-200. AOCS Press, Champaign, IL.

Kepler, C.R., W.P. Tucker and S.B. Tove, (1966). Intermediates and products of the biohydrogenation of linoleic acid by Butyrivibrio fibrisolvens. *J. Biol. Chem.*, 241: 1350-1354.

Khanal, R. C. and Dhiman, T. R. (2004). Biosynthesis of Conjugated Linoleic Acid (CLA): A Review. *Pakistan Journal of Nutrition* 3 (2): 72-81.

Khanal, R. C. and Olson, K.C. (2004). Factors Affecting Conjugated Linoleic Acid (CLA) Content in Milk, Meat, and Egg: A Review. *Pakistan Journal of Nutrition* 3 (2): 82-98.

Kramer, J.K.G., Sehat, N., Dugan, M.E.R., Mossoba, M.M., Yuravetch, M., Roach, J.A.G., Eulitz, K., Aalhus J.L., Schaefer, A.L., Ku, Y. (1998). Distribution of conjugated linoleic acid (CLA) isomers in tissue lipid classes of pigs fed a commercial CLA mixture determined by gas chromatography and silver-ion-high-performance liquid. *Chromatography*. 33: 549-558.

Kritchevsky, D. (2000). Antimutagenic and some other effects of conjugated linoleic acid. *Br. J. Nutr.*, 83: 459-465.

Kritchevsky, D. (2003). Conjugated linoleic acid in experimental atherosclerosis. In J. Sebedio, W.W. Christie and R. Adolf (ed) Advances in Conjugated Linoleic Acid Research, Vol. 2, pp: 292-301. AOCS Press, Champaign, IL.

Millward, D.J. (1999). The nutritional value of plant-based diets in relation to human amino acid requirements. *Proceedings of the Nutrition Society* 58: 249-260.

O'Quinn, P.R., Nelssen, J.L., Goodband, R.D., Unruh, J.A., Woodworth, J.C., Smith, J.S. and Tokach, M.D. (2000). Effects of modified tall oil versus a commercial source of conjugated linoleic acid and increasing levels of modified tall oil on growth performance and carcass characteristics of growing finishing pigs. *J. Anim. Sci.* 78: 2359–2368.

Pariza, M.W. (1999). The biological activities of conjugated linoleic acid. In M. P. Yurawecz, M. M. Mossoba, J. K. G. Kramer, M. W. Pariza and G. J. Nelson (ed) Advances in Conjugated Linoleic Acid Research, Vol. I., pp: 12-20. AOCS Press, Champaign, IL.

Park, Y., Albright, K. J., Liu, W., J. Storkson, . M., Cook, M. E. and Pariza, M.W. (1997). Effect of conjugated linoleic acid on body composition in mice. *Lipids* 32:853–858.

Pisulewski, P. M. (2005). Nutritional potential for improving meat quality in poultry. Institute of Genetics and Animal Breeding, Jastrzêbiec, Poland. *Animal Science Papers and Reports*. 23(4): 303-315.

Simon, O., Männer, K., Schäfer, K., Sagredos, A., Eder, K. (2000). Effects of conjugated linoleic acid on protein to fat proportions, fatty acids, and plasma lipids in broilers. European Journal of Lipid Science and Technology. 102: 402-410.

Sirri, F., Tallarico, N., Meluzzi, A. and Franchini, A. (2003). Fatty acid composition and productive traits of broiler fed diets containing conjugated linoleic acid. *Poult. Sci.* 82: 1356–1361.

Smith S.B., Hively T.S, Cortese G.M., Han J.J., Chung K.Y., Castenada P., Gilbert C.D., Adams V.L., Mersmann H.J. (2002). Conjugated linoleic acid depresses Ä9-desaturase index and stearoyl coenzyme A desaturase activity in porcine subcutaneous adipose tissue. *Journal of Animal Science*. 80: 2110-2115.

Szymczyk, B., Pisulewski, P.M., Szczurek, W. and Hanczakowski, P. (2001). Effects of conjugated linoleic acid on growth performance, feed conversion efficiency, and subsequent carcass quality in broiler chickens. *Br. J. Nutr.*, 85: 465-473.

Watkins, B.A., Li, Y., Romsos, D.R., Hoffman, W.E., Allen, K.G.D. and Seifert, M.F. (2003). CLA and bone modeling in rats. In J. Sebedio, W.W. Christie and R. Adolf (ed) Advances in Conjugated Linoleic Acid Research, Vol. 2, pp: 218-250. AOCS Press, Champaign, IL.

WHO, (2004). Food and Health in Europe; a New Basis for Action. WHO Regional Publications. European Series: no 96. Copenhagen.

WHO/FAO, (2003). Diet, Nutrition and the Prevention of Chronic Diseases. WHO Technical Report Series: no 916. Geneva.

□□□

44

Organic Livestock Farming : Opportunities and Constraints

VISHNU SHARMA AND SANJITA SHARMA
Department of Animal Nutrition, Post Graduate Education and Research Centre for Livestock Health & Production, Rajasthan University of Veterinary & Animal Sciences, Jaipur, Rajasthan-302 020

Introduction

Organic farming seeks to develop sustainable systems of food production, which reduce reliance on external inputs, and emphasizes high standards of animal welfare and care for the environment. Organic term primarily and simply reflects something very close to nature, ethics and tradition in general and involves principles that generate produce of high quality, coherent with environment in particular (Sharma & Sharma,2006). According to the Codex Alimentarius Commission and all existing national regulations, "organic production is a holistic production management system that avoids use of synthetic fertilizers, pesticides and genetically modified organisms, minimizes pollution of air, soil and water, and optimizes the health and productivity of interdependent communities of plants, animals and people". Finally, organic production is not just about production but includes the entire food supply chain, from production and handling, through quality control and certification, to marketing and trade.

Organic agriculture is no longer a phenomenon of developed countries but it is now commercially practiced in 120 countries with greatest share of global organic surface area (IFOAM, 2009) is in Oceania/Australia (37.46%), followed by Europe (24.14%) and Latin America (19.8%), Asia (8.9%), North America (6.8%) and Africa (2.7%). More over, it is widely known that a large part of global food production systems is non-certified organic agriculture, often at subsistence level.

Organic Livestock Production

Livestock farming is an important part of organic farming systems both as a part of the concept and in practice, forming an integrated system with harmony between the land, the animals, and the people. Good animal health and welfare are important parts of an organic animal system (Vaarst and Enevoldsen, 1994) whereas main aspects of criticism were the increasing use of chemical substances, especially mineral fertilizers and pesticides. Organic animal husbandry has developed slower than organic plant production since organic movement has developed primarily from environmental concerns, with an early focus on soil fertility and human health. It is commonly accepted that organic livestock farming systems is associated with improved food quality. Natural pasture based farming systems produce milk rich in fat and in micro-components, which are beneficial to human health (Morand-Fehr *et al*, 2007).

The situation for organic livestock farming has however changed radically during the past decade even though; organic livestock production faces major challenges with regard to harmonization and successful integration of organic animal husbandry into the whole organic production system (Hovi *et al.* 2003). In a recent analysis report (Nykänen and Canali, 2006) on transitional research on organic food & farming in major European countries, Denmark had the largest fraction of Animal husbandry research. The guidelines have been formulated and developed by the International Federation of Organic Agriculture Movements (IFOAM, 1996) and meanwhile have found application all over the world. Furthermore, the basic standards of IFOAM have been used as the baseline for developing the regulation. These standards are then elaborated into more detailed standards by national or local certification organizations.

NPOP guidelines for raising organic livestock

The standards and procedures have been formulated in harmony with international standards such as CODEX and IFOAM. Government of India has launched the National Programme on Organic Production (NPOP) in the year 2000 which provides information on standards for organic production criteria and procedures. National centre for organic farming (NCOF) established at Ghaziabad with its 6 regional centers (RCOF) at Bangalore, Bhubneshwar, Hisar, Imphal, Jabalpur & Nagpur. Few states like

Uttarakhand, Mizoram, Sikkim & Nagaland declared intention of the states to go totally organic. In recently released livestock policy in the state of Rajasthan, thrust has been given on development of organic animal husbandry sector in the state. A number of improvements have been made in the NPOP document keeping international requirements in mind. NPOP standards also take care of the organic livestock production.

Salient features covering organic livestock production standards are as follows-

Breeding

Breeds should be chosen which are adapted to local conditions. A.I. is allowed but ETT is not allowed in organic standards. Hormonal heat treatment and induced birth not allowed.

Feeding

The livestock should be fed 100 % organically grown feed of good quality. Agro-products from organic feed processed industry should be used. In organic production system, use of synthetic livestock feed additives should be avoided (Lampkin, 1990). At least 50 % of the feed should come from the farm itself. Synthetic appetizers, preservatives, colouring agent, urea, abattoir waste, droppings & dung, solvent extracted meal and genetically engineered organism or products shall not be included in feeding programme. Fodder preservatives as bacteria,fungi and bacteria may be used. Molasses are allowed.

Production

Animal product may be sold as organic only after the farm has been under conversion period for at least 12 months and standards have been met for appropriate time. Appropriate time for dairy and egg production is 30 days and for meat production organic standard should be followed for 12 months. All organic animals should be born and raised in organic holdings however when organic livestock is not available, the certification programme brought- in conventional animals.

Management

Animal husbandry management should be governing by physiological and ethological needs of the farm animal so that animal is allowed to conduct basic behavioral needs. Flock size should not adversely affect behavioral pattern and sufficient free movement should be allowed. Land less animal husbandry system shall not be allowed. The concept of organic animal farming can fulfill the criteria for sustainability and to diminish environmental pollution of agricultural production (Sundrum, 2001). Herd/ flocked animals shall not be kept individually. Mutilations not allowed except castration, tail docking of lambs and dehorning. Management practices should be directed to the well being of animal for achieving maximum resistance to the disease and preventing future in infections. Use of natural medicines and methods should be emphasized. Transport and stress should be minimized to slaughter the animal and preferably stunning should be employed before being bled to death.

Opportunities in Indian Context

Livestock practices adopted in the field particularly, by small and medium farmers are more or less organic in nature and therefore, offers a good environment for propagation of organic animal husbandry. Natural breeding is largely practiced with proven males. Farmers rely on traditional or indigenous health care practices. Domestic animals enjoys affectionate behavior and cows treated as mother get full respect and worshiped.

Livestock is an essential part of organic system for nutrient recycling, weed control, pasture establishment, soil fertility and energy use efficiency. These long term goals are necessary to maintain sustainability of the eco system.

S.No.	Existing traditional practice	Score	Relation
1.	Mix-crop Livestock system	High	Recycling of nutrients
2.	Indigenous native germ plasm	High	Biodiversity conservation
3.	Local biomass for feeding	High	Energy use efficiency
4.	Treatment with traditional wisdom and local herbs	High	Avoidance of nuisance element in food chain.

Market Potential & Regulation

Presently, no data base is available specifically for availability of organic animal farms in India. However, all organic producers are directly or indirectly supposed to be linked with livestock farming. India exported 35 organic products worth US$ 21 Million during 2004- 05 (Gouri 2006), but these products did not have any item of animal origin except honey. India is having 1.18 million organic agricultural lands and comes in first 10 countries with the most organic agricultural land. Among top ten countries with the largest numbers of organic producers, India ranked top with 677,257 organic producers. In India, the number of organic producers almost doubled in 2009(Annonymous,2011). Export market for organic farming is clearly growing and presently 40 b US$ market potential with annual growth rate

19 percent. The products are under supply in US & Europe and imports are required. The most popular organic product groups are fresh fruit and vegetables, dairy products, organic eggs and bakery wares.

The NPOP standards for production and accreditation system have been recognized by European Commission and Switzerland as equivalent to their country standards. Similarly, USDA has recognized NPOP conformity assessment procedures of accreditation as equivalent to that of US. With these recognitions, Indian organic products duly certified by the accredited certification bodies of India are accepted by the importing countries.

Constraints and Recommendations

Indian agriculture is characterized by small scale (<2ha), subsistence farming operations under low input low output production systems, where, livestock are essentially integrated with crop farming. Thus, alongside organic crop production, the prospects for organic livestock production are yet to be explored (Chander and Mukherjee, 2005) but mostly these animal husbandry practices in resource deficient areas are by default organic in nature. Practical approaches for organic farming should be based on locally existing animal production systems which already have close resemblance to prescribed organic practices (Sharma & sharma, 2010).

Institutional

Relative to enormous opportunities and inherited favorable points in existing system, very less attention has been given for development of organic livestock systems. Most of the time issues have been raised for only organic agriculture or at the most for cattle welfare, and the issue has not being addressed properly in national bodies and policies. Proper funds should be available for promotional research and awareness regarding organic livestock. The sector needs specific promotion to farmers to cope up transient losses during transition period from conventional to organic one. An all India net work programme on research and extension aspects of small ruminant organic production should be initiated by competent body encompassing various regional centers.

Regulatory

Existing standards for organic livestock needs revision since they are largely adopted from foreign countries where livestock production system, agro-climatic situation and socio-economic condition of farmers vary greatly than to our country. Most of the standards for organic livestock are subjective and vague which needs to be objective and precise. For this, streamline research is required, evolving concrete recommendations, leaving minimum room for discretion of various inspection authorities.

Input supply

Feed availability represents one of the most limiting factor to an organic system (Nardone, 2000). Practical approaches for organic farming should be based and developed from locally existing animal production systems which already have close resemblance to prescribed organic practices. A set of recommendations are required at various levels.

Product Market

Organized marketing system for organic meat, milk, wool, yarn etc. so that farmer can get premium price for the product. Success of milk cooperative societies can be translated in livestock organic cooperatives. Agencies like APEDA can play a big role regarding exploration of foreign market however strict certification measures needs to be implemented.

Research and Extension initiatives

Lack of scientific information from research in organic livestock production is a great limitation. Issues related to organic lamb, organic milk with therapeutic attributes, organic & eco-friendly wool & yarn are few core aspects which are on high priority to address. The biggest hurdle in adoption of organic principles is lack of awareness and sensitization among farmers, consumers and extension workers regarding short term and long term advantages of organic practices. Therefore, tailor-made training programmes are required for different sections of the society and mass campaign needs to initiate with regards to organic livestock products.

Conclusion

In conclusion, organic livestock production has a great potential globally and offers a great market for export. It has advantage in assuring safe food chain and minimizes health risks. Indian practices are quiet organic by default, however there is need to organize this sector to harness benefit out of it. In developed countries organic livestock intends primarily for welfare & ethics but in developing countries, economics has to play a big role. Efforts should make to review existing standards to be in line with local agro-climatic & socio-economic conditions.

References

Annonymous, (2011). The World of Organic Agriculture. Statistics and Emerging Trends 2011. IFOAM & FiBL : Key results from the survey on organic agriculture worldwide, 2011.

Chander M and Mukherjee R. (2005). Organic Animal Husbandry: Concept, Status and Possibilities in India – A review. *Indian Journal of Animal Sciences*, 75 (12): 1460-69.

Gouri P V S M. (2006). Policy issues related to organic farming. In: Sanjay Kumar, R.S.Rathore, Reena Mukherjee, G Das and Mahesh Chander (eds), Organic Animal Husbandry: Concepts, Standards & Practices, Indian Veterinary Research Institute, 166pp.

Hovi, M., Sundrum, A. and Thamsborg, S. M. (2003). Animal health and welfare in organic livestock production in Europe: current state and future challenges. *Livestock Production Science*. 80: 41-53.

IFOAM, (1996). International Federation of the Organic Agricultural Movement: Basic Standards for Organic Agriculture and Food Processing, 10th Edition. SÖL, Bad Dürckheim.

IFOAM, (2009). The World of Organic Agriculture: Statistics and Emerging Trends 2009.

Lampkin, N. (1990). In : Organic Farming, Farming Press Book, IPSWICH, UK.

Morand-Fehr,P., Fedele. V., Decandia,M. and Le Frileux,Y. (2007). Influence of farming and feeding systems on composition and quality of goat and sheep milk. *Small Ruminant Research*, 68: 20-34.

Nardone, A. (2000). Weather conditions and genetics of breeding systems in the Mediterranean area. *Proc. XXXV Intern. Symp. of Societa' Italiana peril Progresso della Zootecnia, Ragusa* (I), 67-91.

Nykänen, A. and Canali, S. (2006). Coordination of European Transnational Research in Organic Food and Farming, Project no. ERAC-CT-2004-011716, Ministry of Agriculture and Forestry in Finland.

Sharma S and Sharma V. (2006). Local biomass use and environment adaptation as pillars of organic animal production in dry regions of India. *In: Proc. 1st IFOAM International Conference on Animals in Organic Production* University of Minnesota, St. Paul, MN, USA.

Sharma,V. and Sharma. S. (2010). Present status and future prospectus of organic farming in small ruminant Production. Invited Lead Paper presented in National Seminar on Stress Management in Small Ruminant Production and Product Processing. Organized by CSWRI & ICAR at Jaipur on January, 29-31, 2010 & chapter was included in edited book on Climate Change & stress Management: Sheep & Goat Production, pp.677-686, Pub. SSPH, Delhi.

Sundrum A. (2001). Organic livestock farming: A critical review. *Livestock Production Science*. 67: 207–15

Vaarst, M. and Enevoldsen, C. (1994). Disease control and health in Danish organic dairy herds. In: Hiusman, E.A. (Ed.), Proceedings. 4th Zodiac Symposium, Biological Basis of Sustainable Animal Production. EAAP, Publ. No. 67: 211–217.

□□□

45

Rural Livestock Production System : Constraints and Opportunities for Economic Sustainability in North Eastern Region of India

R.J. KUKDE AND R. BURAGOHAIN
Department of Animal Nutrition, College of Veterinary Sciences and A.H.
Central Agricultural University, Selesih, Aizawl, Mizoram – 796014

Introduction

The North Eastern Region (NER) of India, of Mystic spenders and rich cultural heritage, spreads over an area of 2, 62,179 sq. Km, stretched 89.46 to 97.30° east longitude, and 21.57 to 29.30° north longitudes. This region has 4500 Km long international border with five countries namely, Bangladesh, Bhutan, China, Nepal and Myanmar, with 39 million people in 890 geographical areas of 4% population, 475 ethnic groups and 400 languages or dialects.

The livestock and poultry are, by and large, inseparably associated with sections of rural society both vertically and laterally contributing for economic sustenance in the NE region of India. Livestock is an integral part of the people in this region since ages and contributes tremendously to nutritional security and poverty alleviation through increased household income. Almost all the domesticated livestock species can thrive well in the agro-climatic environment of the NE India. Farming system differs widely on the basis of culture, food habit, topography of land, soil type, rainfall distribution and several other factors. Cattle and buffalo rearing is the most traditional for the people for milk, meat and work purpose, although most of the people do not have the habit of drinking milk regularly as a part of diet. Mithun is reared in Nagaland, Arunachal Pradesh, Manipur and Mizoram mainly for meat purpose; whereas, yak is unique for Arunachal Pradesh and Sikkim. Pig and poultry rearing is common and goat and sheep are kept by the poorer sections in all the states. Hill farmers have integrated crop farming with a large no. of livestock and this system supports 14.90 million cattle, 4.5 million buffaloes, 2.90 million sheep, 4.80 million goat, 1 million pigs, 0.7 million horses, mules and ponies and 0.15 million other livestock. Improving and sustaining the productivity shall directly benefit around 50 million NER farmers economically.

Mixed crop-livestock farming and pastoralism are the two common production systems found across the North-East India. Farmers derive their livelihood somewhat equally from agriculture and livestock. People maintain their livestock primarily on grazing i.e. on traditional '*No input with or without output*' management system. However, as natural grasses are not available throughout the year, migratory or semi-migratory systems of livestock rearing are practiced particularly in acute water and fodder scarce situations. Semi-migratory or transhumance rearing system is found among the yak farmers of Arunachal Pradesh and Sikkim and also among the mithun rearers in Nagaland.

In recent years, under industrialized systems of production of commercial poultry, dairy as well as goat and pig farms, cost of production has been reduced manifolds than before. However, it necessitates conversion of good agricultural land to fodder plots/animal houses and also in many occasions do not address social, environmental and public health concerns in the long run. For concentrating large numbers of animals in a small area sometimes results accumulation of animal wastes which in turn contaminate air, soil and water increasing the risk of communicable diseases. The process of industrialization is also sometimes considered as one of the probable causes of wiping out poor farmers, small enterprises and local breeds. For Example, broiler and layer chicken in organized farms across the world rely on less than half a dozen breeds, although there are 606 breeds of chicken worldwide. The recent outbreak of bird flu in India demonstrates the pressures of global trade and its impact on small holders. Because for eradication of H1N1, many tribal families were also targeted with meagre compensation, whereas for those poor families poultry was extremely valuable asset reared in the backyard. Thus, the rural breeds of livestock and livestock production system have values in the recent days of "*organic*" concept of livestock farming. Greater emphasis should be laid on the need for substantial increase of total biomass production to be used for the feeding of livestock through better management to supply proper nutrients and also to reduce wastes. No animal production programme could be sustainable without adequate provision of feeds and fodders. In the present study, an attempt was made to review the rural livestock production system of the North East India with reference to constraints of feeding and management and opportunities for economic sustainability of the rural people in the days to come.

Livestock, Poultry Population and Production Scenario in the North East

Although there is a large livestock population in the NE states (Table. 1) however, the productivity is not sufficient to meet the local consumption needs of the people in terms of milk, meat and eggs (Table.2). Being productivity positively correlated with balanced nutrition and scientific management, shortage of concentrates and quality green grasses/fodders in required quantity and awareness in parts of the farmers may be the contributing factors. In this regards, exploitation, nutritional evaluation and characterization of the available feed resources has a significant bearing for sustainability of livestock productivity in the NE region of India.

Table 1 : Livestock population of the NE states (As per livestock census, 2003) in Thousands

State	Cattle	Buffalo	Sheep	Goat	Pigs	Horse	Poultry	Yak	Mithun
Arunachal Pradesh	458	11	19	231	330	7	1743	9	192
Assam	8440	678	170	2987	1543	12	21664	0	0
Meghalaya	767	18	18	327	419	2	2821	0	0
Mizoram	36	6	1	17	248	2	1125	0	2
Tripura	759	14	3	472	209	2	3057	0	0
Sikkim*	159	2	6	124	38	2	322	7	0
Nagaland	451	34	4	175	644	1	2789	0	40
Manipur	418	77	6	33	415	2	2941	0	20

Table 2 : Requirement and availability of livestock products in NE region

Products	Minimum requirement	Availability
Milk	201 g/head/day	100 g/head/day
Meat	7,122 million tones (Annually)	1 million tones (Annually)
Egg	180 eggs/head/year	12 eggs/head/year

Source: NEDFi Databank

Present status of feed and fodder availability in the North east

The climate of the NE region varies from near tropical in the plains to alpine in the hills based on which the region has been classified into six agro-climatic zones (Table 3). On an average, 54.48% of total geographical area is under forest cover out of which about 44.14% comes under protected and reserved area and rest 55.86% comes under unclassified forest, however the net sown area in NE region is only about 12.7%. The soil is acidic in nature and the pH ranges from 4.0 to 6.8. The animal husbandry has tremendous potentiality in this region for the availability of large area of uncultivable and grass land. Fodder cultivation as such is not practiced in this region. Livestock rearers follow the cut and carry methods of feeding their livestock.

Table 3 : Agro-climatic zones of the North East Region of India

Particulars	Climatic Zones	Height from sea level (m)	Crop/ crop sequences
Zone – I	Alpine	More than 3500	Pasture
Zone – II	Temperate and Sub-alpine	1500 – 3500	Potato-rice, rice mono-cropping and vegetable
Zone – III	Sub-tropical hill	1000 – 1500	Rice and maize mono-cropping, maize + ragi mixed, ginger and turmeric
Zone – IV	Sub-tropical plain	400 – 1000	Rice and maize mono-cropping, ginger and turmeric, rice-rice (irrigated condition)
Zone – V	Mild tropical hill	200 – 800	Rice and maize mono-cropping
Zone – VI	Mild tropical plain	0 – 200	Rice-rice (low land), jute / rice / sweet potato mono-cropping

Source: Dairy India Year Book, 2008

Rural Livestock Feeding and Management System in the NE India

Dairy animals

P[illegible]in areas of NER, particularly in Assam and Tripura, semi-intensive type of managemental system in followed for diary animals. The rural farmers generally let their animals loose during the daytime to the field and nearby jungle for grazing and in the evening offer dry roughages, mainly paddy straw, along with some cultivated green grasses or collected pasture grasses. No concentrate ration is prepared by the farmers of their own as per nutritional requirement of the animals. However, offering of home grown cereal by-products like rice polish or rice bran to the productive animal is common in the villages. In the hilly areas of the NE, dairy farming is very much scattered.

As the opportunities for sale of milk and milk products are very limited under rural conditions in the hilly states and drinking of milk is not a regular habit among the people, dairy farming is more or less concentrated in some specific regions only and that to with communities like Nepali people. The jungle grasses and tree leaves comprises of the bulk of the feeds of these animals. The productivity of the animals is less.

Table 4 : Availability, requirement and deficit of feeds and fodders for livestock (Million tonnes).

Feeds	2005	2006
Concentrate		
Availability	54.63	48.27
Requirement	121.90	130.55
Deficit (%)	64.10	63.03
Green fodders		
Availability	743.46	763.23
Requirement	839.07	854.72
Deficit (%)	11.48	10.72
Dry fodder		
Availability	483.46	763.23
Requirement	561.80	562.77
Deficit (%)	13.98	12.27

Pig production system

The pig management system differs in the plain and hilly areas of the North east India. Both scavenging and intensive rearing are common practice among the farmers in Assam and Tripura. The farmers utilize kitchen waste, hotel waste or vegetable waste as the staple feeds of their pig. Thus, practically there is no investment at all for feeding of their pigs. The pig sty is constructed with bamboo/wood and asbestos sheet/dry grasses/straw is used as the roofing materials.

In the hilly region of the North East, the pig farmers construct their pigsty with locally available materials like bamboo and woods generally in road side slope area with a raised platform of about 2-3 feet high from the ground. The farm equipments included mainly iron vessel for boiling feeds, empty mustard oil tin or cut piece of woods or bamboos as feeding and watering troughs.

The farmers prefer to rear crossbred pigs on their farms since they have better growth performance and are healthier than indigenous ones and hence have large litter size, low mortality rate and high back fat thickness. The farmers of the hilly region prefer Hampshire and Saddle Back breed for crossing.

Stall feeding is followed by almost all of the farmers in complete hilly region and this is unlike the scavenging system commonly seen in plain areas. The farmers provide kitchen waste to the pigs with small quantity of concentrates along with various locally available unconventional feeds. Feeds are provided after boiling to the pigs. Feed supplement like mineral mixture, vitamins etc are not added by the farmers.

Vaccination and deworming schedule is followed by only a small section of the farmers. Giving iron injection to the piglets to prevent piglet anaemia and uses drugs for skin diseases and ectoparasite control is very rare. The general care and management practices include cutting of needle teeth, weaning of piglets, castration, care to pregnant sow, care after farrowing, treatment of non-conceived sows, cleaning of pigsty, marketing etc. Castration and weaning are practiced by all the farmers.

Poultry production system

Indigenous poultry occupies a major portion of the total poultry population of the North East for their adoptability to agro-climatic condition and more importantly popularity and preference for meat and egg of indigenous chicken in the region. They are one of the main tools of income generation under rural conditions and closely linked to the religious and socio-cultural lives of the rural people and household food security. They are reared under scavenging by '*No input*' production system. In the hilly regions of the North East, the demand of poultry egg and meat is very high. However, the farmers usually rear very small number of birds and they utilize their kitchen waste for feeding their birds along with home grown cereal by-products like rice bran/ polish or maize grain. The village people usually do not use any concentrate feed mixture. The local poultry birds scavenge throughout the day in and around the farmers' house and at night they take shelter inside the farmers' house or in cages made of bamboo constructed nearby the house.

Managemental and feeding system of Yak and Mithun

The yak (*Poephagous grunniens* L.) is a multi-purpose bovid for the people in high altitude areas of Arunachal Pradesh. It provides milk, meat and hair which are considered as organic. They are found usually between 3000-4500 m above mean sea level (MSL). The rearing system of yak is semi-migratory (transhumance) free range system. The farmers practice two pasture utilization strategies i.e. during summer, yaks are taken to high altitude alpine pasture (4500 m and above MSL) and in winter, they come to pockets near to their villages located at mild altitude (3000 m and above MSL). Grazing in summer pasture is from May to September and from December to February in winter pasture. Thus, the yak production system is a low cost production cycle. Availability of fodder, its growth stage and nutritive value influences the productive performance of yak. A scanty feed resource during the winter period is a major nutritional factor hampering the performance in terms of body weight gain, reproduction and even of their survival. As there is practically no disease management by the yak herdsman, this is also another factor affecting the productivity of yaks.

The mithun (*Bos frontalis*) is another unique species associated with the social, cultural and religious life of hilly tribal people of Nagaland, Arunachal Pradesh, Manipur and Mizoram. It is a valuable source of milk and meat as well as leather to the tribal communities. The farmers rear this animal at various altitudes between 1000 to 3000m MSL and exclusively under free grazing condition. Mithun basically thrives on the jungle forages, tree fodders, shrubs, herbs, and other natural vegetations. Farmers do not provide any additional feeding. The mithun are generally kept under natural forest in a semi-wild state. Owners generally keep mithuns in community herd in fenced hilly jungle area and village council assigns mithun grazers to take care of their animals.

The approach

Sustainable livestock production in the country in general and hill states of NE in particular is confronted with the following problems.

a) Resource degradation and environmental damage caused by deforestation and overgrazing.

b) Utilization of land for alternative enterprises.

c) Poor genetic quality of most of the local breeds/strains of livestock and poultry.

d) Feed and fodder availability.

e) Weak support services (technology transfer/extension, breeding, animal health) mostly due to undulating topography of the hills, remoteness etc.

f) Limited investment in livestock sector.

g) Lack of organised markets.

Constraints Under Rural Livestock Production System

1. With the increasing human population day by day, the grazing land for livestock is also decreasing which in turn increases pressure on the rural livestock rearers, particularly to the small, marginal and landless farmers.

2. The number of processing units of livestock produce is very scanty throughout the North East region.
3. Limited production of conventional feed ingredients of livestock and poultry in the NE region contribute for their higher price for dependence on other states of India for supply.
4. Small farm size presents a serious constraint because of lack of access to resources as well as the difficulties of promoting the application of practical technologies capable of a discernable impact.
5. Lack of awareness about scientific feeding and management of livestock and poultry in parts of the farmers affect productivity and hence economic return.
6. The nutritional deficiencies and imbalances are ignored by the farmers under rural production system.

Strategies for augmenting productivity under the rural feeding and management

a. Creating awareness in regards to scientific feeding and management of livestock and poultry among the rural people with special emphasis on judicious uses of locally available un-conventional feeds and fodders in balancing livestock rations.
b. The small size of the farms determines, to a large extent, to which new technologies can be adopted, and this aspect needs to be considered in the formulation and application of suitable technologies.
c. Small holding size is also a constraint to production and sustainability. The technologies have to be demonstrated on-farm as potentially valuable technologies are also ignored in many occasions at village level.
d. Awareness towards supplementing concentrate ration (based on nutrient availability from grazing forages), prebiotic, probiotic and chelated minerals (to enhance growth and reproduction) and use of urea molasses block (to enhance the nutrient availability from poor forages).
e. Establishment of animal feed/feed and fodder banks and adaptation of fodder preservation measures (i.e. plastic bag silage).
f. Utilization of unconventional feed resources and development of cost effective technologies for detoxifying the incriminating factors present in them.
g. Technologies like total mixed ration or complete feed block incorporating the low cost ecosystem available feed and fodders for the livestock.

h. There is need for a comprehensive policy and proper coordination between the forest officials and the livestock development agencies for effective utilization of available feed resources.

Conclusion

Small farms constitute the backbone of traditional agriculture. Livestock are not only the efficient utilisers of the available biomass to a range of valuable animal products i.e. milk; meat, wool, manure, and draught power but also contribute towards fertilising the soil with their dung and urine. Achievements of sustainable development, food security and economic growth in the NE region will depend on –

- Integrated systems and improved efficiency in management of natural resources.
- Development of environmentally sound, low input and location specific farming systems based on prevalent ecosystems.
- In order to ease out the problem of non-availability of superior germplasm in this region as well as to maintain a steady and sustaining source of quality breeding stock, it will be desirable to establish livestock germplasm banks at least one in each district of the states.
- Improvement of available crop residues by physical, chemical, biological and microbial treatment and their judicious utilization after enrichment.
- Introduction of high yielding cultivated fodder in suitable areas.
- Effective health cover measures of livestock and poultry will be another important area towards achieving sustainable production in NER.
- In NER, there should be co-operative and/or private enterprises for engaging own "Veterinary Service Unit" by the Veterinary graduates under entrepreneurship programme to take care of health as well as artificial insemination and marketing of livestock products.
- Extension services in Animal Husbandry and Veterinary sector in NER is extremely poor. Farmers are not aware about the production and health technology developed for enhancing livestock productivity. A vigorous extension drive for livestock production farming system is necessary.
- Entire NER of the country is facing problem of livestock processing and marketing. NE Hill region essentially needs organized abattoir for processing and marketing of various meat products so that the producers can have easy access to production outlets.

Considering the socio-economic and socio-cultural scenario among the people living in NE region, it could be predicted that the existing mixed farm concept shall continue. Sustaining growth in livestock sector can ensure employment generation and thus reduce poverty. Appropriate feeding and management strategies coupled with comprehensive production policy may help in augmenting productivity under rural livestock production system in the North East region of India.

References

Baruah, K.K. (2007). Scope for utilization of indigenous feed and fodders for augmenting the productivity in Mithun. In: Brain storming session on Sustainable mithun production for economic upliftment of tribal population in NEH region, K.K.Baruah (Ed.), published by Director, NRC-Mithun (ICAR), Nagaland.

Buragohain, R., Ghosh, M.K., Baruah, K.K., Pathak, P.K. and Bhattacharya, M. (2006). Mineral status of feeds, fodder and tree leaves for dairy animals in Jorhat district of Assam. *Animal Nutrition and Feed technology*. 6: 289-293.

Haque, N., Toppo, S., Rahman H. and Bujarbaruah K.M. (2008). Feed and fodder resources of Northeastern India. *In: Dairy Year Book* 2008, pp.146.

Pourouchottamane, R., Ramesha, K.P. and Chatterjee, A. (2004). Status and managemental strategies for yak production. In: Yak Farming, D.K.Sharma and K.P.Ramesha (Ed.), published by Director, NRC-Yak (ICAR), Dirang, Arunachal Pradesh, pp.36-48.

Rajkhowa, C. (2007). Mithun: A promising component for hilly livestock production system. In: Brain storming session on Sustainable mithun production for economic upliftment of tribal population in NEH region, K.K.Baruah (Ed.), published by Director, NRC-Mithun (ICAR), Nagaland.

Sarmah, B.C. (2007). Interventions on reproductive physiology to augment mithun production. In: Brain storming session on Sustainable mithun production for economic upliftment of tribal population in NEH region, K.K. Baruah (Ed.), published by Director, NRC-Mithun (ICAR), Nagaland.

□□□

46

Precision Animal Nutrition for Efficient and Economical Milk Production

D.V. REDDY
Professor & Head, Department of Animal Nutrition
Rajiv Gandhi College of Veterinary and Animal Sciences, Pondicherry-605 009

Introduction

A major advantage of ruminants is their ability to convert vast quantities of otherwise human inedible, low digestibility plant material (forages, crop residues) into high quality human edible food products. However, ruminant animal converts only 4 to 25% of dietary protein into products such as milk, meat and wool, while it is only 2 to 17% for energy.

Prof. R.A.Leng in his lecture "Decline in available world resources - implications for livestock production systems" in FAO/IAEA International Symposium June 2009 held at Vienna, Austria, discussed the three simultaneous and interrelated/interactive crises that the world is facing, one of which is climate change. Increasing temperatures in tropical countries can have a slowing effect on photosynthesis and hence plant growth. Recent models suggest that global warming is likely to reduce world agricultural output by between 16 and 3%. However, the effects will not be spread evenly and productivity in the tropical, developing countries likely to be reduced disproportionately by 21 - 9%.

Environmental issues, animal welfare and safety are particularly important in the knowledge-based economy, and have moved animal production beyond the singular goal of providing animal products and maximizing profit. Therefore, feeding animals is not only a consideration of economic traits but also environmental traits and welfare traits. Producers seeking a fair income for their current work and investment are facing challenges, because feeding animals should not only be environmental friendly and biologically safe, but also be accommodate social ethics. These are achievable by feeding animals in precision animal nutrition mode (Reddy and Krishna, 2009; Reddy, 2011; Reddy and Narahari, 2011).

What is precision animal nutrition?

Precision animal nutrition (PAN) is defined as providing the animal with the feed that precisely meet its nutritional requirements for optimum productive efficiency to produce better quality animal products (milk, meat and eggs) and to contribute cleaner environment and thereby ensure profitability. Cleaner environment means reducing the enteric emission of methane, excretion of nitrogen (ammonia), phosphorus (P) and other compounds into the environment. It is aimed at supplying the nutrients to the animals matching their requirements to improve not only the animal physiology and health but also the enrichment of their products for the well being of the consumer.

Tools to achieve precision animal nutrition

The tools to achieve PAN include more precise ration formulation based on nutritional value of each batch of ingredient, proper weighing and mixing of ingredients, use of nutricines / feed additives and improved feed processing techniques, implementing phase feeding and split-sex feeding.

The lead paper is organized into two parts: Feeding to minimize nutrient requirements for maintenance and Precision feeding of dairy cows to improve nitrogen efficiency.

I. Feeding to minimize nutrient requirements for maintenance

Feed costs represent a large portion of the costs of producing milk. Hence factors that impact the efficiency of conversion of feed to milk are of considerable importance. These include several biological processes, environmental influences, genetic factors. The main components of energy requirements are the costs associated with maintenance, body composition changes, and production (growth, reproduction and lactation). Maintenance energy needs are a priority in the animal. Maintenance is the physiological state in which there is no net change in body energy or alternatively when energy balance is zero. Increased maintenance costs have a direct impact on the efficiency of conversion of feed to milk or tissue deposition. A decrease in maintenance requirements or a dilution of maintenance in dairy cows that are capable of producing greater amounts of milk is, therefore, an important goal in the dairy enterprise.

Components of Maintenance

The components of maintenance include the energy required for basal metabolism; energy of thermal regulation; the energy costs associated with digestion, absorption and assimilation of meals at maintenance intake; and the energy associated with waste production. Basal metabolism is essentially equal to fasting heat production (FHP) or the heat production of an animal in a post-absorptive state in a thermoneutral environment in an inactive (lying or standing with no activity) state (Baldwin, 1995).

Factors that affect FHP are due to differences in sex, breed, physiological state, level of production, and previous plane of nutrition. The importance of plane of nutrition is highlighted in experiments where sheep were shifted from a high nutritional status to low nutritional status. The observed maintenance requirements were 32% greater than when shifting animals to the opposite diet sequence. It can be explained by a high correlation between FHP and weight of the major digestive organs (primarily liver and gastrointestinal tract).

Factors Affecting Maintenance Requirements

The adjustment to maintenance requirements for lactating cows includes the effect of activity, terrain, and level of feed consumption (NRC, 2001). These adjustments recognize the increased overhead maintenance requirements associated with additional physical activity and the energetic costs associated with increased nutrient digestion and absorption. For heifers, the impact of growth, thermal loss due to cooling, body composition, coat condition, and heat stress are all recognized as adjustments to maintenance requirements.

Type of diet

High fibre diets: Animals on diets with high fibre contents spend more time on chewing and rumination than those on diets with less fibre. This would have increased the energy costs of maintenance. Higher maintenance requirements on forage-based diets could result from higher energy requirements (higher heat production) of the gastrointestinal tract to digest the feed. Oxygen consumption in the intestines has been shown to increase on diets rich in forage (Reynolds *et al.*, 1991).

Nitrogen content of the diet: Excess nitrogen content in the diet increases the NE_m requirements. High concentrations of CP may be found in grass, and surpluses of nitrogen have to be excreted. The synthesis and excretion of urea requires 21.8 kJ / g excreted N.

Condition of the cows

The condition of the cows may also play a role in increased maintenance requirements. Lean cows may have higher maintenance requirements than fat cows, because of the higher rate of turnover of protein compared to body fat. Lean body mass is associated with greater metabolic activity and is positively correlated with basal energy expenditure (Speakman *et al.*, 2004).

Breed effect

There is considerable evidence to suggest differences in maintenance requirements among beef breeds (NRC, 1996). A portion of the breed effect on maintenance requirements in beef cattle is due to inherent differences in lean tissue as a fraction of total body weight (BW) among breed types. Early experiments suggested a similar scenario for dairy breeds (Van Es, 1961), but a more recent comparison of Holstein and Jersey cattle indicates that although milk production was greater for Holstein cows, the energy requirements per unit of metabolic weight were the same for both breeds (Tyrrell *et al.*, 1991). Similarities in lean mass percentage among dairy cattle breeds may be one of the underlying biological effects that obviate a breed adjustment for maintenance requirement. The NRC (2001) accepts a lack of variability due to breed in assigning maintenance energy requirements.

Immune challenge

One of the challenges in animal nutrition is in understanding how energy is partitioned among physiological processes. There is a paucity of research that directly examines the impact of immune challenges on maintenance energy expenditure. However, it is well recognized that sub-acute disease affects productivity. Therefore, it is reasonable to assume that a portion of the costs of an immune challenge are reflected in increased maintenance costs.

Visceral organ size

Visceral organ size plays a critical role in determining energy expenditure. Liver represents approximately 1.6% of empty BW but it receives 30% of cardiac output and is responsible for 25% of FHP (Baldwin, 1995). Therefore, a small change in liver size or metabolic activity may have a tremendous impact on maintenance requirements. For example, liver weight is greater in lactating cows compared to nonlactating cows. Most of this 25% increase in liver size is needed to accommodate the increased needs for gluconeogenesis and ureagenesis that accompany lactation. The maintenance requirement for lactating cows are about 10% higher than that for non-lactating cows because of bigger internal organs (heart, lungs, stomach and intestines), and a higher feed consumption in lactating animals.

Relationship between BMR and visceral organ size: The close relationship between basal metabolic rate and visceral organ size is highlighted in laboratory mice that have been subjected to divergent selection for a high and low basal metabolic rate (Ksiazek *et al.*, 2004). Food consumption was greater for high BMR mice, and organ weights were also greater when expressed either as absolute weight or as portion of lean body mass. Greater liver weights were associated with greater BMR. The fact that BW did not differ between these lines of mice but BMR was clearly different indicates the importance of visceral tissue to the whole body maintenance requirement.

Selection of animals for low maintenance requirement

The coefficient of variation for maintenance for cows under controlled conditions is 8 to 10% (Van Es, 1961). Therefore, this variation could represent an opportunity to select animals with an inherently low maintenance requirement, and thus existence of a high potential efficiency for channeling nutrients to milk or tissue gain.

Effects of early life events on maintenance requirements

Considerable data indicate that events during certain critical periods of gestation can have a lasting impact on the metabolism of the offspring (Barker and Clark, 1997; McMillen *et al.*, 2001). The fetal programming hypothesis of metabolic diseases has evolved from epidemiological data that linked low birth weight, maternal nutrition, and increased prevalence of adult disease (Barker and Clark, 1997).

It is becoming increasingly obvious that epigenetic inheritance, or non-DNA based forms of heritability, may also be part of the fetal programming puzzle (Bogdarina *et al.*, 2004). It appears that a portion of these changes may involve alterations in BMR. Although these effects have not been specifically documented for dairy cattle, the available evidence suggests that the potential exists in this regard.

A study in mature human subjects identified a correlation with body composition and energy expenditure that is linked to fetal growth and birth weight (Kensara *et al.*, 2006). Specifically, low birth weight individuals displayed less fat free body mass as adults and had lower resting energy expenditure. Similar programming effects may exist for dairy cattle and may impact requirements for maintenance, production, or both (Donkin, 2008).

II. Precision feeding of dairy cows to improve nitrogen efficiency

Dairy cattle diets can be adjusted to improve nitrogen efficiency. Precision feeding reduces N and P inputs to the levels required to maintain optimum production, resulting in 20-40% reductions in the nutrient content of manure.

It has been demonstrated that through proper feeding management practices and careful nutritional formulation, N inputs can be reduced without compromising animal performance.

A close matching of diet to nutritional requirements of the animal, feeding only enough rumen undegraded protein (RUP) to meet cows' metabolizable protein requirements, reducing particle size to increase ruminal digestion of grain starch and increase microbial protein formation optimizes microbial protein synthesis, maximizes feed N conversion into milk and minimizes urinary N excretion.

Urea-N recycling Process

In animals, ammonia is generated in the gastrointestinal tract (GIT) lumen (rumen, small intestines, lower gut) from microbial activity. In ruminants, however, ammonia-N represents from 37 to 66% of the total N resources (amino acid-N and ammonia-N) absorbed. Absorbed ammonia-N is converted to urea by the liver, with the urea either excreted into urine or recycled to the rumen for use in microbial protein synthesis. The extent that absorbed ammonia is partitioned between these two fates is variable and largely unpredictable. There is much greater potential to improve N efficiency of ruminants through a better understanding of the urea recycling process. Ammonia utilization can be improved and thus urea excretion can be minimized.

Factors that affect urea-N recycling and utilization in ruminants

Urea is recycled to the rumen through plasma, endogenous secretions and saliva and this process of N recycling is of tremendous importance to ruminants. The extent that urea-N recycles 'from rumen to liver to rumen' is highly dependent upon prevailing conditions in the rumen (rumen ammonia concentration and rumen pH), and type of fermentation characteristics promoted by dietary feed ingredients.

Dietary protein intake: In general, at low protein intakes and when low quality roughage diets are fed, ruminants tend to have lower blood concentrations of urea, lower urinary urea excretion and increased transfer of urea to the GIT (Huntington, 1989; Marini and Van Amburgh, 2003). Archibeque *et al.* (2001) evaluated urea kinetics and N metabolism and concluded that the efficiency of N use is greater at low N intakes even though the absolute movements of N through the body (i.e. urea flux) increased with N intake.

Energy intake and fermentability of the diet: Increasing the fermentable carbohydrate fraction of the diet (supplemental grain, starch, dried pulp and sucrose) increases urea recycling to the rumen (Kennedy and Milligan, 1980), since they significantly increase urea degradation in the rumen. This response may be due to a combination of factors including a reduction in rumen ammonia concentration, and an increase in the quantity and rate of fermentation of dietary organic matter in the rumen (Kennedy and Milligan, 1980).

Enhancing nitrogen efficiency in lactating dairy cows

Numerous studies show that dairy cows utilize feed CP (N x 6.25) much more efficiently than other ruminant livestock but still excrete about 2 to 3 times more N in manure than in milk. Inefficient N utilization necessitates feeding large amounts of supplemental protein, increasing milk production costs, and contributing to environmental N pollution (Glen Broderick, 2005).

Several feeding strategies have been evaluated with the focus on improving N efficiency. All these improvements in efficiency should lead to reduce feed costs associated with expensive protein supplements.

Use of milk urea nitrogen (MUN) as a practical tool for monitoring herd performance

The NRC (2001) Dairy publication proposes that metabolizable protein (MP) be used for ration formulation rather than CP. Metabolizable protein is basically the sum of microbial protein and RUP. When supplies of RDP and rumen undegradable protein (RUP) are balanced for milk production, plasma urea will fall within a specific range for a group of cows. In addition, milk urea is as useful as blood urea to monitor protein status. Urea moves into milk via passive diffusion from blood and rapidly equilibrates with blood values.

Factors that affect efficiency of feed N transformation into milk

Ruminants obtain the metabolizable protein (MP) required for maintenance and production from microbial protein synthesized in the rumen plus dietary protein that escapes the rumen undegraded.

1. Optimizing synthesis of microbial protein in the rumen

Ammonia level: Ruminal bacteria utilize peptides, amino acids (AA) and ammonia for protein synthesis. *In vitro* research showed that microbial protein formation was not improved by ammonia-N concentrations greater than 5 mg/dL (Satter and Slyter, 1974). However, *in situ* studies suggested that ammonia-N levels as high as 20 mg/dL (Mehrez *et al.*, 1977) may be required to maximize carbohydrate digestion in the rumen.

2. Optimizing amount and composition of rumen degraded protein: practising phase feeding

Dietary CP that is not utilized by the cow gets excreted largely as urinary N, regardless of whether the CP is digested in the rumen or the intestine. Wu and Satter (2000) conducted a study for the entire lactation period following the phase feeding of protein. They found that the dietary CP regime supporting optimum yield of fat-corrected milk (FCM) over the whole lactation involved feeding 17.4% CP for the first 16-weeks after calving, followed by 16.0% CP for the remaining 28 weeks; greater than those levels of CP reduced the milk and protein yields. Depressed production at higher CP may have occurred because of dilution of dietary energy, and because of the metabolic cost of excreting excess N as urea (NRC, 1989).

3. Feeding enough RUP

Compared to an isonitrogenous diet supplemented with urea, much greater milk production was obtained when 1 of 3 true proteins (cottonseed meal<canola meal<soybean meal) that differed in RUP and AA content (Brito and Broderick, 2007) were fed. Enhanced production on different sources likely was related to the AA pattern of the RUP being complementary to microbial protein (Broderick, 1994).

4. Balancing the rations for amino acids

Nitrogen excretion is a function of protein feeding. Reducing dietary protein decreases nitrogen excretion, and it may—but does not have to—reduce milk yield. Reducing dietary protein, while concomitantly balancing for amino acids, can result in an equivalent or greater milk yield.

Feeding low CP rations to dairy cows without affecting their milk yield: Dairy producers should consider lowering crude protein (CP) levels in rations for two primary reasons. One is to improve profitability by increasing the efficiency of converting feed nitrogen (N) intake to milk N output while maintaining milk production. A second reason is that feeding lower CP rations decreases the excretion of N to the environment. On many of farms, there is an opportunity to lower ration CP by 0.5 to 1.5 units with minimal risk of lowering milk production (Chase *et al.*, 2009). A number of trials testing various levels of CP in diets were conducted and found that, generally, there were no increases in yields of milk, fat-corrected milk, or protein with more than 16.5% dietary CP. In one trial, reducing CP to 15.6%, but adding rumen undegraded protein (RUP) as heated soybean meal (SBM), did not support production equal to 16.6% CP. However, fish meal, especially low soluble fish meal, and canola meal were found to be more effective sources of RUP than SBM or cottonseed meal.

Importance of rumen-protected methionine: Methionine and lysine are the essential AA most often limiting for lactating dairy cows (Schwab, 1996). Responses to rumen-protected methionine (RPM) have been more consistent than to rumen-protected lysine (Armentano *et al.*, 1997). The results of several trials (Broderick *et al.*, 2008; Broderick *et al.*, 2009) confirm that RPM supplements will correct the methionine limitation without adding dietary CP beyond 15.8%.

Milk N efficiency (MNE)

Milk N efficiency (MNE) is one index that can be used to assess the efficiency of N use in the dairy cow. This index is simply the ratio of the quantity of N excreted via the milk as a percent of the quantity of feed N consumed. The MNE values observed in commercial dairy herds usually ranges between 20 and 35%. This implies that 65 to 80% of the consumed N is excreted in the manure. As ration CP increases, the MNE value tends to decrease.

The following salient findings can be drawn from a research trial in which rations ranging from 13.5 to 19.4% CP were fed (Olmos Colmenero and Broderick, 2006).

- The quantity of N excreted in the milk changed very little for all levels of ration CP used in this trial.
- Total manure N excreted per day increased as ration N intake went up.
- The portion of the total manure N found in the faecal portion varied little with increasing ration CP levels.
- As total N excretion went up with higher levels of ration CP, urinary N was the main route of excreting excess N.
- Milk N efficiency decreased as ration CP increased.

Formulating diets for achieving efficient and economical milk production

Formulating diets for specific target levels is a fundamental and practical approach for achieving efficient and economical milk production (Dave Byers, 2007). Formulate for specific nutrients, which can be measured in a laboratory.

1. *Fibre carbohydrates:* The most important nutrient to formulate for in dairy rations is the fibre. It is necessary for the health of the rumen, the health of the animal, and the efficiency of fermentation. Formulate for 32 - 34% NDF. This is higher than many recommendations and slightly higher than the NRC (2001). Furthermore, aim for effective NDF.
2. *Nonfibre carbohydrates (NFC):* After meeting the fibre requirement, the objective is to liberally feed glucose precursors, primarily starches and

sugars, to drive milk production. This produces the following cascade of events: starches & sugars >>> propionate (rumen) >>> glucose (liver) >>> lactose (mammary gland). Milk production varies directly with the production of lactose, because it is the osmotic regulator of milk yield. Optimizing the levels of starch and sugars is necessary for the best possible milk performance (Broderick and Radloff, 2004).

3. *Protein:* Formulate for balancing for three protein fractions. First, balance for RDP: It is as follows: RDP = NFC (lb) / 3.30. Target for a balance of -0.30 to -0.50 lb/d. The reason for a negative balance is that it permits feeding diets lower in crude protein. Second, formulate for the amino acid, lysine. The target level is a balance of +4.0 to +8.0 g/d. Lastly, formulate for the amino acid, methionine. The target level is a balance of -2.0 to -4.0 g/d. The typical strategy is to formulate diets with feeds that are relatively rich in rumen undegraded, lysine, and if necessary or beneficial, supplement with rumen protected, methionine.
4. *Fat:* Since fats are not sources of fermentable energy for rumen microbes, use minimal levels of fat. There is, however, a level of fat needed to support reproductive efficiency (3.0 – 5.0% is adequate). Where possible, follow fat levels in the lower part of this range (3.0 – 4.0%). The literature does tend to show two disadvantages of liberally fat feeding (>5.0%). One, DMI is generally depressed, especially with Ca salts of FA. This seems to be the result of unsaturated fat increasing satiety and reducing gut motility. Two, protein test is generally depressed 1 – 2 points.
5. *Ash:* Try to restrict the level of ash below 7% in rations. This gives ration space in order to feed extra fermentable carbohydrates.

References

Archibeque, S.L., J.C. Burns, and G.B. Huntington. (2001). Urea flux in beef steers: Effects of forage species and fertilization. *J. Anim. Sci.* 79: 193-1943.

Armentano, L.E., S.J. Bertics, and G.A. Ducharme. (1997). Response of lactating cows to methionine or methionine plus lysine added to high protein diets based on alfalfa and heated soybeans. *J. Dairy Sci.* 80: 1194-1199.

Baldwin, R.L. (1995). Modeling Ruminant Digestion and Metabolism. Chapman and Hall, London, UK.

Barker, D.J.P., and P.M. Clark. (1997). Fetal undernutrition and disease in later life. Rev. Reprod. 2: 105–112.

Bogdarina, I., H.C. Murphy, S.P. Burns, and A.J. Clark. (2004). Investigation of the role of epigenetic modification of the rat glucokinase gene in fetal programming. *Life Sci.* 74: 1407-1415.

Brito, A.F. and G.A. Broderick. (2007). Effects of different protein supplements on milk production and nutrient utilization in lactating dairy cows. *J. Dairy Sci.* 90: 1816-1827.

Broderick, G.A. (1994). Quantifying forage protein quality. In G.C. Fahey, Jr., M.D. Collins, D.R.

Mertens and L.E. Moser (ed.) Forage Quality, Evaluation, and Utilization. American Soc. Agron., Madison, WI, pp. 200-228.

Broderick, G.A. (2005). Feeding dairy cows to minimize nitrogen excretion. Page 137. In: 2005 Proceedings Tri-State Dairy Nutrition Conference, Fort Wayne, IN.

Broderick, G.A., and W.J. Radloff. (2004). Effect of molasses supplementation on the production of lactating dairy cows fed diets based on alfalfa and corn silage. *J. Dairy Sci.* 87: 2997-3009.

Broderick, G. A., M. J. Stevenson, R. A. Patton, N. E. Lobos and J. J. Olmos Colmenero. (2008). Supplementing rumen-protected methionine to reduce dietary crude protein in dairy cows. *J. Dairy Sci.* 91: 1092-1102.

Broderick, G. A., M. J. Stevenson and R. A. Patton. (2009). Effect of dietary crude protein, rumen-undegraded protein and rumen-protected methionine on milk production of lactating dairy cows. *J. Dairy Sci.* 92: in press.

Chase, L.E.,R.J.Higgs and M.E.Van Amburgh. (2009). Feeding low crude protein rations to dairy cows-opportunities and challenges. Page 220. In: 2009 Proceedings of Cornell Nutrition Conference For Feed Manufacturers, 71st Meeting: October 20–22, 2009 DoubleTree Hotel Syracuse, East Syracuse, New York.

Dave Byers. (2007). Practically dropping protein of diets to reduce nitrogen excretion.Page 98. In: Proceedings of Four-State Dairy Nutrition and Management Conference, Dubuque, Iowa.

Donkin, S.S. (2008). Feeding to Minimize Nutrient Requirements for Maintenance and Increase Milk Production. Page 91. In: 2008 Proceedings of Tri-State Dairy Nutrition Conference Fort Wayne, IN.

Huntington, G.B. (1989). Hepatic urea synthesis and site and rate of urea removal from blood of beef steers fed alfalfa hay or a high concentrate diet. *Can. J. Anim. Sci.* 69: 215-223.

Kennedy, P.M., and L.P. Milligan. (1980). The degradation and utilization of endogenous urea in the gastrointestinal tract of ruminants: A review. *Can. J. Anim. Sci.* 60: 205-221.

Kensara, O.A., S.A. Wooton, D.I. Phillips, M. Patel, D.J. Hoffman, A.A. Jackson, and M. Elia. (2006). Substrate-energy metabolism and metabolic risk factors for cardiovascular disease in relation to fetal growth and adult body composition. *Am. J. Physiol. Endocrinol. Metab.* 291: E365-371.

Ksiazek, A., M. Konarzewski, and I.B. Lapo. (2004). Anatomic and energetic correlates of divergent selection for basal metabolic rate in laboratory mice. *Physiol. Biochem. Zool.* 77: 890-899.

Lenis, N.P., P. Bikker, J. van der Meulen, J.T. van Diepen, J.G. Bakker, and A.W. Jongbloed. (1996). Effect of dietary neutral detergent fiber on ileal digestibility and portal flux of nitrogen and amino acids and on nitrogen utilization in growing pigs. *J. Anim. Sci.* 74: 2687-2699.

Marini, J.C., and M.E. Van Amburgh. (2003). Nitrogen metabolism and recycling in Holstein heifers. *J. Anim. Sci.* 2003. 81:545-552.

McMillen, I.C., M.B. Adams, J.T. Ross, C.L. Coulter, G. Simonetta, J.A. Owens, J.S. Robinson, and L.J. Edwards. (2001). Fetal growth restriction: Adaptations and consequences. *Reproduction.* 122:195–204.

Mehrez, A. Z., E. R. Ørskov and I. McDonald. (1977). Rates of rumen fermentation in relation to ammonia concentration. *Brit. J. Nutr.* 38: 437-443.

National Research Council. (1989). Nutrient Requirements of Dairy Cattle. 6th rev. ed. Natl.Acad. Sci., Washington, DC.

National Research Council. (1996). Nutrient requirements of beef cattle. 6th rev. ed. Natl. Acad. Sci., Washington, DC.

National Research Council. (2001). Nutrient requirements of dairy cattle. 7th rev. ed. Natl. Acad. Sci., Washington, DC.

Olmos Colmenero, J.J. and G.A. Broderick. (2006). Effect of dietary crude protein concentration on milk production and nitrogen utilization in lactating dairy cows. *J. Dairy Sci.* 89: 1704-1712.

Reddy, D.V. (2011). Precision animal nutrition for pigs: A tool for economic and eco-friendly animal production. Chapter contributed in the book entitled "Advanced Animal Nutrition for developing countries" U.R.Mehra et al.(eds) published by M/s Satish Serial publishing house, Delhi.

Reddy, D. V. and N. Krishna. (2009). Precision animal nutrition: A tool for economic and eco-friendly animal production in ruminants. *Livestock Research for Rural Development. Volume 21, 23 pages Article #36.* Retrieved from http://www.lrrd.org/lrrd21/3/redd21036.htm

Reddy, D.V. and D. Narahari. (2011). Precision Animal Nutrition: A tool for economic and eco-friendly poultry production. *World's Poultry Science Journal* (In Press).

Reynolds, C.K., H.F. Tyrrell, and P.J. Reynolds. (1991). Effects of diet forage-to-concentrate ratio and intake on energy metabolism in growing beef heifers: net nutrient metabolism by visceral tissues. *J. Nutr.* 121:1004-1015.

Satter, L. D. and L. L. Slyter. (1974). Effect of ammonia concentration on rumen microbial protein production in vitro. *Brit. J. Nutr.* 32: 199-208.

Schwab, C.G. (1996). Rumen-protected amino acids for dairy cattle: Progress towards determininglysine and methionine requirements. *Anim. Feed Sci. Tech.* 59: 87-101.

Speakman, J.R., E. Krol, and M.S. Johnson. (2004). The functional significance of individual variation in basal metabolic rate. *Physiol. Biochem. Zool.* 77: 900-915.

Tyrrell, H.F., C.K. Reynolds, and H.D. Baxter. (1991). Utilization of dietary energy by Jerseycompared to Holstein cows during the lactation cycle.

□□□

47

Estimation of Microbial Protein Supply to Ruminants based on Urinary Excretion of Purine Derivatives : Prospects and Limitations

A.K. VERMA
Principal Scientist (Animal Nutrition), Swine Production Farm
Indian Veterinary Research Institute, Izatnagar-243 122, U.P., India

Introduction

The small and medium farmers in developing countries like India have limited available resources for feeding their livestock. Thus, any strategy for improvement in livestock production requires efforts to maximize the efficiency of utilization of available feed resources. The utilization of poor quality roughages as feed for ruminants depends mainly on the efficiency of microbial fermentation in their fore-stomach. Moreover in such roughage-based diets, rumen microbes constitute main source of digestible protein to the host animal (Soejono *et al.*, 1999). Rumen microbial biomass provides the majority of amino acids that are utilized by host ruminants for their tissue maintenance, growth and production (Jayasuriya, 1999). Therefore, knowledge of the microbial contribution to the nutrition of the host animal is essential to develop feed supplementation strategies for improving ruminant production.

It has been extremely difficult to determine the microbial protein contribution to ruminant nutrition (Nolan, 1999). The methods generally used for determining microbial protein production depend on the external markers such as ^{15}N, ^{32}P and ^{35}S, and internal markers such as diamino pimelic acid (DAPA), L-alanine and ribonucleic acid (RNA). However, the need to use post-ruminally cannulated animals, and complicated and error-associated procedures to determine digesta flow are major limitations in these methods. Furthermore, the process of utilizing markers or isotopes is complex, tedious and difficult to practice extensively under field conditions (Broderick and Merchen, 1992). The method based on measurement of purine derivatives (PD) in urine over comes the disadvantages of the above methods. The idea of using microbial purine compounds as a specific marker for the rumen microbial biomass was suggested by McDonald in 1954. It is simple (only requires a total collection of urine) and non invasive (does not require any surgical preparation of the animal) and has the potential to be further simplified for use under farm conditions (Ojeda and Parra, 1999).

Purines are heterocyclic rings with nitrogenous bases with varying functional groups. The purine bases, adenine and guanine are found in both DNA and RNA. Microorganisms have high concentrations of purine containing compounds (RNA and DNA) relative to concentrations in plant and mammalian cells. Furthermore, rumen microbes in general, rapidly degrade purines in diets. They are, therefore, likely to be present in only negligible amounts in digesta leaving the rumen, therefore, the purines present in digesta entering the small intestine is almost totally of microbial origin. These purine components are then metabolised in ruminants to form purine derivatives (PD). The term purine derivatives refer to the sum of allantoin, uric acid, xanthine and hypoxanthine. All four compounds are excreted in the urine of sheep, goat, llamas, red deer and camels; but xanthine and hypoxanthine are virtually absent from urine of cattle, buffaloes and yaks (Chen and Gomes, 1992; Chen *et al.*, 1990). In ruminants hypoxanthine and xanthine are converted to uric acid by xanthine oxidase, and uric acid is further converted to allantoin by uricase. The presence of high activities of xanthine oxidase in cattle and buffalo plasma leads to the complete conversion of hypoxanthine and xanthine to uric acid (Chen *et al.*, 1996). Since microbial enzymes in rumen rapidly degrade purines of dietary and endogenous materials, so any purines present in the digesta in the small intestine can be expected to be only of microbial origin and can be considered to be specific markers for the microbial fraction (Nolan, 1999). Therefore, with an understanding of how urinary excretion response to purine absorption, the microbial purine outflow from the rumen and hence microbial nitrogen supply to the animal can be estimated from the measured excretion of PD in the urine (Chen *et al.*, 1990). Prediction equations based on urinary purine derivatives (PD) excretion rate as an index to predict rumen microbial protein production have been developed for European cattle (Chen *et al.*, 1990; Verbic *et al.*, 1990), sheep (Fujihara *et al.*, 1991; Balcells *et al.*, 1991), Indian buffaloes (Dipu, 2004) and crossbred calves (George, 2004; Singh, 2004). The important parameters required for this are daily PD excretion through urine, endogenous PD excretion and the proportion of plasma PD excreted in the urine, or the recovery of exogenous PD from the urine. However, the relationships between microbial yield of purines from the rumen and urinary excretion of purine derivatives may differ between different breeds and species of ruminants (IAEA, 1999). With estimates of daily urine volume and urinary concentrations of PD, the total daily urinary excretion of PD can be determined and used to predict the rates of absorption of purines from the small intestine using relationships developed for individual ruminant species. Since only urine is needed, an estimation of microbial protein supply can be incorporated into nitrogen balance and digestibility trials without much additional labour inputs. The advantages of this technique are its non-invasive nature and relative ease of use.

Despite major progress having been made in modeling the quantitative response of urinary PD excretion to purine absorption from the small intestine, some factors that affect PD excretion are still not completely understood. Although consistent purine input-output relationships have been observed for European cattle and sheep, there are variations among animal individuals of the same species/breed and much larger variations among different animal species and requires further investigation. More extensive studies are required to examine the effect of renal physiology on PD excretion, with a focus on identifying the factors, which affect the renal excretion of plasma PD. The effect of GFR and tubule exchange may be further studied. The species difference in purine metabolism (including profile of xanthine oxidase) is an interesting subject on its own right. Differences may be viewed in the context of animal adaptation to their environments.

The development of newer methods to help defining the purine input-output relationship is also required. So far techniques based on post-ruminal infusion of purine bases have been used, but these techniques are complex and require surgical intervention of experimental animals. It will be ideal if simpler and more accurate techniques can be developed. The direction shall be to use radioactive or stable isotopic tracers to define the parameters for the already developed models. New techniques for determination of the endogenous contribution of PD in the urine also await development. Again, the use of ^{15}N- tracers may play a role. More work needs to be carried out to validate the results of the estimates of microbial N supply from PD excretion. Moreover, in order to achieve a more accurate estimation ratio of purine-N: total-N in rumen microbes, will need to be defined better under local conditions. A system for the field application of spot urine measurement needs to be developed. Therefore, future research in this area will be in two directions. One direction is to develop methods for field application. Simple, robust and inexpensive methods for determination of PD are required, so that the analysis work can be done in extension or veterinary laboratories. Another direction is to develop methods for purine metabolism studies. The method should be accurate and able to detect concentration of micro gram per litre level.

References

Balcells, J., Guada, J. A., Castrillo, C. and Gasa, J. (1991). Urinary excretion of allantoin and allantoin precursors by sheep after different rates of purine infusion into duodenum. *J. Agri. Sci. Cambridge*. 116: 309-317.

Broderick, G.A. and Merchen, N. R. (1992). Markers for quantifying microbial protein synthesis in the rumen. *J. Dairy Sci.* 75: 2618.

Chen, X. B. and Gomes, M. J. (1992). Estimation of microbial protein supply to sheep and cattle based on urinary excretion of purine derivatives- *An overview of the technical details.* Rowett Research Institue, University of Aberdeen U.K.

Chen, X. B., Orskov, E. R. and Hovell F.D. DeB. (1990). Excretion of purine derivatives by ruminants: endogenous excretion, differences between cattle and sheep. *Brit. J. Nutr.* 63: 121-129.

Chen, X. B., Samarweera, L., Kyle, D. J., Orskov, E. R. and Abeygunawardene, H. (1996). Urinary excretion of purine derivatives and tissue xanthine oxidase activity in buffaloes, with special reference to differences between buffaloes and *Bos taurus*. *Brit. J. Nutr.* 75: 397-407.

Dipu, M.T. (2004). Effect of different levels of feed intake on purine derivative excretion and nutrient utilization in buffaloes. MVSc Thesis. Deemed University, IVRI, Izatnagar, India.

Fujihara, T., Matsui, T. and Harumoto, T. (1991). Urinary excretion of purine derivatives and blood plasma level of allantoin in sheep and goats during fasting. *In: Proceedings of the Sixth International Symposium on Protein Metabolism and Nutrition*, Herning, Denmark. pp. 170-172.

George, S.K. (2004). Effect of plane of Nutrition on purine derivatives excretion and nutrient utilization in crossbred calves. MVSc Thesis. Deemed University, IVRI, Izatnagar, India.

International Atomic Energy Agency (1999). Nuclear based technologies for estimating microbial protein supply in ruminant livestock. International Atomic Energy Agency *(IAEA) -TECDOC*-1093, Vienna. 119p.

Jayasuriya, M. C. N. (1999). Summary of the co-ordinated research project on development, standardization and validation of nuclear based technologies for estimating microbial protein supply in ruminant livestock for improving productivity. *IAEA-TECDOC*-1093. Vienna, pp. 1-6.

Nolan, J. V. (1999). Prediction of rumen microbial outflow based on urinary excretion derivatives. In: Nuclear based technologies for estimating microbial protein supply in ruminant livestock. *IAEA-TECDOC*- 1093. Vienna, pp. 9-19.

Singh, M. (2004). Prediction of microbial protein production from urinary excretion of purine derivatives in crossbred cattle. MVSc Thesis. Deemed University, IVRI, Izatnagar, India.

□□□

48

Clinical Nutrition Approaches for Health and Welfare of Ruminants under Tropical Conditions

A.K. PATTANAIK[1]* S.K. MISHRA[2] AND K. SHARMA[3]
Division of Animal Nutrition
Indian Veterinary Research institute, Izatnagar – 243 122
[1]Senior Scientist, Clinical & Pet Nutrition Laboratory, Division of Animal Nutrition, Indian Veterinary Research institute, Izatnagar – 243 122; [2]Associate Professor, Department of Animal Nutrition, College of Veterinary Science & Animal Husbandry, Orissa University of Agriculture & Technology, Bhubaneswar – 751 003; [3]Assistant Director General (HRD), Indian Council of Agricultural Research, Krishi Anusandhan Bhawan-II, Pusa, New Delhi – 110 012

Introduction

Clinical nutrition is defined as the potential use of diet (and nutritional supplements) as a means to augment health and prevent disease. The prime objective of the clinical nutritionist is to sustain the nutritional health of the animal. This could be achieved by selecting the suitable diet and recommending the most appropriate feeding strategy to suit the animal's physiological state and/or disease. As such clinical nutrition encompasses two areas viz. preventive nutrition and therapeutic nutrition. Preventive nutrition recognizes and compensates for deficiencies of key nutrients that can eventually lead to multiple and possibly irreversible health problems. Correct and balanced nutrition is the foundation for good health of animals. For maximal effectiveness, feeding management must allow for the biochemical individuality of each animal, especially so in situations of illness. Therapeutic nutrition, on the other hand, is the practice of using feed or nutrients such as vitamins, minerals, oils, and amino acids in an attempt to alter the course of a disease process. In other words, it is the dietary management of clinically ill animals, with the primary goal of (a) optimizing nutrient intake, (b) minimizing catabolism (utilization of body stores), and (c) maximizing immune competence and recovery process. To sum up, clinical nutrition of livestock aims at use of principles of nutritional approaches for correction of nutrient deficiency or excess, replacement of nutrients for amelioration, and feeding of nutrients for inhibition of disease. In case of sick animals, it involves provision of nutritional support as adjunct to therapy facilitating replenishment of tissue stores, improvement of immune system, and prevention of death from cachexia.

Clinical Nutrition Scenario in Tropics

Nutrition represents one of the most serious limitations to livestock production in most of the tropics including India as feed resources are inadequate in both quality and quantity. When compared vis-à-vis the trend of availability of feed resources, the enormous ruminant population would be expected to continue to face the deficit of feeds and nutrients in the coming years to the same extent, as it is today. Hence, feed / nutritional security is a serious issue related to animal welfare which could very well be expected to have a confounding effect on the clinical nutrition approaches for farm animals in the tropics. An associated issue, at least in veterinary practice typical to developing countries, is that most of the clients (animal owners) do not have background knowledge of scientific animal production. In this scenario, use of principles of clinical nutrition in veterinary practice to ensure health and welfare of farmed animals requires additional knowledge, skill and logistical preparedness that may seem elementary to veterinarians.

There is at present a strong interest in the relationship between nutrition and health in farm animals. It has been well recognized that activation of the immune system will impact on nutrient use and requirements of animals. However, this knowledge is rarely applied in veterinary practice, more so under Indian conditions. Obviously, the same diet cannot be suggested to animals differing in their health status. In other words, the diet of a diseased animal must not be the same as that of a healthy animal. Proper nutrition can minimize the incidence or help control metabolic, infectious, and reproductive disorders in animals. Accordingly, a number of nutritional supplements and feeding management strategies can be used as supportive treatment for various metabolic and infectious diseases. In this context, the dietary management of animal(s) in potential risks of developing illness or proneness to disease/stress situations is also equally important.

Nutrition for health

Health is a general term that describes the overall well-being and condition of an animal, and can be defined as the absence of disease. It is a subjective matter, typically determined by visual observation of the animal (clinical examinations), and often coupled with various clinical measurements (e.g., rectal temperature or serum clinical profiles) to aid in confirmation of disease states and diagnosis.

The consumers' demand for wholesome food, with limited or no use of antibiotics, growth hormones and synthetic performance enhancers is a challenge to animal scientists in general and nutritionists in particular. Quite appropriately, a healthy food can come only from a healthy animal. And to maintain an animal's health by protecting itself from various infectious and non-infectious health problems is an onerous task. This applies equally to both intensive as well as extensive system of livestock production. Dietary manipulation could constitute one of the important and prime approaches in the control and/or prevention of these non-infectious diseases; formulation and use of appropriate diets fortified with components essential for appropriate defense mechanisms would not only take care of proper maintenance of health but also growth, production and performance in livestock.

Using nutrition to increase animal's defense against infection has been a recent area of research. In this context it is the *feeding for health* rather than *feeding for production* is gradually taking precedence in livestock production systems. It is argued that once the health is assured, the animal can take care of the production, given the fact that it has genetic capability to do so. Another important recent development in this field has been the *welfare* issue of livestock, which is set to become a prime criterion for any production system. In this scenario, ensuring stress-free and disease-free animal production will be the key approach. With the advancement of knowledge, it is becoming increasingly clear that nutrition plays crucial roles in maintaining an efficient immune system which is of paramount importance in maintaining the balance between health (read production) and disease. Hence, nutrition for health and welfare of livestock constitutes an important area in animal science research.

Changing perspective of animal nutrition

Conventional animal nutrition usually considers the dietary inputs in terms of production responses without considering the importance of cellular nutrition and its absolute importance in the animal's life-maintaining metabolic functions, which ultimately ensures effective productive and reproductive performances. The emphasis instead must be on what dietary inputs affect the cells that are ultimately responsible for bringing about the production response. It is no longer adequate to feed the animal for a desired production output without first determining what the implications of the feed and the production activity has on the entire body (health). In many situations performance is achieved by conventional nutritional inputs usually at the expense of creating some dysfunction in some structure, tissue, organ system or metabolic pathway. Hence achieving desirable performance output without a resultant decrease in health or lifespan constitutes a more prudent use of the science of nutrition.

Too often conventional medicine fails to realize that chemical therapy will not work unless body is innately capable of responding appropriately; excellent nutrition and environmental conditions ensure an animal the best possible foundation for an efficient and effective defense strategy against day-to-day challenges. Preventive therapies, practices and factors that deny an invader the opportunity to establish a destructive presence are the best defense against compromised health. The best prevention unquestionably is to optimize the immune system, and this could be best accomplished by appropriate nutrition and feeding strategies.

Consequence of disease on nutrition

Recent research has demonstrated that endemic diseases negatively impact livestock performance without causing obvious clinical signs of disease. Infectious agents induce an immune response designed to remove the offending agent from the body. In turn, the immune system induces a cascade of effects, many of them detrimental to growth, on the animal's metabolic system. It is therefore suggested that technologies that minimize activation of the animal's immune system will enhance the rate and efficiency of growth and improve lean deposition in the carcass (Murphy, 2002). Studies have shown that, during a health challenge, immune substances cause a metabolic response to the infection that shifts nutrients away from tissue growth to support the immune response. Even when the challenge is subclinical in nature, the effect is sufficient to disrupt normal metabolism and cause losses in performance.

Exposure of an animal to any substances, whether pathogenic or nonpathogenic, results in an immune response from the inflammatory cells in the blood and tissues. The substances that are released activate the immune system, causing reduced appetite, an increase in basal metabolic rate, a shift in the use of both ingested and stored nutrients by the body, and the possibility of a slight elevation in body temperature. However, sometimes there is no obvious sign that disease is present.

When animals are challenged by disease, protein synthesis decreases while protein breakdown increases. The balance between synthesis and breakdown shifts toward breakdown as a result of at least three things: (a) reduced feed intake - the body's supplies of amino acids are gradually consumed as the body's defenses fight the infection, (b) the immune response requires the consumption of amino acids to provide the building blocks to make immune compounds, like antibodies, and (c) the amino acid composition of muscle does not match the amino acid needs of immune products, so the body is forced to break down a disproportionate amount of muscle to meet the amino acids needs of the immune system. Consequently, the protein losses during an immunological challenge are greater than what can be maintained by feed intake, an effect that is compounded when feed intake is reduced. In addition to skeletal muscle, the intestinal tract may also provide a source of amino acids to mount an immune response. Research in other animals has shown that the body can initiate protein breakdown to pull nutrients from tissues having a lower priority, making them available for use by the immune system. In essence, the body will literally consume itself in the process of prioritizing resources in its fight against pathogens. In addition to effects on protein synthesis, the processes initiated by an immune challenge also cause major shifts in fat metabolism. Typically, as energy is consumed during periods of immune activation, fat reserves are broken down as a source of energy to feed the immune system.

As a consequence of the metabolic and physiological effects of disease, animals endemically infected with disease agents suffer from poorer growth performance, as reflected in reduced average daily feed intake, average daily gain, and feed efficiency. All pathogens that cause an immune response have the potential to disrupt metabolic processes and interfere with nutrient utilization.

Metabolic effects of host defence in livestock

Exposure of host to infectious agents, trauma or stressors stimulates the immune system. During this defence response, homeostatic balances can be modified through a process called *homeorrhesis*, which redistributes blood flow and mobilizes nutrients to facilitate both whole body and local tissue defence. A central component to this response is the activation of acute phase response (APR); the principal activators being the pro-inflammatory cytokines, interleukin (IL)-1 α/β, IL-6, tumor necrosis factor (TNF) α and the type I interferons (IFN) α / α (Colditz, 2004). An important feature of APR is the overriding effects the pro-inflammatory cytokines on the anabolic effects of insulin, growth hormone and insulin like growth factor (IGF)-1. In the context of livestock production, the activation of APR could lead to reduced utilization of nutrients by tissues producing fibre, meat, milk and skin. In addition to the changed profile of nutrient utilization by production tissues, there can be direct metabolic cost of immune activation. Metabolic rate is elevated by 5-13% per degree of fever, while energy requirements of leukocytes increase

2-3 folds per cell following their activation. Thus a reduction in growth rate during immune activation will depend not only on homeorrhetic responses affecting accretion of nutrients in the production tissues but also on costs associated with pathology during infection. Overall, the competition between the tissues of the immune system and the production tissues for utilization of nutrients, in the resource allocation theory, leads to a negative correlation between production and immune activation or disease resistance.

Clinical nutrition approaches for ensuring health

As already discussed in the introduction section, the scope of clinical nutrition in farm animal practice is far reaching, involving both preventive and therapeutic nutrition. While therapeutic nutrition more or less lies in the domain of medicine specialists, it is the preventive nutrition which can be used as a clinical nutrition tool by animal nutritionists to effectively (a) prevent onset of a disease, (b) moderate the course of an imminent illness, (c) expedite the recovery from a disease, and/or (d) reduce the convalescence period post-recovery. While a detailed discussion on the therapeutic role of nutrients is out of the scope of the present discussion, effort has been made in the following section to highlight some of the preventive approaches which are typical to clinical nutrition issues pertinent to tropical/Indian conditions.

Nutrients as substrates for immune system : Dietary components have an enormous effect upon the immune system. The consequences of an impaired immune function are reduced resistance to infection, higher mortality form infection, poor performance, decreased quality of life and an increased sensitivity to environmental stressors affecting ultimately the production outputs. Proper diets consisting of bioavailable nutrients and essential bioactive molecules in precise relation to one another optimize the immune systems' ability to protect against infections by pathogens as well as non-infectious health hazards.

Table 1 : Specific role of nutrients in the immune system[1]

Nutrients	Mechanism
All nutrients	Substrates for the immune system
Iron, biotin, manganese (nutritional immunity)	Deprivation of nutrients from pathogens
Fatty acids, vitamins A, D, E	Direct regulatory effects on cells of the immune system
Energy, protein	Changing the balance of hormones that regulate immunity
Antioxidants	Reduction of pathology induced by an immune response
Non-starch polysaccharides, lectins, sugars	Physical and chemical actions of feeds in the intestines

[1]Adopted from Klasing (2003)

Although the immune system, taking into consideration the weight of all the leukocytes and their products involved in immune function, constitutes probably less than 2 per cent of the body weight, it is a vital system whose requirements must be met (Klasing, 2003). The development and maintenance of the immune system is dependent upon dietary substrates such as energy and amino acids. These substrates are necessary for the anabolic activity of the immune system's cells (leukocytes), such as proliferation and antibody production as well as the hepatic secretion of a quantum of immunologically active molecules, the acute phase proteins. All the nutrients serve the immune system by way of supplying substrates. Fatty acids and vitamins A, D and E have direct regulatory effects on the cells of the immune system. Similarly, iron, biotin and manganese play a role by being deprived from access to the pathogens. The mechanism by which nutrients modulate immunity is showed in Table 1. More importantly, all the antioxidant nutrients play a significant role by reducing the pathology induced by an immune response. The immune function may be enhanced not only by maintaining appropriate amounts of antioxidants, but also by the involvement of enzymes in aiding the production of energy, proteins, cells and hormones needed in defense mechanisms (Nockels, 1996). The understanding of how the cells of the immune system obtain their nutrients is incomplete. It appears that when leukocytes are activated, they express high levels of nutrient transporters, which allow them to easily obtain necessary nutrients even when they are at low concentrations; from muscle and other tissues. When leukocytes become activated by pathogens, they release a series of pro-inflammatory cytokines (IL-1, TNF and IL-6) that go throughout the body and redistribute nutrients, especially those from the skeletal muscle. While it usually obtains many of the required nutrients over a wide range of dietary levels, some trace nutrients like iron, copper, and zinc besides some vitamins are problematic because of their low concentrations in muscle as well as their relatively high need within the immune system.

Nutrients as antioxidants : Normal aerobic cellular metabolism in mammalians entails continuous production of reactive oxygen species such as superoxide anion radical (O^-_2), hydroxyl radical (HO^-), hydrogen peroxide (H_2O_2). Further, activity of the immune system releases a variety of noxious substances at the site of infection in order to kill the invading pathogens. For example, phagocytic granulocytes undergo respiratory burst to produce oxygen radicals to destroy the intracellular pathogens. However, these oxidative products can, in turn, damage healthy cells if they are not eliminated. Although immune system responds in a controlled way so that lethality is localized to the pathogen and not on surrounding tissues, however collateral damage to the healthy cells surrounding the site of infection is evident in many infections. Antioxidants serve to stabilize the highly reactive free radicals; thereby minimizing the damaging effect by way of maintaining the structural and functional integrity of the cells (Chew, 1995). Therefore, antioxidants are very important to immune defense and health of animals and, consequently, to their productivity.

Cells must maintain a proper balance between the levels of free radicals (pro-oxidants) and antioxidants to ensure the structural integrity of cellular components. If there is an imbalance in favour of free radicals, sensitive biological structures such as DNA, lipids and proteins could be damaged. Leukocytes, the principal cells of the immune system, are particularly more susceptible to damaging effects of free radicals because of high percentage of PUFAs in their plasma membranes an increased production of free radicals as part of their normal function (Heaton et al., 2002). From an immunological point of view, accumulating levels of DNA damage may also cause reduced cellular function that potentially leads to suboptimal immune response towards infection (Barnett and Barnett, 1998).

A variety of components, of both endogenous and exogenous (dietary) origins, make up the body's antioxidants system, matching clearly the diversity of the prooxidants. These include small molecule antioxidants (glutathione) which neutralize free radicals, enzymes which catalyze radical and peroxide quenching reactions viz. catalase, superoxide dismutase (SOD) and glutathione peroxidase (GSH-Px) and, metal binding proteins which sequester iron and copper ions that catalyze oxidative reactions, if free (Jacob, 1995). Catalase, present in peroxisomes of mammalian cells, contains Fe, and serves to destroy H_2O_2 generated by oxidase enzymes. Likewise, Zn and Cu are needed for Cu-Zn-SOD, which converts superoxide to H_2O_2 in cytosol. The H_2O_2 is then reduced to water by Se-dependent GSH-Px. This enzyme may also convert lipid peroxides to alcohols. A similar enzyme, Mn-SOD, is present in mitochondria. The amount and function of these enzymes may be limited not only by the quantity of mineral but also by protein availability; Zn and Cu are bound to the proteins metallothionein and ceruloplasmin, respectively, which have antioxidant capabilities (Nockels, 1996). Thus, essential trace elements like Fe, Cu, Zn, Mn and Se are often classified as antioxidant nutrients. However, an overburden of free metal ions, especially Fe and Cu, can catalyze oxidation of biomolecules (Jacob, 1995). However, the ionic forms of these metals that can generate prooxidants (for example, decomposition of H_2O_2 to OH) are usually in very short supply *in vivo*. This is effectively maintained by the complexation (sequestration) of these metals with transport or storage proteins. Besides these minerals, certain exogenous dietary vitamins also play important roles in antioxidants defense. Vitamin C (ascorbic acid) is an effective quencher of many oxyradicals in the body's aqueous compartments such as the blood plasma and cell cytosol. Vitamin E (tocopherol) provides antioxidant protection in the body lipid phases, especially protection of unsaturated fatty acids cell membranes. Carotenoids in fruits and vegetables are also believed to provide antioxidant protection to lipid rich tissues. Besides, a variety of minor plant constituents such as flavonoides, limnoids and procyanins also exhibit antioxidant action *in vitro*.

Increased susceptibility to infectious disease because of malnutrition in livestock has been recognized for many centuries. Vitamins and minerals, such as vitamin E, selenium, copper, and zinc, when properly supplemented, can enhance an animal's immunity against diseases, such as mastitis, by increasing resistance to infections and by decreasing severity of infections when they do occur. Both trace minerals and vitamins play important roles in the health of livestock. For high producing animals, nutrient supplementation for trace minerals and vitamins go beyond correcting for deficiencies but are aimed rather at minimizing stress and optimizing production efficiency.

Tissue defense mechanisms against free-radical damage generally include vitamin C, vitamin E, and â-carotene as the major vitamin antioxidant sources. In addition, several metallo-enzymes which include glutathione peroxidase, catalase, and superoxide dismutase are also critical in protecting the internal cellular constituents from oxidative damage. The dietary and tissue balance of all these nutrients are important in protecting tissues against free radical damage. Both *in vitro* and *in vivo* studies have shown that these nutrients generally enhance different aspects of cellular and non-cellular immunity. The antioxidant function could, at least in part, enhance immunity by maintaining the functional and structural integrity of important immune cells. A compromised immune system will result in reduced animal production efficiency through increased susceptibility to diseases, thereby leading to increased animal morbidity and mortality.

Animals' requirements for vitamins and minerals are influenced by several factors, including age, stage of production and reproduction. It is now understood that, for some vitamins and minerals, the amount required for optimal immune response is greater than the amount required for growth and reproduction. Animals can have sufficient vitamin and mineral intake for adequate growth and reproductive performance but not have optimal immune performance. By the time clinical signs of deficiency become apparent, immunity, growth, and fertility already may have been compromised.

Nutraceuticals as functional feeds : Functional foods are "those foods that encompass potentially healthful products including any modified food or ingredient that may provide a health benefit beyond the traditional nutrients it contains". Application of the concept of functional foods to animal nutrition for optimizing health and productivity has been the current focus of research worldwide. Although not new, the validation of the processes underlying the beneficial effects can significantly contribute to the animal heath and productivity. The functional feeds may include phytochemicals, prebiotics, probiotics and other health-promoting nutraceuticals, but from animal nutrition point of view phytochemicals constitute the most potential functional feeds.

Phytochemicals, as plant components with discrete bio-activities towards animal biochemistry and metabolism are being widely examined for their ability to provide health benefits. It is important to establish the scientific rationale to defend their use in animal feeds, as potential nutritionally active ingredients. Phytochemicals could provide health benefits as: (1) substrates for biochemical reactions; (2) cofactors of enzymatic reactions; (3) inhibitors of enzymatic reactions; (4) absorbents/ sequestrants that bind to and eliminate undesirable constituents in the intestine; (5) ligands that agonize or antagonize cell surface or intracellular receptors; (6) scavengers of reactive or toxic chemicals; (7) compounds that enhance the absorption and or stability of essential nutrients; (8) selective growth factors for beneficial gastrointestinal bacteria; (9) fermentation substrates for beneficial oral, gastric or intestinal bacteria; and (10) selective inhibitors of deleterious intestinal bacteria (Dillard and German, 2000).

Feeding through life stages : In addition to the basic principles of nutrition, several key areas deserve additional attention to optimize animal health, i.e., to understand the importance of certain phases in the life cycle of animals. Two such important life stages involve birth-to-weaning and periparturient phases. A new-born animal, not having a fully operational immune system, needs extra care to prevent it from health hazards which must start with colostrum feeding. Similarly, the stresses associated with weaning constitute another critical phase so far as nutritional wellbeing is concerned. Nutritional manipulation during this phase involving provision of stress-alleviating nutraceuticals (prebiotics, probiotics) may help overcome the imminent growth depression as well as predisposition to infectious diseases. The transition from pregnant, non-lactating to non-pregnant, lactating is critical for the health of dairy animals. Most of the metabolic diseases of dairy cows - milk fever, ketosis, retained placenta, and displacement of the abomasum - occur within the first 2 weeks of lactation. In addition to metabolic disease, the majority of infectious disease experienced by the dairy cow, especially mastitis, but also diseases such as Johne's disease and salmonellosis, become clinically apparent during the first 2 weeks of lactation. It has been observed that during the transition period, in addition to heightened nutritional demands, cows can experience oxidative stress and certain degree of mmuno-suppression (Bernabucci *et al.*,

2002; Piccinini *et al.,* 2004). Hence, the altered metabolic demand for these stages warrants for special considerations while delineating nutritional management for young animals as well as periparturient animals.

Conclusion

The field of clinical nutrition is rapidly evolving as an emerging area in animal nutrition curriculum, research as well as veterinary practice. Many veterinarians are now trying to incorporate nutritional knowledge into the health management of their patients. However, many of the practitioners have only minimal exposure to nutritional management education. As such, there is a real need for consorted efforts to generate database, instruction materials and research approaches which could ultimately facilitate the practicing veterinarians to incorporate clinical nutrition into their practices. A well-coordinated nutrition, health care, and management program is required to maximize efficiency and productivity. A proper nutrition program is paramount for the animals to have adequate health. Animals fed properly are more resistant to many infectious and non-infectious stressors. This is due to better body tissue integrity, more antibody production, improved immunity to diseases, greater detoxifying ability, increased blood regeneration, and other factors. When proper nutritional programs involving adjustment of nutrient levels for metabolic needs for maintenance, growth, reproduction, and lactation are implemented, greater animal productivity can be ensured.

References

Barnett, Y.A. and Barnett, C.R. (1998). Mech. *Ageing Dev.* 102: 165-175.

Bernabucci, U., Ronchi, B., Lacetera, N. and Nardone, A. (2002). *J. Dairy Sci.* 85:2173-2179.

Chew, B.P. (1995). *J. Nutr.* 125: 1804S-1808S.

Colditz, I.G. (2004). *Aust. J. Exp. Agri.* 44: 453-457.

Dillard, C. J. and German, J. B. (2000). *J. Sci. Food Agric.* 80: 1744-1756.

Galyean, M.L., Perino, L.J. and Duff, G.C. (1999). *J. Anim. Sci.* 77: 1120–1134.

Heaton, P.R., Catrina, F.R., Sarah, J.M., Raymond, *et al.* (2002). *J. Nutr.* 132: 1720S-1724S.

Jacob, A.J. (1995). *Nutr. Res.* 15: 755.

Klasing, K. (2003). In: *Scientific Advances in Animal Nutrition.* Natl. Acad. Press, NY, pp. 13-20.

Nockels, C.F. (1996). *Anim. Feed Sci. Technol.* 62: 59-68.

Piccinini, R., Binda, E., Belotti, M., Casirani, G. and Zecconi, A. (2004). *Vet. Res.* 35: 539–550.

□□□

49

Nutritional Strategies to Mitigate Methane from Ruminants with Special Reference to Enhancement of Reductive Acetogenesis

NISHA JHA, S.S. KUNDU, CHANDER DATT, R.C. UPADHYAY AND PANKAJ JHA
Division of Dairy Cattle of Nutrition, National Dairy Research Institute, Karnal (Haryana)

Abstract

Rumen microbes convert cellulosic materials to volatile fatty acids, synthesize microbial protein and also produce methane concomitantly. Methane production is probably the predominant hydrogen sink during anaerobic organic matter decomposition in the rumen. The two other natural sources of hydrogen sink in the rumen are unsaturated fatty-acids in feeds and propionate formation during the process. Another sink for hydrogen is to divert it for acetic acid synthesis, a process called as reductive acetogenesis. Reductive acetogenesis can be a novel approach to reduce methane production in the rumen. Many chemical compounds have been tested for their effects on methane production in the rumen. More practical approach to reduce methane production under Indian conditions could be selection of low methane yielding feed ingredients and the combinations of such feed ingredients to prepare rations. The addition of feed adjuncts like Ionophores, 2-bromoethanesulphonate, anthraquinone, sulphate source, *Saccharomyces cerevisiae* etc. showed encouraging results on CH_4 inhibition. In conclusion, ruminant feed composition and addition of feed adjuncts offer useful ways of mitigating enteric methane production, thereby, decreasing the level of methane in the atmosphere.

Introduction

The rumen is possibly one of the most characterized gut microbial ecosystems and for many years animal nutritionists, microbiologists, physiologists and biotechnologist have been exploring the possibility to manipulate its ecology with the aim of maximizing animal productivity and improving overall host health. Rumen microbes convert cellulosic materials to volatile fatty acids, synthesize microbial protein and also produce methane (CH_4) concomitantly (Fig. 1). CH_4 producing microbes reside in the reticulo-rumen and large intestine of ruminant livestock. All methanogen species utilize hydrogen ions (H^+) to reduce CO_2 in order to produce CH_4 as this reaction is thermodynamically favorable to the organisms (Fig. 2). Availability of H_2 in the rumen is determined by the proportion of end products resulting from fermentation of the ingested feed. The data showed that cattle selected for high productivity on high concentrate diets produced 8 to 11% less CH_4 as a percentage of gross energy (GE) than animals kept in a pasture based system. The genetic selection of high producing animal using high concentrate diets appears to be promising for mitigation of enteric CH_4 emission.

CH_4 production is probably the predominant H_2 sink during anaerobic organic matter decomposition in the rumen. The two other natural sources of H_2 sink in the rumen are unsaturated fatty-acids in feeds and propionate formation during the process. Obviously, nutrition, especially the type and amount of carbohydrates, plays a very significant role in CH_4 emission. Another sink for H_2 is to divert it for acetic acid synthesis, a process called as reductive acetogenesis or homoacetogenesis. Organisms that are able to reduce CO_2 to acetate via the acetyl coenzyme A (acetyl-CoA) or Wood-Ljungdahl pathway are termed acetogens. The key enzymes involved in Acetyl-CoA pathway are the formyltetrahydrofolate synthetase (FTHFS), Carbonmonoxide dehydrogenase (CODH), and Acetyl CoA synthase (ACS). This metabolic capability differentiates reductive acetogens from organisms that synthesize acetate by other metabolic pathways. Therefore, reductive acetogenesis can be a novel approach to reduce CH_4 production from the rumen. The net amount of CH_4 released from the rumen is determined based on the amounts of CH_4 production and CH_4 oxidation or consumption. The dynamics of CH_4 oxidation in the rumen is poorly understood but CH_4 oxidation has been reported from anaerobic environments (Valentine and Reeburgh, 2000). Many chemical compounds have been tested as potential feed additives for ruminants on the basis of their direct or indirect effect on CH_4 production in the rumen. This review has been dealt with under the following section.

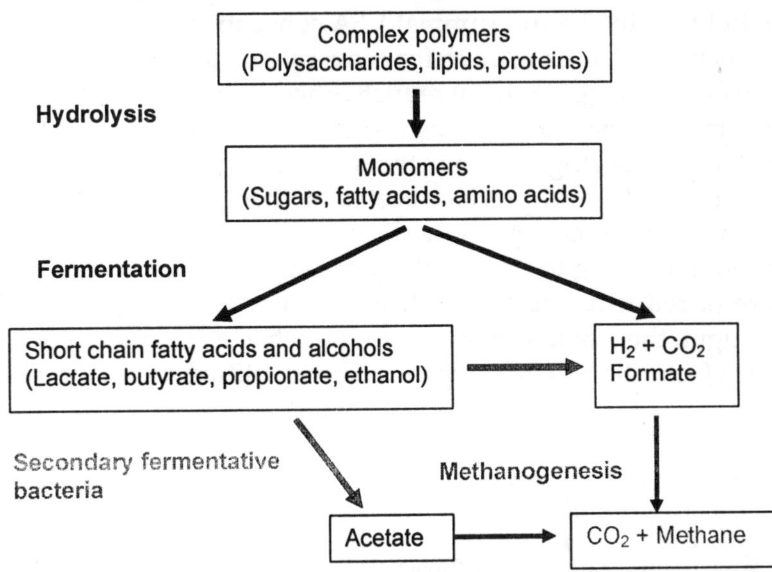

Fig. 1 : Flow chart of methanogenesis

1. Acetogens and reductive acetogenesis in the rumen

1.1 Acetogens in the rumen

Acetogens are extremely heterogenous group of strict anaerobic bacteria with the ability to grow as autotrophs on H_2-CO_2 and as heterotrophs on various carbohydrates. They all reduce CO_2 to acetate for generation of energy by using the Acetyl-CoA pathway. The first recognized ruminal acetogen, *Eubacterium limosum,* was isolated as a methanol utilizing anaerobe from a sheep fed a molasses based diet (Genthner *et al.,* 1981) and later on it was observed that they have the capacity to grow on CO_2 and H_2 to produce acetate. The second ruminal acetogen, *Acetitomaculum ruminis* was isolated from cattle rumen by Greening and Leedle (1989). Later on, acetogenic bacteria like *Peptostreptococcus productus, Ruminococcus shinkii and Clostridium defficile* were isolated from the rumen of lambs fed on milk. Joblin (1999) reported purification of 10 ruminal acetogens and the population density of acetogenic bacteria was variable among the ruminant species and it also depended upon the diet of the animal. Leedle and Greening (1988) found ruminal acetogens in range of >10^8 cells/g digesta of cattle fed either a 3:1 or 1:3, hay: concentrate diet. Little is known about the acetogens in the rumen of grazing animals but in the case of lactating dairy cows, a concentration of upto 10^6/g digesta has been detected by various workers. Fonty *et al.* (2007) reported that a high population density (10^7 to 10^8 cells/g) of ruminal acetogens slowly developed in methanogen-free lambs and ruminal methanogens were not essential for effective fermentation in the rumen. Lambs with a methanogen-free rumen grew well but feed intake and ruminal VFA concentration were lower though not markedly dissimilar from those for conventional lambs reared on the same diet. These findings suggested that reductive acetogens can sustain a functional rumen and replace methanogens as a sink for H_2 in the rumen. Kleive and Joblin (2007) used acetogens from the stomach of marsupials and termite hindguts to utilize H_2 and produce acetate. Other than reductive acetogenic capability, the ruminal acetogens have lot of similar characteristics. The ruminal acetogens do not belong to any single taxonomic group. Taxonomic diversity is a feature of reductive acetogens from other ecosystem (Schink, 1994). In termite hindgut, the major acetogens are spirochaetes (Leadbetter *et al.*, 1999). Spirochaetes from the rumen have yet to be identified as acetogens.

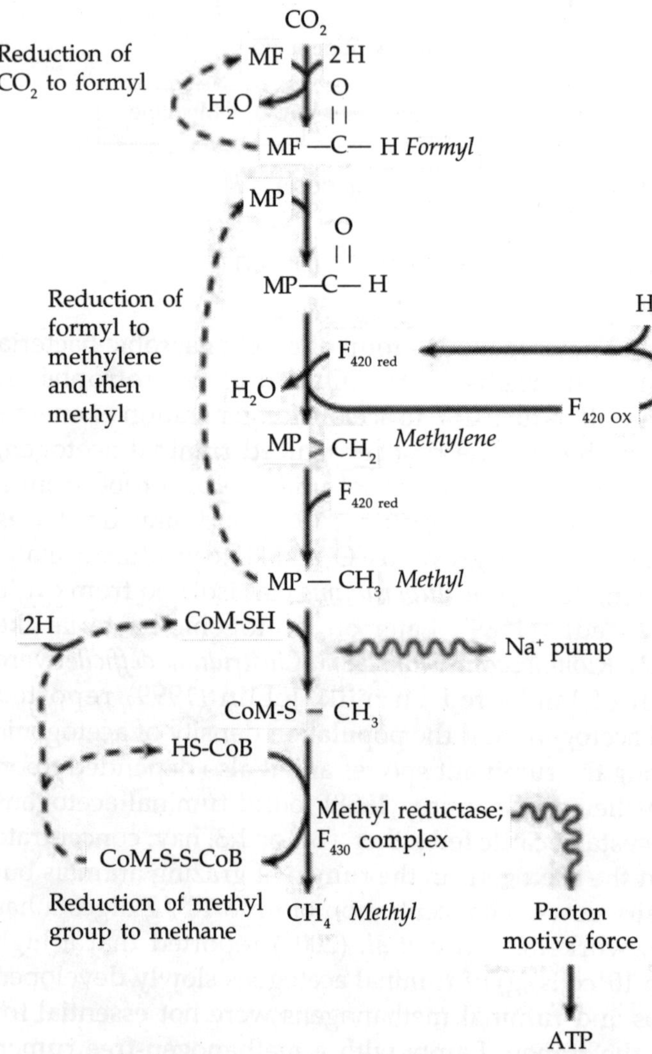

Fig. 2 : Biochemical pathways of methanogenesis by the reduction of CO_2 (Where, *MF: Methanofuran, MP: Methanopterin, CoM: Coenzyme M (Mercapto-ethansulfonat), F420: Factor 420, and F430: Factor 430*)

1.2 Reductive acetogenesis in the rumen

It has been shown that acetogens are present in higher numbers in the rumen of newborn lambs, before establishment of methanogens (Morvan *et al.*, 1994), and also in the rumen of mature animals fed low forage diets (Leedle and Greening, 1988). Acetogenic bacteria could, therefore, be good candidates to compete with methanogens for H_2 utilization, and their acetogenesis could represent a beneficial alternative to methanogenesis. Diversion of energy from CH_4 to acetate by H_2/CO_2-consuming acetogenic bacteria could potentially enhance the energetic efficiency of ruminants and decrease CH_4 emission (Mackie and Bryant, 1994).

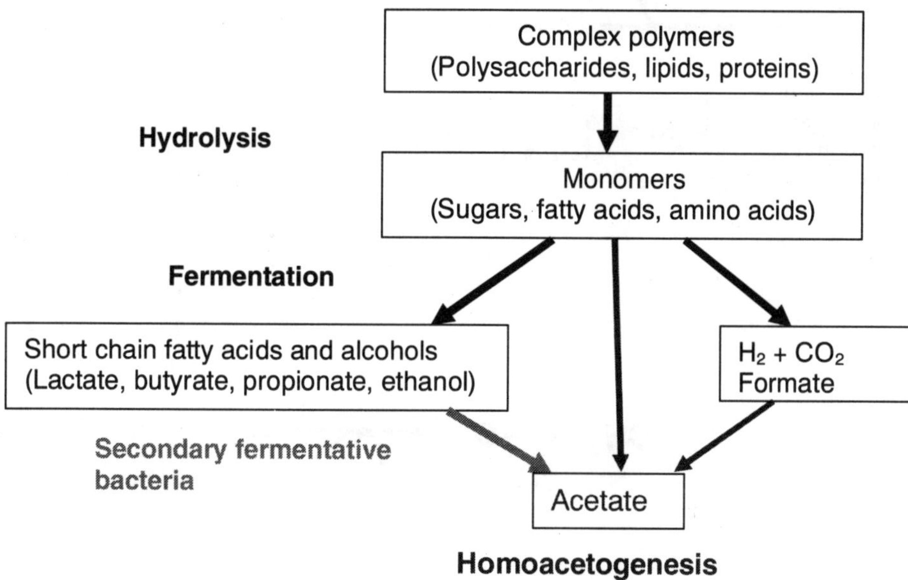

Fig. 3 : Flow chart of reductive acetogenesis (homoacetogenesis)

Although CH_4 generation is often the dominant mechanism for removing H_2 produced in the rumen but this is not the case for all digestive systems. In similar anaerobic ecosystems such as in stomach of kangaroo, termite hindgut, rat caeca and also in the human hindgut, H_2 is removed by reductive acetogenesis (Fig. 3 & 4). In these environments, reductive acetogens replace methanogens and utilize H_2 to produce acetate which is utilized by the host animal. The potential importance of H_2/CO_2-utilizing acetogenic bacteria in the rumen has been described ($2CO_2 + 8H = CH_3COOH + 2H_2O$), however, their capacity to effect a total synthesis of acetate from H_2 and CO_2 in ruminal contents and the factors influencing the magnitude of this activity have not been fully elucidated.

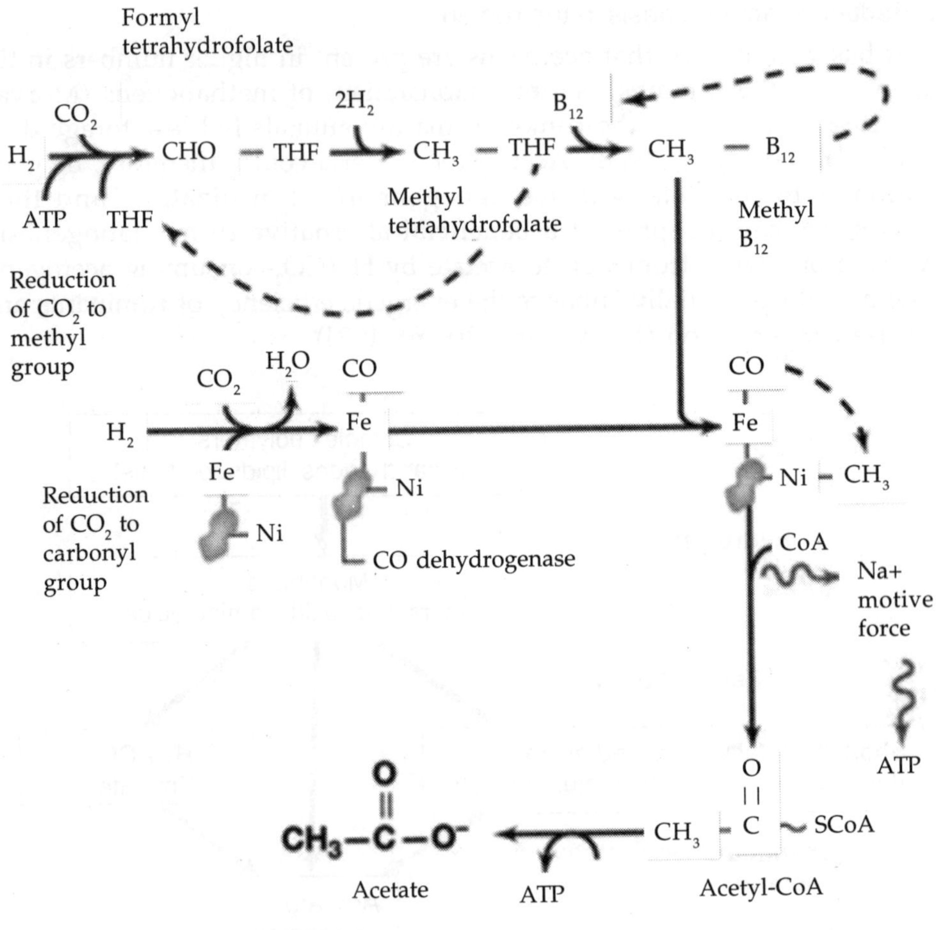

Net : $4\ H_2 + 2\ CO_2$ □ $Acetate^{-} + 2\ H_2O + H^{+}$

Fig. 4 : Biochemical pathway of reductive acetogenesis (acetyl-CoA or Wood-Ljungdahl pathway)

LeVan *et al* (1998) demonstrated that reductive acetogenic bacteria are inhabitants of the rumen ecosystem yet have negligible endogenous H_2/CO_2-consuming activity. From the pure-culture H_2 threshold studies, it was observed that ruminal methanogenic bacteria limited acetogenesis by lowering the H_2 partial pressure to a level insufficient for H_2 utilization by *A. ruminis* 190A4, a strain of ruminal acetogens. Incubations with a nonlimiting concentration of H_2, endogenous acetogenic activity was not detected unless methanogenesis was selectively inhibited by 2-bromoethanesulfonic acid (BES). This activity in the presence of BES could be further enhanced by the addition of an axenic culture of the rumen acetogen, *A. ruminis* 190A4. In absence of BES, reductive acetogenic activity was increased with the concentration of added *A. ruminis* 190A4 under conditions of H_2 excess. Simultaneous activity of acetogenic and methanogenic bacteria was indicated only when the population density of *A. ruminis* 190A4 was 10^7 CFU/ml, nearly approaching the rumen concentration of methanogenic bacteria (10^8 cells/ml). Hence, the population density of *A. ruminis* 190A4 dramatically influenced the accumulation of acetate resulting from H_2/CO_2- utilizing activity. Nollet *et al.* (1997) also reported similar results while using acetogens, *Peptostreptococcus productus.* Authors concluded that redirection of ruminal H_2 disposal seems to require a strategy for compromising H_2 consumption by ruminal methanogens and selection of a ruminal acetogen with a H_2-scavenging ability approaching that of ruminal methanogens.

Studies on *in vitro* incubations of caecal and colonic digesta from cattle and pigs (Demeyer, 1991), suggested that 10 to 15% of the acetate and butyrate may have been derived from reductive acetogenesis. Reductive acetogenesis accounted for 10 to 15% of the acetate produced in sheep with unstable rumen fermentation (Faichney and Graham 1996). Reductive acetogenesis has been reported to be 13% and 16% in lambs given a single meal of medium (300 g/day) and a high level (500 g/day) of dietary DM, respectively (Faichney *et al.*, 1999).

Reductive acetogenesis varied from 15.39 to 27.38% of the acetate among 45 rations under *in vitro* conditions using buffalo rumen fluid (Jha, 2011). In another study, CH_4 production decreased (14.6 to 50.9%) while reductive acetogenesis increased (44.6 to 77.8 %) in Anthraquinone (AQ) added sorghum fodder based rations. Positive effects on *in vitro* digestibility, CH_4 production and reductive acetogenesis were found in Na_2SO_4 added berseem based rations (1 and 2g/kg ration). *In vivo* study also indicated 14.4 to 17.3% reductive acetogenesis in the 3 groups of animals fed on 3 different berseem fodder based TMR and it increased significantly with the addition of Na_2SO_4 @ 1 and 2 g/kg ration.

Fonty *et al.* (2007) opined that reductive acetogenesis was not a significant part of ruminal fermentation in conventional lambs but contributed 21 to 25% to the fermentation in methanogen-free meroxenic animals. Addition of fumarate to rumen contents from methanogen-free lambs increased H_2 utilization. In rumen contents from meroxenic animals lacking ruminal methanogens, the H_2 recovery was less than 50% (28 to 46%) and in conventional lambs it was 90 to 107%. The findings show the effectiveness of methanogens in capturing H_2 in the rumen and proportion of ruminal H_2 in lambs lacking methanogens was captured by processes other than reductive acetogenesis. Alternative H_2 sinks may be associated with the increased propionate and butyrate levels found in incubations. In conventional lambs and in meroxenic lambs containing *M. wolinii*, methanogenesis was the dominant H_2 sink. In all lambs with ruminal methanogens, the amount of CH_4 measured from incubations exceeded that expected from the stoichiometry. Zadbuke *et al.* (2009) reported that the CH_4 production in response to bromochloromethane was reduced by 30% and some reductive acetogenic groups were probably growing in response to inhibition of CH_4 in the rumen.

2. Methanotrophs and CH_4 oxidation in the rumen

2.1 Methanotrophs in the rumen

Methanotrophic bacteria are a physiologically unique group of microorganisms distinguished by their ability to use CH_4 as sole source of carbon and energy (Hanson and Hanson, 1996). Microbial ecologists have long been interested in the methanotrophs due to their key role in the global CH_4 cycle, oxidizing CH_4 to CO_2 (King, 1992). Methanotrophs (CH_4 oxidizing bacteria) are obligate aerobes; often microaerophilic, morphologically diverse, aquatic and terrestrial in habitats, widespread in soil and water. Sometimes they are present at the interface between anoxic zones (where CH_4 is formed) and oxic zones (where O_2 is available for respiration). CH_4 oxidizing bacteria were detected in the cattle and swamps rumen. Little is currently known about methanotrophs in the rumen (Stocks and McCleskey, 1964). Jha (2011) attempted to identify the methanotrophs by PCR using specific primers (Chen *et al.* 2007) in the Murrah buffalo rumen and obtained 16S rDNA sequences showed 97 to 99% sequence similarity with uncultured rumen and non rumen bacteria. Previously, Mitsumori *et al.* (2002) planned to detect the methanotrophic community from the rumen fluid and rumen epithelium of a Holstein cow but its sequencing was not found to be related with methanotrophs.

2.2 Methane oxidation in the rumen

Substantial information regarding CH_4 production in the rumen (Wolin *et al.* 1997) is available; however, there is a very less information about CH_4 consumption, which would be mainly caused by CH_4 oxidation in the rumen. Approximately 20% of the net global CH_4 flux is oxidized before it can enter the atmosphere (Prather *et al.*, 1995), however, other study using an artificial rumen indicated that only 0.3% of CH_4 flux is oxidized (Kajikawa and Newbold, 2000). Although CH_4 oxidation in rumen fluid occurs, the contribution of ruminal methanotrophs to overall ruminal CH_4 metabolism appears only 0.2–0.5% of the CH_4 produced (Kajikawa *et al.*, 2003).

Moss *et al.*, (2001) reported that an aerobic CH_4 oxidising population might be present on the surface of the rumen epithelium, where diffusion from the blood will increase local O_2 concentrations (Czerkawski, 1969), cannot be excluded. Anaerobic CH_4 oxidation must be coupled to an electron sink reaction other than O_2. In this experiment, CH_4 oxidation was inhibited by addition of BES or molybdate but not affected by addition of tungstate. Molybdate and tungstate are known inhibitors of sulphate and nitrate reduction, respectively. Hoehler *et al.* (1994) suggested that in marine sediments, CH_4 could be oxidized by reverse methanogensis of CH_4 to CO_2 and H_2, coupled with sulphate reduction to remove H_2.

3. Type of feedstuffs and CH_4 production

During the microbial fermentation in the rumen, carbohydrates, protein and glycerol are fermented to acetate, propionate, and butyrate, CO_2, NH_3 and CH_4. The CH_4, formed due to reduction of CO_2 by H_2 via methanogenesis cannot be used as an energy substrate and is eructed in the air as green house gas, contributing to environmental pollution. The energy value of CH_4 is 13.15kcal/g and CH_4 formation represents a loss of 5 to 15% of the feed energy to the host animal depending on diet composition and level of feed intake. Blummel and Orskov (1993) recorded the average proportion of CH_4 in wheat and barley straws to be 17.9% of total gas production at 24 h incubation. Srinivas and Gupta (1994) found that the CH_4 in mustard cake, groundnut cake, cottonseed cake, maize, barley grain, and wheat bran was 23.6, 24.6, 39.0, 24.0, 20.7 and 23.5, % of total gas, respectively. CH_4 production was the highest from grains followed by bran and hulls, oil cakes, roughages and lowest from animal by products (Lee *et al.*, 2003).

Ayyappan, (2008) reported that the CH_4 production (as % of total gas during 24 h incubation) from cereal grains and wheat bran ranged from 15.09 to 17.17, from protein sources, 15.17 to 16.55 and from straws 18.13 to 18.24. CH_4 production (ml/200 mg substrate) during 24 h duration ranged from 6.73 to 7.43 from energy sources, 5.32 to 5.64 from oil cakes and 5.94 and 5.98 from straws. Amongst the cereal grains, wheat and barley grains produced similar amount of CH_4, which was higher ($P<0.01$) than the amount produced from other ingredients. When expressed on DOM basis, CH_4 production was the highest from straws and lowest from MC and GNC. Higher CH_4 production from straws than from other feed ingredients may be attributed to their content of higher structural carbohydrates which degrade slowly during fermentation (Singh and Mohini, 2004).

Kamble (2009,) did not find any significant difference in gas production and CH_4 production among green fodders whereas other parameters differed significantly. The TDMD and CH_4 production (ml/g IVTDDM) was the highest in wheat (90.65%) and maize fodder (66.61) and lowest in maize (77.45%) and wheat fodder (50.57). Significant differences among the feedstuffs with regard to CH_4 production and IVTDMD have been reported (Kamble *et al.*, 2009 and 2010; Datt *et al.*, 2009). Thereby, selection of genus/species/varieties on the basis of CH_4 production appears to be attractive proposition for future studies. The study indicated the choice of legume to mitigate CH_4 production in the order chicory> mustard> leuceana> white clover> chinese cabbage> lucerne> turnip> fenugreek> berseem.

TOMD (mg/kg DM) and PF (mg TOMD/ ml gas) of paddy straw, cotton seed, groundnut, mustard cake, maize grain and wheat bran were 494.6 and 3.86; 606.0 and 5.97; 648.2 and 6.31; 825.6 and 3.38 and 658.0 and 4.07, respectively (Kiran and Krishnamoorthy, 2007). Straws possessed high amount of structural carbohydrates such as cellulose and hemi-cellulose with varying level of lignin which are responsible for their low degradability. Straws and wheat bran produced significantly ($P<0.01$) less gas per mg of substrate fermented than other feedstuffs. Higher PF would mean aiming for higher EMPS *in vivo* (Blummel *et al.*, 2003). PF of feedstuffs can theoretically vary from 2.75 to 4.41, reflecting Y_{ATP} of 10 to 40 and PF exceeding 4.41 is likely an analytical artifact and other factors that increases TD, such as soluble unfermented OM or that decreases gas production, such as the degraded protein, contributed to higher PF (Blummel *et al.*, 2003; Kiran and Krishnamoorthy, 2007).

In vitro CH_4 production (g/kg TOMD) ranged from 21.3 to 33.5 in energy sources, 20.5 to 28.1 in protein sources, 18.4 to 26.3 in by-products, 28.4 to 47.0 in green roughages and 34.7 to 48.4 in dry roughages. CH_4 production (g/kg TOMD) was higher and similar in green and dry roughages (36.5 and 40.0), however, energy sources (26.8), protein sources (23.8) and by products (22.9) had similar CH_4 production, but comparatively less values than the roughages. Significant ($P<0.05$) differences were observed within and among the groups indicating that the CH_4 generating potential is an individual characteristics of feed ingredients (Jha, 2011).

Net gas production (ml/ 0.2g DM incubated) varied from 26.84 to 39.44 among the rations incubated in the Murrah buffalo rumen fluid for 24h (Jha, 2011) and *in vitro* TDMD% and TOMD% were highest in the ration consisting of chicory, mustard seed cake and sugar beet root (87.3 and 88.3) and lowest in sorghum fodder, cotton seed cake and red sorghum grain containing ration (52.3 and 50.2) among 45 rations. Different feeds can affect the relative proportion of microbes in the rumen; this may influence the extent of fermentation of feeds (Nagadi *et al.*, 2000).

Singh and Mohini (2004) reported that the proportion of CH_4 in total gas was the highest (43%) when the diet contained straw only and it got reduced gradually with increasing level of concentrate and lowest value (17.4%) was recorded when diet contained concentrate mixture only. TMR containing roughage and concentrate in the ratio of 60: 40 gave IVDMD and IVOMD values of 60.03% and 60.98% at 48 h incubation, whereas same ratio of roughage and concentrate in 45 different rations gave highest and lowest IVTDMD% (87.3 and 52.3) and IVTOMD% (88.3 and 50.2) at 24 h incubation (Jha, 2011). CH_4 production ranged between 13.2 to 19.8% of total gas and it varied from 18.5 to 44.2 g/kg TOMD. The parameter differed significantly in different rations indicated that the selection of feed ingredients to prepare the ration is important for CH_4 mitigation strategies.

4. Feed adjuncts and their effect on CH_4 production

Direct inhibition of methanogenesis by halogenated CH_4 analogues has been demonstrated. Amichloral (a hemiacetal of chloral and starch) increased liveweight gain in sheep (Trei, 1972) but antimethanogenic activity declined with prolonged feeding (Cole and McCroskey, 1975; Johnson, 1975). Similarly, the effects of trichloroacetamide and trichloroethyl adipate on ruminal methanogenesis were apparently transient (Clapperton, 1977; Trei, 1972). The anti-methanogenic activity of bromochloromethane was also reported to be transient (Sawyer, *et al.* 1974), however, other workers suggested that a combination of bromochloromethane and a-cyclodextrin was more stable and capable of suppressing CH_4 emission in sheep and cattle over a prolonged period.

Plant secondary metabolites such as saponins and tannins have been reported to reduce CH_4 emissions (Wallace, 2004; Patra *et al.*, 2006; Kamra and Pawar, 2010). Saponins have been shown to possess strong defaunating properties both *in vitro* and *in vivo* which eventually reduce CH_4 emissions, however, the effect of saponins on protozoa may be transient (Koenig *et al.*, 2007). Beauchemin *et al.* (2008) concluded that there is evidence for a reduction in CH_4 from at least some sources of saponins, but all are not effective. Likewise, some condensed tannins can reduce CH_4 emissions. Two modes of action of tannins on methanogenesis have been proposed (Tavendale *et al.*, 2005) direct effect on ruminal methanogens and an indirect effect on H_2 production due to lower feed degradation. Some legumes contain condensed tannins but unfortunately these may reduce forage digestibility. McAllister and Newbold (2008) reported that extracts from plants such as rhubarb (*Rheum emodi*) and garlic (*Allium sativum*) could decrease CH_4 emissions and garlic oil and some of its components decreased *in vitro* CH_4 production (Busquet *et al.*, 2005, Macheboeuf *et al.*, 2006).

Organic acids are generally fermented to propionate in the rumen and in the process reducing equivalents are consumed. Thus, they can be an alternative sink for H_2 and reduce the amount of H_2 used in CH_4 formation.

Newbold *et al.* (2005) reported fumarate and acrylate to be the most effective in batch culture and artificial rumen. Newbold *et al.* (2002) reported a dose-dependent response to fumarate in sheep. Wallace *et al.* (2006) described a proportional reduction of CH_4 when encapsulated fumaric acid was fed to sheep. While other reports (McGinn *et al.*, 2004; Foley *et al.*, 2007) indicated no or small reductions in CH_4 production when beef cattle were fed malate. The level of reduction in CH_4 emissions that could be achieved is variable and uncertain and the main impediment to this strategy is the high cost of organic acids which makes their use uneconomical.

4.1 Effect of ionophores on methanogenesis.

Ionophores (monensin, salinomycin and lasalosid) are the molecules that are embed in the membranes of gram-positive microorganisms and disrupt ion balances, ultimately destroying the cell. A study by Guan *et al.* (2006) evaluated the efficacy of supplementing cow diets with these molecules in order to decrease H_2 availability to methanogens and thus decrease enteric CH_4 production. The addition of monensin to the cattle diets resulted in a 27-30% decrease in CH_4 emissions for 2-4 weeks only. Methanogens have been observed on the surface of some ciliate protozoa and may account for 9-25% of methanogenesis in the rumen fluid (Kumar *et al.*, 2009). However, the decline in protozoa numbers and CH_4 production was found only to be transitory, and rotation of monensin and lasalocid ionophores every two weeks did not appear to increase the extent or duration of depression in enteric CH_4 emissions. Sirohi *et al.* (2009a) reported that the propionate production increased with the increasing dosage of Ionophores and they (Sirohi *et al.*, 2009b) also found that the monensin supplementation had positive effects on CH_4 reduction and IVDMD remain unchanged. Long term administration of monensin to dairy cattle reduced methane by 7% and that this reduction persisted for 6 months with no adverse effect on milk yield (Odongo *et al.*, 2007).

4.2 Effect of bromoethanesulphonate (BES) on methanogenesis

BES is a potent inhibitor of methanogenesis because it is a structural analogue of the cofactor mercaptoethanesulfonic acid (coenzyme M) and interferes with the final reductive step of methanogenesis. BES is a specific inhibitor of methanogens and does not appear to inhibit the growth of other bacteria. Dong et al. (1997) observed that BES depressed CH_4 production by 71% without significantly affecting OM digestibility and VFA concentrations in the artificial rumen (Rusitec). The reduction in CH_4 was attributed to the toxic effect of BES to methanogenic bacteria. However, its effectiveness persisted for only 3 d in sheep (Immig *et al.*, 1995), suggesting that adaptation of the methanogenic population occurred. While BES is an effective inhibitor of CH_4 production, it may not offer a viable method of reducing CH_4 on a commercial level. Ungerfeld *et al.* (2004) evaluated the sensitivity of representative rumen methanogens to BES and found reduced CH_4 production from *Methanobrevibacter ruminantium, Methanosarcina mazei* and *Methanomicrobium mobile* and the sensitivity of the methanogens to BES was species-dependent.

4.3 Effect of sulphate on methanogenesis.

Sulphate is effective in reducing CH_4 emission by a mechanism: SO_4^{-} + $4H_2$ + $2H^+ \rightarrow H_2S + 4H_2O$. Sulphate reduction to H_2S consumes 8 electrons and thus offers high potential to reduce CH_4 emission. Participation of sulphate in anaerobic CH_4 oxidation has been reported (Devol *et al.* 1984; Iverson and Jorgensen, 1985; Hansen *et al.*, 1998). Sulphate reduction has been reported to occur in the rumen but is considered a minor route of H_2 disposal compared with methanogensis (Ushida *et al.*, 1995). Kajikawa, *et al.* (2003) investigated CH_4 oxidation along with sulphate reduction in the ruminal fluid of sheep. They found that the sulphate-dependent CH_4 oxidation occurred in the rumen but provided no direct evidence for the pathways used and concluded that, CH_4 oxidation occurs anaerobically in rumen fluid in consort with sulphate reduction. Similarly, Valentine and Reeburgh (2000) speculated that reactions in which acetate is formed from either two CH_4 molecules or CH_4 and CO_2, with subsequent consumption of H_2 and acetate to form HCO_3^- and HS^- may be more thermodynamically favourable for sulphate-dependent CH_4 oxidation in anaerobic conditions.

McSweeney *et al.*, (2009) observed increase in DMI in the sulphate-supplemented, diet with no change in the % digestibility of DM and ADF, marked increase in microbial N flow and significant increase in purine levels from the rumen. The *in vivo* study reflected the higher digestibility of nutrients, less CH_4 production and higher reductive acetogenesis in Na_2SO_4 (1 and 2 g/kg ration) supplemented groups as compared to control group (Jha, 2011).

4.4 Effect of Saccharomyces cerevisiae on methanogenesis

In the presence of yeast cells, the acetate concentration increased significantly, indicating that the acetogenic bacterial species was stimulated and more efficient H_2 utilization occurred and 70% of the H_2 was used for acetate production indicating the effect of fungal feed additives on acetogenic bacterial strain (Chaucheyras *et al.*, 1995). The *S. cerevisiae* strain used in the experiment was able to stimulate an acetogenic species even in the presence of methanogens. Some previous reports have evidenced the role of B vitamins and organic acids (Nisbet and Martin, 1992) provided by *S. cerevisiae* in the stimulation of rumen microorganisms.

Eun *et al.* (2003) reported that brewer's yeast culture enhanced the activity of bacteria that convert H_2 to acetate and decreased CH_4 output by 25% in a continuous culture of ruminal microorganisms. Newbold *et al.* (1995) reported that the effects of probiotics on fermentation pattern are not consistent across the experiments and between strains of yeast. Doreau and Jouany (1998) found no effect of *S. cerevisiae* on fermentation in lactating dairy cows, while Takahashi *et al.* (1997) observed that a probiotic preparation significantly increased CH_4 production in sheep. Even on high fibre containing diets, a positive effect on the fibrolytic community has been observed upon the inclusion of yeast due to a stabilization of ruminal pH and a reduction in lactate production. Addition of *S. cerevisiae* @ 1g/kg ration was beneficial in terms of increased digestibility and reduced CH_4 production (Jha, 2011).

4.5 Effect of 9, 10-anthraquinone (AQ) on methanogenesis

AQ is naturally occurring aromatic organic compound found in some plants which has promising effect on methanogens (Garcia-Lopez *et al.*, 1996) without having adaptation or toxic problems (Kung *et al.*, 2003). AQ inhibits methanogenesis by mixed rumen micro-organisms *in vitro* (Garcia-Lopez *et al.*, 1996; Kung, *et al.*, 1998) and to depress CH_4 production in lambs over a 19 day period (Kung *et al.*, 1998). Garcia-Lopez *et al.* (1996) speculated that AQ inhibited the reduction of methyl co-enzyme M to CH_4 by uncoupling electron transfer in methanogens. CH_4 production increased with the increasing levels of AQ in high fibre diet but reduced in the medium and low fiber diets (Sirohi *et al.*, 2009b).

Reduction of CH_4 in culture supplemented with AQ confirmed inhibitory effect of this chemical on methanogens (Garcia- Lopez *et al.* 1996; Hadi, 2010). This effect caused an accumulation of H_2 in treated cultures with AQ (Garcia-Lopez *et al.*, 1996; Kung *et al.*, 2003). It was reported that direct inhibition of methanogens stimulated propionate production (Mohammed *et al.*, 2004). The increase in concentration of propionate due to 4 ppm of AQ could probably be due to utilization of some H_2 which would be accumulated but this process can account for only small proportion of the saved H_2. Perhaps some of excess of H_2 was used for microbial lipid synthesis. Feeding AQ to the sheep did not influence digestibility (Kung *et al.*, 2003) whereas decrease in IVDMD and IVOMD was reported. Reduced CH_4 production (14.6 to 50.9%) along with TOMD (5.9 to 18.2%) but higher reductive acetogenesis (44.6 to 77.8 %) were observed in AQ added sorghum based rations indicating that AQ can be added to the ration along with such type of feed adjunct which have positive effect on digestibility of ration (Jha, 2011).

Conclusion

More practical approach to reduce CH_4 production under Indian conditions could be preparing rations based on selection of feed ingredients having low CH_4 production potential. Creating such an environment in the rumen that promotes reductive acetogenesis while decreasing CH_4 production holds good promise as a CH_4 mitigation strategy, however, it needs. BES appears to be a potent CH_4 inhibitor; however, adaptation of the methanogenic population to BES may occur. Adaptation problems have not been observed in AQ. In most of the studies digestibility also reduced along with CH_4 with the addition of AQ. Therefore, AQ can be used in conjunction with such feed adjunct which has positive effect on digestibility of ration. *In vitro* and *in vivo* studies using Na_2SO_4 and *S. cerevisiae* at lower level are indicative of beneficial effects in terms of digestibility and CH_4 production. Although various feed adjuncts are now available to achieve this aim, the choice of adjuncts must depend on the potency, safety, and expense of the candidate adjunct.

References

Ayyappan, K. (2008). Optimization of energy and nitrogen availability for microbial protein synthesis in the rumen. Ph.D. Thesis, National Dairy Research Institute, Karnal, India.

Beauchemin, K.A., Kreuzer, M., O'Mara.F. and McAllister, T.A. (2008). *Australian Journal of Experimental Agric.* 48: 21-27.

Blummel, M. and Orskov, E.R. (1993). Comparison of in vitro and nylon bag degradability of roughages in predicting feed intake in cattle. *Anim. Feed Sci. Technol.,* 40: 109-119.

Blummel, M., Karsli, A. and Russell, J.R. (2003). Influence of diet on growth yields of rumen micro-organism in vitro and in vivo: influence on growth yield of variable carbon fluxes to fermentation products. *Br. J. Nutr.,* 90: 1-11.

Busquet M., Calsamiglia S., Ferret A., Carro M.D. and Kamel C. (2005). *Journal of Dairy Science.* 88: 4393-4404.

Datt, Chander., Singh, N.P., Aruna Chhabra, Bujarbaruah, K.M., and Dhiman, K.R. (2009). Nutritional evaluation of cultivated fodders grown under agro-climate of Tripura. *Indian J. Anim. Sci.* 79: 1143-1148.

Chaucheyras, F., Fonty, G., Bertin, G. and Gouet, P.(1995). *In vitro* H_2 Utilization by a Ruminal Acetogenic Bacterium Cultivated Alone or in Association with an Archaea Methanogen Is Stimulated by a Probiotic Strain of Saccharomyces cerevisiae. *Appl. Environ. Microbiol.* 61: 3466–3467.

Chen, Y., M.G. Dumont, A. Ce´bron and J.C. Murrell. (2007). Identification of active methanotrophs in a landfill cover soil through detection of expression of 16S rRNA and functional genes. *Environ. Microbiol.* 9: 2855–2869.

Clapperton, J.L. (1977). The effect of a methane-suppressing compound trichloroethyl adipate on rumen fermentation and the growth of sheep. *Anim. Prod.* 24: 169–181.

Cole, N.A. and McCroskey, J.E. (1975). Effects of hemiacetal of chloral and starch on the performance of beef steers. *J. Anim. Sci.* 41: 1735–1741.

Czerkawski, J. W. (1969). Methane production in ruminants and its significance. *World Rev. Nutr. Diet.* 11:240-282.

Demeyer, D.I. and De Graeve, K. (1991). Differences in stoichiometry between rumen and hindgut fermentation, *J. Anim. Physiol Anim. Nutr.* 22: 50–61.

Devol, A.H., Anderson, J.J, Kuivila, K. and Murray, J.W. (1984). A model for coupled sulfate reduction and methane oxidation in the sediments of Saanich Inlet. *Geochimica et Cosmochimica Acta.* 48: 993–1004.

Dong, Y., Bae, H. D., McAllister, T. A., Mathison, G. W. and Cheng, K. J. (1997). Effects of exogenous fibrolytic enzymes, abromoethanesulfonate and monensin on fermentation in a rumen simulation (RUSITEC) system. *Can. J. Anim. Sci.* 79: 491–498.

Doreau, M. and Jouany, J.P. (1998). Effect of Saccharomyces cerevisiae culture on nutrient digestion in lactating dairy cows. *J. Dairy Sci.* 81: 3214–3221.

Eun, J.S., Fellner, V., Whitlow, L.W. and Hopkins, B.A. (2003). Influence of yeast culture on fermentation by ruminal microorganisms in continuous culture. Department of Animal Science Bulletin, North Carolina State University, Raleigh, NC.

Faichney, G. J., and Graham, N. M. (1996). Reduced methane emissions associated with unstable rumen fermentation in sheep. *Proceedings of the Nutrition Society of Australia* 20: 120-123.

Faichney, G.J., Graham, N.M. and Walker, D.M. (1999). Rumen characteristics, methane emissions, and digestion in weaned lambs reared in isolation. *Aust. J. Agric. Res.* 50: 1083–1089.

Foley, P.A., Callan, J., Kenny, D.A., Johnson, K.A. and O'Mara, F.P. (2007). *Proc. of the Agricultural Research Forum*, pp. 112.

Fonty, G., Joblin, K., Chavarot, M., Roux, R., Naylor, G and Michallon, F. (2007). Establishment and development of ruminal hydrogenotrophs in methanogen-free lambs. *Appl. Environ. Microbiol.* 73(20): 6391–6403.

Garcia-Lopez, P.M., Kung, L.Jr. and Odom, J.M.I. (1996). In vitro inhibition of microbial methane production by 9,10- anthraquinone. *J. Anim. Sci.* 74: 2276–2284.

Genthner, B.R.S., Davis, C.L. and Bryant, M.P. (1981). Features of rumen and sewage sludge strains of Eubacterium limosum, a methanol and H_2/CO_2- utilizing species, *Appl. Environ. Microbiol.* 42: 12–19.

Greening, R.C. and Leedle, J.A.Z. (1989). Enrichment and isolation of Acetitomaculum ruminis, gen. nov., sp. nov.: acetogenic bacteria from the bovine rumen, *Arch. Microbiol.* 151: 399–406.

Guan, H., Wittenberg, K., Ominski, K., Krause, D. (2006). Efficacy of ionophores in cattle diets for mitigation of enteric methane. *Journal of Animal Science*. 84: 1896-1906.

Hadi, (2010). Manipulation of rumen microbial ecosystem using feed additives to mitigate methane emission and enhance nutrient utilization in cattle. Ph. D. Thesis, National Dairy Research Institute, Karnal (Haryana), India.

Hansen, L.B., Finster, K., Fossing, H. and Iversen, N. (1998). Anaerobic methane oxidation in sulfate depleted sediments: effects of sulfate and molybdate addition. *Aquatic Microbial Ecology* 14: 195-204.

Hanson, R.S. and Hanson, T.E. (1996). Methanotrophic bacteria. *Microbiol. Rev.* 60: 439-471.

Hoehler, T.M., Alperin, M.J., Albert, D.B. and Martens, C.S. (1994). Field and laboratory studies of methane oxidation in an anoxic marine sediment: evidence for a methanogen-sulfate reducer consortium. *Global Biogeochemical Cycles.* 8: 451–463.

Immig, I., Fielder, D., Van Nevel, C. and Demeyer, D. (1995). Inhibition of methanogenesis in the rumen of a sheep with BES. *Proc. Soc. Nutri. Physiol.* 4: 68–75.

Iverson, N. and Jorgensen, B.B. (1985). Anaerobic methane oxidation rates at the sulfate-methane transition in marine sediments from Kattegat and Skagerrak (Denmark). *Limnology and Oceanography*. 30: 944–955.

Jha nisha, (2011). Dietary manipulation of reductive acetogenesis and methane oxidation in the buffalo rumen. Ph.D. Thesis, National Dairy Research Institute, Karnal (Haryana), India.

Joblin, K.N. (1999). Ruminal acetogens and their potential to lower ruminant methane emission. *Aust. J. Agric. Res.* 50: 1307- 1313.

Johnson, D.E. (1975). Adaptational responses in nitrogen and energy balance of lambs fed a methane inhibitor. *J. Anim. Sci.* 38: 154–157.

Kajikawa, H. and Newbold, C.J. (2000). Methane oxidation in the rumen. *Journal of Animal Science*, 78 (Suppl. 1): 291.

Kajikawa, H., Valdes, C., Hillman, K., Wallace, R.J. and Newbold, C.J. (2003). Methane oxidation and its coupled electron-sink reactions in ruminal fluid. Lett. *Appl. Microbiol.* 36: 354–357.

Kamble, A.B, Kundu, S.S., Chander Datt, Madhu Mohini and Nisha Jha. (2010). Evaluation of carbohydrate and protein fractions in commonly available roughages for cattle and buffaloes. *In Proc.*: VII Biennial ANA Conference" Animal Nutrition Strategies for Environmental Protection and Poverty Alleviation" held at OUAT, Bhubaneswar from December 17 to 19, 2010. p139.

Kamble, A.B. (2009). Evaluation of feeds for carbohydrate, protein fractions and in vitro methane production. M. V. Sc. Thesis, National Dairy Research Institute, Karnal (Haryana), India.

Kamble, A.B., S.S. Kundu, S. K. Shelke, Chander Datt, Nisha Jha. (2010). Evaluation of concentrate feedstuffs for carbohydrate and protein fraction and in vitro methane production. *Indian J. Anim. Nutr.* 27(2): 109-115.

Kamra, D.N. and Pawar, M.M. (2010). Methane mitigation by plant secondary metabolites-an indigenous approach. In: "National Symposium on Climate Change and Livestock Productivity in India" held at NDRI, Karnal from October 7 to 8, 2010. pp. 56-70.

King, G.M. (1992). Ecological aspects of methane oxidation, a key determinant of global methane dynamics. *Adv. Microb. Ecol.* 12:431-468.

Kiran, D. and Krishnamoorthy, U. (2007). Rumen fermentation and microbial biomass synthesis indices of tropical feedstuffs determined by the in vitro gas production techniques. *Anim. Feed Sci. Technol.*, 134: 170-179.

Klieve, A and Joblin, K. (2007). New Zealand Pastoral Greenhouse Gas Research Consortium Report, pp. 34-35.

Koenig, K.M., Ivan, M., Teferedegne, B.T., Morgavi, D.P., Rode, L.M., Ibrahim, I.M. and Newbold, C.J. (2007). *British Journal of Nutrition.* 98: 504-516.

Kumar, S., Puniya, A., Puniya, M., Dagar, S., Sirohi, S., Singh, K., Griffith, G. (2009). Factors affecting rumen methanogens and methane mitigation strategies. *World Journal of Microbiology and Biotechnology.* 25: 1557-1566.

Kung, J.L., Smith, K.A., Smagla, A.M., Endres, K.M., Bessett, C.A., Ranjit, K.N. and Yaissle, J. (2003). Effects of 9,10 anthraquinone on ruminal fermentation, total tract digestion, and blood metabolite concentrations in sheep. *J. Anim. Sci.* 81: 323-328.

Kung, L. Jr., Hession, A.O., Bracht, J.P. (1998). Inhibition of sulfate reduction to sulfide by 9,10- anthraquinone in in vitro ruminal fermentations. *J. Dairy Sci.* 81: 2251–2256.

Leadbetter,J.R., Schmidt,T.M., Graber,J.R. and Breznak,J.A. (1999). Acetogenesis from H_2 plus CO_2 by spirochetes from termite guts. *Science.* 283: 686-689.

Lee, H. J., Lee, S. C., Kim, J. D., Oh, Y. G., Kim, B. K., Kim, C. W. and Kim,. K. J. (2003). Methane production potential of feed ingredients as measured by in vitro gas test. *Asian- Aust. J. Anim. Sci.*, 16: 1143-1150.

Leedle, J.A.Z. and Greening. R.C. (1988). Postprandial changes in methanogenic and acidogenic bacteria in the rumens of steers fed high- or low forage diets once daily. *Appl. Environ. Microbiol.* 54: 502–506.

LeVan,T.D., Robinson,J.A., John Ralph, Greening,R.C., Smolenski,W.J., Leedle, J.A.Z. and Schaefer, D.M. (1998). Assessment of reductive acetogenesis with indigenous ruminal bacterium populations and Acetitomaculum ruminis. *Appl. Environ. Microbiol.*, Sept: 3429–3436.

Macheboeuf, D., Lassalas, B., Ranilla, M.J., Carro, M.D. and Morgavi, D.P. (2006). *Reproduction Nutrition Development* 46: S103.

Mackie, R.I. and Bryant, M.P. (1994). Acetogenesis and the rumen: syntrophic relationships, p. 331–364. In H. L. Drake (ed.), Acetogenesis. Chapman and Hall, New York, N.Y.

McAllister,T.A. and Newbold,C.J. (2008). *Australian Journal of Experimental Agriculture* 48:7-13.

McGinn, S.M., Beauchemin, K.A., Coates, T., Colombatto, D. (2004). *J. Anim. Sci.* 82: 3346-3356.

McSweeney, C.S., Sampath, K.T. and Prasad, C.S. (2009). Final report; increasing the productivity of cattle in India and Australia with rumen fungal treatments. ACIAR, GPO Box 1571, Canberra ACT 2601, *Australia. Report number* FR2009-13.

Mitsumori,M., Ajisaka1,N., Tajima,K., Kajikawa,H. and Kurihara,M., (2002). Detection of Proteobacteria from the rumen by PCR using methanotroph-specific primers. *Letters in Applied Microbiology.* 35: 251–255.

Mohammed, N., Lila, Z.A., Ajisaka, N., Hara, K., Mikuni, K., Kanda, S. and Itabashi, H. (2004). Inhibition of ruminal microbial methane production by β-cyclodextrin iodopropane, malate and their combination *in vitro. J. Anim. Phys. Anim. Nutr.* 88: 188–195.

Morvan,B., Dore,J., Rieu-Lesme,F., Foucat,L., Fonty,G. and Gouet,P. (1994). Establishment of hydrogen-utilizing bacteria in the rumen of the newborn lamb. *FEMS Microbiol. Lett.* 117:249–256.

Moss,A.R., Newbold,J. and Wilkins,D. (2001). Methane oxidation in rumen fluid. Novel feed additives for decreasing methane emissions from ruminants. *MAFF Project Number:* CSA 4320.

Nagadi, S., Herrero, M. and Jessop, N. S. (2000). The influence of the diet of the donor animal on the initial bacterial concentration of the rumen fluid and in vitro gas production degradability parameters. *Anim. Feed Sci. Technol.*, 87: 231-239.

Newbold,C.J., López,S., Nelson,N., Ouda,J.O., Wallace,R.J. and Moss,A.R. (2005). *Brit. J. Nutr.* 94: 27–35

Newbold,C.J., Ouda,J.O., Lopez,S., Nelson,N., Omed,H., Wallace,R.J. and Moss,A.R. (2002). In: Greenhouse gases and animal agriculture, Eds J. Takahashi and B.A. Young, Elsevier, pp 151-154.

Newbold,C.J., Wallace,R.J., Chen,X.B. and McIntosh,F.M. (1995). Different strains of Sacchararomyces cerevisiae differ in their effects on ruminal bacterial numbers in vitro and in sheep. *J. Anim. Sci.* 73: 1811–1819.

Nisbet,D.J., and S.A.Martin. (1992). Effect of direct-fed microbials on rumen microbial fermentation. *J. Dairy Sci.* 75: 1736–1744.

Nollet,L., Demeyer,D. and Verstraete,W. (1997). Effect of 2-bromoethanesulfonic acid and Peptostreptococcus productus ATCC 35244 addition on stimulation of reductive acetogenesis in the ruminal ecosystem by selective inhibition of methanogenesis. *Appl. Environ. Microbiol.* 63:194–200.

Odongo, N. E., R. Bagg, G. Vessie, P. Dick, M. M. Or-Rashid, S. E. Hook, J. T. Gray, E. Kebreab, J. France and B. W. McBride. (2007). Long-term effects of feeding monensin on methane production in lactating dairy cows. *J. Dairy Sci.* 90:1781-1788.

Patra, A.K., Kamra, D.N. and Agarwal, N. (2006). *Animal Feed Science and Technology*. 128: 276-291.

Prather, M., Derwent, R., Ehhalt, D., Fraser, P., Sanhueza, E. and Zhou, X. (1995). Other trace gases and atmospheric chemistry. In: Intergovernmental Panel on Climate Change, Climate Change 1994: Radiative Forcing on Climatic Change ed. Houghton, J.T., Meira Filho, L.G., Bruce, J., Hoesung, L., Callander, B.A., Haites, E, Harris, N and Maskell, K, pp. 77–126. Cambridge: Cambridge University Press.

Sawyer, M.S., Hoover,W.H. and Sniffen,C.J. (1974). Effects of a ruminal methane inhibitor on growth and energy metabolism in the ovine, *J. Anim. Sci.* 38: 908-914.

Schink, B. (1994). Diversity, ecology, and isolation of acetogenic bacteria, p. 197–235. In H. L. Drake (ed.) Acetogenesis. Chapman and Hall, New York, N.Y.

Singh, G. P. and Mohini, M. (2004). Effect of dietary manipulation on methane production in crossbred cattle. *Indian J. Anim. Nutr.*, 21: 95-99.

Sirohi, S.K., Neha Pandey, B. Singh, Madhu Mohini, A.K.Puniya, S.S.Kundu and Nisha Jha. (2009b). Effect of Monensin and Anthraquinone Supplementation on Rumen Fermentation and Methane Production in vitro. *Proc. ANA World Conf.* p 183.

Sirohi, S.K., Neha Pandey, B. Singh, Nisha Jha, Madhu Mohini and Dheer Singh. (2009a). Effect of Monensin and Salinomycin on Rumen Metabolism and Methanogenesis in buffalo Rumen Fluid *in vitro*. *Proc. ANA World Conf.* p 185.

Srinivas, B. and Gupta, B.N. (1994). Rumen degradable protein content and gas production on rumen fermentation of some concentrate ingredients and their relationship. *Indian J. Anim. Nutr.*, 11: 171-175.

Stocks,P.K. and Mc Cleskey,C.S., (1964). Morphology and physiology of Methanomonas methanooxidans. *Journal of Bacteriology* 88: 1071–1077.

Takahashi,J., Chaudhry,A.S., Beneke,R.G. and Young,B.A. (1997). Modification of methane emission in sheep by cysteine and a microbial preparation. *Sci. Total Environ.* 204: 117–123.

Tavendale,M.H., Meagher,L.P., Pacheco,D., Walker,N., Attwood,G.T. and Sivakumaran,S. (2005). *Animal Feed Science and Technology*. 123-124,

Trei,J.E., Parish,R.C., Singh,Y.K. and Scott,G.C. (1972). Effect of methane inhibitors on rumen production by rumen bacteria when methane synthesis is inhibited, *J. Dairy Sci.* 70: 1835–1840.

Ungerfeld, E. M., S. R. Rust, D. R. Boone and Y. Liu. (2004). Effects of several inhibitors on pure cultures of ruminal methanogens. *J. Appl. Microbiol.* 97:520-526.

Ushida,K., Ohashi,Y., Tokura,M., Miyazaki,K. and Kojima,Y. (1995). Sulphate reduction and methanogenesis in the ovine rumen and porcine caecum: a comparison of two microbial ecosystems. *Deutsche tiera¨rztliche Wochenschrift* 102: 154–156.

Valentine, D.L. and Reeburgh, W.S. (2000). New perspectives on anaerobic methane oxidation. *Environ. Microbiol.* 2: 477– 484.

Wallace,R.J. (2004). *Proceedings of the Nutrition Society* 63: 621-629.

Wallace,R.J., Wood,T.A., Rowe,A., Price,J., Yanez,D.R., Williams,S.P. and Newbold, C.J. (2006). In 'Greenhouse Gases and Animal Agriculture: An Update. (Ed. Soliva CR, Takahashi J, and Kreuzer M), pp.148-151 (Elsevier International Congress Series 1293, Amsterdam, The Netherlands).

Wolin, M.J., Miller,T.L. and Stewart,C.S. (1997). Microbe-microbe interactions, p. 467–488. In P. N. Hobson and C. S. Stewart (ed.), the rumen microbial ecosystem. Chapman and Hall, London, United Kingdom.

Zadbuke, S.S.,Denman S.E., Kamra D.N. and McSweeney C.S. (2009). Formyltetrahydrofolate synthetase gene in normal and methane inhibited rumen liquor of cattle. *Proc. ANA World Con.* 14-17 Feb. New Delhi, India: 105-108.

□□□

50

Feeding Strategies to Maintain Livestock Productivity during Natural Calamities

M.P.S. BAKSHI[1] AND M. WADHWA
[1]Former Sr Nutritionist cum Head
Department of Animal Nutrition
Guru Angad Dev Veterinary and Animal Sciences University, Ludhiana-141004, India

Introduction

The impacts of natural disasters such as hurricanes, floods, earthquakes and tsunamis have been increasing steadily since the 1950's, particularly in developing countries (IPCC, 2007). India has traditionally been vulnerable to natural disasters due to its unique geo-climatic conditions. Floods, droughts, cyclones, earthquakes and landslides have been recurrent phenomena. India is one of the most flood prone countries in the world after Bangladesh and accounts for one-fifth of the global death count due to floods. About 60% of the landmass is prone to earthquakes of various intensities. Among various natural calamities, flood is the major devastating natural calamity resulting in heavy loss of vegetation. Twenty-three out of thirty two-states/union territories in the country are subject to floods and 40 million hectares of land, roughly one-eighth of the country's geographical area, is prone to floods. On an average about 50-60 percent of the cropped area in flood affected area remain submerged and it takes at least a minimum of 30 days to bring the field for cultivation purposes.

About 8% of the total area is prone to cyclones, 68% of the area is susceptible to drought. In Indian subcontinent, drought is predominantly characterized by monsoon failure. The summer monsoon accounts for

70-90% of the annual rainfall over major parts of South Asia. In past century, the country has experienced 21 large-scale droughts. In Jaisalmer (Rajasthan) which experiences very high summer temperature (>45°C), there have been 39 drought affected years over a span of 49 years since 1956. The major effects of droughts are widespread crop failures leading to acute shortages of food and fodder, adversely affecting human and livestock health and nutrition; scarcity of drinking water accentuated by deteriorating ground water quality and declining water tables. Therefore, there is a need to formulate feeding strategy for maintenance of animals to ensure its survival during and after the natural calamity. Feeding strategies during scarcity depend on the specific conditions prevailing in any particular area.

Each disaster will present a different set of challenges and issues, and may also affect certain populations more than others. The disasters that can threaten livestock in a given region range from slow onset (chronic) to rapid onset (acute), to complex, and the populations most affected may be pastoralists, small farmers with minimal livestock holdings, or those who manage mixed farming systems. Slow onset disasters may recur yearly, and can often be predicted on the basis of climate shifts and weather patterns. Drought and ensuing famine are perhaps the most serious threats to livestock holdings worldwide. The natural calamities play havoc with the humans and livestock. The worst affected are livestock. The animals are offered what so ever feedstuffs available in small quantity, which cannot meet their nutrient requirements. The larger sufferer would be ruminants as most of them depend on crop residues, pastures and grazing lands. Acute shortage of animal's feeds and fodder is one of the major reasons for low productivity and growth rate of livestock (Bhagwat, 2008).

Severe malnutrition due to natural calamities may cause irreparable damage to the internal organs/tissue and may reduce growth rates due to appetite suppression and also depress productive and reproductive performance. Animal mortalities from malnutrition increase because fodder is insufficient or inappropriate. Endemic diseases increase when herds mix at watering points and weakened animals have low resistance. Livestock losses can be enormous.

When conditions improve, livestock are important assets in helping people to recover nutritionally and economically. In times of insecurity, with displacement of local populations, livestock can provide important support for families allowing them to move away and still maintain some food security because the animals move with them.

Effect of Restricted Feeding / malnutrition during Natural Calamities

Severe malnutrition due to natural calamities may cause irreparable damage to the internal organs/tissue and may reduce growth rates due to appetite suppression and also depress productive and reproductive performance. Keeping in views these issues, this paper will focus on certain effects and their remedies.

Limited feeding did not affect weight gain and skeletal growth of heifers but improved the feed efficiency, resulted in excretion of less dry matter, without affecting the excretion of nitrogen and phosphorus (Hoffman *et al.*, 2007). Calf birth weight, dystocia or lactation performance, initial or final body weight, hip height, heart girth, or body condition score of heifers was not affected by limited feeding. Driedger and Loerch (1999) observed an increased efficiency of N utilization when non lactating cows were limit fed. Limited feeding had no effect on blood profile except increase in BUN in heifers.

Growth results from the differences between tissue synthesis and degradation and losses from the body of energy, nitrogen and minerals due to excretion. During normal development muscle exhibits initially the highest growth rate followed by fat deposition. When growth rates are reduced, there is a coordinate decrease of tissue turnover. However, some tissues react more than others (viscera, adipose tissue, and muscle). The empty visceral fraction decreases (Wester *et al.*, 1995). Animals fed at sub-maintenance levels showed muscle growth close to zero, but fat mobilization continues and decrease in visceral weight, leading sometimes to altered body composition. Some adipose compartments, such as subcutaneous fat, may be mobilized more easily than others (Yambayamba *et al.*, 1996).

Severe feed restriction and weight losses are characterized by a sharp decrease of synthesis, relative to degradation, indicating that the mechanisms of synthesis are much more sensitive to low (and high) feeding intensity than degradation. Tissues are mobilized sequentially. Weight losses result initially from an early mobilization of a very labile protein compartment (Paquay *et al.*, 1972). This lasts for some days until a new equilibrium is reached, paralleled by a decrease of basal metabolism. Then fat is mobilized dependent on the severity of restriction whereas the protein pool is conserved as much as possible. Finally, insufficient amounts of energy associated with excess protein could lead to fat mobilization associated with some muscle deposition (Fattet *et al.*, 1984). However, when lean animals are feed-restricted, muscle constitutes the main source of energy, causing a greater protein than fat losses (Foot and Tulloh, 1977). During severe and prolonged feed restriction, the initial switch from protein to fat mobilization is initially observed but is rapidly followed by combined fat and protein losses. Drouillard *et al.*, (1991) affirmed that tissues are affected by growth restriction dependent on their metabolic activity and metabolically very active tissues or organs (such as liver or intestine) show greater weight losses. As a rule, early maturing body components are less affected by feed restriction, but recover less during refeeding (Kamalzadeh *et al.*, 1998).

During feed restriction basal metabolism is reduced, mainly because of decrease in volume and metabolic activity of the viscera (Ortigues and Durand, 1995). Other tissues also show a shift in the metabolism of nutrients and energy sources. Adipose tissue and liver release enhanced amounts of free fatty acids and ketone bodies, respectively, which are used by muscle and other extra hepatic tissues as energy substrates (Bossart *et al.*, 1985). When feed restriction is severe, a large transfer of nitrogen between liver and kidneys occurs associated with enhanced liver glutamine synthesis (Heitmann and Bergman, 1980). These reactions result from a sharp decrease of the protein synthesis/ degradation ratio owing to the reduction of plasma levels of anabolic hormones and increased levels of catabolic hormones. Blum *et al.* (1985) revealed that in response to reduced feed intake concentrations of thyroxine (T_4), 3,5,3'-triiodothyronine (T_3), insulin (INS), plasma IGF-I concentration, glucose and á-amino-acid nitrogen (AAN) were reduced, those of growth hormone (GH) and nonesterified fatty acids (NEFA) were elevated. Lower concentrations of T_3 and T_4 allow the organism to spare energy by decreasing basal metabolism. In lambs, protein restriction alone exerts a faster decrease of IGF-I concentration than energy restriction. Lower concentrations of T_3 and T_4 allow the organism to spare energy by decreasing basal metabolism. Feed restriction increased the extent of negative energy balance and caused transient increases in concentrations of NEFA, acetate, and ß-hydroxybutyrate in plasma. Concentration of glycogen in liver was less in feed-restricted cows.

Bhardwaj *et al.* (2011[a]) observed the effect of restricted feeding on the performance of buffalo calves. According to them feed restriction by 25 percent resulted in low intakes of dry matter and that of nitrogen, but without affecting the digestibility of nutrients. The low N-excretion observed in animals fed restricted diet indicated improved efficiency of utilization or conservation of nutrients as N-retention observed was same as observed in animals offered standard diet. The levels of total and individual volatile fatty acids produced in rumen were low in animals fed restricted diet. The animals under restricted feeding showed low blood glucose levels. The serum protein (18.8%), globulin (30.9%), BUN and creatinine (31.8%), plasma GH (188%) levels were high, while that of T_3 (-32.4%) and T_4 (-15.9%) levels were low in animals fed restricted diet. The animals under restricted feeding showed lower urinary excretion of total purine derivatives, absorption of purine derivatives and microbial N synthesis in comparison to those offered normal diet. The final weight of animals under restricted feeding was less than that observed for animals fed normal diet. On an average the animals in control group gained 482g/d in comparison to loss of 138g/d in animals fed restricted diet.

Feeding Strategies during Natural Calamities

During natural calamities, feed security should be considered as important as food security, because keeping animals alive ensures families' survival after the occurrence of drought or disaster. The biggest challenge is to averse the acute shortage of feed stuffs in order to avoid the adverse effect of restricted feeding/malnutrition. The following feeding strategies should be followed without delay. The safe centers/states should be ready with complete feed blocks, urea molasses mineral blocks and bales of straws (untreated/urea treated) etc.

Complete feed block (CFB) : is the best way to supply all the required nutrients to farm animals. The CFBs can be easily transported to the site of natural calamities. CFBs may contain forage, crop residues, agro-industrial by products, non-conventional feeds, concentrate ingredients and other supplementary nutrients in desired proportions. The rice straw (a pollutant in certain areas like Punjab/Haryana, where 80% of the straw is burnt in the field) can be effectively used in making complete feed blocks. The chaffed untreated or urea treated rice straw can be used as basal roughage supplemented with ingredients like mustard cake, rice bran, molasses and binder, with or without hay. A block weighing around 15 kg (dimension of 0.5 cubic feet) containing about 13% proteins and 50 to 55% total digestible nutrients is sufficient to meet the daily requirements of an adult large ruminant. The nutritive value is 33% higher than common feed. The cost of the block varies with the quality e.g. from Rs 75-115 for low to high yielders. Complete feed blocks are prepared by using block making machine (costing around Rs 5 lakhs).

Inclusion of cotton stalks, maize cobs and sunflower heads in complete feed blocks resulted in increased milk yield by 11.3, 11.5, 23.5 percent and less intake of dry matter by 28.2, 26.7 and 15.0 percent in comparison to the conventional diet, thereby reducing the cost of feed/kg milk by 21.5, 23.4 and 25.2 percent, respectively. Anandan *et al.*, (2010) reported milk yield of 16.7 and 11.4 litres/day on feed blocks produced from premium and lower-quality sorghum stover, respectively indicating the feasibility of medium levels of milk production on crop-residue-based complete feeds.

The complete feed blocks containing cotton stalks, maize cobs and sunflower heads supported 87–108 g average daily gains (ADG) in Nellore ram lambs and 71 to 81 g ADG in local male kids in intensive-feeding system. The higher ADG on supplementing complete feed blocks and lower dry matter intake/kg gain (20 percent in sheep and 15 percent in goats) resulted in decreased cost of feed/kg gain by 13 to 32 percent in lambs and 13 to 22 percent in kids compared with the conventional diet. Dressing percentage and meat: bone ratio was optimum and almost similar for complete and conventional diets in sheep and goats.

In addition, enteric methane production can be reduced considerably by formulating a balanced complete-diet/feed block with different concentrate ingredients and crop residues. Gross energy lost as methane reduced from 5.64 to 4.90 percent and from 5.85 to 5.14 percent in buffalo and cows, respectively (Kannan and Garg, 2009). This energy can definitely be diverted for recouping the loss caused by malnutrition/restricted feeding.

These results, if translated for natural calamities, can prove to be a boon for animals and mankind suffering through hands of nature.

Urea molasses multinutrient blocks (UMMB) : is a blend of energy, protein and minerals for strategic supplementation in the diet of ruminants. The UMMB is a convenient and inexpensive method of providing a range of nutrients to the animals. It can improve the utilization of low quality roughages by satisfying the requirement of the rumen microorganisms, creating a better environment for the fermentation of fibrous material and increasing production of microbial protein and volatile fatty acids. The conventional UMMB weighing 3.0 kg contains (g): molasses 900, urea 300, mustard cake 300, de-oiled rice bran 300, wheat flour 450, mineral mixture 450, calcium oxide 120, salt 120 and guar gum 60. Two to eight UMMBs can be prepared at a time, either in a manually operated (for small/marginal/landless dairy farmer) or electrically operated (for commercial production) block-making machine (Wadhwa and Bakshi, 2011). On an average, an animal licks about 500-700 g UMMB/day, but some of the animals can lick as much as 1.25 kg/day without any deleterious effect on their health.

The blocks can also be prepared by using non-conventional feed resources. Iso-nitrogenous and iso-energetic UMMBs were prepared by replacing: a) wheat flour with waste bread (an excellent source of by-pass starch containing 11–12% crude protein) and b) oiled mustard cake with tomato pomace (20–22% CP, 10–11% ether extract and a 'good' amount of lycopene, an antioxidant and pigment that gives colour to meat). Adult male Murrah buffalo consumed 1.08 kg of conventional block compared with 1.32–1.84 kg experimental blocks, over and above normal diet. The UMMB supplementation improved intake of wheat straw, CP digestibility and N-retention. The use of such wastes can reduce the cost of producing UMMB (Chobey *et al.*, 2011). The cost of molasses can be reduced by using spent sugar syrup available at nominal charges or free from the 'Muraba' (fruits preserved in sugar syrup) manufacturing industry. Bakshi, Wadhwa and Parmar (unpublished) used spent sugar syrup in place of molasses for manufacturing UMMB. The results were comparable with those recorded for UMMB containing molasses.

Due to mineral deficiencies, pica is a common problem in almost all the animals during natural calamities. Pica was effectively reduced by UMMB supplementation. In some cases, animals suffering from haemoglobinurea due to phosphorus deficiency recovered when supplemented with UMMB. Farmers reported animals to be better general body condition, with glossy coats and healthier appearance. Cows that had not shown oestrus signs for a long time (presumably due to inadequate nutrition) resumed cycling when given mineral-rich blocks. Increases in milk production due to UMMB supplementation have generated additional income whilst improving reproductive performance, leading to more calves. These improvements have undoubtedly improved the socio-economic status of farmers.

UMMB supplementation of early-calved buffalo induced a higher proportion (71 vs. 14 percent) exhibiting oestrus during the first 50 days post-partum compared to controls. Pre-partum UMMB supplementation improved milk yield, and peak milk yield was maintained longer during the post-partum period. UMMB supplementation for 30 days in delayed-puberty buffalo heifers induced oestrus in 33 percent of cases in summer, and in 93 percent of cases in winter. Similarly in anoestrous buffalo, UMMB supplementation induced ovarian activity in 40 percent of buffalo during the summer season and in 90 percent during the winter season. In addition, UMMB supplementation was shown to increase the effect of pregnant mare serum gonadotropin used to induce oestrus in anoestrous and delayed-puberty buffalo.

Additional benefit of these UMMBs is that certain medicines can be incorporated to decrease the productive and reproductive problems of animals. A study conducted by Brar *et al.*, (2006) revealed that supplementary feeding in recently calved buffalo with medicated UMMB - 'Replanta' (an indigenous herbal preparation) decreased the time for shedding of placenta (5.75 vs 4.40 h) and the days to first post-partum oestrus (42.5 vs. 36 day) for treated and control group, respectively. UMMB containing anthelmintic has been successfully used for controlling nematode parasites.

The blocks may be specially formulated to provide energy, nitrogen, and important vitamins and minerals to enable animals to survive until pasture conditions improve.

Urea treated/Naturally fermented straws/stovers : is the most economical way to conserve the nutrients and to improve the quality/nutritive value of poor quality crop residues. More than 80% of surplus rice straw is burnt in Punjab, Haryana and Eastern UP, causing environmental pollution/global warming. The straw if used judiciously can save livestock population suffering through the cruel hands (floods/draughts) of nature.

The urea: rice straw (3.5:96.5), moistened to 40% and fermented by open stacking method for 9 days. It was observed that more than 85 per cent of the added urea was hydrolysed by 9th day, thereby eliminating the chances of urea toxicity to animals fed urea treated straw (Bakshi *et al.*, 1986, 1987; Wadhwa and Bakshi, 2011). The method proved to be highly applicable under field conditions. It has universal application in improving the nutritive value of many cereal (wheat, rice, barley, oat) straws, maize stovers, sorghum and pearl millet stalks (Bakshi and Langar, 1994). Pathogenic microbes like *Salmonella* or *E. coli* were never detected in any of the stacks (Gangwar and Bakshi, 2000). The fermentation process could be hastened by using freshly prepared 9 day fermented wheat/rice straw as a natural crude inoculum (5% DM basis). The 6-9 day inoculated straw preparation had significantly higher nutritive value (NV) than non-inoculated fermented straw (Bakshi and Langar, 1989; Bakshi and Wadhwa, 2001). The shelf life of the fermented straw is more than one year without any deterioration in the quality. After the stipulated period of 9days, the stack should not be dismantled; rather the quantity required for feeding should be taken from one side of the stack.

Natural fermentation of rice straw involves physical, chemical and biological processes. During natural fermentation, addition of urea solution activates microbes, which results in breakdown of urea to ammonia. Growth (catabolic activities) of microbes (biological treatment) increases the temperature of stack to 50-55°C (physical treatment) and enrich the rice straw with microbial protein. The rise in stack temperature facilitates the penetration of ammonia in the cell wall of straw. Ammonia, being a weak alkali, breaks down the lingo-cellulosic bonds (chemical treatment), thereby free cellulose is available for the microbial fermentation in the rumen (Bakshi and Wadhwa, 1999). This improves the availability of nutrients from fermented straw in comparison to untreated straw. It was concluded that 9 day naturally fermented urea rice straw, daily supplemented with mineral mixture and vitamin A (or carotene), could meet both energy and protein requirements for maintenance of adult buffaloes (Kaur *et al.*, 2008).

The FRS based ration had higher TDN (7.1 vs. 6.0) and lower DCP (3.6 vs. 5.5) values in comparison the RS based rations. The better utilization of nutrients resulted in higher gain in weight (250 vs. 167 g/d) in buffalo calves fed FRS (Bakshi and Langar,1990; Wadhwa *et al.*, 2010). The FRS supplemented with concentrate mixture containing urea, uromol bran or deep stacked poultry litter had no adverse effect on the productive performance of young calves (Bakshi *et al.*, 1996). The feeding of FWS could sustain the productive and reproductive performance of lactating buffalo (Lamba *et al.*, 2002) even when supplemented with either a lesser quantity of concentrate or concentrate mixture with low-protein content.

Spent straws : is the residue left after the harvest of *mushrooms- a delicacy* for human beings, posing a threat to the environment for its' disposal. Reports from this laboratory revealed that *Agaricus bisporus* harvested wheat straw (Bakshi and Langar, 1985; 1991), *Pleurotus* harvested wheat straw (Bakshi *et al.*, 1985) and *Volveriella diplacia* harvested rice straw (Langar and Bakshi, 1986) could be used as livestock feed. The *Volveriella* SRS had higher CP content (8.2%) than the RS (4.3%) based ration. The growth of *Volveriella* on RS increased the lignin content of the spent straw; however the oxalate content of straw decreased considerably, with no difference in the digestibility of nutrients. Rice straw can be used with wheat straw (50:50) for the cultivation of *Pleurotus florida*. Spent WS-RS had lower nutritional worth than WS-RS but could be incorporated in the complete feed of ruminants provided it is compensated for OM. The spent WS-RS based diet did not have any adverse effect on voluntary DM intake, palatability, digestibility of nutrients, blood profile and N-utilization (Kaur *et al.*, 2010). Above all the conventional protein supplements could be spared for other species. The spent straw can be baled for easy transportation to the needy site.

Densified and Enriched Rice Straw

Baled rice straw: The rice straw can be baled by using a fully automatic field/stationary baler like that developed by the Department of Farm Power and Machinery at Punjab Agricultural University. The machine is manufactured in the State and costs around Rs.2.5Lakh. Each bale has the dimension of 3'x1.5'x1.25' and weights around 28-35 kg (Fig. 1). The bales can be transported to drought and flood prone areas. The baled rice straw can be enriched by sprinkling urea solution and keeping the bales in the form of a stack for 9 days, before transporting. Such value addition would not only increase the nutritive value and palatability of crop residues (Kaur *et al.*, 2007) but also save storage space and reduce transport costs and wastage.

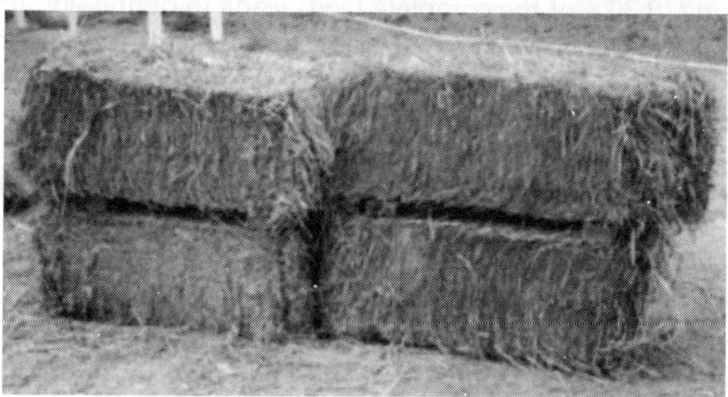

Fig. 1 : Baled rice straw

Use of Bypass Feed Supplements

Bypass protein: Studies have shown that the feeding by-pass protein to growing animals increased growth rate (25–30%), reduced rearing costs and resulted in earlier maturity of calves. Feeding by-pass protein also improved the reproductive efficiency of breeding bulls (Walli, 2008, 2009). The daily milk yield in animals supplemented with bypass protein was more by 1.0 to 1.5 litres. Supplementation with by-pass protein feed was found to be economical in lactating animals yielding on average 5–8 litres of milk daily (Garg, 2009). Because of the faster growth rate, calves attain early maturity leading to an early age at first calving. In young bulls, by-pass protein feeding resulted in increased libido and better semen quality, possibly due to enhanced amino acid supply. The lower plasma ammonia levels due to bypass protein feeding also lessened the interfering effect on embryonic/fetal growth in cows and buffalo, which resulted in better conception rates.

Histopathological studies on growing goats were also conducted to prove that the technology is safe and has no adverse effect on the health of animals. The untreated mustard seed cake fed to goats resulted in cellular damage in various organs, especially liver. This could possibly be due to glucosinolate present in the cake which is converted to isothiocyanate, causing adverse effects. The treatment of cake by formaldehyde also protects glucosinolate from being converted to isothiocynate. This was demonstrated by the higher plasma thyroxine levels and lower isothiocynate levels in the milk of goats fed formaldehyde-treated mustard seed cake. Formaldehyde was not detected in the milk of these animals. Also the urea content in milk was reduced following the feeding of by-pass protein, suggesting that the quality of milk is also improved after feeding formaldehyde-treated oilseed cakes (Sahoo, *et al*, 2006).

Bypass fat: It may or may not have its direct effect on daily DM intake in beef/ dairy cattle, but its' level of supplementation affects DMI. High level of incorporation (10-30% of the complete feed) leads to depression in DMI. The supplemental CaSFA showed no deleterious effect on the rumen fermentation or VFA production. The supplemented fat/ oil formed coating around the fibrous particles thereby preventing microbial breakdown, resulting in depression in CF digestibility. No such depression was observed when fats were protected. The total tract digestibility of nutrients was not influenced by protected fat. The plasma concentration of free FA (during early lactation only), triglycerides, phospholipids and cholesterol (beef cattle as well) increased significantly in lactating cows fed CaSFA. The supplementation of protected fat may or may not affect the daily milk yield, as it depends on stage of lactation (early, middle or late lactation) and genetic potential (high, medium or low yielders) of cows. However, milk composition showed some response, the

FCM, and fat content in the milk increased, the milk protein and SNF depressed.

Wadhwa *et al.* (2011[a]) conducted a 180 days field trial on 15 crossbred cows in early lactation, producing more than 10 kg milk/d. The bypass fat (150-200g BPF) supplementation showed no adverse effect on blood profile, except an increase in triglyceride (TG) level. The plasma progesterone concentration was higher on day 15 of the observed oestrus cycle (7.50 vs. 6.15 ng/dl) as well as at 30 days of pregnancy (9.18 vs.6.93 ng/dl) in BPF supplemented group as compared to control group. The average daily milk yield was improved by 1.13 kg/d (21.55 vs. 20.42 kg/d) in BPF supplemented group as compared to control group with an increase in protein, lactose and SNF content in milk, but without effecting milk fat content as compared to control group. Supplementation of BPF showed no effect on milk urea nitrogen (MUN). The body weight of the animals was improved considerably in BPF group as compared to control (551 vs. 508 kg) group. Daily supplementation of 150-200g bypass fat improved the milk yield, its composition and health of the high yielding crossbred cattle Wadhwa *et al.* (2011[a]).

Bypass protein and fat: In another 180 day field trial, the diet of lactating crossbred cows was supplemented daily with 200g each of bypass protein and bypass fat. The protein in the soybean meal was protected by using 1% formaldehyde and protected fat by making Ca salt of rice bran fatty acid oil by fusion method. The body weight estimated from the body length and heart girth revealed that there was no significant effect of feed supplements. The milk yield (kg/animal/day) and fat content (%) of milk of the animals fed diet supplemented with bypass nutrients was higher than those fed unsupplemented (control group) or the diet supplemented with chelated minerals. The MUN was comparable in all the groups and the range of MUN indicated that the animals in all the groups were well fed. The other constituents of milk were comparable in all the groups (Wadhwa *et al.*, 2011[b]). These bypass nutrients can be included in complete feed blocks or UMMB, for special category of animals.

Fodder Banks should be Established in the Region

Keeping in view of flood and drought situations, there is a need to establish feeds and fodder banks at non-affected areas. Ministry of Agriculture and Cooperation has a scheme with the name of Gramin Bhandaran Yojana. Similar programmes may be proposed for feeds and fodder to encourage farmers to contribute in such banks. These banks are necessary to meet the emergency needs of livestock during floods and other natural calamities.

These strategies need to be translated and transferred in order to prevent the losses caused by natural calamities.

Post Natural Calamities-Nutritional Management

Before discussing the nutritional managements to bring the animals to normal conditions it important to know how animals will respond to normal feeding schedule. There are few apprehensions like, will the animals be able to regain the normal growth pattern/ productivity levels etc. or not?

Effect of Compensatory Feeding

Compensatory growth describes the ability of animals to exhibit, after feed restriction, a higher growth rate than unrestricted animals of the same chronological age (O'Donovan, 1984). It is a complex biological event associated with factors such as higher feed intake (Wright *et al.*, 1986), increase in gut fill and high efficiency of feed use (Carstens *et al.*, 1991), changes in the composition of tissue gained (Baker *et al.*, 1985) and/or alteration in endocrine status (Blum *et al.*, 1985). Compensatory (or catch-up) growth may be defined as a physiological process whereby an organism accelerates its growth after a period of restricted development (Hornick *et al.*, 2000). Compensatory growth requires an adaptation period whose duration varies from one species to another. In ruminants it takes about one month. The response to compensatory growth may also vary depending on the duration or intensity of under-nutrition before re-alimentation (Wilson and Osbourn, 1960), and breed (Tesfaye, 2000) in which slower maturing type of cattle respond better in terms of compensatory growth after a period of under-nutrition than fast maturing cattle. In some cases an enhanced feed intake is also observed, adding to catch-up growth. Improvements in nutrient digestibility have also been reported (Williams and Macdearmid, 1985). Verma *et al.* (2000) reported that when the animals were shifted to revival diet, the intake and digestibility of all the nutrients were similar between the groups. The loss in body weight during survival was compensated during revival feeding with an average daily gain of 449.9 (restricted) and 337.5g (normal) in corresponding groups.

Only few reports are available on the changes in live weight gain and metabolic adaptations during the compensatory growth phase in cattle (Hays *et al.*, 1995; Hornick *et al.*, 1998[a,b]). When growth restriction is moderate (e.g., about 300 g/d in cattle), catch-up growth rate increases during about one month and reaches a maximum close to 2 kg/d in cattle. The maximal growth rate lasts for approximately another month and is followed by a sharp decrease to reach a minimum at about 4m after the beginning of refeeding. At the initial stage of compensatory growth, deposited tissue is mostly muscle and protein and carcass composition is close to that of the restriction phase (Wright and Russel, 1991). Thereafter, fat deposition takes over and the final body composition depends on refeeding duration. When lean meat growth potential is limited, in dairy breeds or in adults, fat deposition predominates from the beginning. Sometimes, fat deposition is confined to some of the body compartments. Fat deposition may even coincide with intramuscular fat reduction, probably as a result of fast muscle growth (Hornick *et al.*, 1999).

Yambayamba *et al.* (1996) showed that the growth of intramuscular fat was lower than that of subcutaneous fat during compensatory growth in heifers. Drew and Reid (1975) also found more protein, less fat and less energy in the empty body of compensating animals. Compensatory growth possibly increased the proportion of peripheral fat but decreased intramuscular fat in muscle tissue. Fox *et al.* (1972) found that gain of compensating steers contained more protein and less fat up to 364 kg body weight. However, when extended to 454 kg, no differences were observed.

Energy deficient animals that are re-fed tend to express a similar response pattern to feeding as controls. Thus, one of the first features of re-feeding within days is the normalization of plasma insulin levels. This is surprising because the lower weight and fatness of the animals at the beginning of compensatory growth would have been associated with relatively low insulin levels since this hormone is positively correlated with these parameters. Occasionally, during the initial phase of refeeding the secretion of insulin may be transiently enhanced and greater than in controls. This phenomenon may appear within days or weeks (Blum *et al.*, 1985; Wester *et al.*, 1995). According to Blum *et al.* (1985) it could represent a signal for the initiation of anabolic processes. Later during compensatory growth, high plasma insulin are also found (Blum *et al.*, 1985) and may contribute to enhanced deposition of fat in compensating animals. The relatively high concentrations of insulin may stimulate the uptake of metabolites (such as glucose) by the hypothalamus, leading to a decrease of the production and secretion of GH (Buonomo and Baile, 1990). In response to refeeding, concentrations of T_4, T_3 and INS increased within days. In contrast, GH decreased whereas rT_3 did not change Within 2 d of refeeding there was a rapid fall of NEFA and an increase of glucose, and â-hydroxybutyrate within 2 and 12 d, respectively (Blum *et al.*, 1985). One of the characteristics of compensatory growth is thus a sharp decrease of the ratio GH to insulin.

Bhardwaj *et al.* (2011[b]) studied the effect of realimentation (to 100 or 125% NRC) on restricted (75% NRC) fed buffalo calves and observed that DM intake, digestibility of nutrients, and nitrogen retention were not affected. However, rumen fermentation pattern (TVFAs, acetate, total-N, TCA-N and amminical-N) on the realimentation to 100 or 125% NRC improved in comparison to that in animals that never faced feed restrictions. The urinary excretion of purine derivatives, absorption of purine derivatives and microbial nitrogen synthesized in the rumen were comparable indicating recoupment of digestive and absorptive processes. Booster feeding (125% NRC) offered to animals suffered from feed restriction resulted in increased blood glucose and IGF levels, whereas serum IGF level in animals on compensatory feeding (100% NRC) was low. On realimentation to 100 or 125% NRC after feed restriction (75% NRC) buffalo calves showed a remarkable recovery and reached close to the animals under normal (100% NRC) feeding schedule and never faced feed restriction. However the animals, even on realimentation, could not achieve the same BW as those offered normal diet throughout the experiment. Bhardwaj *et al.* (2011[b]) revealed that animals which were on restricted feeding could recoup from the negative effects, during realimentation phase (compensatory or booster feeding), but failed to show the performance equivalent to that shown by the animals on normal diet during the experimental period.

This paper emphasize that feed restrictions/malnutrition caused due to natural calamities results in certain adverse effects, which could not be reversed even after providing the booster feeding, which may result in poor productive and reproductive efficiency of animals. Since during natural calamities, priority is to sustain the animals on basic feeding schedule, the co-operative societies, krishi vigyan kendras, and NGOs should have the banks for complete feed blocks, UMMB, bales (naturally urea fermented, spent and or ensiled straws), bypass nutrients etc. so as to ensure the feed security.

But one must ensure that animals are not allowed to graze in water logged areas. There should be provision of clean drinking water to animals. Feed is free from fungal contamination and wet feeds should be dried before feeding. Provide 40-50g of salt per adult animal and 10-20g for small ruminants and calves daily through feed if UMMB is not available. Complete feed blocks should be provided particularly to the pregnant and lactating animals. Requirement of energy may be met by providing molasses. Top feeds/tree leaves available in the area should be provided to meet the dry matter requirement.

References

Baker, R. D., Young, N. E. and Laws, D.A. (1985). *Anim. Prod.* 41: 309–321.

Bakshi, M.P.S. and Langar P.N. (1985). *Indian J. Anim. Sci.* 55: 1060-63.

Bakshi, M.P.S. and Langar, P.N. (1989). *Indian J. Anim. Sci.* 59: 846-50.

Bakshi, M.P.S. and Langar, P.N. (1990). Effect of feeding naturally fermented wheat straw on the availability of nutrients and growth of buffalo calves. Proc. Natl. Symp. Buff. Dev. for Econ. Returns. (Ed. J.S. Dhillon) pp. 23-27 held at New Delhi.

Bakshi, M.P.S. and Langar, P.N. (1991). *Indian J. Anim. Sci.* 61: 653-54.

Bakshi, M.P.S. and Langar, P.N. (1994). *Buffalo J.* 10: 19-27.

Bakshi, M.P.S. and Wadhwa, M. (1999). Feeding strategies for incorporating crop residues in ruminants ration. *In* K.K. Singhal & S.N. Rai, eds. *Proc Animal Nutrition Workers Conference*, pp. 52–58. Hyderabad, Animal Nutrition Society of India, India.

Bakshi, M.P.S. and Wadhwa, M. (2001). *Indian J. Anim. Sci.*, 71: 710–711.

Bakshi, M.P.S., Gupta, V.K. and Langar, P.N. (1985). *Agric. Wastes*, U.K. 13: 51-57.

Bakshi, M.P.S., Gupta V K and Langar P N. (1986). *Agric. Wastes*, 16: 37–46.

Bakshi, M.P.S., Gupta, V.K. and Langar, P.N. (1987). *Biol. Wastes*, 21: 283–289.

Bakshi, M.P.S., Wadhawan, V.M., Wadhwa, M. and Langar, P.N. (1996). *Bubalus bubalus. J. Buffalo Sci. Tech.*, 2: 57–62.

Bakshi, M.P.S., Wadhwa, M., Gangwar, M. and Lamba, J.S. (2011). *Indian J. Anim. Nutr.* (in press).

Bhagwat, S. R. (2008). Deptt. Anim. Nutr. COVSc. Sdau, Sardarkrushinagar Dairy Year Book.

Bhardwaj, R., Wadhwa, M. and Bakshi, M. P. S. (2011a). *Indian J. Anim. Sci.* (in press).

Bhardwaj, R., Wadhwa, M. and Bakshi, M. P. S. (2011b). *Indian J. Anim. Sci.* (in press).

Blum, J. W., Schnyder, W., Kunz, P. L., Blom, A. K., Bickel, H. and Schürch A. (1985). *J. Nutr.* 115: 417–424.

Bossart, M. A., Leuenberger, H., Kuenzi, N. and Blum, J. W. (1985). *Zschr Tierz Züchtungsbiol.* 102: 23–33.

Buonomo, F. C. and Baile, C. A. (1990). *Domestic Animal Endocrinology.* 7: 435–450.

Brar, P. S., Nanda, A. S. and Juyal, P. D. (2006). Reproductive performance of dairy buffalo receiving supplements of urea molasses multinutrient block (UMMB). *In Improving animal productivity by supplementary feeding of multinutrient blocks, controlling internal parasites and enhancing utilization of alternate feed resources*, pp. 39–50, Vienna, IAEA-TECTOC-1495, International Atomic Energy Agency, Vienna, Austria.

Choubey, M., Wadhwa, M. & Bakshi, M.P.S. (2011). *Indian J. Anim. Sci.*, (in press).

Drew, K. R. and Reid, J. T. (1975). *J. Agric. Sci.* 85: 193-204.

Driedger, L. J. and Loerch, S. C. (1999). *J. Anim. Sci.* 77: 967- 972.

Drouillard, J. S., Ferrell, C. L., Klopfenstein, T. J. and Britton, R. A. (1991). *J. Anim. Sci.* 69: 811-818.

Fattet, I., Hovell, F. D. B., Orskov, E. R., Kyle, D. J., Pennie, K. and Smart, R. I. (1984). *Br. J. Nutr.* 52: 561–74.

Foot, J. Z. and Tulloh, N. M. (1977). *J. Agric. Sci.* 88: 135–142.

Fox, D. G., Johnson, R. R., Preston, R. L., Dockerty, T. R. and Klosterman, E. W. (1972). *J. Anim. Sci.* 34: 310-318.

Gangwar, M. and Bakshi, M.P.S. (2000). *Indian J. Anim. Sci.* 70: 871-73.

Garg, M.R. (2009). Bypass protein technology for enhancing milk production. *9th National Seminarfor popularisation of oilmeal usage in compound cattle, poultry and aqua feeds.* Lucknow (UP), Organised by the Solvent Extractors' Association of India, India.

Hays, C. L., Davenport, G. M. and Osborn, T. G. (1995). *J. Anim. Sci.* 73:589 -97.

Heitmann, R. N. and Bergman, E. N. (1980). *American J. Physiol.* 239: E248 -254.

Hoffman, P. C., Simson, C.R. and Wattiaux, M. (2007). *J. Dairy Sci.* 90: 946-954.

Hornick, J. L., Van Eenaeme, C., Clinquartm A., Diez, M. and Istasse, L. (1998a). *J. Anim. Sci.* 76: 249 -259.

Hornick, J. L., Van Eenaeme, C., Diez, M., Minet, V. and Istasse, L. (1998b). *J. Anim. Sci.* 76: 260-271.

Hornick, J. L., Van Eenaeme, C., Clinquart, A., Gerard, O. and Istassem L. (1999). *Anim. Sci.* 69: 563-72.

Hornick, J. L., Van Eenaeme, C., Ge´rard, O., Dufrasne, I. and Istasse, L. (2000). *Domes. Anim. Endoc.* 19: 121-132.

IPCC. (2007). Climate Change: The Physical Science Basis. Extracts from the IV Assessment Report. Intergovernmental Panel on Climatic Change. Survey of the Environment 2007, *The Hindu*, pp147-155.

Kamalzadeh, A., Koops, W. J. and Van Bruchem, J. (1998). *Livest. Prod. Sci.* 5: 57– 67.

Kannan, A. and Garg, M.R. (2009). Effect of ration balancing on methane emission in lactating

Jaffarabadi buffaloes and Gir cows under field conditions. *In Proc. Animal Nutrition Association World Conference*, p. 211 (volume I), New Delhi, India.

Kaur, K., Kaur, J., Wadhwa, M. and Bakshi, M.P.S. (2007). *Indian J. Anim.Nutr.*24:88-91.

Kaur, K., Kaur, J., Wadhwa, M., Balwinder Kumar and Bakshi, M.P.S. (2008). *Indian J. Anim. Nutr.* 25: 195-200.

Kaur, K., Wadhwa, M. and Bakshi, M.P.S. (2010). *Indian J. Anim. Sci.* 80:750–753.

Lamba, J.S., Wadhwa, M. and Bakshi, M.P.S. (2002). *Bubalus bubalis, J. Buffalo Sci. Tech.* 8: 72–79.

Langar, P.N. and Bakshi, M.P.S. (1986). *Agril. Waste.* U.K. 15: 309-11.

O'Donovan, P. B. (1984). *Nutr. Abstr. Rev.* 54: 389–410.

Ortigues, I. and Durand, D. (1995). *Br. J. Nutr.* 73: 209-226.

Paquay, R., De Baere, R. and Lousse, A. (1972). *Br. J. Nutr.* 27: 27-37.

Tesfaye A. A. (2000). Effects of duration of feed restriction on compensatory growth of crossbred bulls. In: Proceeding of Seventh Annual Conference of Ethiopian Society of Animal Production (ESAP), Addis Ababa, Ethiopia, 26–27 May 1999, pp. 89–95.

Verma, A. K., Dass, R. S. and Mehra, U. R. (2000). *Anim. Feed Sci. Technol.* 87:253-261.

Wadhwa, M. and Bakshi, M. P. S. (2011a). Urea molasses multi-nutrient blocks/licks - a blend of nutrients for ruminants. In Proc. Successes and failures with animal nutrition practices and technologies in developing countries. FAO Electronic Conference, 1-30 September 2010, Rome, Italy. Ed. Harinder P.S. Makkar. Pp 35-40.

Wadhwa, M. and Bakshi, M. P. S. (2011b). Processing and evaluation of poor-quality crop residues as livestock feed. In Proc. Successes and failures with animal nutrition practices and technologies in developing countries. FAO Electronic Conference, 1-30 September 2010, Rome, Italy. Ed. Harinder P.S. Makkar. Pp 51-56.

Wadhwa, M., Grewal, R.S. and Bakshi, M.P.S. (2011a). *Indian J. Anim. Sci.* 81 (In press)

Wadhwa, M., Hundal, J.S. and Bakshi, M.P.S. (2011b). *Indian J. Anim. Sci.* 81 (In press)

Wadhwa, M., Kaur, K. and Bakshi, M.P.S. (2010). *Indian J. Anim. Sci.* 80: 249–252.

Walli, T.K. (2008). Densified TMR–A newer nutrient delivery system for feeding dairy animals in tropics. *In Proc. XXXVI Dairy Industry Conference*, pp. 74–79. Varanasi, India.

Walli, T.K. (2009). Crop residue based densified feed block technology for improving ruminant productivity. *In* Compendium T.K. Walli ed., *Satellite Symposium on Fodder Block Technology*, pp. 67–73. New Delhi, ILDEX India.

Wester, T. J., Britton, R. A., Klopfenstein, T. J., Ham, G. A., Hickok, D. T. and Krehbiel, C. R. (1995). *J. Anim. Sci.* 73: 1674–88.

Williams, P. E. V. and Macdearmid, A. (1985). *Anim. Prod.* 44: 474.

Wilson, P. N. and Osbourn, D.F. (1960). *Biol. Rev.* 35:324-363.

Winchester, C. F., Davis, R. E. and Hiner, R. L. (1967). Malnutrition of young cattle: Effect on Feed utilization, eventual body size and meat quality.*USDA Tech. Bull.* 1374: 26.

Wright, I. A. and Russel, A. J. F. (1991). *Anim. Prod.* 52: 105–113.

Wright, I.A., Russel, A.J., Hunter, E.A. (1986). *Anim. Prod.* 43: 211–223.

Yambayamba, E. S. K., Price, M. A. and Jones, S. D. M. (1996). *Livest. Prod. Sci.* 46:19-32.

□□□

About the Editors

Dr. S.P.Tiwari is Professor and Head, Department of Animal Nutrition at College of Veterinary Science and Animal Husbandry, Anjora, Durg, under the aegis of Indira Gandhi Krishi Viswavidyalaya, Raipur, Chhattisgarh. Dr. Tiwari did his BVSc & AH from College of Veterinary Science and Animal Husbandry, Mhow, in 1981 and received Maj. Juneja Trophy for getting highest marks in the faculty as "Best out going student". Dr. Tiwari did his MVSc in Animal Nutrition from Haryana Agriculture University, Hissar in 1983. He has completed his PhD in Animal Nutrition from Indian Veterinary Research Institute, Izatnagar in 1988. He started his career as Assistant Professor in Himachal Pradesh Agriculture University, Palampur from 1988 to 1991 and subsequently Associate Professor at Rajasthan Agriculture University, Bikaner from 1991 to 1993. Thereafter, he joined in the same capacity at Indira Gandhi Agriculture University, Raipur from 1993 to 1999. Dr. Tiwari joined the same University as Professor of Animal Nutrition in 1999 and Head of the Department in 2004 and continuing in the same capacity at the College of Veterinary Science & AH, Anjora, Durg. Dr. Tiwari is a distinguished Animal Nutritionist and contributed significantly in the area of strategic supplementation, integrated farming system, Medicated urea molasses mineral blocks and clinical nutrition. He received ND Kehar Award for the best PhD thesis. He has guided 20 MVSc and 3 PhD students. Dr. Tiwari was PI and Co-PI of many ICAR adhoc research projects besides NARP, NATP and State and other University level projects. He has published about 110 research papers and three book chapters on various aspects of animal nutrition. He was awarded with Merit scholarship during undergraduate and Junior and Senior Research Fellowships during masters and doctorate degree programme by Indian Council of Agriculture Research, New Delhi. He is life member of ANA, ANSI, ISNA, IPSA, IAVNAW and many other scientific societies. He is Fellow of Animal Nutrition Association and Fellow of Indian Poultry Science Association. He is member of Academic council and Administrative council of the university.

Dr. P.K. Sanyal graduated from Bengal Veterinary College, Bidhan Chandra Krishi Viswa Vidyalaya, West Bengal in the year 1976 and subsequently obtained MVSc in Veterinary Parasitology in the year 1980 from the same university with Teaching Asstt. Fellowship. Following award of ICAR Senior Fellowship, he continuously persuaded for PhD in Veterinary Parasitology from Haryana Agricultural University, Hisar under the guidance of Dr. N.S. Ruprah and graduated in the year 1984.

Subsequently Dr. Sanyal joined Central Sheep & Wool Research Institute as Scientist S-1 through Agricultuarl Research Service and served there for around six years both at Avikanagar and its Southern Regional Centre, Mannavanur, Kodaikanal. He then joined National Dairy Development Board as Scientist-III in R&D wing (Biotechnology Laboratory) in the year 1990 and subsequently promoted to Sr. Scientist in the year 1995. In the year 2003, Dr. Sanyal left NDDB and joined Indira Gandhi Krishi Viswavidyalaya as Professor & Head, Deptt. of Veterinary Parasitology, College of Veterinary Science &AH, Anjora, Durg and continuing thus far.

He has published 53 papers in peer reviewed International and 116 in National journals, 9 popular articles, 5 chapters in books, 4 conference proceedings, 1 laboratory manual. He has presented 98 papers in different conferences and 9 papers are awaiting publication. He is a member of Board of Editors of 3 Indian journals and member of panel of referee of 3 international and 5 national journals.

A fellow of National Academy of Veterinary Sciences, India and Indian Association for the Advancement of Veterinary Parasitology, Dr. Sanyal is the recipient of The Rafi Ahmed Kidwai Award of ICAR for the triennium 1993-1995, Sir B.V. Rao Gold Medal and Shri S.M. Ismail Oration Award, 2004 of IAAVP. He is now a member of Research Advisory Committee of Central Sheep & Wool Research Institute, Avikanagar.